PSYCHOLOGY OF PHYSICAL ACTIVITY AND SEDENTARY BEHAVIOR

Ryan E. Rhodes, PhD
University of Victoria
Victoria, British Columbia, Canada

Heather A. Hausenblas, PhD
Jacksonville University
Wellness Discovery Labs
Jacksonville, Florida

Amanda L. Rebar, PhD
Central Queensland University
Rockhampton, Australia

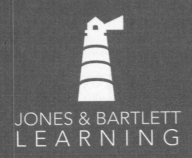

JONES & BARTLETT
LEARNING

World Headquarters
Jones & Bartlett Learning
25 Mall Road
Burlington, MA 01803
978-443-5000
info@jblearning.com
www.jblearning.com

Jones & Bartlett Learning books and products are available through most bookstores and online booksellers. To contact Jones & Bartlett Learning directly, call 800-832-0034, fax 978-443-8000, or visit our website, www.jblearning.com.

25738-0

Production Credits
Vice President, Product Management: Marisa R. Urbano
Vice President, Content Strategy and Implementation:
    Christine Emerton
Director, Product Management: Matthew Kane
Product Manager: Whitney Fekete
Director, Content Management: Donna Gridley
Content Strategist: Carol Brewer Guerrero
Content Coordinator: Samantha Gillespie
Director, Project Management and Content Services: Karen Scott
Manager, Program Management: Kristen Rogers
Manager, Project Management: Jackie Reynen
Project Manager: Roberta Sherman
Senior Digital Project Specialist: Angela Dooley

Senior Marketing Manager: Susanne Walker
Content Services Manager: Colleen Lamy
Product Fulfillment Manager: Wendy Kilborn
Composition: Exela Technologies
Project Management: Exela Technologies
Cover Design: Michael O'Donnell
Senior Media Development Editor: Troy Liston
Rights & Permissions Manager: John Rusk
Rights Specialist: Benjamin Roy
Cover & Title Page Images: © Norbert9/Shutterstock;
    © sergeymansurov/Shutterstock
Printing and Binding: Lakeside Book Company

Library of Congress Cataloging-in-Publication Data
Names: Rhodes, Ryan E., 1973- author. | Hausenblas, Heather A., author. | Rebar, Amanda L., author.
Title: Psychology of physical activity and sedentary behavior / Ryan E. Rhodes, PhD, Heather A. Hausenblas, PhD,
    Amanda L. Rebar, PhD.
Other titles: Exercise psychology
Description: Second edition. | Burlington, MA : Jones & Bartlett Learning, [2023] | Revised edition of: Exercise psychology /
    Heather Hausenblas, Ryan E. Rhodes. [2017]. | Includes bibliographical references and index.
Identifiers: LCCN 2022038307 | ISBN 9781284248517 (paperback)
Subjects: LCSH: Physical fitness–Psychological aspects. | Exercise–Psychological aspects. |
    Sedentary behavior. | BISAC: HEALTH & FITNESS / Exercise / General
Classification: LCC RA781 .H367 2023 | DDC 613.7/1–dc23/eng/20221223
LC record available at https://lccn.loc.gov/2022038307

6048

Printed in the United States of America
27 26 25 24 23   10 9 8 7 6 5 4 3 2 1

Dedication

We dedicate this book to you—the reader. Be well, be kind, make change.

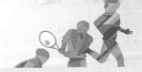

Brief Contents

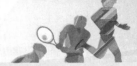

Contents

SECTION 4 Theoretical Models for Physical Activity and Sedentary Behavior 287

CHAPTER 14 Social Cognitive Theory and Theory of Planned Behavior

CHAPTER 15 Motivational Theories

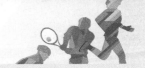

Foreword

Ryan Rhodes, Heather Hausenblas, and Amanda Rebar each bring a wealth of knowledge, expertise, and experience in the psychology of physical activity and sedentary behavior area to the table. They grasp the bigger picture, synthesize information, articulate concepts, and come up with important and meaningful research questions. They are established and well-respected leaders in our field. Just as important, we have collaborated on many projects and papers, and I have rarely come across three more positive, productive, and thoughtful individuals whom I am proud to call my colleagues.

In this timely second edition, Ryan, Heather, and Amanda have integrated important updates reflecting the progress our field has made. In addition, they have logically restructured the book facilitating an understanding of the important concepts—which will help you, the reader, build the foundation of knowledge in this area. This should enable you to become informed on what is known about physical activity and sedentary behavior, why physical activity and sedentary behaviors are important, why and how to change physical activity and sedentary behaviors, and how to use this knowledge in research and application.

Important and exciting new themes to this second edition:

"We need to increase physical activity and decrease sedentary behavior to promote health."

The increased focus on sedentary behavior is warranted due to its now well-documented independent effects on health outcomes and increased research on determinants and interventions targeting sedentary behavior. It is, however, equally important to consider physical activity alongside sedentary behavior as we strive to understand the effect and interaction these behaviors have on each other; thus, it is a strength of this book that it addresses both behavioral domains.

"The digital environment may be a curse or a blessing for health— the choice which it will be is ours to make."

The addition of the digital environment reflects the increased global digitalization, which includes, but is not limited to, wearables, smartphones, social media, and the Internet of things. It is at this point difficult to imagine life without these electronic gadgets and it has opened a new "environment" that presents both facilitators and barriers to physical activity and sedentary behavior, along with an unprecedented reach and speed of information/intervention dissemination. Although the digital environment may frequently be blamed for the increase in chronic diseases, it is up to us to realize that the digital environment is an unprecedented opportunity to positively impact human health behavior.

"Human decision making is only partially based on logic and forethought."

This edition also features a new chapter on dual-process models. This reflects a development that the predominantly social-cognitive theories/ models do not seem to explain behavior (physical activity or sedentary behavior) very well. Dual process models incorporate subconscious or unconscious automatic related processes, which have an important role to play in our everyday decision making and thus in health behavior change. It is vital for us to understand what role these factors have and how we can incorporate these factors into our intervention approaches to more effectively promote physical activity and decrease sedentary behavior.

Ryan, Heather, and Amanda have taken a conversational approach to this book, which makes it easy to read and facilitates understanding. This includes providing learning objectives, critical thinking activities, vignettes, and review questions. Such interactive writing engages the reader and enhances learning. This text is very valuable to motivate practitioners, researchers, professors, and students to push their contributions to the next level. In so doing, the book will be a catalyst to our field.

—Claudio R. Nigg, PhD, FSBM
Professor and Head, Department of Health
Sciences, Institute of Sport Science
University of Bern
Bern, Switzerland

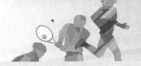

Preface

What contributes to our overall health? What might surprise you is that our behavior—that is, what we are actually doing (or not doing)—has the most significant impact on our overall health. According to the U.S. Department of Health and Human Services (2022), our behavior has more of an impact on our health than our genetics, our environment, and our access to medical care.

If we break our behavior down even further, physical activity has one of the biggest impacts on our overall health. The science is clear—every system of the body benefits when a person is physically active. Physical activity is highly effective for preventing and treating many of our most prevalent chronic diseases, including coronary heart disease, hypertension, heart failure, obesity, depression, and diabetes. Additionally, physical activity can help improve how we feel, with both immediate and long-term impacts on our well-being and mental health. The bottom line is that physical activity is very (very) good for our health. In fact, people who are regularly physically active have a 33% lower risk of all-cause mortality than those who are not physically active, and, excitingly, health benefits start to be gained with any increase of moderate- or vigorous-intensity physical activity (2018 Physical Activity Guidelines Advisory Committee, 2018).

Physical activity by itself, however, isn't enough to achieve overall health because it needs to be paired with a reduction in sedentary behavior. Sedentary behavior includes activities undertaken in either a sitting or reclined position, such as watching TV, reading, and engaging in activities on the computer. Too much sitting appears to be a health risk that is additional to, and interactive with, too little physical activity. We need to not only move more at a moderate and/or vigorous pace, but we also need to stand up more during the day.

In the July 2012 issue of *The Lancet*, which was dedicated to physical activity and health, the journal's editor concluded with the following statement: "In view of the prevalence, global reach, and health effect of physical inactivity, the issue should be appropriately described as pandemic, with far-reaching health, economic, environmental, and social consequences" (July 2012). This powerful conclusion has now led to two additional special issues in 2016 and 2021 on physical activity, which reveal that more than ever, the field of physical activity and sedentary behavior psychology is of great importance.

How can we get people to move more and sit less? In this book we have tackled this question by exploring the research, summarizing the key areas in this increasingly significant area of scientific inquiry to shed light on possible answers to this question. Our main goal in writing this book was to produce the first targeted book to bring the research examining the psychology of both physical activity and sedentary behavior together in a comprehensive, educational, and informative format with a socioecological scope.

This book is intended for health professionals, researchers, professors, and students who are interested in learning more about the psychological basis of exercise and sedentary behavior. It is our hope that it will stimulate continued interest and research in these important aspects of human behavior.

Organization of the Book

In all areas of science, the first general stage is description. This stage is essential because it informs us about "what is." A large proportion of the research in the psychology of exercise and sedentary behavior has been descriptive in nature. **Section 1** is devoted to the introductory material describing exercise psychology (Chapter 1) and the psychology of sedentary behavior (Chapter 2).

Section 4 in the first edition has moved to become **Section 2** in this edition, to discuss environmental factors that influence individual behavior before exploring the resulting effects. Section 2 provides an overview of research that has centered on an individual's social, physical, and digital environments. Chapter 3 focuses on the social environment (e.g., family, friends, and teammates). Chapter 4 outlines aspects of the physical environment (e.g., neighborhoods, parks, green spaces) that are important influences on physical activity and sedentary behavior. New to this edition, Chapter 5 discusses the digital environment—from the increase of technology-based platforms and screen time, to the role of exergames, health and fitness tracking applications, and social media.

Section 3 provides an overview of research that has centered on the relationships between physical activity and sedentary behavior and various health outcomes. Considerable research has identified a number of psychological benefits of being physically active, including reduced anxiety and depression, improved stress reactivity, enhanced self-esteem, increased body satisfaction, and improved cognitive functioning. In Chapter 6, we examine how physical activity and sedentary behavior affect overall health-related quality of life and positive mood states such as vigor and happiness in the general population as well as special populations, such as cancer patients, pregnant women, and individuals with obesity. In Chapter 7, we examine how personality traits affect our exercise and sedentary behaviors and our levels of happiness.

In Chapter 8, we examine the mind-body connection between physical activity and sedentary behavior and cognition. Chapter 9 explores how physical activity and sedentary behavior affect our sleep and considers whether sleep may impact physical activity or sedentary behavior. In Chapter 10, we explore how physical activity and sedentary behavior affect depressed mood and clinical mood disorders. Chapter 11 covers the relationship between these topics and anxiety and stress. In Chapter 12, we discuss the effect of physical activity and sedentary behavior on self-esteem and the related construct of body image. Finally, a number of potential exercise-related disorders and negative behaviors have been associated with exercise, such as exercise dependence, steroid use, muscle dysmorphia, and eating disorders. The final chapter in this section, Chapter 13, focuses on disorders and addictions related to excessive exercise.

In **Section 4** (formerly Section 2), various theoretical models that have been advanced to explain and predict involvement in exercise and sedentary behavior are discussed. Chapter 14 deals with one of the most extensively used theoretical models to understand human behavior—social cognitive theory—and this new edition adds discussion of the theory of planned behavior to this chapter. In Chapter 15, motivational theories are examined, including the health belief model, self-determination theory, and protection motivation theory. The transtheoretical model, a popular approach to the study of involvement in exercise, is discussed in Chapter 16; this chapter also has significant new content on action control theories that focus on the translation of positive intentions into behavior. Finally, Chapter 17 is new to this edition and discusses dual process theories, which include focus on nonconscious, automatic influences on our behavior, such as habit and identity.

The fourth stage of science is intervention. Essentially, the description stage provides a basis for the explanation stage (theory), the prediction stage involves a test of theory, and the intervention stage involves the application of what has been learned from the other three stages.

Because the benefits of more physical activity and less sedentary behavior are so important for the individual and society in general, numerous attempts have been made to develop effective intervention strategies to not only increase physical activity behavior but also reduce sedentary behavior. Strategies on how to promote physical activity involvement and reduce sedentary behavior, including those that have focused on the individual level, social level, policy level, and environment, are integrated within each of the chapters.

Key Features

- **Learning Objectives.** Each chapter begins with a list of goals to focus the reader's learning and engagement with the content.

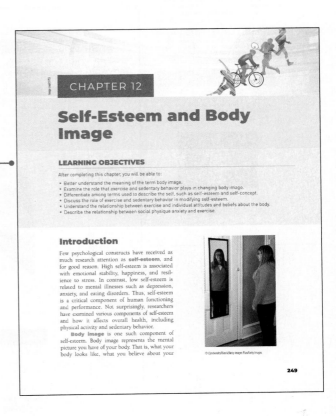

- **Critical Thinking Activities.** Short questions and activities are included throughout each chapter to present opportunities for the reader to challenge and delve deeper into the theories, concepts, and research presented.

Systematic Reviews and Meta-Analyses   **7**

3. Are People Physically Active?

The final part of the tomato effect courthouse steps, question pertains to whether people are eating the tomatoes or not. Or, is physical activity being embraced by a large portion of the world's population? Unfortunately, the answer is a qualified no. Only about half of North American adults are regularly engaging in aerobic physical activity, and only 20% engage in regular aerobic and muscle-strengthening activity (2018 Physical Activity Guidelines Advisory Committee, 2018; Clarke et al., 2019). Globally, more than 25% of the population (1.4 billion adults) are not engaging in regular physical activity, with more women (1 in 3) than men (1 in 4) at risk of negative health consequences as a result (World Health Organization, 2018). Additionally, more than 80% of adolescents do not engage in regular physical activity (Guthold et al., 2019). Despite the universal understanding of the benefits of physical activity, there has been no improvement in levels of physical activity since 2001, and in high-income countries, physical inactivity has increased by 5% since then (World Health Organization, 2018).

So, the answer to the first question of this chapter—"Does participation in physical activity show evidence of a tomato effect?"—seems to be a qualified yes:

1. Yes, physical activity is good for us.
2. Yes, most people are aware and accepting that physical activity is good for them.
3. Generally, people are not physically active.

CRITICAL THINKING ACTIVITY 1-3

What is another example of the tomato effect that has occurred or is occurring?

CRITICAL THINKING ACTIVITY 1-2

If you were asked to plan an intervention to reduce the gap of inequality in levels of physical activity between women and men, what intervention would you design and how would it help reduce the gap?

© Spectral-Design/Getty Images.

---

108   **Chapter 5** Digital Environment

CRITICAL THINKING ACTIVITY 5-1

Have you downloaded fitness or other health behavior change apps on your smartphone? Do you use them regularly? Why or why not?

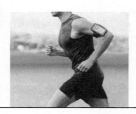

While the findings of Mhealth studies have been promising, some of these results may be a result of weaker study designs and biases in measurement. For example, Mönninghoff and colleagues (2021) highlighted that many of the studies in their review (80%) had study designs with considerable biases. Primally, Romeo and colleagues and meta-tiveness of objectively As we have self-reported measurement assessment improve the authors ide-ria and con-duced a ne that studies results we periods ra of Mhealth dren have 2019). The to be taken tions, and experimen Consi on physica appraise t in decreas early revie tive in som reviewed (interventio a small ove ham et al. ined Mhea behavior i

---

Physical Activity, Sedentary Behavior, and Clinical Sleep Disorders   **203**

© averna/ShutterStock.

CRITICAL THINKING ACTIVITY 9-4

What would you tell someone who believes exercise at night would make it difficult for them to fall asleep? In other words, is this really a valid reason to not exercise?

Sedentary Behavior and Sleep

Emerging research is revealing that sedentary behavior is negatively related to sleep quality in a variety of populations and age groups. Yang and colleagues (2017) conducted a systematic review and meta-analysis of the evidence for the association between sedentary behavior and sleep problems. 16 studies were reviewed, and it was found that sedentary behavior was associated with a 38% increase in the risk of sleep disturbances, but sedentary behavior was not found to increase the risk of daytime sleepiness or poor sleep quality. The authors concluded that,

although the evidence suggests that prolonged sedentary behavior may have detrimental effects on sleep, more studies with longer follow-up periods, and experimental designs are needed to establish these effects more conclusively.

A review of screen time, sedentary behavior, physical activity, and sleep in children younger than 5 years old covered evidence from 31 studies (Janssen et al., 2020). They concluded that screen time is associated with poorer sleep outcomes in infants, toddlers, and preschoolers, recommending that parents, clinicians, and educators should promote less evening screen time for children under age five to enhance sleep outcomes. A review of screen-based sedentary behavior among adolescent girls also reported that more screen-based sedentary time was associated with more sleep problems, noting however that most studies do not account for physical activity, which may serve to buffer from some of these effects (Costigan et al., 2013). Although not nearly as comprehensive as the body of evidence surrounding the benefits of physical activity on sleep, these three reviews demonstrate that sedentary behavior, and screen-time in particular, may be detrimental to sleep. Given that daytime sleepiness can make sedentary behaviors more tempting, people can easily get into a bad cycle of a night of poor sleep leading to a sedentary day, leading to another night of poor sleep, and so on. Most people have personally experienced the negative effects that a night or two of poor sleep can have on all aspects of your life; however, some people have persistent negative consequences of poor sleep from clinical disorders.

Physical Activity, Sedentary Behavior, and Clinical Sleep Disorders

Historically, research investigating physical activity, sedentary behavior, and sleep has focused on people without sleep disorders. But more recently, researchers have begun to examine the effects of these behaviors on people with sleep disorders.

- **Vignettes.** At the end of each chapter, a fictional vignette is presented to depict how a person might encounter that chapter's topic in real life and its impact on that person's health.

---

hormones, in response to continuous stressors people experience, can result in hormonal imbalances and adrenal dysfunction. The ultimate result of the release of these stress hormones over time has negative effects on people's overall health such as sleep, mood disturbances, and suppressed immune system.

Psychosocial Effects

Potential psychosocial mechanisms include improved self-regulation or self-control (Oaten & Cheng, 2005), improved sleep, aggregated positive effects of acute exercise on mood (Reed & Buck, 2009), reduced tension, and increased feelings of control (Salmon, 2001). Several explanations have been advanced, but most likely, the effects of physical activity and sedentary

> CRITICAL THINKING ACTIVITY 11-4
>
> Can you describe some reasons why physical activity and sedentary behavior may impact stress or anxiety? Make sure you think about some psychosocial and neurobiologic explanations.

behavior on stress, anxiety, and anxiety disorder symptoms are the result of complex interactions between neurobiologic and psychosocial processes. (Asmundson et al., 2013; Landers & Arent, 2007).

Summary

Feelings of stress arise when we perceive an imbalance between the demands of the situation and our ability to meet those demands. The body responds with a "flight-or-fight" response and changes in the autonomic nervous system: increased heart rate, increased blood pressure, and so on. Sometimes, these stress responses can include feelings of anxiety—the worry and anticipation of a threat. Some people are more prone than others to feeling anxiety more often and some have stress and anxiety interfere so much with daily life that it is a diagnosable anxiety disorder. The good news, however, is that increases in physical activity and reductions in sedentary behavior likely enhance our ability to deal with stress and to prevent and manage anxiety disorder symptoms.

Vignette: Wáng

Everyone keeps telling me how good my life is and how lucky I am to have this life. And sometimes I feel the same way—I am lucky. I got into a great University, I'm doing well in school, and I work really hard to be competitive for graduate programs through my volunteering program and part-time gig at the café. But every once in a while, I feel like giving it all up. Sometimes I wake up in the night and just feel so overwhelmed with my never-ending to do list that I just feel like I don't even know where to begin. But then I get so worried about what my Dad will think if I don't get into grad school and how disappointed my professors will be if I don't live up to their expectations—so I keep going. Even though my heart races and I feel like I can't take a deep breathe, I keep going. Eventually, I'll catch

up with things enough to take a break, but it sure can't be for the next 4 years!

Last night, I had such a horrible sense of things piling up high and a lack of control that I had to get help. I called the University's student support services and I've got an appointment to meet with them next week. Just calling for help makes me feel better even though they haven't even done anything yet. Well, that's not right. They did tell me to get outside and go for a run. I haven't run in so long and it felt so good. My heart was beating fast while I was doing it and my breathe was quick, but once I was done, I had these realizations that the things I was worrying about don't seem so bad anymore. I feel like I can cope. Although it doesn't solve any of my problems necessarily, at least I know I can

---

- **Review Questions.** At the end of each chapter, Review Questions allow readers to evaluate the achievement of the objectives outlined at the start of the chapter.

- **Applying the Concepts.** At the end of each chapter, readers are asked questions that tie the knowledge gained in the chapter to real-world scenarios.

---

xiety and Stress

...to get my stress under...
...n high school but I just...
...with University studying...
...t a priority for me any-...
...s and anxiety were my...
...s time to do things for...
myself again. Maybe it's time to make running a

priority. Even though it takes an hour every day to get ready for the run, run, then shower and dress afterward, it surprisingly hasn't put me behind on anything. It seems like I'm more productive after a run then if I had just sat and powered through my work and skipped a run. It's definitely not a cure-all, but it's a cure-some for my worries and some days, that's huge!

Key Terms

anxiety A cognitive and emotional stress response that includes anticipation of a future threat.

anxiety disorders Diagnosable health conditions, distinct from feelings of anxiety or stress, characterized by a range of psychological and physiologic symptoms including excessive rumination, worrying, uneasiness, and fear about future uncertainties.

fight-or-flight response The response of the sympathetic nervous system to a stressful event, preparing the body to fight or flee, associated with the release of stress hormones.

homeostasis The natural state of our body and mind, characterized by calmness and balance that is disrupted by stress responses.

non-clinical populations consisting of people who have not been diagnosed with a clinical disorder.

state anxiety Temporary state of high anxiety.

stress The process by which we perceive and respond to events, called stressors, that we appraise as threatening or challenging.

stress hormones such as cortisol and epinephrine released by the body in situations that are interpreted as being potentially dangerous.

stressor Any event or situation that triggers coping adjustments.

trait anxiety Individual differences in tendencies to experience frequent high levels of state anxiety.

Review Questions

1. What is the difference between stress and anxiety?
2. What is the distinction between anxiety and clinical anxiety disorders?
3. Describe the proposed mechanisms of how physical activity is associated with stress and anxiety. Does physical activity impact stress and anxiety? Does stress and anxiety impact physical activity?
4. What type of study could you set up to investigate whether time spent being sedentary influences daily anxiety? How

would that study be different if you wanted to investigate whether time spent being sedentary influenced your risk of being diagnosed with a clinical anxiety disorder?
5. Describe three clinical anxiety disorders and how they are distinct.
6. How would you describe the evidence about whether physical activity is a good treatment option for clinical anxiety disorders? What about the literature about sedentary behavior and clinical anxiety disorders?

Applying the Concepts

1. What do you think Wáng is experiencing when he runs? How is that helping how he feels and what is the scientific explanation behind it?

2. Will Wáng's stress get better if he runs regularly compared with just when he feels overwhelmed? Why or why not?

Student Resources

A Navigate eBook comes with each new purchase of this textbook, and includes:

- Knowledge check questions—students may test their knowledge at the end of each section
- Quizzes—gradable quizzes at the end of each chapter
- Practice Activities—writeable PDFs that can be assigned for student practice
- Flashcards—students may check their knowledge of key terms
- Interactive glossary

The Navigate eBook can be read online or offline through the Navigate app.

Instructor Resources

The following resources are available to instructors to aid in teaching the content:

- Test Bank—including in LMS-compatible formats
- Slides in PowerPoint format—ready and customizable for instructor presentations
- Chapter Projects—in-class activities for each chapter
- Instructor Manual—for selected chapters, tips, and grading rubrics for the additional chapter projects provided
- Lecture Outlines—an outline of each chapter's content
- Answer Key to In-Text Questions—answers to the textbook chapter Review Questions
- Answer Key to Practice Activities—instructors may provide these to students for their self-study or may assign the Practice Activities as homework
- Sample Syllabus—how to teach the textbook's topics in a typical course
- Image Bank—slide deck including key images from the text

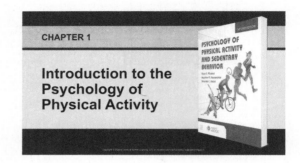

References

Physical Activity 2012. Series for the Lancet Journals. July 18, 2012. Volume 380, Issue 9838, https://www.thelancet.com/series/physical-activity

Physical Activity 2016: Progress and Challenges. *The Lancet.* Copyright © 2022 by Elsevier. Published July 27, 2016. Retrieved August 13, 2022 from https://www.thelancet.com/series/physical-activity-2016

Physical Activity 2021. *The Lancet.* Copyright © 2022 by Elsevier. Published July 21, 2021. Retrieved August 13, 2022 from https://www.thelancet.com/series/physical-activity-2021

Physical Activity Guidelines Committee. (2018). *2018 Physical Activity Guidelines for Americans.* U. S. Department of Health & Human Services.

U.S. Department of Health and Human Services. (2022). Determinants of health. Healthy People 2020. Site last updated February 6, 2022. Retrieved August 13, 2022, from https://www.healthypeople.gov/2020/about/foundation-health-measures/Determinants-of-Health

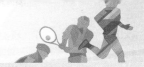

About the Authors

Ryan E. Rhodes

Ryan E. Rhodes, PhD, is a professor in the School of Exercise Science, Physical and Health Education, cross-appointed in the Department of Psychology, and Director of the Behavioral Medicine Laboratory at the University of Victoria, in Victoria, British Columbia, Canada. He has taught both undergraduate and graduate courses on the psychology of physical activity and sedentary behavior for over 20 years. His research includes the psychology of physical activity with an applied focus on promotion during critical life transitions such as parenthood, early family development, and retirement. Dr. Rhodes is also one of the world's experts on the intention-behavior gap, which was made popular by New Year's resolutions that people struggle to enact every year. He has held over 100 grants for this research and he has contributed over 500 publications, 35 book chapters, and three books. Dr. Rhodes is a Fellow of the Canadian Academy of Health Sciences, Society of Behavioral Medicine, Academy of Behavioral Medicine, American Psychological Association, and a College Member of the Royal Society of Canada. He is also the Co-Editor-in-Chief of *Psychology and Health*, and Associate Editor of *Exercise and Sports Sciences Reviews*.

Heather A. Hausenblas

Heather Hausenblas, PhD, believes we can have healthy and happy lives through simple wellness habits. She is a health psychology expert, international award-winning scientist, public speaker, and best-selling author. Her research focuses on how our health habits affect our well-being. Dr. Hausenblas has published seven books and over 100 scientific articles. Even with her vast education on wellness, Heather's outlook shifted when her eldest son was diagnosed with an autoimmune disease in 2018. Her journey is captured in her best-selling new book, *Invisible Illness*, a guide to reducing overwhelm and achieving optimal health while living with an autoimmune disease. Dr. Hausenblas obtained her PhD from Western University in Canada. She was a faculty member and the Director of the Exercise Psychology Lab at the University of Florida, and she has served as a scientific advisor for nutrition, health, and wellness companies. She is currently a professor of Health Sciences at Jacksonville University. Heather is the CEO and Founder of Wellness Discovery Labs, a health behavior research company, and she is the co-founder of Healthy Moves Journaling, a wellness company that focuses on small changes for big health improvements. When Heather is not walking the family dog, cooking with natural ingredients, watching her sons play sports, or exercising outdoors with friends, she's researching wellness. She is a health and science nut—it's her career, hobby, and passion. She resides in Jacksonville, Florida, with her husband and three boys.

Amanda L. Rebar

Amanda L. Rebar, PhD, believes that the most effective way to help people live healthier lives is by making the healthy options fun, efficient, and satisfying. Amanda is a self-proclaimed theory and statistics nerd, with more than 160 peer-reviewed scientific publications. Dr. Rebar has received national fellowships, grants, and honors for her work investigating motivation of physical activity. She consults with industries, government agencies, and the public health sector to promote enhancing the long-term outcomes of public health initiatives. She is a science award recipient from Queensland and the Australian Institute of Policy and Science and has received four awards commending her work to advocate for women in science. Dr. Rebar obtained her Masters (2010) and PhD (2013) from Pennsylvania State University, with specialization in sport and exercise psychology. She is currently an associate professor of psychology and Director of the Motivation of Health Behaviours Lab at Central Queensland University, Australia. Dr. Rebar is an advocate of open science and has a passion for data analysis and the data analysis program, R. While at work, Dr. Rebar spends her time learning from her students. Outside of work, Amanda loves playing on the beach with her two young boys, Drew and Max, and trying not to get seasick on their boat with her partner, Andy.

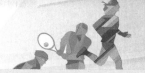

Reviewers

Jedediah E. Blanton, PhD
Assistant Professor of Practice
University of Tennessee
Knoxville, Tennessee

Tim Dasinger, PhD
Assistant Professor
University of Tennessee at Martin
Martin, Tennessee

Brenda A. Riemer, PhD
Eastern Michigan University
Ypsilanti, Michigan

J. P. Willow, PhD
Assistant Professor of Applied Exercise Science
Gannon University
Erie, Pennsylvania

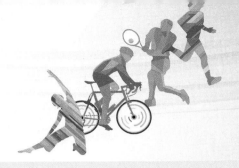

SECTION 1

Introduction to the Psychology of Physical Activity and Sedentary Behavior

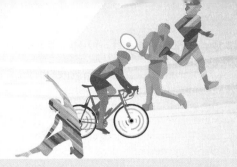

CHAPTER 1

Introduction to the Psychology of Physical Activity

LEARNING OBJECTIVES

After completing this chapter, you will be able to:

- Describe what the tomato effect is and whether physical activity could be considered a tomato effect.
- Recognize the difference between systematic reviews and meta-analyses.
- List at least four correlates of physical activity.
- Report the current Physical Activity Guidelines for Americans.

Introduction

Lao Tzu was a famous ancient Chinese philosopher who is quoted as saying that "the journey of a thousand miles begins with a single step." This proverb means that even the longest and most difficult ventures or journeys have a starting point. From the perspective of personal fitness and well-being, we know that the road to physical fitness and a healthy lifestyle is a lifetime journey with many obstacles. In fact, participation in physical activity might show signs of a "tomato effect". You might rightly ask, "What's a tomato effect?"

The tomato effect is a term James and Jean Goodwin (1984) used to describe a phenomenon whereby highly efficacious therapies are either ignored or rejected. Generally, the reason is that these therapies are not well-received in light of popular beliefs or common understandings. A tomato effect, however, can also occur if people simply ignore or otherwise not act in line with the evidence available.

The term "tomato effect" is derived from the history of the tomato in North America. The tomato was discovered in Peru and then transported to Spain, from where it made its way to Italy, France, and most of the rest of Europe. By 1560, the tomato played a major role in the diet of most Europeans. In North America, however, tomatoes were avoided because they were considered poisonous. The basis for this belief was that they belong to the nightshade family of plants, and some fruits from the nightshade family can cause death if eaten in large quantities. Thus, throughout the 18th century, tomatoes were not grown in North America. In fact, the turning point did not occur until 1820. Apparently, in a dramatic gesture, Robert Gibbon Johnson ate a tomato on the courthouse steps in Salem, New Jersey, and survived! According to legend, he stood on the courthouse steps and ate tomatoes in front of a large, amazed crowd that had assembled to watch him. When he neither dropped dead nor suffered any apparent ill effects, witnesses of his "experiment" slowly began to open their minds. By the end of the decade, American gardeners were growing tomatoes for food. Subsequently, tomatoes began to be accepted as a nutritious food source. It was not until the 20th century, however, that commercial marketing of the tomato began in earnest. Today, it represents one of the largest commercial crops in North America (Goodwin & Goodwin, 1984).

Tomato effects have three characteristics: First, there must be evidence that the treatment is beneficial; second, people must have awareness of the benefits of the treatment; and third, despite this awareness, people are not using the treatment. So, to answer the question "Does physical activity show a tomato effect?" we need to address the following three questions:

1. Is physical activity good for us?
2. Are people aware and accepting that physical activity is good for them?
3. Are people physically active?

Physical Activity and the Tomato Effect

1. Is Physical Activity Good for Us?

According to Goodwin and Goodwin (1984), the use of aspirin for the alleviation of pain, swelling, and stiffness of rheumatoid arthritis also is characterized by a tomato effect. They noted that high doses of aspirin only became an accepted treatment about 70 years after initial studies demonstrated that aspirin is effective in treating some arthritis symptoms. What about physical activity? Is a tomato effect toward physical activity prevalent in our society?

One part of the answer to this question, of course, pertains to whether physical activity is

beneficial or not. Scientists spent a large portion of the previous century conducting research on the physiological benefits of both acute and chronic physical activity. Since then, our understanding of the benefits of physical activity have expanded beyond physiological reactions to activity and include mental health and wellbeing benefits. Basically, every system of the body and mind benefit when a person exercises regularly. In fact, regular physical activity is likely the single best prescription that people of all ages can take for a host of health benefits (Church & Blair, 2009). Physical exercise, although not a drug, possesses many traits of a powerful pharmacological agent. Indeed, the saying "exercise is medicine" is supported by scientific evidence of the benefits of physical activity. Notably, however, physical activity is quite different from "medicine" when it comes to adherence to prescriptions. Starting and maintaining a physically active lifestyle is definitely not as simple as taking a pill. It is important we tackle these issues in understanding how to help people engage in more activity because a routine of daily physical activity stimulates a number of beneficial physiological changes in the body and it can be highly effective for the prevention and treatment of many of our most prevalent chronic diseases, including coronary heart disease, hypertension, heart failure, obesity, depression, and type 2 diabetes. In fact, being regularly physically active increases how long you live and how good you feel while you're alive.

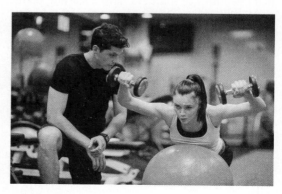

© wavebreakmedia/Shutterstock.

In 2018, Physical Activity Guidelines for Americans were developed based on a massive effort of scientists to conglomerate evidence of the health benefits of physical activity (2018 Physical Activity Guidelines Advisory Committee, 2018; Piercy et al., 2018). This huge set of reviews established that physical activity has multiple health benefits for people of all ages, regardless of age, sex, race, ethnicity or body size. They found that some of these benefits are experienced quickly after starting physical activity, such as reduced anxiety, improved sleep and cognitive function, and reduced blood pressure; while others are gained months or years after regular engagement in physical activity, such as cardiorespiratory fitness, increased strength, and decreased depressive symptoms. The overwhelming evidence for the health benefits of physical activity led the Advisory Committee to conclude that people who are physically active for approximately 150 min a week have a 33% lower risk of all-cause mortality than those who are not physically active, and excitingly, health benefits start to be gained with any increase of moderate- or vigorous-intensity physical activity (2018 Physical Activity Guidelines Advisory Committee, 2018). The bottom line is that physical activity is very good for our physical health, mental health, and wellbeing. See **Table 1-1** for a summary of the health benefits of physical activity surmised by the Physical Activity Guideline Advisory Committee. Several additional systematic reviews were

---

Table 1-1 Health Benefits of Physical Activity

Children and Adolescents

- Improved bone health (ages 3–17 years)
- Improved weight status (ages 3–17 years)
- Improved cardiorespiratory and muscular fitness (ages 6–17 years)
- Improved cardiometabolic health (ages 6–13 years)
- Reduced risk of depression (ages 6–13 years)

Adults and Older Adults

- Lower risk of all-cause mortality
- Lower risk of cardiovascular disease mortality
- Lower risk of cardiovascular disease (including heart disease and stroke)
- Lower risk of hypertension
- Lower risk of type 2 diabetes
- Lower risk of adverse blood lipid profile
- Lower risk of cancers of the bladder, breast, colon, endometrium, esophagus, kidney, lung, and stomach
- Improved cognition
- Reduced risk of dementia (including Alzheimer's disease)
- Improved quality of life
- Reduced anxiety
- Reduced risk of depression
- Improved sleep
- Slowed or reduced weight gain
- Weight loss, particularly when combined with reduced calorie intake
- Prevention of weight regain following initial weight loss
- Improved bone health
- Improved physical function
- Lower risk of falls (older adults)
- Lower risk of fall-related injuries (older adults)

U.S. Department of Health and Human Services. Physical Activity Guidelines for Americans, 2nd edition. Washington, DC: U.S. Department of Health and Human Services; 2018. https://health.gov/sites/default/files/2019-09/Physical_Activity_Guidelines_2nd_edition.pdf

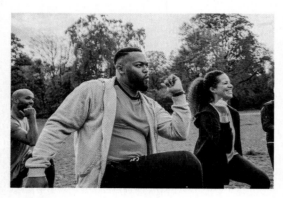

© Maskot/DigitalVision/Getty Images.

commissioned for the Canadian guidelines, which supplement and support the American Physical Activity guidelines, contributing to the overwhelming evidence base for the health benefits of physical activity (Ross et al., 2020).

All of these health risks aggregated from physical inactivity result in a significant amount of healthcare costs for individuals and nations. An economic analysis of the burden of physical inactivity revealed the direct healthcare costs, including **productivity losses** (i.e., loss of revenue due to unavailability of employees), and **disability-adjusted life years** (DALYs; i.e., the combination of years of life lost to premature death and years of life lost to time lived in poor health or in disability) attributable to physical inactivity across 142 countries (Ding et al., 2016). They estimated that globally, physical inactivity costs health-care systems $53.8 billion in 2013, most of that paid by the public sector. Deaths from physical inactivity contributed to $12.9 billion in productivity losses. Physical activity was also found to result in losses of 13.4 million DALYs globally, with 75% of DALYs lost within low- and middle-income countries.

CRITICAL THINKING ACTIVITY 1-1

Why do you think the impact of physical activity on DALYs is so much more prevalent in low- and middle-income countries compared to high-income countries?

These substantial physiological benefits of physical activity are no secret and have been endorsed through national and global initiatives. For example, the World Health Organization (WHO, 2018) has estimated that more than 5 million deaths per year could be averted if the global population were more physically active and it has put out recommendations that people regularly engage in physical activity from birth to death.

2. Are People Aware and Accepting that Physical Activity is Good for Them?

As discussed earlier, scientists, healthcare professionals, and government health agencies are aware of the benefits of physical activity. A second part of the question pertaining to whether a tomato effect toward physical activity exists in society is whether the population has a full understanding of the benefits of a physically active lifestyle.

For at least 20 years, most Americans have reported being aware that physical activity has health benefits. In a study of more than 2,000 Americans households, 94% of people reported that physical activity provides health benefits (Morrow et al., 2004). In a study of 615 Australian adults, people's detailed knowledge of the benefits of physical activity were investigated (Fredriksson et al., 2018). Almost all (99.6%) participants strongly agreed that physical activity was good for their health, and many people even overestimated how many diseases and conditions are preventable through regular physical activity. Nearly 100% of mothers acknowledge that physical activity is important for their child's health too (Rhodes et al., 2013). That more than 90% of people polled agree that physical activity is good for health is pretty outstanding when you put it in perspective. For example, only 68% of Americans polled know that oil, natural gas, and coal are fossil fuels, and only 79% of Americans are aware that antibiotic resistance is a major concern of antibiotics overuse (Kennedy & Hefferon, 2019). The near universal awareness that physical activity is good for us should translate into most everyone being regularly physically active… right?

3. Are People Physically Active?

The final part of the tomato effect courthouse steps. question pertains to whether people are eating the tomatoes or not. Or, is physical activity being embraced by a large portion of the world's population? Unfortunately, the answer is a qualified no. Only about half of North American adults are regularly engaging in aerobic physical activity, and only 20% engage in regular aerobic and muscle-strengthening activity (2018 Physical Activity Guidelines Advisory Committee, 2018; Clarke et al., 2019). Globally, more than 25% of the population (1.4 billion adults) are not engaging in regular physical activity, with more women (1 in 3) than men (1 in 4) at risk of negative health consequences as a result (World Health Organization, 2018). Additionally, more than 80% of adolescents do not engage in regular physical activity (Guthold et al., 2019). Despite the universal understanding of the benefits of physical activity, there has been no improvement in levels of physical activity since 2001, and in high-income countries, physical inactivity has increased by 5% since then (World Health Organization, 2018).

CRITICAL THINKING ACTIVITY 1-2

If you were asked to plan an intervention to reduce the gap of inequality in levels of physical activity between women and men, what intervention would you design and how would it help reduce the gap?

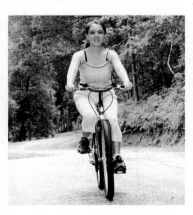

© Spectrelabs/iStock/Getty Images.

So, the answer to the first question of this chapter—"Does participation in physical activity show evidence of a tomato effect?"—seems to be a qualified yes:

1. Yes, physical activity is good for us.
2. Yes, most people are aware and accepting that physical activity is good for them.
3. Generally, people are not physically active.

CRITICAL THINKING ACTIVITY 1-3

What is another example of the tomato effect that has occurred or is occurring?

So, it remains an important global issue that people know the benefits of physical activity, but most are not regularly engaging in physical activity. When it came to tomatoes, the solution was a compelling presentation of evidence that contradicted people's fears and concerns—Johnson eating a tomato surrounded by people in courthouse steps. Could an appealing display of scientific evidence work the same in ridding physical activity of its "tomato effect"? Scientists focusing on the psychology of physical activity and sedentary behavior are trying to do just that. Physical activity psychology researchers conduct studies to provide evidence to inform the world about physical activity and to help people become more active. Then, when enough studies have been conducted, generalized conclusions can be drawn using scientific methods called systematic reviews and meta-analyses.

Systematic Reviews and Meta-Analyses

Continually throughout this book, you will read about the findings of systematic reviews and meta-analyses. We tend to lean on reviews and meta-analyses because they provide an overview perspective of the state of evidence on a particular issue of effect. Whereas a single study finding may be the result of specific design features or random chance, reviews and meta-analyses aggregate evidence from many studies to come to a general consensus across the evidence, and so are less prone to error. A **systematic review** is a literature review focused on a particular research question that tries to identify, appraise, select, and synthesize all high-quality research evidence relevant to that question. A **meta-analysis** is a statistical method of reviewing a body of research evidence that is both systematic and quantitative. **Quantitative research** refers to the systematic empirical investigation of a phenomena via statistical, mathematical, or numerical data or computational techniques. There are many other ways that scientists analyze and report evidence and more methods continue to emerge with innovations in technology and knowledge (Coffee & Tod, 2022). Some approaches are more relevant when new questions emerge in the field, and studies are conducted to determine what types of measures and quantitative studies should be considered, while other approaches such as reviews or meta-analyses are more appropriate when there already is a large body of existing evidence addressing a specific question. There are even umbrella reviews—systematic review of other systematic reviews and **meta-syntheses**—meta-analyses of other meta-analyses (Faulkner, Fagan, & Lee, 2021)! As you read the book, keep an eye out for mention of different types of methods used in the studies that have produced evidence within our field.

Research Integration Through a Meta-Analysis

Consider the following question: Is physical fitness related to anxiety? Across different studies, the operational definition of anxiety could vary markedly. For example, participants' anxiety might be tested with a single self-report question, such as "I feel very anxious." Responses could then be obtained on a nine-point scale containing anchor statements such as "Strongly Disagree" and "Strongly Agree," or it might be tested with a psychometrically sound inventory containing 20 anxiety-relevant questions to which the individual responds "True" or "False," or it might even be assessed using a physiological measure

such as heart rate with responses indicated in beats per minute.

Across that same cross-section of studies, the operational definition of fitness also could vary. For example, fitness might be assessed through the self-reported amount of time spent running per week. Then, responses could be obtained in minutes and/or hours per week, or, fitness might be defined through measures of muscular strength and responses expressed in grams or kilograms (or ounces or pounds) lifted. Finally, fitness might even be assessed using a physiological measure such as maximal oxygen uptake with responses stated in milliliter per kilogram of body weight.

Imagine carrying out a literature review focusing on the question of the relationship between fitness and anxiety. If 50 studies were located, they might vary in the operational definitions used for anxiety, the operational definitions used for fitness, the size of the samples tested, and the nature of the samples tested by, for example, age, gender, physical health status, and mental health status. Also, the 50 studies might vary in their findings relative to the question. That is, 35 studies might show that fitness is associated with reduced anxiety, 10 studies might find that fitness is unrelated to anxiety, and 5 studies might conclude that fitness is associated with increased anxiety. Any scholar attempting to summarize this body of research with a systematic review would be forced to conclude that the results were either mixed or unclear.

In 1976, Gene Glass introduced a protocol for conducting a meta-analysis whereby the magnitude of the treatment effects in individual studies were quantified and the results of several studies were averaged. As Glass, McGaw, and Smith (1981) stated, the essential characteristic of a meta-analysis is that it "is the statistical analysis of the summary findings of many empirical studies" (p. 21). In other words, in statistics a meta-analysis refers to methods focused on contrasting and combining results from different studies in the hope of identifying patterns among study results, sources of disagreement among those results, or other interesting relationships that may come to light.

In essence, the result from an individual study is converted to a standard score, which is called an effect size. Because effect sizes are standard scores, the measures (and the units used to express those measures) in the various studies are not relevant. A percentile is another example of a standard score. Moreover, standard scores can be added and then averaged to draw conclusions about the overall impact of a particular treatment.

Finally, and this is also important, the possible influence of what are called moderator variables should be examined. Moderator variables directly influence the relationship of an independent variable to a dependent variable. So, returning to our example, it would be possible to assess statistically through a meta-analysis whether age is a moderator variable in the fitness–anxiety relationship. If increased fitness is associated with reduced anxiety, does that relationship hold across the age spectrum from adolescents to older adulthood?

Meta-analysis is particularly useful in areas of research where a large number of studies are available, not all the studies are of uniform quality, there is wide variability in the operational definition of the variables, there are differences in the nature of the subjects or differences in designs, and the results have not been completely consistent. Meta-analysis offers the opportunity to statistically average the effects from various studies in order to come to some conclusion for the population as a whole. It is also possible, of course, to subdivide the pool of studies and examine conditions that might serve to moderate the basic relationship.

Interpretation of Effect Sizes

Most of us can easily interpret quantities or amounts when commonly used measures such as inches, feet, seconds, and kilograms are used. Most of us also have a common understanding of the meaning of standard statistical scores such as a percentile (e.g., you scored in the 85th percentile on your SAT). However, interpretation of an effect size is not as intuitively obvious.

Fortunately, Cohen (1992) has provided some guidelines that are useful for understanding the results from a meta-analysis. Thus, the descriptive term "small" can be used for any effect size within the range of $d = 0.20$ to 0.49. Also, the descriptive term "medium" can be used for effect sizes in the range of $d = 0.50$ to 0.79. Finally, the descriptive term "large" can be used for any effect size that is greater than $d = 0.80$.

Another statistical way to interpret an effect size is also available. Consider, for example, the differences in anxiety scores in an experimental group exposed to 16 weeks of exercise versus the improvement in anxiety scores in a control group that simply met and talked for the 16 weeks. An effect size of $d = 0.33$ for the improvement (i.e., reduction) in anxiety scores in the experimental group over that in the control group would mean that the average experimental person improved in (showed a reduction for) anxiety one-third of a standard deviation more than was the case for the average control person. Most people find it easier to use the descriptive terms small, medium, and large for effect sizes of 0.20, 0.50, and 0.80, respectively, although these are relatively arbitrary cutoffs. Using these cutoffs, we would describe effects that are quite distinct using the same descriptive – an effect of 0.50 and 0.79 are both 'large', while an effect of 0.49 is 'small' but one of 0.50 is 'medium'. There are clear limitations to this approach, and there are other ways to interpret effects such as benchmarking.

Benchmarking is a way of interpreting effect sizes that does not rely on the arbitrariness of effect size descriptives. It allows us to describe effects in "real-world" terms. For example, a meta-synthesis of previous meta-analyses used benchmarking to describe the size of effects of physical activity interventions with meaningful metrics of energy expenditure (Wright et al., 2021). They found that overall, physical activity interventions from 2,762 trials had a median effect size of $d = .21$ (small), which equated to an increase of 1,320 steps per day, 15.6 additional minutes of daily moderate-to-vigorous physical activity, and a 4.3% increase in the proportion of participants engaging in regular physical activity.

Physical Activity Psychology

If physical activity is efficacious, one important challenge facing scientists, health professionals, and governments is to help large segments of the population become more physically active. How this will be achieved is not likely to come through additional research in exercise physiology, although that discipline will undoubtedly provide answers to important questions, such as how much activity is necessary to obtain the physiological benefits described earlier. As a science, exercise physiology does not concern itself with general issues associated with understanding and modifying behavior, influencing public opinion, motivating people, and changing people's attitudes. Nor is it a concern of the biomechanics, historians, or sociologists of sport and physical activity. Questions concerning human attitudes, moods, cognitions, and behavior fall directly under the mandate of psychology.

Psychology is a science devoted to gaining an understanding of human behavior. In turn, the area of science we refer to in this text as physical

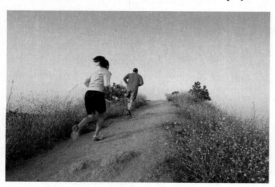

© Logoboom/Shutterstock.

activity psychology (also called exercise psychology) is devoted to gaining an understanding of (1) individual attitudes, moods, feelings, cognitions, and behaviors in the context of physical activity, and (2) the social, environmental, and physical factors that influence those attitudes, feelings, cognitions, and behaviors. In other words, **physical activity psychology** is defined as the study of psychological issues and theories related to physical activity. Physical activity psychology is a subdiscipline within the field of psychology, as well as a subdiscipline within the field of kinesiology.

Individual Correlates of Physical Activity

To understand, promote, and maintain physical activity and decrease sedentary behavior, we need to examine determinants and correlates of these behaviors. In the case of physical activity, a **correlate** is a variable that is associated with either an increase or decrease of physical activity. Importantly, correlates are only statistical associations, rather than evidence of a causal relationship between a factor and physical activity (Bauman, et al., 2002). In comparison, when a variable has been assessed in a longitudinal observational study or an experimental design it is called a determinant. Thus, a **determinant** is a variable that has a causal association with physical activity. Given that the research examining physical activity determinants has largely been generated in either cross-sectional or retrospective studies, the implicit suggestion of causation often is not appropriate (Bauman et al., 2012; Rhodes et al., 2017).

For ease of interpretation, we will use the term correlate in this section because most often this is the more accurate term for physical activity adherence. For example, it is well documented that as we get older, we tend to be less active. It is not true, however, that advancing age causes people to be less active. All of us know older people who are very physically active and younger individuals who are inactive. Also, there is no single variable that explains all physical activity behavior.

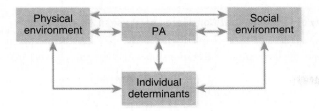

Figure 1-1 A Conceptualization of the Social Ecological Framework for Physical Activity (PA).

Reproduced from Nigg, C. R., Rhodes, R., & Amato, K. R. (2013). Determinants of physical activity: Research to application. In J. M. Rippe (Ed.), *Lifestyle medicine* (pp. 1435–1446). Taylor & Francis Group.

Different variables exert different degrees of influence on different people. For example, spousal support may be important for some people to exercise, but not others. Also, the strength of spousal influence for each person may vary during different stages of their married life. Spousal support for physical activity may be relatively unimportant in early adulthood but important in older adulthood.

Another way to look at individual correlates is to ask the question, "Why are some people physically active and not others?" This is a difficult question to answer. Because physical activity is affected by diverse factors, behavioral theories and models (such as the theory of planned behavior and the transtheoretical model) are used to guide the selection of variables to study. Integration of ideas from several theories into an **ecological model** (including inter-relations between individuals and their social and physical environments) is now becoming more commonplace (Sallis, Owen, & Fisher, 2008). An ecological approach uses a comprehensive framework to explain physical activity, which proposes that determinants at all levels (i.e., individual, social, environmental, and policy) contribute to or influence whether someone engages in exercise. A key principle is that knowledge about all types of influence can inform development of multilevel interventions to offer the best chance of success.

Figure 1-1 presents a social ecological framework for physical activity (see Nigg, Rhodes, & Amato, 2013). This ecological framework highlights people's interactions with their physical and social/interpersonal environments, with individuals shaping their environments, as well as being shaped by them (McLeroy et al., 1998). The focus of this section is on the individual correlates of physical activity. The list of physical activity correlates is long, and individual-level factors such as age, sex, health status, self-efficacy, and previous physical activity are correlated with physical activity levels (Bauman et al., 2012). **Table 1-2** summarizes some of the main individual correlates of

Table 1-2 Summary of the Individual Correlates of Physical Activity

Correlate Category	Specific Correlate	Relationship with Physical Activity (PA)
Demographic	Age	Negative: PA levels continually decline as we get older.
	Socioeconomic status	Positive: Higher socioeconomic status associated with higher PA levels.
	Gender	Male populations exercise more than female populations.
	Health status	Healthy people are more active than persons with medical and psychological conditions.
	Education level	Positive: Higher education level correlated with higher PA levels.

(continues)

Table 1-2 **Summary of the Individual Correlates of Physical Activity**   *(continued)*

Correlate Category	Specific Correlate	Relationship with Physical Activity (PA)
	Weight	Negative: People in the overweight or obese range exercise less than healthy-weight people.
	Marital status	Unrelated. No relationship with marital status and PA levels.
Behavioral	Previous PA	Positive: Previous PA is positively related to future/current PA behavior.
	Smoking	Negative: Negative relationship between cigarette smoking and PA.
Psychological	Self-efficacy	Positive: Higher self-efficacy (confidence in the ability to be physically active in specific situations) correlated with higher PA levels.
	Barriers	Negative: Negative relationship between an individual's perception that there are barriers to PA participation and that individual's actual PA behavior.
	Attitude	Positive: Attitude (overall appraisal or evaluation of PA) positively related with PA intention and behavior.
	Enjoyment	Positive: Enjoyment positively related to PA.

physical activity into categories of demographic, psychological, and behavioral (Bauman et al., 2012; Nigg et al., 2013).

There is also evidence emerging about correlates of physical activity for specific groups of people. For example, Sterdt et al. (2014) conducted a review of systematic reviews investigating correlates of physical activity for children and adolescents. Nine reviews and one meta-analyses

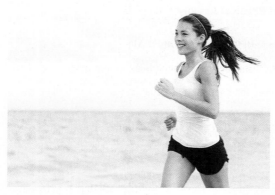

were included which identified 16 correlates consistently associated with more physical activity for children and youth, including demographic factors such as gender, age, ethnicity, and family income, individual cognitive factors such as how good individuals perceived themselves to be at physical activity; as well as social and environmental factors such as participation in community sports, time spent outdoors, and support from parents/guardians. Vancampfort et al. (2012) reviewed correlates of physical activity in patients with schizophrenia and found 25 studies which provided evidence that, for this population, more engagement in physical activity was associated with fewer negative symptoms and medication side effects and social isolation, as well as several other medical, cognitive, social, and environmental factors. In low- and middle-income countries, it was found that older age, unemployment, pain and health problems as well as slow gait and weak grip strength were associated with lower levels of physical activity in adults and older adults (Koyanagi et al., 2017), and less participation in physical education, higher food insecurity, less parental monitoring, fewer friends, and experiences of bullying were associated with lower activity levels in youth (Vancampfort et al., 2019).

Correlates Are Just the Beginning

Investigation of correlates of physical activity is important because we need to understand what factors are associated with physical activity, so we start to determine how to help people engage in more physical activity. However, there are several limitations to this approach to physical activity psychology. First, as we mentioned before, an association between two variables does not mean one causes the other. So, we cannot take it for granted that each of these correlates can and should be changed as a means to enhance people's physical activity levels. Unless major advancements have been made since we've authored this book, we'd have a tough time making people younger!

Second, physical activity and many of the factors that influence our physical activity behavior are **dynamic** – that is, they change over time. So, while it is a good starting point to assess people's physical activity levels and correlates at a single point in time, that is probably not sufficient to adequately capture these factors (Ruissen et al., 2021). I bet just in the last few weeks, you can remember days when you were really active and motivated and times when you were really not motivated and not active. To make real-world changes, scientists are now using more methods to investigate the real-world dynamics of physical activity psychology, which we'll bring up throughout this book.

Finally, a list of correlates only gets us so far in understanding the complex reality that is how and why a person is or is not physically active. Some of these correlates are more meaningful than others, some will be more relevant for some people than for others, and some will only be relevant under some circumstances. Let's face it – physical activity psychology is complex. The benefits we get from physical activity and the factors that lead us to be physically active or inactive are not as simply stated as a grocery list. That's why, in this book, you will be reading a lot about theories and models pertinent to physical activity psychology. We'll revisit these later in the book, but for now, it's important to remember that correlates and determinants are an important starting point for understanding physical activity psychology, but they're just that – a starting point. They can be building blocks for the basis of our understanding. Speaking of building blocks, to this point, we've largely omitted one of the most important pieces of knowledge to know before digging more deeply into the field of physical activity psychology. Before we drill into how and why people should be physically active, we need to understand what we mean by "physically active". How much physical activity should people be striving for? Fortunately, there are guidelines for that.

Guidelines for Physical Activity

The latest iteration of the Physical Activity Guidelines for Americans (2018 Physical Activity Guidelines Advisory Committee, 2018) provides recommendations for physical activity from people aged 3 years to older adults and includes recommendations for specific groups of people, including women during pregnancy and the postpartum period, adults with chronic health conditions, and adults with disabilities. They also put forth recommendations for safe physical activity to reduce risk of injuries and other adverse events. These guidelines are presented in **Table 1-3**. Beyond these specific guidelines for the amount and types of activities that one should be engaged in, the recommendations provide advice on how this can be implemented. The guidelines were written for a professional audience (such as students in a physical activity and sedentary behavior psychology course), so it is recommended that a plain language translation should be used for individuals, families, and communities. There are campaign resources, including interactive tools, fact sheets,

Table 1-3 2018 Physical Activity Guidelines for Americans

Key Guidelines for Preschool-Aged Children

- Preschool aged children (3 -5 years) should be physically active throughout the day to enhance growth and development.
- Adult caregivers of preschool-aged children should encourage play that includes a variety of activity types.

Key Guidelines for Children and Adolescents

- It is important to provide young people opportunities and encouragement to participate in physical activities that are appropriate for their age, that are enjoyable, and that offer variety.
- Children and adolescents (6 – 17 years) should do 60 min (1 hour) or more of moderate-to-vigorous physical activity daily:
  - **Aerobic:** most of the 60 min or more per day should be either moderate- or vigorous-intensity aerobic physical activity and should include vigorous-intensity physical activity on at least 3 days a week.
  - **Muscle-strengthening:** As part of their 60 min or more of daily physical activity, children and adolescents should include muscle-strengthening physical activity on at least 3 days a week.
  - **Bone-strengthening:** As part of their 60 min or more of daily physical activity, children and adolescents should include bone-strengthening physical activity on at least 3 days a week.

Key Guidelines for Adults

- Adults should move more and sit less throughout the day. Some physical activity is better than none. Adults who sit less and do any amount of moderate-to-vigorous physical activity gain some health benefits.
- For substantial health benefits, adults should do at least 150 min (2 hours and 30 min) to 300 min (5 hours) a week of moderate-intensity, or 75 min (1 hour and 15 min) to 150 min (2 hour and 30 min) a week of vigorous-intensity aerobic physical activity, or an equivalent combination of moderate- and vigorous-intensity aerobic activity. Preferable, aerobic activity should be spread throughout the week.
- Additional health benefits are gained by engaging in physical activity beyond the equivalent of 300 min (5 hours) of moderate-intensity physical activity a week.
- Adults should also do muscle-strengthening activities of moderate or greater intensity that involve all major muscle groups on 2 or more days a week, as these activities provide additional health benefits.

Key Guidelines for Older Adults

The key guidelines for adults also apply to older adults. In addition, the following key guidelines are just for older adults:

- As part of their weekly physical activity, older adults should do multicomponent physical activity that includes balance training as well as aerobic and muscle-strengthening activities.
- Older adults should determine their level of effort for physical activity relative to their level of fitness.
- Older adults with chronic conditions should understand whether and how their conditions affect their ability to do regular physical activity safely.
- When older adults cannot do 150 min of moderate-intensity aerobic activity a week because of chronic conditions, they should be as physically active as their abilities and conditions allow.

Key Guidelines for Women During Pregnancy and the Postpartum Period

- Women should do at least 150 min (2 hours and 30 min) of moderate-intensity aerobic activity a week during pregnancy and the postpartum period. Preferably, aerobic activity should be spread throughout the week.
- Women who habitually engaged in vigorous-intensity aerobic activity or who were physically active before pregnancy can continue these activities during pregnancy and the postpartum period.
- Women who are pregnant should be under the care of a health care provider who can monitor the progress of the pregnancy. Women who are pregnant can consult their health care provider about whether or how to adjust their physical activity during pregnancy and after the baby is born.

Key Guidelines for Adults with Chronic Health Conditions and Adults with Disabilities

- Adults with chronic conditions or disabilities who are able, should do at least 150 min (2 hours and 30 min) to 200 min (5 hours) a week of moderate-intensity, or 75 min (1 hour and 15 min) to 150 min (2 hours and 30 min) a week of vigorous-intensity aerobic physical activity, or an equivalent combination of moderate- and vigorous-intensity aerobic activity. Preferably, aerobic activity should be spread throughout the week.
- Adults with chronic conditions or disabilities, who are able, should also do muscle-strengthening activities of moderate or greater intensity and that involve all major muscle groups on 2 or more days a week, as these activities provide additional health benefits.
- When adults with chronic conditions or disabilities are not able to meet the above key guidelines, they should engage in regular physical activity according to their abilities and should avoid inactivity.
- Adults with chronic conditions or symptoms should be under the care of a health care provider. People with chronic conditions can consult a health care professional or physical activity specialist about the types and amounts of activity appropriate for their abilities and chronic conditions.

Key Guidelines for Safe Physical Activity

To do physical activity safely and reduce risk of injuries and other adverse events, people should:

- Understand the risks, yet be confident that physical activity can be safe for almost everyone.
- Choose types of physical activity that are appropriate for their current fitness level and health goals, because some activities are safer than others.
- Increase physical activity gradually over time to meet key guidelines or health goals. Inactive people should "start low and go slow" by starting with lower intensity activities and gradually increasing how often and how long activities are done.
- Protect themselves by using appropriate gear and sports equipment, choosing safe environments, following rules and policies, and making sensible choices about when, where, and how to be active.
- Be under the care of a health care provider if they have chronic conditions or symptoms. People with chronic conditions and symptoms should consult a health care professional or physical activity specialist about the types and amounts of activity appropriate for them.

U.S. Department of Health and Human Services. Physical Activity Guidelines for Americans, 2nd edition. Washington, DC: U.S. Department of Health and Human Services; 2018. https://health.gov/sites/default/files/2019-09/Physical_Activity_Guidelines_2nd_edition.pdf

videos, and graphics at: https://www.health.gov/PAGuidelines/ such as **Figure 1-2**.

Previous American Physical Activity Guidelines

Some people may have a misperception that the health benefits of physical activity can only be achieved by strenuous sustained aerobic activity such as a vigorous 45-minute run. Such perceptions were fostered by the original exercise guidelines established by the American College of Sports Medicine in 1978 (See **Table 1-4** for a description of these 1978 guidelines). These guidelines were based on the improvement of cardiovascular fitness; however, they were often applied to general health (Haskell, 1994). These original guidelines were very specific and led to somewhat regimented thinking about how much physical activity should be recommended. This caused many people to think that physical activity amounts that did not meet these specific criteria would be of either limited or no value (Blair, LaMonte, & Nichaman, 2004).

The next guidelines established by the American College of Sports Medicine and the Centers for Disease Control in 1996 stated that adults should accumulate a minimum of 30 minutes of moderate-intensity physical activity on most, if not all, days of the week (U.S. Department of Health and Human Services, 1996; see Table 1-4). Moderate-intensity physical activity, for example, could include brisk walking at a pace of 3 to 4 miles per hour, climbing stairs, and doing heavy housework. The recommendation for accumulation of physical activity indicated that people can engage in shorter bouts of activity spread out over the course of the day. For example, a person

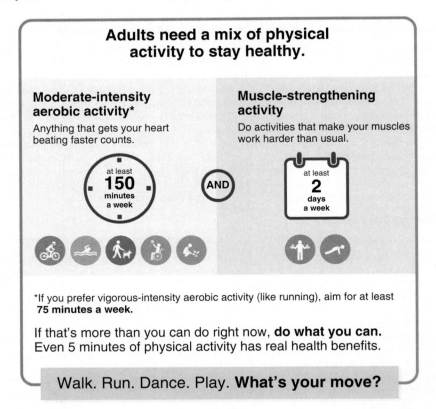

Figure 1-2 Move Your Way Graphic from the U.S. Department of Health and Human Services' Physical Activity Campaign.

U.S. Department of Health and Human Services, https://health.gov/moveyourway.

could go for a 10-minute brisk walk in the morning, afternoon, and evening to reach the daily goal of 30 minutes. The suggestion that physical activity can be accumulated over the course of the day, rather than performed continuously in a single session, was motivated by the difficulties reported by numerous individuals in trying to find a block of 30 minutes per day for physical activity. A main goal of these guidelines was to show people that they do indeed have the time to exercise.

Table 1-4 Former Adult Guidelines for Physical Activity

Activity Characteristics	American College of Sports Medicine (1978)	U.S. Department of Health and Human Services (1996)
Frequency	3–5 times per week	Most (preferably all) days of the week
Intensity	Vigorous	Moderate
Duration	20–45 minutes	Accumulation of ⩾ 30 minutes of daily activity in bouts of at least 10 minutes
Type	Aerobic activity	Any activity that can be performed at an intensity similar to that of brisk walking

Even though lack of time is the most reported barrier to physical activity, adding more time to the day likely wouldn't increase physical activity levels (Rebar et al., 2019). Research findings challenged the guidelines that physical activity bouts must be at least 10 minutes in duration to achieve health benefits. A systematic review of 29 articles tested the association between length of bouts of physical activity and health outcomes. They found evidence that physical activity in bouts <10 min in duration were associated with several health outcomes (Jakicic et al., 2019). One study of more than 4,000 participants showed that the impact of moderate-to vigorous-intensity physical activity on all-cause mortality was not dependent on whether people got their minutes of physical activity in many 5 min bouts or fewer bouts of 10 or more min (Saint-Maurice et al., 2018). These results provide compelling evidence that there are health benefits from engaging in bouts of physical activity that last less than 10 min, especially if that means overall you "move more". This shift in evidence was taken into consideration in the changes from the 2008 to 2018 Physical Activity Guidelines via the omission of the recommendation that activity should be accumulated in bouts of 10 min or more.

Overall, the first version of the Physical Activity Guidelines (Physical Activity Guidelines Committee, 2008) read very similar to the 2018 iteration. This was a major advancement in national guidelines for the country in that a group comprising of 13 leading experts in the field of exercise science and public health provided specific recommendations for different groups of people and different age groups based on the evidence of the health benefits of physical activity at that time. The 2018 edition of the guidelines built on this previous version by integrating the

In a special series, Warburton and Bredin (2019) argued that the way we promote physical activity in guidelines could be improved with a strengths-based approach. They argue that generic threshold-based recommendations such as "at least 150 min of MVPA per week" focus attention on deficits and can be discouraging for people. A strengths-based approach may be more appropriate because the focus is on positivity and hope for change at the individual, community, and population levels. Such an approach is argued to encourage more physical activity through self-empowerment and self-determination. (See **Figure 1-3**).

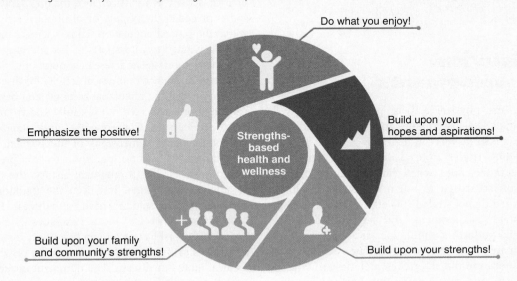

Figure 1-3 Strengths-Based Health and Wellness.

Warburton, D. E., & Bredin, S. S. (2019). Health benefits of physical activity: A strengths-based approach. *Journal of clinical medicine, 8*(12), 2044. https://www.researchgate.net/figure/Strengths-based-health-and -wellness-promotion-through-physical-activity_fig1_337461785 latest scientific evidence in the reported benefits of and recommendations for physical activity. Beyond the elimination of the requirement for physical activity to occur in bouts of at least 10 min, changes to the guidelines included risks of sedentary behavior and their relationship with physical activity, as well as reporting of tested strategies that could be used to get populations more active (2018 Physical Activity Guidelines Advisory Committee, 2018). In a systematic review of people's perceptions of physical activity and sedentary behavior guidelines, it was revealed that people want guidelines that are simple and include good examples and implementation strategies (Hollman et al., 2022). That behavior change approaches have been integrated into the guidelines for the U.S. speaks to the ever-increasing demand to help understand how and why people should engage in regular physical activity. The field of physical activity psychology has an important job ahead of us!

CRITICAL THINKING ACTIVITY 1-5

What do you think about a strengths-based approach to physical activity? Do you think it would be more effective at changing your behavior than specific recommended guidelines? Why or why not?

Historical Developments

The first physical activity psychology (as well as first social psychology and sport psychology) research study was conducted by Norman Triplett in 1898. Triplett noticed that cyclists tended to have faster times when riding against another person compared to when cyclists rode alone. He then demonstrated this effect in a controlled, laboratory experiment, and he concluded that people perform a simple lab task faster in pairs compared with performing it alone.

For example, in one research design, Triplett had children play a game that involved turning a small fishing reel as quickly as possible. He found that the children who played the game in pairs turned the reel faster than those who played

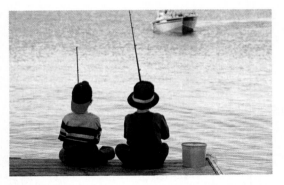

© Sonya etchison/Shutterstock.

alone. These findings were termed social facilitation, which is the tendency for people to do better on simple tasks when in the presence of others. This implies that whenever people are being watched by others they will do well on things that they are already good at doing.

Rejeski and Thompson (1993) noted that although interest has been directed toward the psychology of physical activity since Triplett's (1898) social facilitation studies, most of the research has appeared since the early 1970s. Several reasons were advanced by Rejeski and Thompson for the relatively slow development of the psychology of physical activity as a science. First, the popularity of sports preceded the popularity of physical activity within the general population. Thus, scientists inevitably gravitated toward sports to ask and attempt to answer sports-related research questions. Second, the importance of physical activity for disease prevention and the maintenance of general health has long been suspected but not fully known until relatively recently. Consequently, understanding the psychological dimensions of involvement in physical activity was not perceived to be a pressing priority. Finally, throughout history, the use of a biomedical model has been the traditional approach to understanding health and disease. The **biomedical model of illness** excludes psychological and social factors and includes only biological factors in an attempt to understand a person's medical illness or disease. The dominant concern of the biomedical model is with the treatment of disease as opposed to its prevention. It has only been relatively recent that the importance of a bio-psychosocial approach to disease prevention has been acknowledged. The biopsychosocial model acknowledges that the mind and the body together determine health and illness. As its name implies, the biopsychosocial model's fundamental assumption is that health and illness are the consequences of the interplay of biological, psychological, and social factors. Since these early days, physical activity psychology has grown substantially and now involves investigations of many topics.

Topics of Interest

When research into the psychological aspects of involvement in physical activity increased in the 1970s, it tended to focus on the first portion of the definition outlined above; namely, gaining an understanding of correlates of physical activity and human attitudes, feelings, cognitions, and behaviors in the context of physical activity. Rhodes and Nasuti (2011) examined trends and changes in psychology of physical activity research across 20 years (i.e., 1990–2008) by auditing leading journals where physical activity psychology research is often published. They found that the volume of physical activity psychology research tripled between the 1990s and 2000s. Since then, the field continues to grow with more submissions to most journals in the field. In this book, we will discuss common physical activity psychology research topics outlined in **Table 1-5**.

Table 1-5 **Common Physical Activity Psychology Research Topics**

Topic	Description
Section 2	
Social environment	The perceived and real support we get from the groups and communities we are a part of has an impact on our physical activity and sedentary behavior.
Physical environment	Our physical activity and sedentary behavior are dependent on the opportunities and access we have around us where we live, play and work.
Translational and digital health	Changes in the world, such as our reliance on technology, influence our physical activity and sedentary behavior, as well as the way we can intervene with these behaviors.
Section 3	
Health-related quality of life and positive psychology	Physical activity and sedentary behavior can impact our wellbeing and quality of life.
Personality	Certain aspects of our personality have implications for how much physical activity and sedentary behavior we engage in.
Cognition	Physical activity and sedentary behavior impact how our mind works and the way we think. Physical activity is an important preventative measure and treatment for dementia.
Sleep	Physical activity and sedentary behavior impact our sleep and our sleep impacts how much physical activity and sedentary behavior we engage in.
Depression	Engaging in physical activity decreases our risk of depression and reduces depressive symptoms. It is likely that depression may impact motivation for physical activity and sedentary behavior.

(continues)

Table 1-5 **Common Physical Activity Psychology Research Topics**   *(continued)*

Topic	Description
Anxiety and Stress	Engaging in physical activity can help reduce long-term and acute bouts of stress and anxiety symptoms. Physical activity also reduces the risk of anxiety disorders.
Self-esteem and body image	Engaging in physical activity can improve self-esteem and body image. Self-esteem and body image can impact how and why we engage in physical activity and sedentary behavior.
Section 4	
Social cognitive theories	Much of what we know about motivation of physical activity and sedentary behavior is about our values and expectations about these behaviors and how and why people make strong or weak plans/intentions to change behavior.
Motivational theories	Changes in our physical activity and sedentary behaviors are influenced by why we are motivated to change behavior. Enjoyment is a key factor.
Stage-based and action control theories	What motivates us when we first start physical activity or reduce sedentary behavior is different than what helps us maintain these behavior changes long-term.
Dual process theories	Not all of what dictates our movement behavior is rational or goal-driven. Automatic processes such as habits and our feelings impact our physical activity and sedentary behavior too.

Terminology

Physical Activity and Exercise

A variety of related terms has been the focus of research under the umbrella term physical activity or exercise psychology. Researchers and practitioners, operating under the assumption that definitional clarity is essential for effective communication, have taken care to draw a distinction among terms. Though people use physical activity and exercise interchangeably (Rebar et al., 2017), the terms have different definitions. **Physical activity** is an umbrella term used to describe any body movement produced by skeletal muscles that requires energy expenditure (World Health Organization, 2018). In other words, physical activity refers to any body movement that burns calories, whether from work or

play, daily chores, engaging in a competitive sport, or a daily commute.

Traditionally, exercise, a subcategory of physical activity, was defined as planned, structured, and repetitive activities aimed at improving physical fitness and health (Caspersen, Powell, & Christenson, 1985); however, this definition is controversial as it infers that for a behavior to be "exercise," it must have the end-goal of fitness (Rebar & Rhodes, 2018). Given advancements in our understanding of the complexities of motivation for physical activity behaviors, it is likely more valuable to describe exercise in terms of behavioral characteristics instead of motivational determinants. For example, characteristics that may help distinguish exercise from physical activity may include any or all of the following: frequency, intensity, type, and time (often called the FITT principle; see **Table 1-6** for a description).

Table 1-6 The FITT Principle Defined

Principle	Definition	Example
Frequency	How often you exercise	Five times per week
Intensity	How hard you work during exercise	Moderate intensity
Type	The type of activity you're doing	Brisk walk
Time	How long you exercise	30 minutes

CRITICAL THINKING ACTIVITY 1-6

If it were up to you, how would you define *physical activity* vs *exercise*?

Overall, the field is a bit loose in its terminology for describing physical activity behavior. Researchers sometimes use the terms leisure-time physical activity or recreational physical activity as synonyms for exercise. Others only refer to exercise for moderate- to vigorous-intensity physical activity. Other terms focus on the modality of physical activity such as sport, occupational physical activity, household physical activity, self-care physical activity, and transportation physical activity. We wish that there was more consistency and clarity in the definitions of these terms. For the purposes in this book, we've tended to use "physical activity," with exceptions for specific study or descriptions of the behaviors in certain areas of the field where "exercise" is more commonplace.

Other Terminology Within Physical Activity Psychology

Physical activity psychology has also been referred to as a component of behavioral medicine. **Behavioral medicine** is an interdisciplinary field of medicine concerned with the development and integration of knowledge in the biological, behavioral, psychological, and social sciences relevant to health and illness. The practice of behavioral medicine also includes applied psychophysiological therapies such as biofeedback, hypnosis, and biobehavioral therapy of physical disorders, aspects of occupational therapy, rehabilitation medicine, and psychiatry, as well as preventive medicine.

Health may be viewed as a human condition with physical, social, and psychological dimensions, each characterized by a continuum varying from positive to negative poles. As defined by the World Health Organization over a half century ago (1946), **health** is a state of complete physical, mental, and social well-being and not merely the absence of disease or infirmity. Physical activity, along with a number of other activities, such as maintaining a proper diet and refraining from smoking, contribute to the development and maintenance of health on the positive end of the continuum. Although every health behavior is important in its own right, this textbook concentrates on physical activity and sedentary behavior.

Health psychology is the study of the psychological and behavioral processes in health, illness, and healthcare (Johnston, 1994). It is concerned with understanding how psychological, behavioral, and cultural factors are involved in physical health and illness, in addition to the biological causes that are well understood by medical science. Health psychologists take a biopsychosocial approach; that is, they understand health to be the product not only of biological processes (e.g., a virus, tumor), but also of psychological processes (e.g., stress, thoughts and beliefs, behaviors such as smoking and exercise) and social processes (e.g., socioeconomic status, culture, and ethnicity).

Finally, **sport psychology** is the study of the how psychological factors affect athletes' performance and well-being. Some sport psychologists work with professional athletes and coaches to improve the performance and increase the motivation of athletes. Although sport psychology is commonly referred to as sport and exercise psychology, it is important to understand the distinction between these two related fields.

Summary

Is there a tomato effect—a tendency for people to avoid beneficial activities—insofar as physical activity is concerned? A large number of benefits are associated with physical activity. Furthermore, most people are aware that physical activity is good for them. Despite the known risks of inactivity, in general, throughout the world physical inactivity levels are still unacceptably high. Changes in physical activity behavior and motivation are necessary. To help investigate physical activity behavior, its outcomes, and motivation for physical activity, scientists have investigated the determinants and correlates of physical activity behavior and used systematic reviews and meta-analyses to overview states of evidence from many studies.

A set of recommended guidelines has been made and updated both nationally and globally to suggest amounts and types of physical activity. Generally, adults should aim for 150 min of moderate intensity physical activity or 75 min of vigorous intensity of physical activity per week, although notably any increase in physical activity is beneficial with the key promoted message being, "Move More".

This textbook focuses on the area of science referred to as the psychology of physical activity and sedentary behavior. A variety of diverse behaviors has been the focus of research under the umbrella term psychology of physical activity. Physical activity represents bodily movements produced by skeletal muscles that lead to substantial increases in energy expenditure. This textbook centers on physical activity and sedentary behavior, not other areas such as rehabilitation psychology, sport psychology, or health psychology. What this means, essentially, is that this text incorporates information from research where physical activity or sedentary behavior are the focus.

Vignette: Henry

My parents were not paragons of healthy living. I was in elementary school the day Mom returned from the doctor with a type 2 diabetes diagnosis. The doctor said it was because of all the weight she'd gained after pregnancy as well as her diet. (Her favorite activity was watching daytime television on the couch, and if she ever ate a vegetable, it was soaked in butter and salt.) Since giving birth to me she'd developed back problems and found it painful to walk for more than 5- to 10-minute stretches at a time, so implementing the doctor's recommended 30 minutes of movement a day struck her as impossible. (Needless to say, she didn't follow his advice.)

Dad also had health issues while I was still young. I can't remember a time when he wasn't complaining about the blood pressure pills he needed to take for hypertension. He'd injured his ACL in college playing sports and was afraid to exercise, lest he hurt himself again. Plus, he barely had the time. He worked a demanding job and often worked without enough sleep.

Obviously, physical activity wasn't a priority in my family. Sure, some of my classmates did various activities outdoors to get their blood pumping like biking, hiking, and kayaking in the summers. But I didn't have the money to afford all the gear, and I also worked at the local gas station to save up for college, so I usually met up with my friends after they'd finished these activities so we could play video games at my house or drive into town for a movie.

I have to admit that my more athletic peers intimidated me. I was never picked first in physical education class and I never played sports because I didn't think I was good enough. I tried to stand out, instead, as someone who uses his brain instead of his body. The time I might have spent attending practice for a soccer, baseball, or basketball team I preferred to devote to studying. (If I wasn't hunched over my books, I'd try to pick up an extra shift at work.)

I got into engineering school through early decision. I was thrilled to start working toward my degree. It's something I'd wanted since the third grade. But once I moved to campus and started classes, the stress of having to work part-time and meeting all my academic deadlines became overwhelming. I didn't have an outlet to burn off the mounting stress.

My roommate, an avid exerciser who woke up early to squeeze in his morning runs, suggested I try jogging. "It'll help you relax," he kept trying to convince me, but I kept turning down his invitations to run with him. Then, one Friday afternoon, when neither of us had plans and midterms were almost finished, he asked me to take a walk with him to the college's fitness center. Not having anything better to do , I (reluctantly) agreed.

To be honest, I was humiliated to walk into a gym looking so out of shape. I was already sweating at the thought of other students staring at me and rolling their eyes. I wasn't even sure that my shoes were appropriate for the gym. I tiptoed from one machine to the other in high-tops with holes in the heels. Catching glimpses in the mirrors of students who could have very well been professional weightlifters, I felt out of place. But my roommate urged me to just try a few machines. "You'll be better able to focus on your work," he reassured me.

So, I went on the treadmill. He plugged in a few numbers and forward I went, walking at an incline (and trying not to fall over). The first 5 minutes were rough, but once I got into the swing of things the movement actually felt good. At the 10-minute mark my roommate chided me, "Is that a smile I see?" (I couldn't deny that this wasn't so bad after all.).

After about 15 minutes of walking, he brought me over to the weight rack to show me how to do some basic bicep curls and overhead presses. ("Don't compare yourself to the other people in here," he kept telling me, when I'd looked in shame at the other exercisers who were so much stronger than I was. "Everyone has to start somewhere.").

I didn't tell him then but the reason I persisted at our first gym session was the fear of becoming like my parents. They'd always encouraged me to be better than they were. And though it hurt me to hear in their voices a certain sense of self-defeat—of giving up on taking care of their health—I felt that by exercising I'd be make them proud. (While at the same time avoiding the health issues they'd faced throughout adulthood.)

I've been regularly exercising ever since that day—I'm about to graduate, and am not sure I would have been able to make it this far without the added health boost of exercising regularly.

No, I'll never be a bodybuilder. Or a marathon runner. Or someone with six-pack abs. But had you told me fitness didn't require any of the above—that it could be a lot simpler, entailing a 30-minute walk once or twice a day or a light jog a few times a week with some basic weight training sprinkled throughout, I probably would have started sooner.

Being active isn't as hard as I thought it would be. I just never had a healthy amount of physical activity modeled for me by my parents, and the athletes in my high school, as well as the exercisers I saw in workout videos on social media, seemed to be doing things that were just way out of my range of possibility.

But I've found what works for me. It isn't an exorbitant amount of activity. Rather, it's just enough. And I think it's incredible that a few weekly trips to the gym, a stroll or two around campus each day, and the occasional bike ride on weekends have improved my ability to focus on schoolwork while making me feel stronger, more energetic, and even less stressed. Perhaps best of all, I've gained the confidence to ask someone out on a date!

Key Terms

behavioral medicine An interdisciplinary field of medicine concerned with the development and integration of knowledge in the biological, behavioral, psychological, and social sciences relevant to health and illness.

benchmarking A way of interpreting effect sizes that does not rely on the arbitrariness of effect size descriptives.

biomedical model of illness A model traditionally used to understand health and disease that excludes psychological and social factors and focuses only on biological risk factors.

correlate A variable that is associated with either an increase or decrease of another variable, such as physical activity.

determinant A variable that has a causal association with an outcome, such as physical activity.

disability-adjusted life years (DALYs) The combination of years of life lost to premature death and years of life lost to time lived in poor health or in disability.

dynamic A characteristic of a variable that describes change over time.

ecological model The integration of ideas from several theories, including interrelations between individuals and their social and physical environments.

health A state of complete physical, mental, and social wellbeing.

health psychology The study of the psychological and behavioral processes in health, illness, and health care.

meta-analysis A statistical method of reviewing a body of research evidence that is both systematic and quantitative.

meta-synthesis Meta-analytic approach to synthesizing results of meta-analyses using quantitative methods.

physical activity An umbrella term for any body movement produced by skeletal muscles that requires energy expenditure.

physical activity psychology The study of psychological issues and theories related to physical activity.

productivity loss Loss of revenue as a result of unavailability of employees.

quantitative research The systematic empirical investigation of a phenomenon via statistical, mathematical, or numerical data or computational techniques.

sport psychology The study of the how psychological factors affect athletes' performance and well-being.

systematic review A review of scientific literature focused on a particular research question to identify, appraise, select, and synthesize all high-quality research evidence relevant to that question.

Review Questions

1. List three health benefits of physical activity.
2. What are disability-adjusted life years (DALYs) and how are they influenced by physical activity?
3. Why is it that most people know physical activity is good for them but tend not to engage in it regularly?
4. What is the difference between a systematic review and a meta-analysis?
5. How would you describe the field of physical activity psychology to a friend?
6. What is the distinction between correlates and determinants of physical activity?
7. List four correlates or determinants of physical activity.
8. What are the current recommended guidelines of physical activity for Americans?
9. What is behavioral medicine?

Applying the Concepts

1. List three correlates or determinants of Henry's physical activity.
2. If you were creating an intervention to help Henry become more physically active, what would it entail and why?

References

2018 Physical Activity Guidelines Advisory Committee. (2018). *2018 Physical activity guidelines advisory committee scientific report*. U.S. Department of Health and Human Services.

American College of Sports Medicine. (1978). Position statement on the recommended quantity and quality of exercise for developing and maintaining fitness in healthy adults. *Medicine and Science in Sports and Exercise, 10*, vii–x. https://pubmed.ncbi.nlm.nih.gov/723501/

Bauman, A. E., Reis, R. S., Sallis J. F., Wells, J. C., Loos, R. J., & Martin, B. W. (2012). Correlates of physical activity: Why are some people physically active and others not? *The Lancet, 380*(9838), 258–271.

Bauman, A. E., Sallis, J. F., Dzewaltowski, D. A., & Owen, N. (2002). Toward a better understanding of the influences on physical activity: The role of determinants, correlates, causal variables, mediators, moderators, and confounders. *American Journal of Preventive Medicine, 23*(2), 5–14.

Blair, S. N., LaMonte, M. J., & Nichaman, M. Z. (2004). The evolution of physical activity recommendations: How much is enough? The *American Journal of Clinical Nutrition, 79*(5), 913S–920S.

Church, T. S., & Blair, S. N. (2009). When will we treat physical activity as a legitimate medical therapy … even though it does not come in a pill? *British Journal of Sports Medicine, 43*(2), 80–81.

Clarke, J., Colley, R., Janssen, I., & Tremblay, M. S. (2019). Accelerometer-measured moderate-to-vigorous physical activity of Canadian adults, 2007 to 2017. *Health Reports, 30*(8), 3–10.

Coffee, P., & Tod, D. (2022). Introduction to IRSEP special issue: Research review methodologies in sport and exercise psychology. *International Review of Sport and Exercise Psychology, 1*, 1–4. https://doi.org/10.1080/1750 984X.2021.2014101

Cohen, J. (1992). A power primer. *Psychological Bulletin, 112*, 155–159.

Ding, D., Lawson, K. D., Kolbe-Alexander, T. L., Finkelstein, E. A., Katzmarzyk, P. T., van Mechelen, W., & Pratt, M. (2016). The economic burden of physical inactivity: A global analysis of major non-communicable diseases. *The Lancet, 388*(10051), 1311–1324. https://doi.org/10.1016 /S0140-6736(16)30383-X

Faulkner, G., Fagan, M. J., & Lee, J. (2021). Umbrella reviews (systematic review of reviews). *International Review of Sport and Exercise Psychology, 15*(1)73–1890. https://doi.org/10 .1080/1750984X.2021.1934888

Fredriksson, S. V., Alley, S. J., Rebar, A. L., Hayman, M., Vandelanotte, C., & Schoeppe, S. (2018). How are different levels of knowledge about physical activity associated with physical activity behaviour in Australian adults? *PLOS ONE, 13*(11), e0207003. https://doi.org /10.1371/journal.pone.0207003

Glass G. V. (1976). Primary, secondary, and meta-analysis of research. *Educational Researcher, 5*(10), 3–8.

Glass, G. V., McGaw, B., & Smith, M. L. (1981). Meta-analysis in social research. Beverly Hills, CA: Sage.

Goodwin, J. S., & Goodwin, J. M. (1984). The tomato effect: Rejection of highly efficacious therapies. *The Journal of the American Medical Association, 251*(18), 2387–2390.

Guthold, R., Stevens, G. A., Riley, L. M., & Bull, F. C. (2019). Global trends in insufficient physical activity among adolescents: a pooled analysis of 298 population-based surveys with 1·6 million participants. The *Lancet Child and Adolescent Health. 4*(2), 23–35. https://doi.org/10.1016 /S2352-4642(19)30323-2

Haskell, W. L. (1994). J. B. Wolffe Memorial Lecture. Health consequences of physical activity: Understanding and challenges regarding dose-response. *Medicine and Science in Sports and Exercise, 26*, 649–660.

Hollman, H., Updegraff, J. A., Lipkus, I. M., & Rhodes, R. E. (2022). Perceptions of physical activity and sedentary behaviour guidelines among end-users and stakeholders: A systematic review. *International Journal of Behavioral Nutrition and Physical Activity, 19*(21), 1–13.

Jakicic, J. M., Kraus, W. E., Powell, K. E., Campbell, W. W., Janz, K. F., Troiano, R. P., Sprow, K., Torres, A., & Piercy, K. L. (2019). Association between bout duration of physical activity and health: Systematic review. *Medicine and Science in Sports and Exercise, 51*(6), 1213–1219. https://doi.org/10.1249/MSS.0000000000001933

Johnston, M. (1994). Current trends in health psychology. *The Psychologist, 7*, 114–118.

Kennedy, B., & Hefferon, M. (2019, March 28). What Americans know about science: Science knowledge levels remain strongly tied to education; republicans and democrats are equally knowledgeable. *Pew Research Center Science & Society*. https://www.pewresearch.org/science/2019/03/28 /what-americans-know-about-science/

Koyanagi, A., Stubbs, B., Smith, L., Gardner, B., & Vancampfort, D. (2017). Correlates of physical activity among community-dwelling adults aged 50 or over in six low- and middle-income countries. *Public Library of Science ONE, 12*(10), e0186992. https://doi.org/10.1371 /journal.pone.0186992

McLeroy, K. R., Bibeau, D., Steckler, A., & Glanz, K. (1988). An ecological perspective on health promotion programs. *Health Education & Behavior, 15*(4), 351–377.

Morrow, J. R., Krzewinski-Malone, J. A., Jackson, A. W., Bungum, T. J., & FitzGerald, S. J. (2004). American adults' knowledge of exercise recommendations. *Research Quarterly for Exercise and Sport, 75*(3), 231–237. https:// doi.org/10.1080/02701367.2004.10609156

Nigg, C. R., Rhodes, R., & Amato, K. R. (2013). Determinants of physical activity: Research to application. In J. M. Rippe (Ed.), *Lifestyle medicine* (pp. 1435–1446). New York, NY: Taylor & Francis Group.

Physical Activity Guidelines Committee. (2008). *2008 Physical Activity Guidelines for Americans*. U. S. Department of Health & Human Services.

Piercy, K. L., Troiano, R. P., Ballard, R. M., Carlson, S. A., Fulton, J. E., Galuska, D. A., George, S. M., & Olson, R. D. (2018). The physical activity guidelines for Americans. *The Journal American Medical Association, 320*(19), 2020–2028. https://doi.org/10.1001/jama.2018.14854

Rebar, A. L., Schoeppe, S., Alley, S., Short, C. E., Dimmock, J. A., Jackson, B., Conroy, D. E., Rhodes, R. E., & Vandelanotte, C. (2017). Automatic evaluation stimuli – The most frequently used words to describe physical activity and the pleasantness of physical activity. *Frontiers in Psychology 7*(1277). https://doi.org/10.3389/fpsyg.2016.01277

Rejeski, W. J., & Thompson, A. (1993). Historical and conceptual roots of exercise psychology. In P. Seraganian (Ed.), *Exercise psychology: The influence of physical exercise on psychological processes* (pp. 3–35). New York, NY: Wiley.

Rhodes, R. E., & Nasuti, G. (2011). Trends and changes in research on the psychology of physical activity across 20 years: A quantitative analysis of 10 journals. *Preventive Medicine, 53*, 17–13.

Ross, R., Chaput, J-P., Giangregorio, L. M., Janssen, I., Saunders, T. J., Kho, M. E., Poitras, V. J., Tomasone, J. R., El-Kotob, R., McLaughlin, E. C., Duggan, M., Carrier, J., Carson, V., Chastin, S. F., Latimer-Cheung, A. E., Chulak-Bozzer, T., Faulkner, G., Flood, S. M., Gazendam, M. K., Healy, G. N., Katzmarzyk, P. T., Kennedy, W., Lane, K. N., Lorbergs, A., Mzclaren, K., Marr, S., Powell, K. E., Rhodes, R. E., Ross-White, A., Welsh, F., Willumsen, J., & Tremblay, M. S. (2020). Canadian 24-hour movement guidelines for adults aged 18–64 years and adults aged 65 years or older: An integration of physical activity, sedentary behaviour, and sleep. *Applied Physiology, Nutrition, and Metabolism, 45*, S57–S102.

Ruissen, G. R., Zumbo, B. D., Rhodes, R. E., Puterman, E., & Beauchamp, M. R. (2021). Analysis of dynamic psychological processes to understand and promote physical activity behaviour using intensive longitudinal methods: A primer. *Health Psychology Review, Available Online*, 1–34. https://doi:10.1080/17437199.2021.1987953

Saint-Maurice, P. F., Troiano, R. P., Matthews, C. E., & Kraus, W. E. (2018). Moderate-to-vigorous physical activity and all-cause mortality: Do bouts matter? *Journal of the American Heart Association, 7*(6), e007678.

Sallis, J. F., Owen, N., & Fisher, E. B. (2008). Ecological models of health behavior. In K. Glanz, B. K. Rimer, and K. Viswanath (Eds.), *Health behavior and health education: Theory, research, and practice* (pp. 465–486). San Francisco, CA: Jossey-Bass.

Sterdt, E., Liersch, S., & Walter, U. (2014). Correlates of physical activity of children and adolescents: A systematic review of reviews. *Health Education Journal, 73*(1), 72–89. https://doi.org/10.1177/0017896912469578

Rebar, A. L., Johnston, R., Paterson, J. L., Short, C. E., Schoeppe, S., & Vandelanotte, C. (2019). A test of how Australian adults allocate time for physical activity. *Behavioral Medicine, 45*(1), 1–6. https://doi.org/10.1080/08964289.2017.1361902

Rebar, A. L., & Rhodes, R. E. (2018). Progression of motivation models in exercise science: Where we have been and where we are heading. In G. Tenenbaum & R. C. Eklund (Eds.), *The Handbook of Sport Psychology* (Vol. 4). John Wiley & Sons, Inc.

Rhodes, R. E., Berry, T., Craig, C. L., Faulkner, G., Latimer-Cheung, A., Spence, J. C., & Tremblay, M. S. (2013). Understanding parental support of child physical activity behavior. *American Journal of Health Behavior, 37*(4), 469–477. https://doi.org/10.5993/AJHB.37.4.5

Rhodes, R. E., Bredin, S. S. D., Janssen, I., Warburton, D. E. R., & Bauman, A. (2017). Physical activity: Health impact, prevalence, correlates and interventions. *Psychology and Health, 32*(8), 942–975. https://doi.org/10.1080/08870446.2017.1325486

Triplett, N. (1898). The dynamogenic factors in pacemaking and competition. *American Journal of Psychology, 9*(4), 507–533.

U.S. Department of Health and Human Services. (1996). *Physical activity and health: A report of the Surgeon General*. Atlanta, GA: U.S. Department of Health and Human Services, Centers for Disease Control and Prevention, National Center for Chronic Disease Prevention and Health Promotion.

Vancampfort, D., Knapen, J., Probst, M., Scheewe, T., Remans, S., & De Hert, M. (2012). A systematic review of correlates of physical activity in patients with schizophrenia. *Acta Psychiatrica Scandinavica, 125*(5), 352–362. https://doi.org/10.1111/j.1600-0447.2011.01814.x

Vancampfort, D., Van Damme, T., Firth, J., Smith, L., Stubbs, B., Rosenbaum, S., Hallgren, M., Hagemann, N., & Koyanagi, A. (2019). Correlates of physical activity among 142, 118 adolescents aged 12–15 years from 48 low- and middle-income countries. *Preventive Medicine, 127*, 105819. https://doi.org/10.1016/j.ypmed.2019.105819

Warburton, D. E., & Bredin, S. (2019). Health benefits of physical activity: A strengths-based approach. *Journal of Clinical Medicine, 8*(12), 2044. https://doi.org/10.3390/jcm8122044

World Health Organization. (1946). *Preamble to the constitution of the World Health Organization as adopted by the International Health Conference*, New York, 19–22 June 1946, and entered into force on 7 April 1948.

World Health Organization. (2018). Physical inactivity. World Health Organization.

Wright, C. E., Rhodes, R. E., Ruggiero, E. W., & Sheeran, P. (2021). Benchmarking the effectiveness of interventions to promote physical activity: A meta-synthesis. *Health Psychology, 40*(11), 881–821. https://doi.org/10.1037/hea0001118

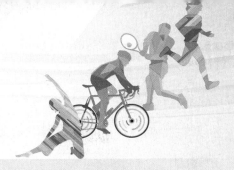

CHAPTER 2

Introduction to the Psychology of Sedentary Behavior

LEARNING OBJECTIVES

After completing this chapter, you will be able to:

- Describe what sedentary behavior is and how it is distinct from physical inactivity.
- Estimate the number of people who are sedentary.
- Describe the attributes of sedentary behavior.
- Differentiate among key terms such as *inactive, screen time*, and *sedentary*.
- Identify individual correlates of sedentary behavior.
- Understand the health effects of sedentary behavior.

Introduction

The health benefits of moderate to vigorous physical activity on a regular basis are well documented and our findings of their benefits continue to increase. The science clearly shows that regular physical activity is associated with the reduction of more than 25 chronic diseases (Rhodes et al., 2017). Today; however, there is a rapid rise in research examining how **sedentary behavior**, as opposed to physical activity, affects our health (Tremblay et al., 2017). Sedentary behavior includes waking activities undertaken in a sitting or reclined position, such as watching TV, reading, playing video games, and engaging in computer activities. Because sedentary behavior is so prevalent and has so many negative

health effects, experts are now beginning to ask the question: "Is sitting the new smoking of our generation?" An interesting question indeed.

CRITICAL THINKING ACTIVITY 2-1

What is meant by the statement: "Is sitting the new smoking of our generation?" Do you think this is true?

The scientific study of sedentary behavior is recent. Within the last 20 years, an explosion of research has occurred even though we have known since the 1950s that sitting too much is hazardous to our health (Morris et al., 1953). In a landmark series of studies, Morris and his

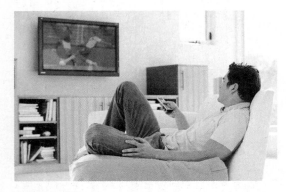

© Monkey Business/Fotolia.

colleagues (1953) examined the activity levels among different occupations. For instance, their seminal study revealed that the sedentary drivers of London's double-decker buses had higher rates of cardiovascular disease than the conductors who climbed the stairs and walked around the bus collecting tickets from passengers. The data were so compelling because the bus drivers and the conductors were similar demographically; that is, the bus drivers and the conductors were the same age and social class. There was only one obvious difference between these two groups—the drivers were sedentary and the conductors were not. In fact, the conductors

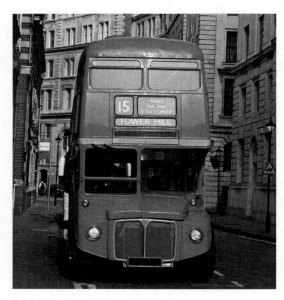

© AnnSteer/iStockPhoto.

ascended and descended 500 to 750 steps per working day. And they were half as likely as the drivers to die of a sudden heart attack.

Morris and his colleagues extended their study findings to other populations, and they noticed that postmen who delivered the mail by either bike or on foot had fewer heart attacks than the sedentary postal men who either served behind the counters or as the telephone switchboard operators. Although, collectively, these early studies provided evidence for the role of physical activity in averting premature mortality, it has only recently been hypothesized that some of these observed associations may be explained by differences in time spent sitting; that is, the bus drivers sat more than the conductors, and the telephone switchboard operators and clerks sat more than the postmen. Unfortunately, the independent roles of sitting vs. physical activity cannot be determined from these early studies. However, they do provide an intriguing look into the potential health effects of sitting too much.

CRITICAL THINKING ACTIVITY 2-2

Why were the independent roles of sitting vs. physical activity not examined in these landmark studies?

Traditionally, physical activity studies have focused on activities performed at moderate to vigorous intensities, rather than sedentary behavior or even mild intensity physical activity. In health guidelines, physical activity of at least moderate intensity has been the critical target, and often the mode has been a focus on vigorous intensity exercise, prolonged in duration. Thus, there is a dearth of research on sedentary behavior, in general, and even less on the psychology of sedentary behavior. The main purpose of this chapter is to examine this emerging field of scientific inquiry. In this chapter, we will define and describe how sedentary behavior is distinct from physical inactivity, examine the sedentary behavior guidelines, discuss the health effects of sedentary behavior, outline individual correlates of sedentary behavior, and determine how sedentary behavior is measured.

Defining Sedentary Behavior

Too much sitting (or being sedentary) appears to be a health risk, particularly when combined with too little moderate-to-vigorous intensity physical activity. What exactly does this mean? Even if people are meeting the physical activity guidelines of, for example, exercising at a moderate intensity for 150 minutes per week, yet spend most of the remaining waking hours left in sedentary activities, this has a negative impact on their health. Thus, not only should people be meeting the physical activity guidelines, but they should also reduce the time they spend sitting during the day (Chaput et al., 2020; 2018 Physical Activity Guidelines Advisory Committee, 2018). This is an emerging area of inquiry, with most research findings illustrating that sedentary behavior has negative health effects independent of physical activity (Saunders et al., 2020). In other words, we need to not only move more at a moderate and/or vigorous pace, but we also need to stand up more during the day. There is some evidence that higher levels of moderate-to-vigorous physical activity (i.e., >60 min per day) can have protective effects against the additional health detriments of sedentary behavior (Ekelund et al., 2016, 2019); however, most people struggle to be physically active at this intensity and duration and stand more during the day (see **Figure 2-1**).

But how does sedentary behavior differ from light activity? Sedentary behavior refers to any waking activity characterized by little physical movement and an energy expenditure of ≤1.5 **metabolic equivalents (METs)** in either a sitting or reclining position (Tremblay et al., 2012). This means that any time a person is either sitting or lying down, that person is engaging in sedentary behavior. Sleeping does not count as sedentary behavior—remember, you must be awake. Sedentary behavior encompasses many activities that often include technology (TV, computer use, video games), socializing (sitting, talking, texting), travel (car, train), work/school (desk job, studying), and leisure activities (reading, listening to music). The collective term of **screen time** is often used to refer to TV watching, playing

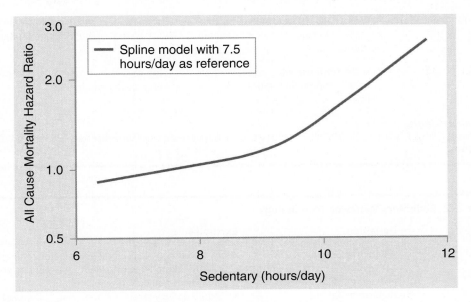

Figure 2-1 Dose-Response between Sedentary Time and All-Cause Mortality.

Reproduced from Ekelund, U., Tarp, J., Steene-Johannessen, J., Hansen, B. H., Jefferis, B., Fagerland, M. W., Whincup, P., Diaz, K. M., Hooker, S. P., Chernofsky, A., Larson, M. G., Spartano, N., Vasan, R. S., Dohrn, I-M., Hagstromer, M., Edwardson, C., Yates, T., Shiroma, E., Anderssen S. A., & Lee, I. M. (2019). Dose-response associations between accelerometry measured physical activity and sedentary time and all cause mortality: systematic review and harmonised meta-analysis. *BMJ, 366*, l4570.

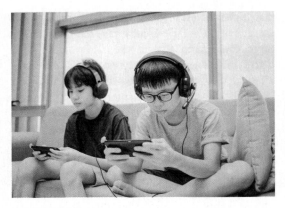

© Edwin Tan/E+/Getty Images.

passive video games, and using mobile devices and computers that can include sitting, standing or moving for multiple purposes. In comparison, **recreational screen time** refers specifically to TV watching, video game playing, using the computer, or use of other screens during leisure time specifically.

Light or mild physical activity, which often is incorrectly grouped with sedentary behavior, involves energy expenditure at the level of 1.6 to 2.9 METs. Mild physical activities include, for example, slow walking, cooking food, and washing dishes. For clarification, **Table 2-1** provides the categories and descriptions of the various physical activity intensities and **Table 2-2** highlights the terminologies for different forms of sedentary behaviors.

Is **sedentarism** different from just not getting enough physical activity? Yes! The term **inactive behavior** or **physical inactivity** typically describes those who are performing insufficient amounts of moderate to vigorous physical activity (van der Ploeg & Hillsdon, 2017). In other words, those people who are not

Table 2-1 **Categories of Physical Activity Intensity**

Intensity	METs	Description	Examples
Light	1.6 to <3	Aerobic activity that does not cause noticeable changes in breathing rate.	Standing, light walking, washing dishes, folding laundry.
Moderate	3 to 6	Aerobic activity that is able to be conducted while having an uninterrupted conversation.	Brisk walking, mopping, water aerobics, easy biking, riding, doubles tennis.
Vigorous	6 to <9	Aerobic activity in which a conversation generally cannot be maintained uninterrupted.	Singles tennis, running, high impact aerobics, biking uphill.

METs = metabolic equivalents.
Data from Norton, K., Norton, L., & Sadgrove, D. (2010). Position statement of physical activity and exercise intensity terminology. *Journal of Science and Medicine in Sport, 13,* 496–502.

Table 2-2 **Sedentary Behavior Terminology**

Term	Definition	Examples
Physical Inactivity	An insufficient physical activity level to meet present physical activity recommendations	▪ Children and youth (5–17 years): Not achieving 60 min of moderate- to vigorous-intensity physical activity per day. ▪ Adults (≥ 18 years): Not achieving 150 min of moderate-to-vigorous-intensity physical activity per week or 75 min of vigorous-intensity physical activity per week.

Term	Definition	Examples
Sedentary Behavior	Any waking behavior characterized by an energy expenditure ≤1.5 metabolic equivalents (METs), while in a sitting, reclining or lying posture	■ Children and youth (5–17 years): Use of electronic devices (e.g., television, computer, tablet, phone) while sitting, reclining or lying; reading/writing/drawing/painting while sitting; homework while sitting; sitting at school; sitting in a bus, car or train. ■ Adults (≥ 18 years): Use of electronic devices (e.g., television, computer, tablet, phone) while sitting, reclining or lying; reading/writing/talking while sitting; sitting in a bus, car or train.
Screen Time	Screen time refers to the time spent on screen-based behaviors. These behaviors can be performed while being sedentary or physically active.	■ All age and ability groups: Watching TV, using a smartphone/tablet, using a computer. ■ Active screen time: Playing active video games, running on a treadmill while watching television.

Tremblay, M. S., Aubert, S., Barnes, J. D., Saunders, T. J., Carson, V., Latimer-Cheung, A. E., Chastin, S. F., Altenburg, T. M., & Chinapaw, M. J. M. (2017). Sedentary Behavior Research Network (SBRN) – Terminology Consensus Project process and outcome. *International Journal of Behavioral Nutrition and Physical Activity, 14,* 75.

meeting specified physical activity guidelines. Lynette Craft and her colleagues (2012) illustrated that the time we spend sitting is independent of the amount of time we spend engaged in moderate to vigorous physical activity. In their study, 91 healthy women between the ages of 40 to 75 years wore an activity monitor for 1 week. The researchers then determined the time (i.e., minutes per day) these women spent sitting, standing, stepping, and in bouts of moderate to vigorous physical activity that was at least 10 minutes in duration.

They found that the time spent sitting, standing, and in incidental physical activities did not differ between women who either met or exceeded the physical activity guidelines compared to those with either no or minimal levels of physical activity (see **Figure 2-2**). These results show that our time spent in moderate to vigorous physical activity does not replace significant periods of sitting time. In other words, physical activity and sedentary behaviors are independent classes of behavior. In fact, some people who meet the physical activity guidelines may spend a great deal of their remaining waking time sitting. This is an excellent example of what is meant by "the active couch potato" (Owen, Healey, & Dunstan, 2010).

CRITICAL THINKING ACTIVITY 2-3

Describe what is meant by "the active couch potato." Do you know anyone who is an active couch potato? How does this affect that person's health?

Thus, there is a need to examine not only how to make a physically inactive public more active but how to also make a sedentary public stand more. Most of society sits for prolonged periods almost every day. The healthy and relatively very active women in the aforementioned study sat about 9 hours a day, which is more than the average adult sleeps. As Craft and colleagues

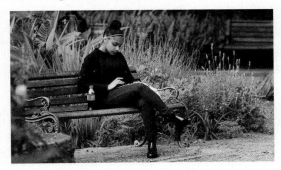

© Michael de Nysschen/Shutterstock.

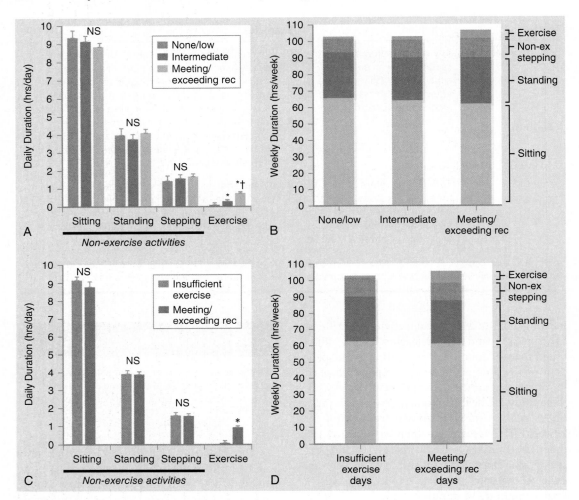

Figure 2-2 Time Spent Sitting, Standing, Incidental Stepping When Not Exercising (Non-exercise Stepping), and Exercising as Defined by the Federal Physical Activity Guidelines. Panels A and B illustrate the results for a cross-sectional comparison between subjects for the mean daily duration of each behavior (A) and the sum of all behaviors accumulated over an entire week (B) for the three groups stratified by time spent exercising. Panels C and D illustrate the within subject analysis results comparing the days that people had insufficient exercise (< 30 minutes) compared to days where they perform at least 30 minutes of aerobic exercise. Values are expressed as means with SEM bars.*p <0.001 vs. None/Low Exercise or Insufficient Exercise; † p < 0.001 vs. Intermediate.

Reproduced from Craft, L. L., Zderic, T. W., Gapstur, S. M., VanIterson, E. H., Thomas, D. M., Siddique, J., & Hamilton, M. T. (2012). Evidence that women meeting physical activity guidelines do not sit less: An observational inclinometry study. *International Journal of Behavioral Nutrition and Physical Activity, 9,* 122. https://doi.org/10.1186/1479-5868-9-122

(2012) noted, sitting is now more abundant than sleeping, which is likely an important development in human history. Public health recommendations and interventions aimed at increasing physical activity behavior are unlikely to impact how much time people spend sitting because they are independent behaviors and the promotion of one (e.g., reducing sedentary behavior) does not necessarily lead to the follow-through of the other (e.g., moderate intensity exercise). As seen in **Table 2-3**, sedentary behavior may operate in a different way from physical activity; thus, sedentary behavior is in need of its basic research inquiry and interventions (Spence et al., 2017).

Table 2-3 **Key Properties Applied to Physical Activity and Sedentary Behavior**

	Physical Activity Behavior	Sedentary Behavior
Motivation	High: Intentional activity with some habitual elements	High: Powerful motivational elements, which appear to include habitual and intentional elements with a strong attitudinal and hedonic base (i.e., affect).
Capability	High: Requires considerable behavioral regulation	Low: Some heightened awareness may be needed but likely not a major property of the behavior.
Opportunity	Moderate: Influenced by select social and environmental aspects	High: Likely heavily influenced by physical and social environments.

Data from Spence, J. C., Rhodes, R. E., & Carson, V. (2017). Challenging the dual-hinge approach to intervening on sedentary behavior. *American Journal of Preventive Medicine, 52,* 403–406.

Health Significance of Sedentary Behavior

Emerging research is finding a relationship between sedentary behavior and the risk of mortality and several chronic diseases (Biswas et al., 2015; Dempsey et al., 2020; Patterson et al., 2018; Saunders et al. 2020). For example, in a meta-analysis and systematic review, Biswas and colleagues (2015) reviewed 47 studies that examined the association of sedentary time with multiple health outcomes. They found that higher levels of sedentary behavior were associated with all-cause mortality, cardiovascular disease mortality, cardiovascular disease incidence, cancer mortality, cancer incidence, and type 2 diabetes incidence. While these associations between sedentary time and health outcomes were generally more pronounced at lower levels of physical activity, sedentary time was still independently associated with deleterious health outcomes regardless of physical activity.

The researchers concluded the existence of a consistent association between sedentary time and diabetes, cancer, cardiovascular disease, and all-cause mortality. Other systematic and meta-analytic reviews have confirmed that prolonged sedentary behavior is associated with poor mental health outcomes. For example, Rodriguez-Ayllon and colleagues (2019) conducted a review of 114 papers on child and youth mental health and sedentary behavior. The authors concluded there were significant associations between greater amounts of sedentary behavior and both increased psychological ill-being (i.e., depression) and lower psychological well-being (i.e., satisfaction with life and happiness) in children and adolescents.

One of the most interesting areas of research in sedentary behavior, physical activity, and health is through analyses of what happens to health outcomes when people substitute the time allotted to these behaviors. For example, Janssen and colleagues (2020) reviewed eight studies of >12,000 unique participants on how behavior composition of sleep, moderate-vigorous physical intensity activity, and sedentary behavior interacted with all-cause mortality, body composition, and cardiovascular health markers. The authors found that reallocating time into physical activity from sleep/sedentary behavior was associated with favorable changes to all of these health outcomes. Taking time from sedentary behavior and reallocating it into physical activity or sleep was associated with favorable changes to all-cause mortality. A similar review of 56 studies found similar results (Grgic et al., 2018). Specifically, the authors found that reallocations of sedentary time to higher intensities of physical activity was associated with a significant reduction in mortality risk. The findings of these studies highlight that the amount of time we allocate to different behaviors matters and that prioritizing regular moderate-to-vigorous intensity physical activity is of critical importance to one's health.

Guidelines for Sedentary Behavior

The current model of physical activity and health is well supported by over 70 years of scientific inquiry, and the beneficial effects of moderate to vigorous intensity physical activity have been more clearly defined in recent years. As Peter Katzmarzyk (2010) noted, if we are complacent with the existing paradigm—that increasing levels of moderate to vigorous physical activity will result in the greatest improvements in public health—we may not obtain the full return on investment with respect to improving quality of life and life expectancy through human movement.

Researchers, healthcare professionals, and government agencies have realized the health importance of limiting people's sedentary behavior in addition to trying to increase their physical activity levels. Some countries, such as Australia and Canada, have been leaders in advancing guidelines on how to reduce sedentary behavior and screen time (Australia Department of Health and Aging, 2012). Because the research is still in its developmental stage, the current sedentary behavior guidelines are considered consensus "sensible" guidelines. This means that as more science emerges on the health effects of sedentary behavior, the guidelines will be updated to reflect the new knowledge.

In 2011, the Canadian Society for Exercise Physiology released sedentary behavior guidelines for children and youth. These guidelines were rolled into 24-hour guidelines that encompassed sleep and physical activity in 2016, with the addition of guidelines for children in the early years (aged 0–4) in 2017 (Tremblay et al., 2016, 2017). These sedentary behavior guidelines were developed with the goal of getting the well-known, yet undervalued, statement across: "Move more and sit less every day." The children and youth guidelines recommend that, for health benefits, children and youth should minimize the time that they spend being sedentary each day. This may be achieved by the following two general categories of (1) limiting recreational screen time to no more than 2 hours per day (with lower levels of screen time associated with additional health benefits) and (2) limiting sedentary (motorized) transport, extended sitting time, and time spent indoors throughout the day. The sedentary behavior guidelines for children in the early years recommends 1) no screen time for children under two and less than one hour for children 3–4 years of age, and 2) no restrained movement or sitting for over an hour at a time. In 2020, Canada completed its 24-hour movement suite of recommendations to include sedentary behavior guidelines for adults and older adults. These recommendations included 1) sitting that should not exceed an accumulation beyond eight hours per day and 2) less than 3 hours of that time should be recreational screen viewing (Ross et al., 2020). **Table 2-4** provides a more detailed description

Table 2-4 Canadian Sedentary Behavior Guidelines

Infants and Young Children 0–4 Years	Children and Youth 5–17 Years	Adults 18+
Not being restrained for more than 1 hour at a time (e.g., in a stroller or car seat) or sitting for extended periods.	Minimize time spent being sedentary.	Limiting sedentary time to 8 hours or less.
For children under 2, screen time is not recommended.	Limit screen time to less than 2 hours a day.	No more of the 8 hours being sedentary should include 3 hours of recreational screen time.
For children 2–4 years, screen time should be limited to under 1 hour per day; less is better.	Limit sedentary (motorized) transport, extended sitting, and time spent indoors throughout the day.	Breaking up long periods of sitting as often as possible.

Data from the Canadian Society of Exercise Physiology (2020): https://csepguidelines.ca/

Table 2-5 Ways to Reduce Children's Sedentary Behavior Time

Early Years (0–4 years)	Children (5–17 years)
Limit the use of playpens and infant seats when baby is awake.	Turn the TV off.
Explore and play with your child.	Hide the remote.
Stop during long car trips for playtime.	Reduce the number of TVs in the home. Take TVs out of kitchens and bedrooms.
Set limits and have rules about screen time.	Plan outdoor family time.
Keep TVs and computers out of bedrooms.	Create a TV watching and computer schedule.
Take children outside every day.	

Data from Salmon, J., Tremblay, M. S., Marshall, S. J., & Hume, C. (2011). Health risks, correlates, and interventions to reduce sedentary behavior in young people. *American Journal of Preventive Medicine, 41,* 197–206.

of the sedentary guidelines for children. See **Table 2-5** for recommendations on how young people should limit their involvement in sedentary pursuits to reduce health risks (Tremblay et al., 2011; Tremblay et al., 2012; Canadian Society of Exercise Physiology, 2020).

While Canada has been the only country thus far to have specific sedentary behavior guidelines for health across all age groups, most countries, including the U.S. (2018 Physical Activity Guidelines Advisory Committee, 2018) and Australia (Australian Government Department of Health, 2014), encourage adults to sit less. This approach was also recently adopted by the World Health Organization (2020). The differences in providing

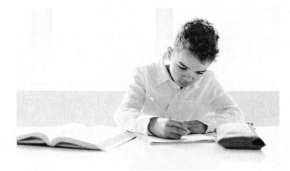

© Lopolo/Shutterstock.

specific guidelines, such as no more than eight hours a day of sitting, compared to a more generic "sit less" form of messaging largely stems from differences in opinion among researchers in terms of what guidelines should represent, given the current state of the evidence. Specifically, it is acknowledged that sedentary behavior is linked to deleterious health outcomes, but many in the international scientific community believe it is still premature to fully describe the dose-response relationship (Stamatakis et al., 2019; Dempsey et al., 2020), while others suggest that some benchmark guideline is better than nothing at all (Chaput et al., 2019). Clearly, all countries will move toward specific sedentary behavior guidelines as this research evolves.

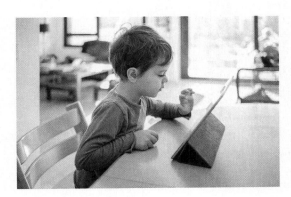

© Westend61 GmbH/Alamy Stock Photo.

CRITICAL THINKING ACTIVITY 2-4

How would you expand on the sedentary guidelines to other populations, including pregnant women, disabled adults, and older adults?

Prevalence of Sedentary Behavior

In addition to the promotion of moderate to vigorous intensity physical activity, people should not sit for extended periods of time. Unfortunately, people, regardless of their age, spend too much time in sedentary activities. Based on the following quote it is likely that the former American educator Robert Maynard Hutchins (1899–1977) also spent a large portion of his day sitting: "The secret of my abundant health is that whenever the impulse to exercise comes over me, I lie down until it passes away" (McEvoy, 1938, p. 482). How many people today hold his view of physical activity and sedentary behavior? In other words, just how sedentary are we? To answer this question, let's take a closer look at the prevalence of sedentary behavior in a variety of populations.

Both children and adults spend a large portion of their day being sedentary. The average child spends about 5 to 10 hours a day being sedentary. Of this sedentary time, young people typically spend 4 hours a day in screen-based behaviors, such as watching video-based programming on TVs, tablets and smartphones, playing video games, and using the computer (Thomas et al., 2020). And the average adult spends more than 9 hours a day in sedentary behaviors (Gennuso et al., 2013; Healy, Matthews, Dunstan, Winkler, & Owen, 2011), which equates to over 60% of their waking time (Prince et al., 2019). Older adults are among the most sedentary. For example, a review by Harvey et al. (2015) that included measurements across 10 countries showed that older adults spend an average of 9.4 hours a day sedentary, equating to 65–80% of their waking day. There is also considerable evidence that sedentary behavior has increased for people of all ages during the COVID-19 pandemic (Stockwell et al., 2021). **Figure 2-3** illustrates the typical adult pattern of daily activities when categorized in terms of intensity level (based on the percentage of a 24-hour day; Norton, Norton, & Sadgrove, 2010). This figure reveals graphically that most of our time during the day is spent engaged in sedentary activities.

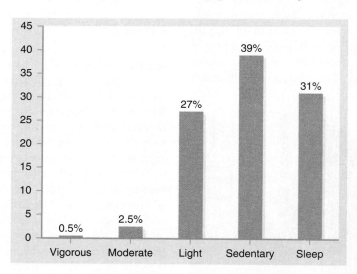

Figure 2-3 Typical Adult Pattern of Daily Activities (percentage of a 24-hour day).

Data from Norton, K., Norton, L., & Sadgrove, D. (2010). Position statement of physical activity and exercise intensity terminology. *Journal of Science and Medicine in Sport, 13*, 496–502.

Based on the quote from Robert Hutchins, it is likely that if he were alive today, he would not be meeting either the physical activity or sedentary behavior guidelines. Research is revealing that very few people are meeting both health guidelines. Canadian researchers found that only 15% of 3- to 4-year-olds and 5% of 5-year-olds are meeting both the physical activity and sedentary behavior guidelines (Colley et al., 2013). These findings are a wake-up call that we need to stand up and get moving.

As another example, sedentary behavior and physical inactivity have increased significantly among American mothers over the last four decades. Edward Archer and his colleagues (2013) analyzed 45 years of national data (from 1965 to 2010) on the following two groups of mothers: (1) those with children 5 years or younger and (2) those with children aged 6 to 18 years. Physical activity was determined by the amount of time allocated to housework, childcare, laundry, food preparation, postmeal cleanup, and exercise. Sedentary behavior was the sum of time spent in a vehicle and using screen-based media.

The researchers found that with each passing generation, mothers have become more physically inactive, sedentary, and obese. From 1965 to 2010, the average amount of physical activity among mothers with younger children fell from 44 hours a week to less than 30 hours a week, resulting in a decrease in energy expenditure of 1,573 calories per week. In comparison, the average amount of physical activity among mothers with older children decreased from 32 hours to less than 21 hours a week, with a reduction in energy expenditure of 1,238 calories per week.

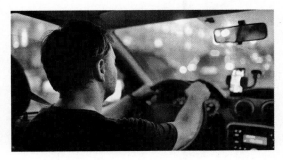

© Maria Sbytova/Shutterstock.

Focus on College Students

What about college students? Newly-found independence often allows college students to make decisions and choices that were previously made for them by their parents/guardians. A review of 125 studies assessing the sedentary behaviors of college students was published recently (Castro et al., 2020). Most studies were cross-sectional (84%) and reported screen time of 61% or total sitting time 39%. The results of self-reported sedentary behavior showed that university students spend 7.29 hours per day being sedentary, but this was considerably higher when students were measured with objective accelerometers (9.82 hours per day average!). Computer use was the most common sedentary behavior and there were no major demographic differences in sedentary behavior (e.g., gender, ethnicity). These results are alarming because they suggest students may engage in more sedentary time compared to the general young adult population. The study also showed evidence that sedentary behavior may be on the rise among university students, further complicating long-term health outcomes.

This finding means that mothers in 2010 would have to eat 175 to 225 fewer calories per day to prevent weight gain than mothers in 1965.

Not surprising, these significant declines in physical activity corresponded with large increases in sedentary pastimes such as watching TV. On average, sedentary behaviors increased from 18 hours a week in 1965 to 25 hours a week in 2010 among mothers with older children, and from 17 hours a week to nearly 23 hours a week among mothers with younger children. Finally, compared to mothers who work outside the home, mothers who did not work outside the home had about twice the decrease in physical activity and a much larger increase in sedentary behavior (see **Figures 2-4** and **2-5**).

In short, the prevalence of sedentary behavior is rapidly increasing across the globe in all age demographics and may have increased even further because of the COVID-19 pandemic. The increased prevalence in sedentary time is largely driven by reductions in movement at work, at

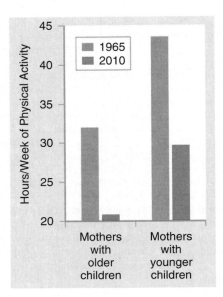

Figure 2-4 Time Allocated to Physical Activity in Mothers by Year. Note: From 1965 to 2010, the time allocated to physical activity decreased in mothers. Specifically, the time allocated to physical activity decreased by 11.1 hours/week (from 32.0 to 20.9 hours/week) in MOC and by 13.9 hours/week (from 43.6 to 29.7 hours/week) in MYC.

Data from Archer, E., Lavie, C. J., McDonald, S. M., et al. (2013). Maternal inactivity: 45-year trends in mothers' use of time. *Mayo Clinic Proceedings, 88*, 1368–1377.

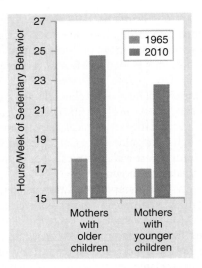

Figure 2-5 Time Allocated to Sedentary Behavior in Mothers by Year. Note: From 1965 to 2010, the time allocated to physical activity decreased in mothers. Specifically, the time allocated to physical activity decreased by 11.1 hours/week (from 32.0 to 20.9 hours/week) in mothers with older children (between the ages of 6 and 18 years) and by 13.9 hours/week (from 43.6 to 29.7 hours/week) in mothers with younger children (i.e., children 5 years of age or younger).

Data from Archer, E., Lavie, C. J., McDonald, S. M., et al. (2013). Maternal inactivity: 45-year trends in mothers' use of time. *Mayo Clinic Proceedings, 88*(12), 1368–1377.

home, and in travel. In particular, the rapid and dramatic changes in the workforce over the last century have resulted in increased sedentary behavior at work (Kirk & Rhodes, 2011; Prince, 2019). Current estimates reveal that people today spend about 80% of their working day sitting (Smith et al., 2016). Because people spend a large

portion of their waking hours at work, it provides an ideal environment to intervene to get people to stand and move more. Research is revealing that active workstations such as treadmill desks and pedal desks can increase energy expenditure without affecting work performance (Prince et al.,

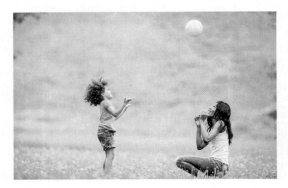

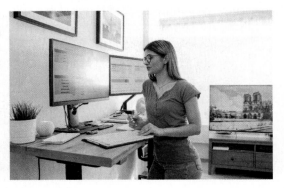

2017). In other words, replacing traditional office chair and desktop computer workstations with active workstations may be a strategy for mitigating the low energy expenditure inherent to contemporary office workstations.

Individual Correlates of Sedentary Behavior

While the health benefits of meeting the physical activity guidelines are well established, the health risks of sedentary behavior, independent of meeting the physical activity guidelines, are evolving. Studies have shown that prolonged sedentary behavior, independent of physical activity level, is associated with various negative health conditions, such as cardiovascular disease, obesity, type 2 diabetes, cancer, metabolic syndrome, and psychological distress. From this evidence, it is essential to identify correlates of sedentary behavior so that interventions can target those individuals at a higher likelihood for engaging in sedentary behaviors.

Several studies have examined correlates of sedentary behavior (e.g., Castro et al., 2018; Chastin et al., 2015; Dogra & Stathokostas, 2014; Dunlop et al., 2014; Harrington, Barreira, Staiano, & Katzmarzyk, 2013; Mielke, da Silva, O'Donoghue et al., 2016; Owen, & Hallal, 2014; Prince et al., 2017; Rhodes, Mark, & Temmel, 2012; Temmel & Rhodes, 2013). Most of the research examining the correlates of sedentary behavior has focused on demographic factors. Thus, we know little about personal motives or environmental and social correlates of sedentary behavior, although what information we do know about these correlates is included in later chapters in this textbook. A summary of emerging findings on the correlates of sedentary behavior is presented in **Table 2-6**. This is a developing area of research, and further study is needed to

Table 2-6 Individual Correlates of Sedentary Behavior

Correlate Category	Specific Correlate	Relationship with Sedentary Behavior
Demographic	Age	Positive: Sedentary behavior increases as we get older.
	Ethnicity	Mixed evidence. No definitive association.
	Socioeconomic status	Negative: Higher socioeconomic status is associated with more general sedentary behavior, while lower socioeconomic status is associated with more leisure-time screen-based sedentary behavior.
	Gender	Mixed evidence. No definitive association.
	Health status	People with chronic diseases, disabilities, and mood disorders are more sedentary than healthy persons.
	Children in the home	Negative: Those with dependent children in the home tend to have less sedentary behavior.
	Weight	Positive: Obese and overweight people sit more than those who are at the recommended weight/BMI for their height.
	Retirement status	People who are retired sit more than people who are not retired.
	Employment status	People who are unemployed are more sedentary than people who are employed. White collar employees are more sedentary than blue collar employees.

(continues)

Table 2-6 **Individual Correlates of Sedentary Behavior**   *(continued)*

Correlate Category	Specific Correlate	Relationship with Sedentary Behavior
Behavioral	Physical activity behavior	People who are physically active tend to be less sedentary.
	Smoking	People who smoke are more sedentary than people who do not smoke.
	Diet	Those who eat a less healthy diet (e.g., high consumption of energy-dense snacks and fast food) are more sedentary.
	Alcohol consumption	No relationship.
	Screen viewing	Positive: TV viewing positively related to sedentary behavior.

substantiate these correlates in high-quality studies with standardized and objective measures of sedentary behavior.

Of interest is the use of technology and how it affects sedentary behavior. In other words, is technology a correlate of sedentary behavior? Today's college students are a unique population to examine the effects of technology on activity levels because they are the first cohort of young people raised entirely in the **digital age** (also

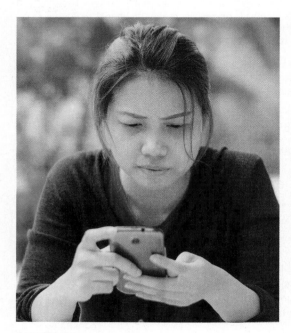

© Inabanz/Shutterstock.

known as the new media or information age). These **digital natives** have interacted with technology from an early age and are often described as "hyperconnected" to their cell phones and other electronic devices (Anderson & Rainie, 2012).

Andrew Lepp and his colleagues (Lepp, Barkley, Sanders, Rebold, & Gates, 2013) examined the relationship between cell phone use and college students' levels of sedentary behavior and physical activity. In the first part of their study, 305 college students completed a self-report questionnaire measuring cell phone use in the following three ways: (1) total cell phone use per day, (2) total number of text messages sent per day, and (3) total number of calls made per day. In the second part of their study, 49 students were interviewed regarding their cell phone use and physical activity behavior; they also completed a progressive treadmill exercise test to exhaustion to assess cardiorespiratory fitness (i.e., VO_2 max test).

The researchers found that students averaged just over 300 minutes (5 hours) of cell phone use per day. In addition, 88.2% of participants reported using the cell phone primarily for leisure. No significant gender differences were found for cell phone use (see **Table 2-7**). The researchers, however, found that cell phone use was negatively related with cardiorespiratory fitness; that is, high-frequency cell phone users tended to be less physically fit than low-frequency cell phone users.

Table 2-7 Self-Reported Cell Phone Use by Gender

Cell Phone Use	Men (n = 134)	Women (n = 168)
Total use per day (minutes)	299	313
Text messages sent per day	214	158
Calls made per day	6.7	5.0

Data from Lepp, A., Barkley, J. E., Sanders, G. J., Rebold, M., & Gates, P. (2013). The relationship between cell phone use, physical and sedentary activity, and cardiorespiratory fitness in a sample of U.S. college students. *International Journal of Behavioral Nutrition and Physical Activity, 21.* https://doi.org/10.1186/1479-5868-10-79

The researchers concluded that cell phone use is associated with physical activity and fitness in a manner similar to other types of sedentary behaviors, such as watching TV and using a computer. Although cell phones provide many of the same temptations as TV and Internet-connected computers, the main difference is that cell phones fit in our pockets and purses and are with us wherever we go. Thus, they provide an ever-present invitation to "sit and play." It appears that compared to low-frequency cell phone users, high-frequency cell phone users are more likely to forgo being physically active to use their cell phones for more sedentary activities, such as using social media, playing video games, and surfing the Internet.

CRITICAL THINKING ACTIVITY 2-5

Compare and contrast the correlates for sedentary behavior and physical activity. What are the main differences? What are the main similarities?

Measures of Sedentary Behavior

Many self-report instruments have been used to detect sedentary behavior, although fewer measures have undergone extensive evidence for validity. Ecological momentary assessment methods to assess sedentary behavior have also become common in research but lack tests of validation (DeGroot et al., 2020; see Chapter 10 for a details on ecological momentary assessment). Recent advances in objective measurement devices (**accelerometers**, inclinometers) have made it possible to measure the full range of movement levels, from sedentary to vigorous physical activity, with a single instrument. Although accelerometers can accurately classify participants' behavior as sedentary, they do not provide information about either the type of sedentary behavior or the context (Prince et al., 2017). In other words, an accelerometer, for example, can tell us if someone is sedentary, but we do not know if the person is sitting and watching TV at home or sitting at a computer at work. Thus, it is recommended that objective measures of sedentary behavior such as accelerometers be used in conjunction with context in specific subjective measures (e.g., self-reports) to assess both the type and context of the sedentary behavior.

Recent research on how people conceptualize sedentary behavior is also important to consider during measurement. Gardner and colleagues (2019) showed that people tend to think of the higher-order activity or goal (e.g., reading a book, driving a car, watching a program, etc.) rather than the act of sitting. These findings highlight the importance of the sedentary activity rather than the behavior of sitting itself. This is particularly important to self-report measures of sedentary behavior. Research has shown that self-report sedentary behavior measures that involve questions on multiple domains and sedentary activities are superior measures of sedentary behavior than general estimates of sitting or single item measures (Dall et al., 2017; Prince et al., 2017; Prince et al., 2020). For example, the Sedentary Behavior Questionnaire is a brief, yet comprehensive, assessment of sedentary behavior in adults. The questionnaire assesses the time that people spend in the following nine sedentary behaviors: watching TV, playing computer/video games, sitting while listening to music, sitting and talking on the phone, doing paperwork or office work,

Table 2-8 Sedentary Behavior Questionnaire

SEDENTARY BEHAVIOR: Weekday

On a typical WEEKDAY, how much time do you spend (from when you wake up until you go to bed) doing the following?

	None	15 min. or less	30 min.	1 hr	2 hrs	3 hrs	4 hrs	5 hrs	6 hrs or more
1. Watching television (including videos on VCR/DVD).	O	O	O	O	O	O	O	O	O
2. Playing computer or video games.	O	O	O	O	O	O	O	O	O
3. Sitting listening to music on the radio, tapes, or CDs.	O	O	O	O	O	O	O	O	O
4. Sitting and talking on the phone.	O	O	O	O	O	O	O	O	O
5. Doing paperwork or computer work (office work, emails, paying bills, etc.)	O	O	O	O	O	O	O	O	O
6. Sitting reading a book or magazine.	O	O	O	O	O	O	O	O	O
7. Playing a musical instrument.	O	O	O	O	O	O	O	O	O
8. Doing artwork or crafts.	O	O	O	O	O	O	O	O	O
9. Sitting and driving in a car, bus, or train.	O	O	O	O	O	O	O	O	O

Rosenberg, D. E., Norman, G. J., Wagner, N., Patrick, K., Calfas, K. J., & Sallis, J. F. (2010). Reliability and validity of the Sedentary Behavior Questionnaire (SBQ) for adults. *Journal of Physical Activity and Health, 7,* 697–705.

sitting and reading, playing a musical instrument, doing arts and crafts, and sitting and driving/riding in a car, bus, or train (see **Table 2-8**).

When participants are completing the Sedentary Behavior Questionnaire, they are asked to report their sedentary time separately for weekdays versus weekend days. Wording for weekday reporting is: "On a typical weekday, how much time do you spend (from when you wake up until you go to bed) doing the following?" In comparison, the wording for weekend day reporting is: "On a typical weekend day, how much time do you spend (from when you wake up until you go to bed) doing the following?"

Summary

Sedentary behavior has become a popular area of research in the psychology of physical activity, and for good reason. The prevalence of sedentary behavior is increasing rapidly across the globe, and it is negatively affecting our health. Some examples of sedentary behavior are sitting for prolonged periods watching television, playing passive video games, and using motorized transport (such as sitting on a bus or in a car). One of the key challenges is to improve our knowledge of how to change sedentary behavior at a unique time in history when our physical and social environment encourages and reinforces sedentary behavior.

Thus, a main question within the psychology of sedentary behavior is how to get people to sit less during the day. This is different from engaging in physical activity. This means that, in addition to promoting regular physical activity, behavioral scientists must find ways to change people's behavior so that they are doing more mild activities, such as standing or moving with light intensity.

The take-home message is that most people need to engage in more moderate to vigorous physical activity and also stand and move more. Future studies should measure sedentary and light activity to determine their independent and joint contributions to various health outcomes. Because this field of inquiry is developing, additional high-quality studies using valid measures of sedentary behavior are needed to further our understanding of the psychology of sedentary behavior.

Vignette: Sam

I wake up around 6:30 a.m. each morning to give myself enough time to shower and get dressed and ready before starting my hour commute via car to work. Most mornings, I'm lucky if I grab a muffin to eat while I drive. It's rare that I have time to sit down for a full breakfast.

I arrive at the office at around 8:45, sometimes a bit after 9:00, if traffic is bad. As an executive assistant to the CEO of a small insurance company, the majority of my day is spent fielding phone calls and emails from clients, scheduling the boss's meetings and travel plans, coordinating with our account director to manage billing inquiries, and organizing reports from the focus groups my company conducts on a monthly basis.

Needless to say, most of this requires me to stay seated. I'd say the most physical activity I get during normal business hours depends on how many times I walk to the copy machine down the hallway and how often I make trips to the restroom throughout the day.

I know that I'm supposed to get more exercise. And the need's especially strong considering that my cholesterol levels were higher than normal on my most recent blood test. I try to watch what I eat so as to control my weight, but I'm well aware health isn't just about being able to fit into a size 4.

I've tried joining a gym before but my commitment to training usually lasts only a few months—often around New Year's or during the first few weeks of spring, when I'm getting ready to be seen in less clothing come summer. The trouble with me is that I just don't feel like I have the energy or the time to commit to working out. Going to the gym adds time to my already lengthy commute to and from work. And, honestly, by the time I leave the office I'm completely exhausted. On particularly stressful days, I'm more likely to come home, order takeout, and watch Netflix for the few hours I have to myself before bedtime rather than going to my local fitness center.

I'm single now and I don't have kids, so I am at an advantage in terms of being able to squeeze a few sessions of exercise in during a week. I've tried recently to commit to doing a few at-home yoga and Pilates routines that I learned online. But it's frustrating to me that physical activity simply isn't built into the typical workday—and also that my commute saps the time and energy I'd have to really put more effort into a legitimate workout.

I've considered getting a treadmill or elliptical machine for my home. But I rent a small apartment and worry about the noise it would make for the neighbors below as well as how much space it would take up. (Not to mention the machine's cost.) I want to imagine there's an easier way to fit it all in. But while I'm working to repay my student loans, make rent each month, and put money into a savings account, the prospect of keeping in shape just seems completely out of reach. Sometimes I wonder: Would I need to go part time just to make room in my life for the gym?

Key Terms

accelerometer A device that detects and quantifies physical activity and movement via an electronic sensor. Records body acceleration minute to minute, providing detailed information about the frequency, duration, intensity, and pattern of movement. The data provided often are used to estimate energy expenditure.

digital age Refers to an economy based on the digitization of information and widespread use of computers. Also known as the computer age or information age.

digital native A person who was born during or after the general introduction of digital technologies and is therefore familiar with computers and the internet from an early age.

inactive behavior Performing insufficient amounts of moderate and/or vigorous physical activity (i.e., not meeting specified physical activity guidelines).

metabolic equivalent (MET) A physiological measure used to express the energy cost of physical activities. It is the ratio of metabolic rate (i.e., the rate of energy consumption) during a specific physical activity to a reference metabolic rate.

physical inactivity The absence of physical activity, usually reflected as the proportion of time not engaged in physical activity of a predetermined intensity.

recreational screen time Activities such as watching television, playing video games, using the computer, or using other screens during discretionary time (i.e., nonschool or work-based use) that are practiced while sedentary.

screen time The amount of time people spend in sedentary behaviors such as playing video games, using the computer, watching television, or using mobile devices.

sedentarism Engagement in sedentary behaviors characterized by minimal movement, low energy expenditure, and rest.

sedentary behavior Any waking activity characterized by an energy expenditure of less than or equal to 1.5 metabolic equivalents (METs) in a sitting or reclining posture.

Review Questions

1. What are the sedentary guidelines for children aged 0 to 4 years?
2. What is the difference between sedentary behavior and inactive behavior?
3. What are some of the health implications of sedentary behavior?
4. Describe the prevalence of sedentary behavior in children, adults, and older adults.
5. How much time do college students spend on cell phone use daily?
6. How does this affect their levels of physical activity and sedentary behavior?
7. Describe two correlates of sedentary behavior.
8. How has sedentary behavior and physical inactivity changed among American mothers over the last four decades? What role do children play?
9. Is sitting the new smoking of our generation? Describe your answer in detail using information provided in this chapter.

Applying the Concepts

1. How has Sarah's sedentary lifestyle affected her health?
2. Why is Sarah so sedentary? What factors in Sarah's life contribute to her sedentary lifestyle?

References

2018 Physical activity guidelines advisory committee. (2018). *Physical Activity Guidelines Advisory Committee Scientific Report.*

Anderson, J., & Rainie, L. (2012). Millennials will benefit and suffer due to their hyperconnected lives. *The Pew Research Center's Internet and American Life Project.* Retrieved from https://www.pewresearch.org/internet/2012/02/29/millennials-will-benefit-and-suffer-due-to-their-hyperconnected-lives/

Archer, E., Lavie, C. J., McDonald, S. M., Herbert, J. R., Taverno Ross, S. E., McIver, R. M., & Blair, S. N. (2013). Maternal inactivity: 45-year trends in mothers' use of time. *Mayo Clinic Proceedings, 88*(12), 1368–1377.

Australian Government Department of Health. (2014). Physical activity and sedentary behavior guidelines. Retrieved March 2014 from https://www.health.gov.au/health-topics/physical-activity-and-exercise/physical-activity-and-exercise-guidelines-for-all-australians#:~:text=combination%20of%20both.-,Be%20active%20on%20most%20(preferably%20all)%20days%2C%20to%20weekly,most%20(preferably%20all)%20days.&text=At%20least%202%20days%20a%20week

Biswas, A., Oh, P. I., Faulkner, G. E., Bajaj, R. R., Silver, M. A., Mitchelle, M. S., & Altern D. A. (2015). Sedentary time and its association with risk of disease incidence, mortality, and hospitalization in adults: A systematic review and meta-analysis. *Annals of Internal Medicine, 162*, 123–132.

Canadian Society for Exercise Physiology. (2011). Canadian physical activity guidelines for adults 18–64 years [Electronic Version]. Retrieved from https://www.physio-pedia.com/Canadian_Physical_Activity_and_Sedentary_Behaviour_Guidelines

Castro, O., Bennie, J., Vergeer, I., Bosselut, G., & Biddle, S. J. H. (2020). How sedentary are university students? A systematic review and meta-analysis. *Prevention Science, 21*, 332–343.

Castro, O., Bennie, J., Vergeer, I., Bosselut, G., & Biddle, S. J. H. (2018). Correlates of sedentary behaviour in university students: A systematic review. *Preventive Medicine, 116*, 194–202.

Chaput, J.-P., Olds, T., & Tremblay, M. (2020). Public health guidelines on sedentary behaviour are important and needed: a provisional benchmark is better than no benchmark at all. *British Journal of Sports Medicine, 54*(5), 308–309.

Chaput, J. P., Willumsen, J., Bull, F., Chou, R., Ekelund, U., Firth, J., Jago, R., Ortega, F. B., & Katzmarzyk, P. T. (2020). 2020 WHO guidelines on physical activity and sedentary behaviour for children and adolescents aged 5–17 years: summary of the evidence. *International Journal of Behavioral Nutrition and Physical Activity, 17* (141).

Chastin, S. F. M., Buck, C., Freiberger, E., Murphy, M., Brug, J., Cardon, G., O'Donoghue, G., Pigeot, I., & Oppert, J. M. (2015). Systematic literature review of determinants of sedentary behaviour in older adults: a DEDIPAC study. *International Journal of Behavioral Nutrition and Physical Activity, 12*, 127.

Colley, R. C., Garriquet, D., Adamo, K. B., Carson, V., Janssen, I., Timmons, B. W., & Tremblay, M. S. (2013). Physical activity and sedentary behavior during the early years in Canada: A cross-sectional study. *International Journal of Behavioral Nutrition and Physical Activity, 10* (epub).

Craft, L. L., Zderic, T. W., Gapstur, S. M., Vanlterson, E. H., Thomas, D. M., Siddique, J., & Hamilton, M. T. (2012). Evidence that women meeting physical activity guidelines do not sit less: An observational inclinometry study. *International Journal of Behavioral Nutrition and Physical Activity, 9*(122).

Dall, P. M., Coulter, E. H., Fitzsimons, C. F., Skelton, D. A., & Chastin, S. F. M. (2017). Taxonomy of Self-reported Sedentary behaviour Tools (TASST) framework for development, comparison and evaluation of self-report tools: content analysis and systematic review. *British Medical Journal Open, 7*(4), e013844.

Degroote, L., DeSmet, A., De Bourdeaudhuij, I., Van Dyck, D., & Crombez, G. (2020). Content validity and methodological considerations in ecological momentary assessment studies on physical activity and sedentary behaviour: a systematic review. *International Journal of Behavioral Nutrition and Physical Activity, 17*(35).

Dempsey, P. C., Biddle, S. J., Buman, M. P., Chastin, S., Ekelund, U., Friedenreich, C. M., Katzmarzyk, P. T., Leitzmann, M. F., Stamatakis, E., van der Ploeg, H. P., Willumsen, J., & Bull, F. (2020). New global guidelines on sedentary behaviour and health for adults: broadening the behavioural targets. *International Journal of Behavioral Nurtrition and Physical Activity, 17*(151).

Dogra, S., & Stathokostas, L. (2014). Correlates of extended sitting time in older adults: An exploratory cross-sectional analysis of the Canadian Community Health Survey Healthy Aging Cycle. *International Journal of Public Health, 59*, 983–991.

Dunlop, D., Song, J., Arnston, E., Semanik, P., Lee, J., Chang, R., & Hootman, J. M. (2014). Sedentary time in U.S. older adults associated with disability in activities of daily living independent of physical activity. *Journal of Physical Activity and Health, 12*(1), 93–101.

Ekelund, U., Steene-Johannessen, J., Brown, W. J., Fagerland, M. W., Owen, N., Powell, K. E., & Bauman, A. (2016). Does physical activity attenuate, or even eliminate, the detrimental association of sitting time with mortality? A harmonised meta-analysis of data from more than 1 million men and women. *The Lancet, 388*(10051), 1302–1310.

Ekelund, U., Tarp, J., Steene-Johannessen, J., Hansen, B. H., Jefferis, B., Fagerland, M. W., Whincup, P., Diaz, K. M., Hooker, S. P., Chernofsky, A., Larson, M. G., Spartano, N., Vasan, R. S., Dohrn, I-M., Hagstromer, M., Edwardson, C., Yates, T., Shiroma, E., Anderssen S. A., & Lee, I. M. (2019). Dose-response associations between accelerometry measured physical activity and sedentary time and all cause mortality: systematic review and harmonised meta-analysis. *British Medical Journal, 366* (14570).

Gardner, B., Flint, S., Rebar, A. L., Dewitt, S., Quail, S. K., Whall, H., & Smith, L. (2019). Is sitting invisible? Exploring how people mentally represent sitting. *International Journal of Behavioral Nutrition and Physical Activity, 16* (85).

Gennuso, K. P., Gangnon, R. E., Matthews, C. E., Thraen-Borowski, K. M., & Colbert, L. H. (2013). Sedentary behavior, physical activity, and markers of health in older adults. *Medicine and Science in Sports and Exercise, 45*(8), 1493–1500.

Grgic, J., Dumuid, D., Bengoechea, E. G., Shrestha, N., Bauman, A., Olds, T., & Pedisic, Z. (2018). Health outcomes associated with reallocations of time between sleep, sedentary behaviour, and physical activity: a systematic scoping review of isotemporal substitution studies. *International Journal of Behavioral Nutrition and Physical Activity, 15*(69).

Harrington, D. M., Barreira, T. V., Staiano, A. E., & Katzmarzyk, P. T. (2013). The descriptive epidemiology of sitting among U.S. adults, NHANES 2009–2010. *Journal of Science and Medicine in Sport.* https://doi.org/10.1016/j.jsams.2013.07.017

Harvey, J. A., Chastin, S. F. M., & Skelton, D. A. (2015). How sedentary are older people? A systematic review of the amount of sedentary behavior. *Journal of Aging & Physical Activity, 23*(3), 471–487.

Healy, G. N., Matthews, C. E., Dunstan, D. W., Winkler, E. A. H., & Owen, N. (2011). Sedentary time and cardio-metabolic biomarkers in U.S. adults: NHANES 2003–06. *European Heart Journal, 32*(5), 590–597.

Janssen, I., Clarke, A. E., Carson, V., Chaput, J. P., Giangregorio, L. M., Kho, M. E., Poitras, V. J., Ross, R., Saunders, T. J., Ross-White, A., & Chastin, S. F. M. (2020). A systematic review of compositional data analysis studies examining associations between sleep, sedentary behaviour, and physical activity with health outcomes in adults. *Applied Physiology, Nutrition and Metabolism, 45*, S248–S257.

Katzmarzyk, P. T. (2010). Physical activity, sedentary behavior, and health: Paradigm paralysis or paradigm shift? *Diabetes, 59*(11), 2717–2725.

Kirk, M. A., & Rhodes, R. E. (2011). Occupation correlates of adults' participation in leisure-time physical activity: A systematic review. *American Journal of Preventive Medicine, 40*(4), 476–485.

Lepp, A., Barkley, J. E., Sanders, G. J., Rebold, M., & Gates, P. (2013). The relationship between cell phone use, physical and sedentary activity, and cardiorespiratory fitness in a sample of U.S. college students. *International Journal of Behavioral Nutrition and Physical Activity, 10* (79). https://doi.org/10.1186/1479-5868-10-79

McEvoy, J. P. (1938, December). Garlands for the living: Young man looking backwards. American Mercury, 482.

Mielke, G. I., da Silva, I. C., Owen, N., & Hallal, P. C. (2014). Brazilian adults' sedentary behaviors by life domain: Population-based study. *PLoS One, 9*(3): e91614. https://doi.org/10.1371/journal.pone.0091614

Morris, J. N., Heady, J. A., Raffle, P. A., Roberts, C. G., & Parks, J. W. (1953). Coronary heart disease and physical activity of work. *The Lancet, 262*(6796), 1111–1120.

Norton, K., Norton, L., & Sadgrove, D. (2010). Position statement of physical activity and exercise intensity terminology. *Journal of Science and Medicine in Sport, 13*, 496–502.

Nq, S. W., & Popkin, B. M. (2012). Time use and physical activity: A shift away from movement across the globe. *Obesity Reviews, 13*(8), 659–680.

O'Donoghue, G., Perchoux, C., Mensah, K., Lakerveld, J., van der Ploeg, H., Bernaards, C., Chastin, S. F., Simon, C., O'gorman, D., & Nazare, J. A. (2016). A systematic review of the correlates of sedentary behaviour in adults aged 18–65 years: a socio-ecological approach. *BioMed Central Public Health, 16*, 163. https://www.ncbi.nlm.nih.gov/pmc/articles/PMC4756464/

Owen, N., Healy, G. N., & Dunstan, D. W. (2010). Too much sitting: The population-health science of sedentary behavior. *Exercise and Sport Sciences Reviews, 38*(3), 105–113.

Patterson, R., McNamara, E., Tainio, M., de Sa, T. H., Smith, A. D., Sharp, S. J., Edwards, P., Woodcock, J., Brage, S., & Wijndaele, K. (2018). Sedentary behaviour and risk of all-cause, cardiovascular and cancer mortality, and incident type 2 diabetes: a systematic review and dose response meta-analysis. *European Journal of Epidemiology, 33*, 811–829.

Prince, S. A., Reed, J. L., McFetridge, C., Tremblay, M. S., & Reid, R. D. (2017). Correlates of sedentary behaviour in adults: a systematic review. *Obesity Reviews, 18*(8), 915–935.

Prince, S. A., Elliott, C. G., Scott, K., Visintini, S., & Reed, J. L. (2019). Device-measured physical activity, sedentary behaviour and cardiometabolic health and fitness across occupational groups: a systematic review and meta-analysis. *International Journal of Behavioral Nutrition and Physical Activity, 16* (30).

Rhodes, R. E., Bredin, S. S. D., Janssen, I., Warburton, D. E. R., & Bauman, A. (2017). Physical activity: Health impact, prevalence, correlates and interventions. *Psychology & Health, 32*, 942–975.

Rhodes, R. E., Mark, R. S., & Temmel, C. P. (2012). Adult sedentary behavior: A systematic review. *American Journal of Preventive Medicine, 42*(3), e3–e28.

Rodriguez-Ayllon, M., Cadenas-Sánchez, C., Estévez-López, F., Muñoz, N. E., Mora-Gonzalez, J., Migueles, J., Molina-García, P., Henriksson, H., Mena-Molina, A., Martínez-Vizcaíno, V., Catena, A., Löf, M., Erickson, K. I., Lubans, D. R., Ortega, F. B., &Esteban-Cornejo, I. (2019). Role of physical activity and sedentary behavior in the mental health of preschoolers, children and adolescents: A systematic review and meta-analysis. *Sports Medicine, 49*, 1383–1410.

Ross, R., Chaput, J., Giangregorio, L., Janssen, I., Saunders, T. J., Kho, M. E., Poitras, V. J., Tomasone, J., El-Kotob, R.,

McLaughlin, E. C., Duggan, M., Carrier, J., Carson, V., Chastin, S., Latimer-Cheung, A., Chulak-Bozzer, T., Faulkner, G., Flood, S. M., Gazendam, M. K., Healy, G. N., Katzmarzyk, P. T., Kennedy, W., Lane, K., Lorbergs, A., Maclaren, K., S., M., Powell, K. E., Rhodes, R. E., Ross-White, E., Welsh, F., Willumsen, J., & Tremblay, M. S. (2020). Canadian 24-hour movement guidelines for adults aged 18–64 years and adults aged 65 years or older: An integration of physical activity, sedentary behaviour, and sleep. *Applied Physiology, Nutrition, and Metabolism, 45*(10), S57–S102.

Saunders, T. J., McIsaac, T., Douillette, K., Gaulton, N., Hunter, S., Rhodes, R. E., Ross-White, A., Tremblay, M. S., & Healy, G. N. (2020). Sedentary behaviour and health in adults: an overview of systematic reviews. *Applied Physiology, Nutrition and Metabolism, 45*(10), S197–S217.

Smith, L., McCourt, O., Sawyer, A., Ucci, M., Marmot, A., Wardle, J., & Fisher, A. (2016). A review of occupational physical activity and sedentary behaviour correlates. *Occupational Medicine, 66*(3), 185–192.

Spence, J. C., Rhodes, R. E., & Carson, V. (2017). Challenging the dual-hinge approach to intervening on sedentary behavior. *American Journal of Preventive Medicine, 52*(3), 403–406.

Stamatakis, E., Ekelund, U., Ding, D., Hamer, M., Bauman, A. E. & Lee, I. M. (2019). Is the time right for quantitative public health guidelines on sitting? A narrative review of sedentary behaviour research paradigms and findings. *British Journal of Sports Medicine, 53*(6), 377–382.

Stockwell, S., Trott, M., Tully, M., Shin, J., Barnett, Y., Butler, L., McDermott, D., Schuch, F., & Smith, L. (2021). Changes in physical activity and sedentary behaviours from before to during the COVID-19 pandemic lockdown: a systematic review. *British Medical Journal Open Sport & Exercise Medicine, 7*, e000960.

Temmel, C., & Rhodes, R. E. (2013). Correlates of sedentary behavior in children and adolescents aged 7–18: A systematic review. *The Health & Fitness Journal of Canada, 6*(1), 118–136.

Thomas, G., Bennie, J.A., De Cocker, K. et al. A Descriptive Epidemiology of Screen-Based Devices by Children and Adolescents: a Scoping Review of 130 Surveillance Studies Since 2000. *Child Indicators Research, 13*, 935–950 (2020).

Tremblay, M. (2012). Reply to the discussion of "Letter to the editor: Standardized use of the terms sedentary and sedentary behaviours"–Sitting and reclining are different states. *Applied Physiology Nutrition and Metabolism, 37*(6), 540–542.

Tremblay, M. S., Leblanc, A. G., Janssen, I., Kho, M. E., Hicks, A., Murumets, K., Colley, R. C., & Duggan, M. (2011). Canadian sedentary behaviour guidelines for children and youth. *Applied Physiology, Nutrition, and Metabolism, 36*(1), 59–64.

Tremblay, M. S., Lablanc, A. G., Carson, V., Choquette, L., Connor Gorber, S., Dillman, C., Duggan, M., Gordon, M. J., Hicks, A., Janssen, I., Kho, M. E., Latimer-Cheun, A. E., LeBlanc, C., Murumets, K., Okely, A. D., Reilly, J. J., Stearns, J. A., Timmons, B. W., & Spence, J. C. (2012). Canadian sedentary behaviour guidelines for the early years (aged 0–4 years). *Applied Physiology, Nutrition, and Metabolism, 37*(2), 370–391.

Tremblay, M. S., Chaput, J. P., Adamo, K. B., Aubert, S., Barnes, J. D., Choquette, L., Duggan, M., Faulkner, G., Goldfield, G. S., Gray, C. E., Gruber, R., Janson, K., Janssen, I., Janssen, X., Jaramillo Garcia, A., Kuzik, N., LeBlanc, C., MacLean, J., Okely, A. D., Poitras, V. J., Rayner, M. E., Reilly, J. J., Sampson, M., Spence, J. C., Timmons, B. W., & Carson, V. (2017). Canadian 24-hour movement guidelines for the early years (0–4 years): An integration of physical activity, sedentary behaviour, and sleep. *BioMed Central Public Health, 17*(874).

Tremblay, M. S., Carson, V., Chaput, J. P., Connor Gorber, S., Dinh, T., Duggan, M., . . Faulkner, G., Gray, C. E., Gruber, R., Janson, K., Janssen, I., Katzmarzyk, P. T., Kho, M. E., Latimer-Cheung, A. E., LeBlanc, C., Okely, A. D., Olds, T., Pate, R. R., Phillips, A., Poitras, V. J., Rodenburg, S., Sampson, M., Saunders, T. J., Stone, J. A., Stratton, G., Weiss, S. K., & Zehr, L. (2016). Canadian 24-hour movement guidelines for children and youth: An integration of physical activity, sedentary behaviour, and sleep. *Applied Physiology, Nutrition and Metabolism, 41*(6), S311–S327.

Tremblay, M. S., Aubert, S., Barnes, J. D., Saunders, T. J., Carson, V., Latimer-Cheung, A. E., Chastin, S. F., Altenburg, T. M., & Chinapaw, M. J. M. (2017). Sedentary Behavior Research Network (SBRN) – Terminology consensus project process and outcome. *International Journal of Behavioral Nutrition and Physical Activity, 14*(75).

van der Ploeg, H., & Hillsdon, M. (2017). Is sedentary behaviour just physical inactivity by another name? *International Journal of Behavioral Nurtrition and Physical Activity, 14*(142).

World Health Organization. (2020). Physical activity. *14*(142) https://www.who.int/news-room/fact-sheets/detail/physical -activity

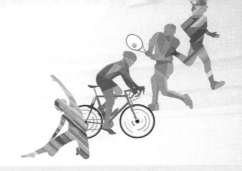

SECTION 2

Environmental Effects of Exercise and Sedentary Behavior

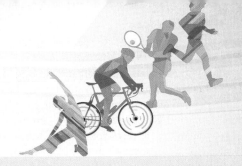

CHAPTER 3

Social Environment

LEARNING OBJECTIVES

After completing this chapter, you will be able to:

- Differentiate between social integration and social network.
- Describe how social inequality, income inequality, and racial discrimination may impact physical activity and sedentary behavior.
- Provide advice about how program developers may measure and enhance social support for their clients or group members.
- Give examples of how social environment can have both positive and negative impacts on physical activity and sedentary behavior.

Introduction

Humans are social beings. In fact, our need to form and maintain strong social attachments with other people is fundamental to our overall health and well-being (Baumeister & Leary, 1995). C. S. Lewis, a famous novelist, illustrated the importance of our social relations in the following quote: "Those who are enjoying something, or suffering something together, are companions" (1945, p. 145). Indeed, social relationships—whether they are positive or negative—influence our thoughts, emotions, and behavior.

Moreover, the absence of supportive social relationships can have a detrimental impact on our physical and psychological health. A lack of social support is associated with higher morbidity and mortality (Tay, Tan, Diener, & Gonzalez, 2013). For example, divorce (where there is a disruption to social support) leads to an early death. How much earlier than married people? The risk

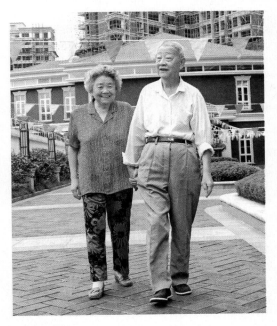

© Jack.Q/Shutterstock.

of dying early is 23% greater among divorced adults than married couples. And the health risk associated with divorce is similar to other well-established risk factors, such as smoking up to 15 cigarettes a day, doing insufficient physical activity, being overweight, and drinking alcohol heavily (Sbarra, Law, & Portley, 2011).

The **social environment** comprises the physical surroundings, social relationships, and cultural milieu within which people function and interact (Barnett & Casper, 2001). The social environment refers to the environment developed by people such as your family, friends, physicians, peers, classmates, neighbors, teachers, and others who you come into contact with regularly. In this chapter, we will examine how our social environment affects physical activity and sedentary behavior by focusing on social support, social identity, and the group dynamics variables of cohesion and leadership.

Social Support

Social support is a complex phenomenon. One measure of that complexity is the number of perspectives adopted in an attempt to define it. In one general perspective, the role of information is emphasized. Cobb (1976), for example, defined social support as information that leads the individual to feel: (1) cared for; (2) loved, esteemed, and valued; and (3) a sense of belonging to a reciprocal network. In another similar perspective, the role of emotion is emphasized. For example, Cassel (1976) proposed that social support reflects the gratification of an individual's basic needs.

In yet another perspective, social support is viewed as a process. As an example of this perspective, Vaux (1992) suggested that social support is a dynamic process that involves transactions between individuals within a specific social context. Finally, yet another perspective draws upon the idea of networks of support. From this perspective, the individual is seen as the focus of networks (collection) of people—networks that can vary in structure (e.g., size, number of links), nature of the linkages (e.g., frequency, intensity of interactions), and the function(s) provided (e.g.,

instrumental, emotional support; Israel, 1982). Perhaps the complexity of social support was best summed up by Alan Vaux (1988) who stated that social support represents a wide cross section of concepts, including "belonging, bonding, and binding; attributes of groups, relationships, and persons; and processes that are social, behavioral, and affective in nature" (p. 33).

Taxonomies for Social Support

A second manifestation of the complexity of social support is the variety of terms that are used interchangeably. In an attempt to distinguish among social support–related concepts, Anton Laireiter and Urs Baumann (1992) proposed a taxonomy. One of the components, **social integration** (also known as social embeddedness), represents the degree to which the individual participates in and is involved in family life, the social life of the community (e.g., churches, community events), and has access to resources and support systems. Social integration is similar to **social networks**; it is the extent that the individual has regular contact with friends, neighbors, and family.

A second component, **support networks** (also known as network resources), represents the individual's social network from a functional perspective. Who does the individual turn to for assistance or emotional support? Who are the individual's potential supporters? Who are the individual's actual supporters? The people an individual routinely turns to for support represent their network resources. As the term implies, support networks represent the pool of support resources available to the individual.

Supportive climates (or supportive environments) represent the quality of social relationships and systems. Is the family unit cohesive? To what extent is there frequent conflict in the family? As might be expected, cohesive families, workgroups, and friendship groups are perceived by the individual to be more supportive.

A fourth component of the taxonomy, **received and enacted support**, represents two aspects of the social support exchange. When social support is viewed as a process, two

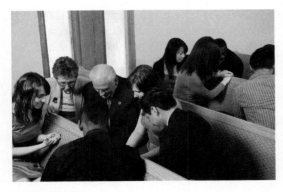

© FatCamera/E+/Getty Images.

individuals are involved. One, the provider of social support, represents enacted support; the other individual in the exchange, the recipient, represents received support.

Another component, **perceived support**, represents the individual's cognitive appraisal. Support received is not synonymous with support perceived. An individual might receive advice, encouragement, and financial assistance from a large network of people, including family, close friends, fellow workers, and health and business professionals. Yet that same individual could perceive that they are socially isolated or have been abandoned insofar as access to support is concerned. Thus, social support cannot simply be

determined by counting the number of contacts between a focal person and their social network.

According to Laireiter and Baumann (1992), the complex phenomena in their taxonomy are related to one another in a hierarchical manner. As **Figure 3-1** shows, social integration represents the broadest, most fundamental category. Without social integration, there could be no support networks, supportive climates, enacted and received support, and/or perceived support. In turn, support networks are a necessary precondition before questions of supportive climate, received and enacted support, or perceived support can arise. As Figure 3-1 shows, the hierarchy continues until, finally, received and enacted support serve as a precondition for perceived support.

Building on the work of Laireiter and Baumann (1992), McNeill, Kreuter, and Subramanian (2006) described five dimensions of the social environment relevant to physical activity and sedentary behavior.

The first dimension, social support and social networks, describes the resources provided by other persons and the structure of social relationships that surround an individual. When applied to physical activity or sedentary behavior interventions, this dimension of social support may be targeted through the use of "buddy systems" or connections to engage with other people.

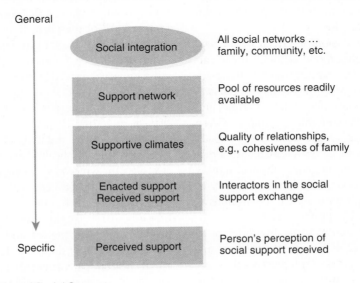

Figure 3-1 Hierarchy of Social Support.

The dimension of **social inequality** and **income inequality** describes the unequal distribution of resources based on social status or income and it influences health behaviors through creating divides between people in terms of what resources they have access to and the degrees of stressors placed on them. Evidence suggests it is not necessarily income amount that is associated with health outcomes, but rather the equality of how resources are distributed in society (Auerbach et al., 2000). Targeting this dimension of social support in physical activity or sedentary behavior interventions could include reducing the unequal distribution of physical activity resources between rich and poor neighborhoods, for instance.

The third dimension is **racial discrimination**, which manifests as different treatment from people or organizations/systems between people of different races or ethnicities. Similar to the dimension of social inequality and income inequality, racial discrimination can lead to uneven distribution of opportunities for physical activity and reducing sedentary behavior and enhanced distress from experiencing racial discrimination, which may lead people to be less likely to engage in health behaviors such as physical activity. To target racial discrimination in physical activity and sedentary behavior interventions, focus would be needed to correct unequal distribution of stressors and physical activity opportunities between people of different races and ethnicities.

The fourth dimension described by McNeill et al. (2006) is neighborhood factors, a broad category which includes characteristics of the place where you live, such as community social services, home ownership, perception of crime, and neighborhood socioeconomic positions. Given that people's access to physical activity likely depends on nearby social resources, it seems pertinent for interventions targeting physical activity and sedentary behavior to address availability of safe, comfortable physical activity environments with good community support services.

The last dimension of social environment as per McNeill et al. (2006) is social cohesion and social capital. This dimension represents the connectedness and solidarity of societies and the resources available to individuals and to society through social relationships. When communities have shared beliefs and expectations, it can be hugely impactful on individuals' behaviors, including their physical activity and sedentary behavior. These external pressures on our behavior need to be accounted for and potentially intervened with so that they reinforce, rather than discourage, physical activity behavior. Some recommend then, that it is more effective to intervene with physical activity and sedentary behavior at the community level, rather than focusing exclusively on individuals.

Negative Aspects of Social Support

A third reflection of the complexity of social support is the fact that the implicit assumption that social support is always positive is not true (e.g., Chogahara et al.,1998; Rafaeli et al., 2008). For example, Chogahara and his colleagues (1998) noted that there have been numerous negative social influences identified in fields such as health psychology. The labels attached to those negative social influences include, for example, social hindrance, social rejection, social inhibition, unsupportive behaviors, unhelpful behaviors, negative social ties, social strain, negative social interactions, social pressure, social disapproval, and stereotypes. All of these can have negative impacts on our healthy movement behaviors. There is building evidence, for example, showing the negative impact that weight stigma in the gym and on reality television shows has on people's physical activity motivation and behavior (Rich & Mansfield, 2019).

Positive social reactions are associated with more psychological health benefits and fewer negative health symptoms, whereas negative social reactions are associated with increased negative psychological health symptoms (Sylaska & Edwards, 2014). Negative social support also has a stronger immediate impact, and it retains its influence over a longer duration. Thus, a supportive statement from parents/guardians to their children such as "you can do it" could positively influence physical activity involvement. However, the negative impact of statements such as "act your age" and "you're too old to ride a bike" would likely carry more weight initially and persist as an influence on activity behavior over a longer period of time.

Social Support as a Personality Trait

A final reflection of complexity lies in the fact that although social support is by its very definition a social construct, there is also evidence that it is an individual construct. In their research, Sarason and colleagues (Sarason et al., 1983; Sarason et al., 1990; Sarason et al., 1991; Sarason et al., 1992) observed that perceptions of the availability of social support represent a stable personality trait. We possess an enduring disposition to see ourselves as being supported by others. Some people, of course, may see themselves as the chronic recipients of considerable support from others (even in the presence of evidence to the contrary). Conversely, some people may have the tendency to see themselves as receiving minimal or no support from others (again, even in the presence of evidence to the contrary). The tendency to perceive oneself as being supported is positively related to both self-concept and self-esteem (Sarason et al., 1992).

Measurement of Social Support

Given the complex nature of social support, it is not surprising that a number of approaches have been taken in its measurement. Generally, these different approaches have reflected differences in the specific research question asked. Who gives the person social support? What type(s) of social support does an individual receive? What is the quantity and quality of that social support?

Essentially, the measurement of social support has taken three general approaches (see **Table 3-1**).

Table 3-1 Typical Approaches in the Measurement of Social Support

Approach	Concept	Example of Possible Measures
Social network resources	Significant others available to provide support	Size of the network Density of the network
Support appraisal	Satisfaction, sufficiency, or helpfulness of support in important domains	Attachment (emotional support) Social integration (network support) Opportunity for nurturance (self-worth from assisting others) Reassurance of worth (esteem support) Reliable alliance (tangible aid) Guidance (information support)
Support behavior	Frequency of occurrence or likelihood of behavior	Financial assistance Practical assistance Emotional support Advice or guidance Positive social interactions

Data from Vaux, A. (1992). Assessment of social support. In H. O. F. Veiel & U. Baumann (Eds.), *The meaning and measurement of social support* (pp. 193–216). New York, NY: Hemisphere Publishing.

One approach is concerned with determining an individual's social network resources (Vaux, 1982). Throughout the school year, for example, a student might have the need for financial assistance (e.g., money to pay for books and tuition), practical assistance (e.g., for a ride to school), emotional support (e.g., for love, affection), advice or guidance (e.g., in course selection), and positive social interactions (e.g., someone to go to coffee with). Measures of social network resources are concerned with who that student could go to for support. There could be more than one person in any or all of the categories, of course. When social support is assessed through measures of social network resources, the focus is on questions of size and density. The index or measure could be in the form of global estimates (e.g., how many people in total are available to provide support) or domain-specific estimates (e.g., how many people are available to provide financial assistance).

A second approach is concerned with determining an individual's support appraisal (Russell & Cutrona, 1984). In this approach, the focus is on satisfaction, sufficiency, and/or help-fulness of the support. The prototypical student introduced above can serve as an example to illustrate support appraisal. The student might have a number of individuals available for positive social interactions (e.g., to have coffee with). However, the student's support appraisal—that is, the satisfaction expressed with their positive social interactions—could be either moderate or low. The appraisal of support could be "I have support but it's just not very good."

Support appraisal has been examined frequently insofar as its relationship to issues such as self-efficacy for physical activity in elderly populations (e.g., Duncan et al., 1993). Generally, the appraisal of social support has centered on six important social needs identified by Weiss (1974). These are attachment, which reflects emotional support; social integration, which reflects network support; opportunity for nurturance, which reflects increased self-worth from assisting others; reassurance of worth, which reflects esteem support; sense of reliable alliance, which reflects tangible aid; and obtaining of guidance, which

reflects information support. The relationship of these various forms of social support to physical activity and sedentary behavior is discussed later in the chapter.

A third, somewhat related approach is concerned with determining support behavior (Barrera, Sandler, & Ramsay, 1981). In this approach, the focus is on the frequency of occurrence or the likelihood that others will provide the behavior. Again, it might be useful to use the prototypical student to illustrate the approach taken. Although the student might have a large number of individuals available for coffee, they might rate the frequency of social interactions as minimal over a month-long period.

The three approaches are similar in that they are designed to assess some manifestation of social support. However, it should be apparent that there are subtle differences as well. Thus, the specific approach taken would depend upon the question asked. Is the health professional or researcher interested in whether the person has a large number of people available for social support? If so, social network resources would be assessed. Is the health professional or researcher interested in whether the person's social support is either frequent or infrequent? If so, support behavior would be assessed. Finally, is the interest in whether the social support available to the person is either more or less satisfying? If so, support appraisal would be assessed.

In summary, although there are a variety of instruments used to assess social support, there is no single, "best" measure. This situation may be partially due to the fact that a wide range of different measurement strategies have yielded "scores" that have successfully been related to a variety of health outcomes. Measures range from single items used to assess whether or not types of social support (e.g., emotional, instrumental) are available (using yes/no responses) to more extensive measures that include multiple items asking about various types of social support.

See **Table 3-2** for a measure of the functional components of social support developed by

Table 3-2 Measuring the Functional Components of Social Support

Instructions: This scale is made up of a list of statements, each of which may or may not be true about you. For each statement circle (4) "definitely true" if you are sure it is true about you and (3) "probably true" if you think it is true but are not absolutely certain. Similarly, you should circle (1) "definitely false" if you are sure the statement is false and (2) "probably false" if you think it is false but are not absolutely certain.

1	2	3	4
definitely false	probably false	probably true	definitely true

1. If I wanted to go on a trip for a day (for example, to the country or mountains), I would have a hard time finding someone to go with me.

2. I feel that there is no one I can share my most private worries and fears with.

3. If I were sick, I could easily find someone to help me with my daily chores.

4. There is someone I can turn to for advice about handling problems with my family.

5. If I decide one afternoon that I would like to go to a movie that evening, I could easily find someone to go with me.

6. When I need suggestions on how to deal with a personal problem, I know someone I can turn to.

7. I don't often get invited to do things with others.

8. If I had to go out of town for a few weeks, it would be difficult to find someone who would look after my house or apartment (the plants, pets, garden, etc.).

9. If I wanted to have lunch with someone, I could easily find someone to join me.

10. If I was stranded 10 miles from home, there is someone I could call who could come and get me.

11. If a family crisis arose, it would be difficult to find someone who could give me good advice about how to handle it.

12. If I needed some help in moving to a new house or apartment, I would have a hard time finding someone to help me.

Scoring:
Items 1, 2, 7, 8, 11, 12 are reverse scored.
Items 2, 4, 6, 11 make up the Appraisal Support subscale.
Items 1, 5, 7, 9 make up the Belonging Support subscale.
Items, 3, 8, 10, 12 make up the Tangible Support subscale.

Data from Cohen, A., Mermelstein, R., Kamarck, T., & Hoberman, H. M. (1985). Measuring the functional components of social support. In I. G. Sarason & B. R. Sarason (Eds.), *Social support: Theory, research, and applications*. The Hague, Netherlands: Martinus Niijhoff.

Cohen and colleagues (1985). This questionnaire has three different subscales designed to measure the following dimensions of perceived social support: appraisal support, belonging support, and tangible support. Each item is measured by four items on a 4-point scale ranging from "definitely true" to "definitely false."

Social Support, Physical Activity, and Sedentary Behavior

The degree to which people sense that they receive the support of others will influence the development of cognitions associated with their involvement in exercise. Carron, Hausenblas, and Mack (1996) statistically summarized available research on the relationship between social support and intention to be physically active through the use of a meta-analysis. They found that social support from family members has a moderate effect (ES = .49) on an individual's intention to engage in physical activity. In addition, important others—physicians, work colleagues, for example—also have a moderate effect on intention (ES = .44), although their influence is slightly lower than that of the family. So, social support has an important role to play in terms of its impact on people's intentions to be physically active.

Social support from important others (e.g., work colleagues) has an even more important role to play than family in terms of the positive affect people develop around physical activity (Carron et al., 1996). Why this is the case is uncertain. Possibly, it is related to the informational and motivational aspects of social reinforcement. Social reinforcement from people who are not intimates can be more motivating because it is generally less frequent and more selective and therefore provides more information to the recipient.

A systematic review of prospective associations between social support and physical activity in healthy adults found 20 studies that had inconsistent findings, but overall, they calculated that there was a small positive association between social support from friends and future physical activity behavior (Scarapicchia et al., 2017). A systematic review and meta-analysis of evidence of social support and physical activity in adolescents also found support for small positive cross-sectional associations of social support and physical activity (Laird et al., 2016). When considering this association in older adults, a review by Smith and colleagues (2017) also found from 27 studies evidence of a positive association between social support and physical activity. Notably, an inverse association was found for loneliness and physical activity. An example would be older adults who felt lonelier tended to be less physically active than those who

Women and Men React Differently to Weight Stigma

Sometimes the people around us can have negative impacts on our motivation. For example, **stigma** is when someone has negative views about you because of a characteristic you have, and evidence shows stigma can negatively impact our motivation for physical activity. In a study of more than 400 individuals with overweight and obesity, it was found that:

- Women experienced more weight stigma than men
- Men with overweight and obesity who experience more weight stigma tend to engage in more physical activity
- Women with overweight and obesity who experience more weight stigma tend to engage in less physical activity (Sattler et al., 2018)

It may be that these individuals are avoiding judgment from others while they exercise. Evidence also suggests weight stigma negatively impacts our self-efficacy and self-determined motivation to be physically active.

CRITICAL THINKING ACTIVITY 3-2

What do you think might explain these different findings on how women and men are impacted by their experienced weight stigma?

did not feel lonely. Social support can help us to be regularly physically active across the lifespan, but this relationship is complex.

A large-scale study by Anne Kouvonen and her colleagues (2012) illustrates the complex effects social support can have on physical activity. They conducted a prospective cohort study of 5,395 adults (mean age = 55.7 years) who completed measures of their confiding/emotional support (e.g., wanting to confide, sharing interests) and practical support, as well as exercise behavior at baseline assessment. At the follow-up assessment 5 years later, the participants' exercise behavior was reassessed. The researchers found that among the participants who reported the recommended levels of exercise at baseline, those who experienced high confiding/emotional support were more likely to report participating in recommended levels of exercise at follow-up. Among those participants who did not meet the recommended target of exercise at baseline, high confiding/emotional support was not associated with improvement in activity levels. High practical support was associated with both maintaining and improving exercise levels. The researchers concluded that emotional and practical support from those closest to the person may help the individual to maintain the recommended level of exercise. Practical support also predicted a change toward a more active lifestyle.

Throughout the lifespan, our physical activity behavior seems to be impacted by our social experiences. Although the evidence is not as comprehensive for sedentary behavior, there is building evidence to suggest that our social environment can impact our sedentary behavior. For example, a study of more than 12,000 Canadian adults revealed that being married leads to less extensive computer use sedentary time, and people with more social support tend to engage in less extensive computer use sedentary time, especially amongst men (Huffman & Szafron, 2017). University students report that sedentary behavior is impacted by their social connections and social environment (Deliens et al., 2015). When asked about the determinants of sedentary behavior at university, students mentioned things like, "If your friends show a lot of sedentary behavior, you will too," and "When I wake up, the first thing I do is check Facebook."

Although most sedentary behavior research considers technology use as a risk factor for more sedentariness, technology can be used as a delivery means of interventions to reduce sedentary behavior. A meta-analysis of interventions aimed at reducing sedentary behavior in healthy adults shows that computer, mobile, and wearable technology tools can be used to reduce sedentary behavior, with a mean reduction across studies of −41.28 min per day of sitting time, although notably, this effect seems to dissipate over time, down to only −1.65 min per day at 6 months postintervention (Stephenson et al., 2017). Hopefully, this evidence highlights that the technology that is gradually becoming more and more prevalent throughout our lives does not necessarily have to lead to us becoming more sedentary, but rather may be a means to help us avoid extensive sedentary behavior (See also Chapter 5).

Social Support During Pregnancy

A study using accelerometry of more than 350 pregnant women found that women participated in 12 min per day of moderate physical activity and 0.3 min per day of vigorous physical activity, and not surprisingly, women tended to engage in the least amount of physical activity during the third trimester – the last months of pregnancy before giving birth (Evenson & Wen, 2011). Additionally, the study revealed that, on average, pregnant women spent more than half of their time in sedentary behavior (Evenson & Wen, 2011). From a social environment perspective, it is notable that pregnant women with higher household income tended to engage in more physical activity than those with a lower household income. Additionally, social support from significant others has shown to impact the physical activity and sedentary behavior of pregnant and postpartum women. Pregnant and postpartum women who perceive greater levels of social support are more likely to be physically active than women who perceive they have less social support during this transitional time into motherhood (McIntyre & Rhodes, 2009). Social support can also help buffer pregnant women from negative mental health impacts of long, sedentary vehicle commutes (MacLeod et al., 2017). Given the importance of maintaining a healthy level of physical activity throughout and following pregnancy and the evidence showing the impact that social environment has on activity levels of pregnant women, it is clear that this is a key time to intervene with improved accessibility of physical activity opportunity and to enhance social support for physical activity and reducing sedentary behavior.

Social Support for People with Chronic Illnesses

When people are diagnosed and living with chronic illnesses, social environment can be instrumental for supporting more physical activity. For example, when cancer survivors are under stress, they tend to not engage in physical activity; however, support group involvement can buffer from this effect (Brunet et al., 2014). Additionally, a study of more than 2,500 patients with coronary artery disease revealed that low social support and more time spent in sedentary behavior is predictive of all-cause mortality, and that sedentary behavior may partially explain this reductive effect of social support on early mortality (Brummett et al., 2005). Social support also has been shown to be imperative for enhancing the physical and mental health benefits of physical activity for those with multiple sclerosis (Motl et al., 2009), Parkinson's disease (Ravenek & Schneider, 2009) and schizophrenia (Gross et al., 2016). Clearly, the social environment has significant impact on movement behaviors of those living with chronic illnesses and should be considered in the healthcare plans of patients. Next, we'll consider how social support may impact physical activity differently, depending on who is providing the support.

Family

Based on a strong body of evidence, a recent consensus statement declared that family is important for the support and promotion of healthy movement behaviors of children and youth (Rhodes et al., 2020). Underpinning this statement is an evaluation of systematic reviews that found substantial evidence of the impact of family support on children's physical activity and sedentary behavior. This evaluation concluded that through encouragement, providing easy access to physical activity opportunities, modelling physical activity behavior, setting expectations, and engaging in physical activity with children, family members can help children and youth engage in more physically active lifestyles (Rhodes et al., 2020). Evidence is also emerging regarding why and how family impacts children's' physical activity.

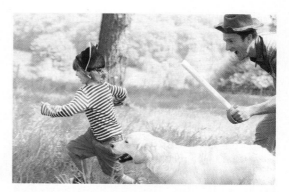

© Monkey Business Images/iStock/Getty Images Plus/Getty Images.

A meta-analysis investigating what factors may explain the impact of parental behaviors on their children's physical activity behavior revealed that there was a medium association between parental support and child physical activity ($r = 0.38$) and a weak association between parental modeling of physical activity and children's physical activity behavior ($r = 0.16$; Yao & Rhodes, 2015). Interestingly, the review found that the effect of parental modelling on children's physical activity behavior differed by gender: The impact of fathers' modelling of physical activity behavior on their sons' physical activity was stronger ($r = 0.29$) than the impact of mothers' modelling of physical activity to sons' behavior ($r = 0.19$). There was no difference, however, between parental gender in the effects of physical activity modelling on girls' behavior.

With regard to sedentary behavior, higher parental television viewing is associated with an increased risk of high levels of television viewing for both boys and girls (Jago et al., 2010). Children are more likely to watch television with their parents and siblings than to engage in physical activity with them (Tandon et al., 2012). In another study, Springer and his colleagues (2006) examined the associations of two types of social support (i.e., social participation in and social encouragement for physical activity) and two social support sources (i.e., family and friends) with self-reported daily minutes of physical activity and sedentary behavior (television/video viewing and computer/video game play) among 718 sixth-grade girls. Students were asked to rate four items that assessed social support. Students were asked to report how often during the past month their (1) family did physical activities with them; (2) family encouraged them to be physically active; (3) friends did physical activities with them; and (4) friends encouraged them to be physically active.

They found that friend physical activity participation and friend and family encouragement were positively related to moderate to vigorous physical activity. Family participation in physical activity had the strongest negative correlation with total minutes of television/video viewing and computer/video game play. The researchers concluded that social support is an important correlate of physical activity among adolescent girls but suggest that the source and type of social support may differ for physical activity and sedentary behaviors. Overall, the evidence indicates that parental support is important for encouraging youth to become more active. Also, an evaluation of reviews found that family-support, including parental support, is an essential component of intervening with sedentary behavior (Biddle et al., 2014).

Peers

While parents are the most important influence early in a child's life, parental influence on the child's day-to-day behavior becomes less evident as the child matures (Rhodes et al., 2019). Children and adolescents spend a significant portion of their time at school with friends and peers. Thus, it is not surprising that their friend's health behaviors influence their individual health behaviors, such as diet. What role do friends play in influencing physical activity and sedentary behavior?

Friendship networks are associated with physical activity and sedentary behavior among children and adolescents (Prochnow et al., 2020; Sawka et al., 2013). When your friends are active, you tend to be active too; whereas, if most of your friends spend time being sedentary, so will you. Existing research has found that playing video games with friends is related to decreased physical activity and increased

sedentary behavior in children (Marques et al., 2014). There is a mutually dependent relationship between adolescent friendship networks and physical activity (de la Haye et al., 2011). Involvement in physical activity plays an important role in adolescents' friendship choices, with youth showing a preference for friends whose activity levels are similar to their own. Friends also influence changes to physical activity over the course of the school year, evidenced by friends' engagement in leisure-time exercise becoming increasingly similar. Beyond the impact of friends' behavior on your own, friends can impact your physical activity and sedentary behavior through encouragement and support (Maturo & Cunningham, 2013; Vancampfort, Damme, et al., 2019). As children and adolescents, not having social support from your peers and friends to be active can make it easy to remain sedentary and avoid opportunities to become more physically active.

Teasing and Bullying

Teasing and bullying reflect negative aspects of social support, and not surprisingly, it has a negative effect on young people's physical activity (Roman & Taylor, 2013). Children who are teased during physical activity or physical education class are less likely to participate in exercise a year later (Jensen, Cushing, & Elledge, 2014). The negative impact of teasing during gym class was found in both overweight children as well as those who were of a healthy weight. However, children with overweight or obesity who experienced teasing during physical activity had a lower perceived health-related quality of life (referring to physical, social, academic, and emotional functioning) 1 year later.

Another study of 7,786 American middle school children found that bullying was associated with fewer days in physical education classes and lower odds of meeting the physical activity guidelines of exercising at least 60 minutes each day (Roman & Taylor, 2013). Adolescents with disabilities may be at particular risk of the negative impacts of bullying. Evidence from Israel

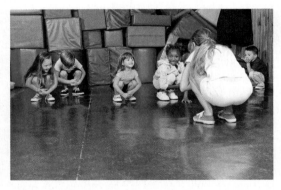

© Robert Kneschke/Alamy Stock Photo.

found that adolescents in grades 6 and 8 with disabilities experienced more bullying and were less physically active than their peers without disabilities (Hutzler et al., 2021). Notably, there is evidence suggesting that social support from parents can help to ensure bullying doesn't translate into lower levels of physical activity amongst school-aged children (Pulido et al., 2019).

What type of perceptions do students and teachers have about bullying in physical education and about both peer and adult support? O'Connor and Graber (2014) used a qualitative interview design to ask these questions of sixth-grade teachers and students. The researchers found that adults acculturate students to support a bullying climate by providing mixed information regarding social interactions, ignoring non-physical instances of bullying and promoting inappropriate curricular selections. The students reported that perceived differences such as appearance, body size, physical ability, and personal attire start most episodes of harassment or bullying in their physical education classes. As well, students perceive fear that prevents many of them from following up on important issues, such as reporting instances of bullying to those in authority, assisting bullied friends, and feeling safe in certain physical education locations. Not surprisingly, bullying negatively impacts the students' desire to engage in physical education classes. Children must be encouraged to engage in physical activity at school in a safe and friendly environment (Jensen et al., 2014).

CRITICAL THINKING ACTIVITY 3-3

Why do you think bullying can have such a long-term effect on people's physical activity behavior?

Healthcare Providers

Physicians and other healthcare providers have an ethical, and some would even say legal, obligation to assess and recommend physical activity to their patients. Physicians are in a critical position to help patients develop healthy lifestyles by actively counseling them on physical activity (Joy et al., 2013). Research indicates that physicians can influence patients to improve their health through proactive advising on the positive health impacts of physical activity during an office visit (Orrow, Kinmonth, Sanderson, & Sutton, 2012).

Unfortunately, many physicians are not talking to their patients about physical activity and are missing a unique opportunity to raise awareness about its benefits (Short et al., 2016). Physicians report several barriers that make it difficult for them to counsel their patients on exercise. Some of these barriers include time demands, insufficient reimbursement, lack of education on the benefits of physical activity, lack of knowledge on how to write an effective exercise prescription, and limited support systems for patient education (McKenna et al., 1998). One study found that more than half of the physicians trained in the United States receive no formal education in

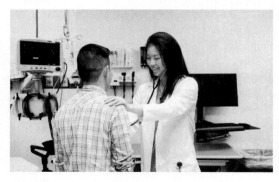

© 4x6/iStock/Getty Images Plus/Getty Images.

physical activity (Cardinal et al., 2014). Lastly, physically active physicians are more likely to counsel patients to be active. Thus, a key message for the healthcare provider community is the importance of serving as a positive physical activity role model.

Dogs

In most developed countries, rates of dog ownership are high. For example, about 40% of Australian and 38.4% of U.S. households own at least one dog (American Veterinary Medical Association, 2022; Animal Medicines Australia, 2019). This high level of dog ownership shows the deep attachment that exists between people and their dogs. In fact, most dog owners consider their pets to be family members. A common activity for dog owners is to walk their dog.

However, is dog ownership related to physical activity? The answer is a clear yes! People who own a dog are more likely to be physically active (Christian et al., 2013; Christian et al., 2016; Rhodes et al., 2020). Dog owners tend to be more physically active than those who do not own a dog (Toohey & Rock, 2011). Christian and her colleagues (2013) conducted a review of 29 studies that compared the physical activity levels of dog owners to those without dogs. They found small to moderate effect sizes that showed that dog owners engaged in more walking and physical activity than people without dogs. More specifically, they found that about 60% of dog owners walked their dog with a median duration and frequency of 160 minutes a week, roughly four walks per week. Dog walking has significant potential to increase the proportion of people to be physically active, either by encouraging those who do not walk their dog to do so or by increasing the amount of walking owners do with their dog (Christian et al., 2016). Interestingly, people who do not own dogs have greater risk of diabetes, hypertension, hypercholesterolemia, and depression compared with those who regularly walked their dogs (Lentino et al., 2012). Because of the health benefits associated with dog walking, it has been suggested that dog walking should be encouraged within communities as a method of promoting and sustaining a healthy lifestyle.

Leading on from this type of research, Rhodes and colleagues (2020) reviewed 13 interventions that involved dog interactions. Intervention approaches include loaning people dogs and intervening with new dog owners and existing dog owners to encourage more dog walking. In 83% of the studies, there were positive outcomes when people became more active as a result of the dog-based intervention, although it may be that the effects are short-lived.

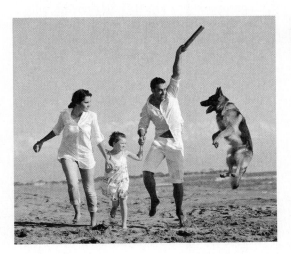

© Shock/iStock/Getty Images.

CRITICAL THINKING ACTIVITY 3-4

Do you think that owning other types of pets besides dogs can result in increased physical activity?

Group Dynamics

Group dynamics include the study of the nature of groups, individual relationships within groups, and group members' interactions with each other. Group dynamics can be defined as the positive and negative forces at play within a group of people. Within the domain of physical activity, a number of variables in group dynamics has been related to sustained behavior (Carron, Hausenblas, & Estabrooks, 1999). In this section, the following group dynamics topics are examined in more detail: social identity, cohesion, and leadership.

Social Identity

Your decisions and how you feel about physical activity or sedentary behavior can be impacted by what is going on in your social groups and how similar or dissimilar you perceive yourself to be. We are all involved in social groups and some of us are even involved in the same groups (students in the same class, for example), but the way we identify with these groups can be different. **Social identity** is the way we identify with our social groups (Beauchamp & Rhodes, 2020). Our social identities impact our decisions through our inferences about what others in our social groups do or think and whether we want to be associated more strongly with that group or not (Beauchamp, 2019). For example, you may strongly identify yourself as a sorority or fraternity member. If you value this social identity and assume that most sorority or fraternity members play sports, you will be more likely to take up opportunities to play sports. However, if you are aversive to the notion of being a typical sorority or fraternity member, you may avoid behaviors that seem like the norm for this group – and therefore avoid sports. How strongly you are influenced by your social identity depends on many factors, including how similar the members of the group are, group cohesion and group leadership (Beauchamp, 2019).

Cohesion

The degree to which a group is cohesive determines the individuals' level of success as a group. When examining the forces that bind individuals together, a logical starting point is the cohesive nature of the physical activity group. Physical activity groups, like other action-based groups (e.g., sports, work, or military groups), become bound together based upon the task and social components of the environment. This bond is

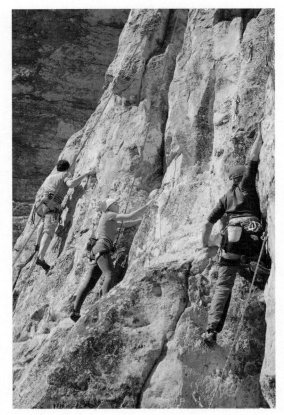

© Vitalii Nesterchuk/Shutterstock.

referred to as **cohesion**, and it is defined as "a dynamic process that is reflected in the tendency for a group to stick together and remain united in pursuit of its instrumental objectives and/or for the satisfaction of member affective needs" (Carron, Brawley, & Widmeyer, 1998, p. 213).

Cohesion is often conceptualized as a multidimensional model (Carron, Widmeyer, & Brawley, 1985) that consists of four dimensions distinguished on two levels. The first level is the individual versus group basis for cohesion. For example, an individual has personal attractions to the group as well as perceptions regarding the collectivity of the group. Simply said, the individual basis for cohesion is exemplified by "I" and "me" statements (e.g., "I like the exercises I do in this class"), whereas the group basis for cohesion is exemplified by "we" and "us" statements (e.g., "We all like the exercises we do in this class").

The second level of group cohesion is based on a distinction between the task and social aspects of group involvement. For example, both individually and as a group there are social outcomes (e.g., activities related to the development and maintenance of social relations) and task outcomes (e.g., activities related to accomplishing a task, productivity, and performance). A social outcome of physical activity classes could be the development of friendships. A task outcome could be the increased attraction to the exercises done in class.

Based upon these two levels of distinction (i.e., individual versus group and social versus task), the following four dimensions of group cohesion are conceptualized: individual attractions to the group–task, individual attractions to the group–social, group integration–task, and group integration–social (see **Figure 3-2**; Carron et al., 1985). Carron and his colleagues hypothesized that people can feel personally attracted to the specific physical activity offered in the class (i.e., individual attractions to the group–task) and to the people who attend the class (i.e., individual attractions to the group–social). People may also perceive that the physical activity group as a whole interacts with one another to get the best work out (i.e., group integration–task) or to socialize (i.e., group integration–social). Within exercise class settings, social cohesion changes over time, whereas task cohesion remains steadier (Dunlop, Falk, & Beauchamp, 2013).

Participating in a physical activity group can help people stay motivated. A review of 52 studies found that in 92% of them, group-based physical activity programs significantly increased physical activity (Harden et al., 2015). Importantly, a strong group connection is important for maintaining the motivation to continue. A large body of research has revealed a positive relationship between group cohesion and physical activity adoption and maintenance (Burke, Carron, Eys, & Estabrooks, 2006; Estabrooks, 2000; Smith-Ray et al., 2012). More specifically, people who have strong perceptions of group cohesion attend group sessions more often, are late less often, and drop out less frequently. Group cohesion also has a positive relationship with attitudes toward physical activity and enhanced perceptions of self-efficacy and personal control (**Table 3-3**).

As well, neighborhood social cohesion is positively related to physical activity participation (Cradock, Kawachi, Colditzm, Gortmaker, & Buka, 2009), and for older adults, neighborhood social cohesion can lead to more physical activity, which in turn enhances mental health (Kim et al., 2020). Parent-reported neighborhood social cohesion is positively associated with weekday and weekend physical activity in youth (Pabayo, Belsky, Gauvin, & Curtis, 2011). This association

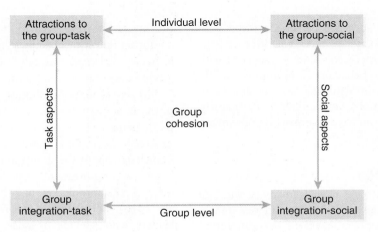

Figure 3-2 Group Cohesion.

Data from Carron, A. V., Widmeyer, W. N., & Brawley, L. R. (1985). The development of an instrument to assess cohesion in sport teams: The Group Environment Questionnaire. *Journal of Sport Psychology, 7*(3), 244–266.

Table 3-3 Sample Items from the Physical Activity Group Environment Questionnaire

Scale	Sample Item
Individual attractions to the group–task	I like the amount of physical activity I get in this program.
Individual attractions to the group–social	I enjoy my social interactions within this physical activity group.
Group integration–task	Members of our group are satisfied with the intensity of physical activity in this program.
Group integration–social	We spend time socializing with each other before or after our activity sessions.

Data from Burke, S. M., Carron, A. V., Eys, M. A., & Estabrooks, P. A. (2006). Group versus individual approach? A meta-analysis of the effectiveness of interventions to promote physical activity. *Sport and Exercise Psychology Review, 2*(1), 19–35.

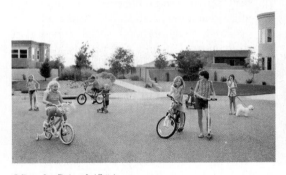

© Shannon Fagan/The Image Bank/Getty Images.

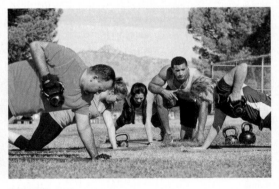

© CREATISTA/Shutterstock.

is most pronounced for boys. For those with depression, anxiety, or mild cognitive impairment, a lack of social cohesion is associated with more sedentary behavior (Vancampfort et al., 2018; Vancampfort, Stubbs, Lara, et al., 2019; Vancampfort, Stubbs, Smith, et al., 2019). Clearly, social cohesion can have an impact on how much we move and sit.

Leadership

A lot of people get physical activity through exercise programs and classes, and researchers and program planners have long been interested in the role that leaders play in participants' attitudes toward and adherence to physical activity programs. A review revealed that leadership has an impact on physical activity behavior, and this is likely explained through leaders' impact on group cohesion and autonomy supportive leadership styles (Gray & Rhodes, 2019). Effective physical activity leaders are those whom the participants feel are properly qualified, are able to develop a personal bond with, and use their knowledge about the group to demonstrate collective accomplishments and a positive social identity (Estabrooks et al., 2004; Stevens et al., 2018). For example, knowledgeable group leaders who provide a sense of mastery and autonomy are important for fostering quality experiences for people with a physical disability

(Shirazipour et al., 2020). It is important to have effective leaders because they influence participants' attitudes, cognitions, and behaviors toward physical activity. Indeed, a meta-analysis by Carron, Hausenblas, and Mack (1996) on social influences in exercise adherence showed that there is a small effect for the influence that exercise leaders have on adherence behavior.

Fox and her collaborators (Fox, Rejeski, & Gauvin, 2000) investigated the impact of leadership style and group dynamics on intention to return to a structured fitness class. Each participant completed a single program session under four conditions in which both leadership style (i.e., an enriched versus a bland leadership style) and group environment (i.e., an enriched versus a bland class environment) were systematically varied. **Table 3-4** provides an overview of the approach taken in each instance. The enriched group environment was manipulated with the use of trained confederates.

At the completion of the session, the participants completed assessments of their intention to return to a similar class and enjoyment of the previous session. Interestingly, a positive effect was found for the interaction between the leadership style and the group environment for enjoyment of the aerobics session. In other words, the participants enjoyed the class more when the environment had both enriched leadership and group dynamics. A positive relationship was also found between the group environment and intention.

Table 3-4 Bland vs. Enriched Leadership Styles and Group Environment

Leadership Style		Group Environment	
Socially Enriched	*Bland*	*Socially Enriched*	*Bland*
Use participants' names.	Do not use participants' names.	Introduce themselves to others as soon as they arrive in class.	Do not introduce themselves to others at any time in class.
Engage participants in general conversation before, during, and after class.	Do not engage in general conversation before, during, or after class.	Initiate casual interactions with other members early in each session.	Do not initiate or promote casual interactions with other members at any time in the class.
Provide specific reinforcement for positive behaviors.	No reinforcement or praise for positive behaviors.	Be compliant with the instructor's wishes.	Be compliant but not enthusiastically.
Give encouragement before and after a skill or mistake.	Fail to follow up with praise after a skill or encouragement after a mistake.	Provide encouragement to the group as a whole.	No encouragement to others or the instructor.
Focus on positive comments during instruction.	Focus on negative comments during instruction.	Respond to all questions the leader directs to the group.	Do not respond to questions the leader directs to the group.
Verbal reward of effort and ability immediately after the exercise and ignore mistakes.	Verbally note mistakes and do not reward effort and ability after the exercise.	Make positive and encouraging remarks to the instructor about the class in general.	No remarks to the instructor even if they directed instructions or corrections toward an individual.

Fox, L. D., Rejeski, W. J., & Gauvin, L. (2000). Effects of leadership style and group dynamics on enjoyment of physical activity. *American Journal of Health Promotion, 14*(5), 277–283.

So, those participants in the enriched group environments intended to return to a similar exercise session, regardless of leadership style. We rely on our leaders to help maintain our motivation, to ensure we can do the activity correctly, and to make us feel like a cohesive group. The more leaders understand about motivation of physical activity and sedentary behavior, the better able they will be to encourage clients, patients, and group members to start and continue to engage in physical activity programs.

Summary

The individuals, groups, communities, and society around us impact how we think, feel, and behave. Our social environment plays important roles in many aspects of our lives, and our physical activity and sedentary behavior are no exception. According to the scientific literature, social support is a complex phenomenon, defined and measured in many different ways. What holds true across these many conceptualizations and operationalizations is that when people around us support our efforts to be physically active and limit our time spent being sedentary, it becomes much easier to have healthy movement values, beliefs, and behavior. During certain life stages such as pregnancy or chronic illness, the effects of social environment can become particularly potent; however, the impact of social environment on our movement behavior starts from childhood and continues well into later life.

Vignette: Madeline

I'm embarrassed to run outside or on a treadmill. Any time I've tried, I just think of the bright purple track suits my parents would go jogging in around our neighborhood in West Virginia when my older sister and I were kids. They may have been fitter than most parents in our Huntington school district, but they were also the laughingstock of most kids I knew.

My mom was the one who really pushed fitness on our family. She implored my sister and me to join her on jogs, harangued us for watching too much television, and gave us a disapproving look when we'd come home with ice cream stains on our clothes or sticky fingers from furtive trips to the bakery after school. My sister had a much harder time with Mom's insistence on eating healthy and exercising every day. She went on to develop an eating disorder and had to drop out of college temporarily to get treatment.

I, on the other hand, avoided fitness trends, gyms, or involvement in team sports as long as I could. That's not to say I didn't get any physical activity. I would go on bike rides, walks, and the occasional hike. But if ever my activities of choice were associated with willful physical activity—that is, the kind people rely on to "get in shape"—my interests immediately shifted to secluding myself at home or in a library with a thick, heavy book.

Of course, as I've gotten older and settled into the working world, I don't have as much time to exercise leisurely. My fiancé has asked me numerous times to join him in CrossFit, but the intensity of that exercise intimidates me. I also don't really see how being able to do 10 push-ups in a row would benefit me.

One thing that has helped me stay active, however, is the Siberian husky my fiancé and I adopted shortly after we moved in together 6 months ago. I don't consider taking the energetic young pup out two—sometimes more—times a day as formal exercise. But I will say that being dragged around by this tireless fur ball keeps me on my toes. (It also happens to be the closest I'll come to running—ever. At least, I hope.)

Acquiring the dog has benefitted my social life. My future husband and I are new to Portland, Oregon—where we were both able to secure jobs, buy a sizable house, and still have some savings left over to start our lives together—and I've found it slightly challenging to make friends.

What's more, a lot of employees at the graphic design office where I work are huge fans of the outdoors. Like me, many of them also eschew the rigidity of most fitness programs marketed by gyms. And so, although I scaled back my time spent moving around when I was first settling in, 9 months into this job I've felt encouraged by my coworkers to get back out there and explore. (Many of them have some great hiking trips, and I've gone out with a couple of them on some nice outdoor walks.)

I've been incredibly lucky to escape that lingering sense of shame I felt for not forcing myself to jog or be on some sports team. Maybe being thousands of miles away from Mom helps. (Though I still worry about my sister, who continues to live at home.)

Part of my desire to be active is the social aspect. Even if I decide to take a bike ride or a hike by myself, I can still share my experience with friends at work who are genuinely interested in my experiences—and have their own to share and compare. And since my dog shows me so much more love when I bring him along for a leisurely outdoor adventure, it makes me even happier.

Key Terms

cohesion A dynamic process that is reflected in the tendency for a group to stick together and remain united in pursuit of its instrumental objectives and/or for the satisfaction of member affective needs.

enacted support The support given by the provider of a social exchange.

group dynamics The nature of groups, individual relationships within groups, and the group members' interactions with each other.

income inequality An unequal distribution of resources based on income.

perceived support An individual's cognitive appraisal of support.

racial discrimination Different treatment from people or organizations/systems between people of different races or ethnicities.

received support The support received from the recipient of a social exchange.

social environment The physical surroundings, social relationships, and cultural milieu within which people function and interact.

social identity The degree to which a person identifies with a social group.

social inequality An unequal distribution of resources based on social status.

social integration The degree to which the individual participates and is involved in family life, the social life of the community and has access to resources and support services.

social networks A person's connectedness to other people.

stigma When people have negative views of a person as a result of associations between characteristics of that person and negative attributes.

support network An individual's social network from a functional perspective. Also known as network resources.

supportive climate The quality of social relationships and systems.

Review Questions

1. What are three components of your social environment?
2. Describe two different perspectives of social support and compare and contrast them.
3. What is social integration?
4. How might perceived support differ from actual support?
5. How could social inequality or income inequality impact physical activity behavior?

6. Describe a way social environment might negatively impact your physical activity or sedentary behavior.
7. What is one way to measure social support?
8. Describe a situation in which group dynamics might influence an individual's movement behaviors.
9. What makes for an effective leader for physical activity?

Applying the Concepts

1. What aspects of Madeline's social environment are facilitative of her being regularly physically active?
2. What aspects of Madeline's social environment might inhibit her physical activity behavior? What changes could she make to her social environment that would make it easier to live a physically active lifestyle?

References

American Veterinary Medical Association. (2019). U.S. *Pet ownership and demographic sourcebook*. https://www.avma.org/KB/Resources/Statistics/Pages/Market-research-statistics-US-pet-ownership.aspx

Animal Medicines Australia. (2019). *Pet ownership in Australia 2019*. https://animalmedicinesaustralia.org.au/wp-content/uploads/2019/10/ANIM001-Pet-Survey-Report19_v1.7_WEB_high-res.pdf

Auerbach, J. A., Krimgold, B. K., & Lefkowitz, B. (2000). *Improving health: It doesn't take a revolution* (Health and Social Inequality). Kellogg Foundation.

Barnett, E., & Casper, M. (2001). A definition of "social environment." *American Journal of Public Health, 91*(3), 465.

Barrera, M., Jr., Sandler, I. N., & Ramsay, T. B. (1981). Preliminary development of a scale of social support: Studies on college students. *American Journal of Community Psychology, 9*(4), 435–447.

Baumeister, R. F., & Leary, M. R. (2007). The need to belong: Desire for interpersonal attachments as a fundamental human motivation. *General Psychology*, (1st Ed.), 497–529.

Beauchamp, M. R. (2019). Promoting exercise adherence through groups: A self-categorization theory perspective. *Exercise and Sport Sciences Reviews, 47*(1), 54–61.

Beauchamp, M. R., & Rhodes, R. E. (2020). A group-mediated approach to precision medicine-social identification, prevention, and treatment. *The Journal of the American Medical Association Psychiatry, 77*(6), 555–556. https://doi.org/10.1001/jamapsychiatry.2020.0024

Biddle, S. J. H., Petrolini, I., & Pearson, N. (2014). Interventions designed to reduce sedentary behaviours in young people: A review of reviews. *British Journal of Sports Medicine, 48*(3), 182–186. https://doi.org/10.1136/bjsports-2013-093078

Bort-Roig, J., Gilson, N. D., Puig-Ribera, A., Contrera, R. S., & Trost, S. G. (2014). Measuring and influencing physical activity with smartphone technology: A systematic review. *Sports Medicine, 44*, 671–686.

Brummett, B. H., Mark, D. B., Siegler, I. C., Williams, R. B., Babyak, M. A., Clapp-Channing, N. E., & Barefoot, J. C. (2005). Perceived social support as a predictor of mortality in coronary patients: Effects of smoking, sedentary behavior, and depressive symptoms. *Psychosomatic Medicine, 67*(1), 40–45. https://doi.org/10.1097/01.psy.0000149257.74854.b7

Brunet, J., Love, C., Ramphal, R., & Sabiston, C. M. (2014). Stress and physical activity in young adults treated for cancer: The moderating role of social support. *Supportive Care in Cancer, 22*, 689–695. https://doi.org/10.1007/s00520-013-2023-0

Burke, S. M., Carron, A. V., Eys, M. A., Ntoumanis, N., & Estabrooks, P. A. (2006). Group versus individual approach? A meta-analysis of the effectiveness of interventions to promote physical activity. *Journal of Sport & Exercise Psychology, 2*, 19–35.

Cardinal, B. J., Park, E. A., Kim, M., & Cardinal M. K. (2014). If Exercise is Medicine®, where is exercise in medicine? Review of U.S. medical education curricula for physical activity-related content. *Journal of Physical Activity and Health, 12*(9), 1336–1343. https://doi.org/10.1123/jpah.2014-0316

Carron, A. V., Brawley, L. R., & Widmeyer, W. N. (1998). The measurement of cohesiveness in sportgroups. In J. L. Duda (Ed.), *Advances in sport and exercise psychology measurement* (pp. 213–226). Morgantown, WV: Fitness Information Technology.

Carron, A. V., Hausenblas, H. A., & Estabrooks, P. A. (1999). Social influence and exercise involvement. In S. Bull (Ed.), *Adherence issues in sport and exercise* (pp. 1–17). New York, NY: John Wiley & Sons.

Carron, A. V., Hausenblas, H., & Mack, D. A. (1996). Social influence and exercise: A meta-analysis. *Journal of Sport and Exercise Psychology, 18*(1), 1–16.

Carron, A. V., Widmeyer, W. N., & Brawley, L. R. (1985). The development of an instrument to assess cohesion in sport teams: The group environment questionnaire. *Journal of Sport and Exercise Psychology, 7*(3), 244–266.

Cassel, J. (1976). The contributions of the social environment to host resistance: the Fourth Wade Hampton Frost lecture. *American Journal of Epidemiology, 104*(2)107–123.

Chogahara, M., O'Brien Cousins, S., & Wankel, L. M. (1998). Social influence on physical activity in older adults: A review. *Journal of Aging and Physical Activity, 6*(1), 1–17.

Christian, H., Bauman, A., Epping, J. N., Levine, G. N., McCormack, G., Rhodes, R. E., Richards, E., Rock, M., & Westgarth, C. (2018). Encouraging dog walking for health promotion and disease prevention. *American journal of lifestyle medicine, 12*(3), 233–243.

Christian, H., Trapp, G. (2013). Understanding the relationship between dog ownership and children's physical activity and sedentary behaviour. *Journal of Science and Medicine in Sport, 15*(Suppl. 1), S275. https://doi.org/10.1016/j.jsams .2012.11.666

Cobb, S. (1976). Social support as a moderator of life stress. *Psychosomatic Medicine, 3B,* 300–314.

Cohen, A., Mermelstein, R., Kamarck, T., & Hoberman, H. M. (1985). Measuring the functional components of social support. In I. G. Sarason & B. R. Sarason (Eds.), *Social support: Theory, research, and applications, 24,* 73–94. The Hague, Netherlands: Martinus Niijhoff.

Conroy, D. E., Yang, C. H., & Maher, J. P. (2014). Behavior change techniques in top-ranked mobile apps for physical activity. *American Journal of Preventive Medicine, 46*(6), 649–652.

Cradock, A. L., Kawachi, I., Colditz, G. A., Gortmaker, S. L., & Buka, S. L. (2009). Neighborhood social cohesion and youth participation in physical activity in Chicago. *Social Science & Medicine, 68*(3), 427–435.

De la Haye, K., Robins, G., Mohr, P., & Wilson, C. (2011). How physical activity shapes, and is shaped by, adolescent friendships. *Social Science & Medicine, 73*(5), 719–728.

Deliens, T., Deforche, B., De Bourdeaudhuij, I., & Clarys, P. (2015). Determinants of physical activity and sedentary behaviour in university students: A qualitative study using focus group discussions. *BioMed Central Public Health, 15*(201), 1–9. https://doi.org/10.1186/s12889-015-1553-4

Duncan, T. E., Duncan, S. C., & McAuley, E. (1993). The role of domain and gender-specific provisions of social relations in adherence to a prescribed exercise program. *Journal of Sport and Exercise Psychology, 15*(2), 220–231.

Dunlop, W. L., Falk, C. F., & Beauchamp, M. R. (2013). How dynamic are exercise group dynamics? Examining changes in cohesion within class-based exercise programs. *Health Psychology, 32*(12), 1240–1243.

Estabrooks, P. A. (2000). Sustaining exercise participation through group cohesion. *Exercise and Sport Science Reviews, 28*(2), 63–67.

Estabrooks, P. A., Munroe, K. J., Fox, E. H., Gyurcsik, N. C., Hill, J. L., Lyon, R., Rosenskranz, S., & Shannon, V. R. (2004). Leadership in physical activity groups for older adults: A qualitative analysis. *Journal of Aging and Physical Activity, 12,* 232–245.

Evenson, K. R., & Wen, F. (2011). Prevalence and correlates of objectively measured physical activity and sedentary behavior among US pregnant women. *Preventive Medicine, 53*(1–2), 39–43. https://doi.org/10.1016/j.ypmed.2011 .04.014

Fox, L. D., Rejeski, W. J., & Gauvin, L. (2000). Effects of leadership style and group dynamics on enjoyment of physical activity. *American Journal of Health Promotion, 14,* 277–283.

Gray, S. M., & Rhodes, R. E. (2019). Leadership approaches in group physical activity: A systematic review. *Leisure/Loisir, 42*(4), 505–527. https://doi.org/10.1080/14927713.2019 .1581993

Gross, J., Vancampfort, D., Stubbs, B., Gorczynski, P., & Soundy, A. (2016). A narrative synthesis investigating the use and value of social support to promote physical activity among individuals with schizophrenia. *Disability and Rehabilitation, 38*(2), 123–150. https://doi.org/10.3109 /09638288.2015.1024343

Harden, S. M., McEwan, D., Sylvester, B. D. et al. Understanding for whom, under what conditions, and how group-based physical activity interventions are successful: a realist review. BioMed Central Public Health 15(958), (2015). https://doi.org/10.1186/s12889-015 -2270-8

Huffman, S., & Szafron, M. (2017). Social correlates of leisure-time sedentary behaviours in Canadian adults. *Preventive Medicine Reports, 5,* 268–274. https://doi.org/10.1016/j .pmedr.2017.01.007

Hutzler, Y., Tesler, R., Ng, K., Barak, S., Kazula, H., & Harel-Fisch, Y. (2021). Physical activity, sedentary screen time and bullying behaviors: Exploring differences between adolescents with and without disabilities. *International Journal of Adolescence and Youth, 26*(1), 110–126. https:// doi.org/10.1080/02673843.2021.1875852

Israel, B. A. (1982). Social networks and health status: Linking theory, research, and practice. *Patient Counseling and Health Education, 4*(2), 65–69.

Jago, R., Fox, K. R., Page, A. S., Brockman, R., & Thompson, J. L. (2010). Parent and child physical activity and sedentary time: Do active parents foster active children. *BioMed Central Public Health, 10*(1), 1–9. https://doi.org /10.1186/1471-2458-10-194

Jensen, C. D., Cushing, C. C., & Elledge, A. R. (2014). Associations between teasing, quality of life, and physical activity among preadolescent children. *Journal of Pediatric Psychology, 39*(1), 65–73.

Joy E. L., Blair, S. N., McBride, P., & Sallis, R. (2013). Physical activity counseling in sports medicine: A call to action. *British Journal of Sports Medicine, 47*(1), 49–53.

Kim, J., Kim, J., & Han, A. (2020). Leisure time physical activity mediates the relationship between neighborhood social cohesion and mental health among older adults. *Journal of Applied Gerontology, 39*(3), 292–300. https://doi .org/10.1177/0733464819859199

Kouvonen, A., De Vogli, R., Stafford, M., Shipley, M. J., Marmot, M. G., Cox, T., Vahtera, J., Väänänen, A., Heponiemi, T., Singh-Manoux, A., & Kivimaki, M. (2012). Social support and the likelihood of maintaining and improving levels of physical activity: The Whitehall II study. *European Journal of Public Health, 22*(4), 514–518.

Laird, Y., Fawkner, S., Kelly, P., McNamee, L., & Niven, A. (2016). The role of social support on physical activity behaviour in adolescent girls: A systematic review and meta-analysis. *International Journal of Behavioral Nutrition and Physical Activity, 13*(1), 1–14. https://doi.org/10.1186/s12966-016-0405-7

Laireiter, A., & Baumann, U. (1992). Network structures and support functions—theoretical and empirical analyses. In H. O. F. Veiel & U. Baumann (Eds.), *The meaning and measurement of social support* (pp. 33–55). New York, NY: Hemisphere Publishing.

Lentino, C., Visek, A. J., McDonnell, K., & DiPietro, L. (2012). Dog walking is associated with a favorable risk profile independent of moderate to high volume of physical activity. *Journal of Physical Activity and Health, 9*(3), 414–420.

Lewis, C. S. (1945). *That hideous strength.* New York, NY: Scribner.

Lindsay Smith, G., Banting, L., Eime, R., O'Sullivan, G., & van Uffelen, J. G. Z. (2017). The association between social support and physical activity in older adults: A systematic review. *International Journal of Behavioral Nutrition and Physical Activity, 14*(1), 1–21. https://doi.org/10.1186/s12966-017-0509-8

Luo, T. C., Aguilera, A., Lyles, C. R., & Figueroa, C. A. (2021). Promoting physical activity through conversational agents: Mixed methods systematic review. *Journal of Medical Internet Research, 23*(9), e25486. https://doi.org/10.2196/25486

MacLeod, K., Shi, L., Zhang, D., Chen, L., & Chao, S. (2017). 1756 - Vehicle Time during Pregnancy and Post-Partum Depressive Symptom: Does Social Support Provide a Buffer? *Journal of Transport & Health, 5,* S5–S6. https://doi.org/10.1016/j.jth.2017.05.282

Maher, C., Ryan, J., Kernot, J., Podsiadly, J., & Keenihan, S. (2016). Social media and applications to health behavior. *Current Opinion in Psychology, 9,* 50–55.

Marques, A., Sallis, J. F., Martins, J., Diniz, J., & Carreiro Da Coasta, F. (2014). Correlates of urban children's leisure-time physical activity and sedentary behaviors during school days. *American Journal of Human Biology, 26*(3), 407–412.

Maturo, C. C., & Cunningham, S. A. (2013). Influence of friends on children's physical activity: A review. *American Journal of Public Health, 103*(7), e23–e38.

McIntyre, C. A., & Rhodes, R. E. (2009). Correlates of leisure-time physical activity during transitions to motherhood. *Women & Health, 49*(1), 66–83.

McKenna, J., Naylor, P. J., & McDowell, N. (1998). Barriers to physical activity promotion by general practitioners and practice nurses. *British Journal of Sports Medicine, 32*(3), 242–247.

Motl, R. W., McAuley, E., Snook, E. M., & Gliottoni, R. C. (2009). Physical activity and quality of life in multiple sclerosis: Intermediary roles of disability, fatigue, mood, pain, self-efficacy and social support. *Psychology, Health & Medicine, 14*(1), 111–124. https://doi.org/10.1080/13548500802241902

O'Connor, J. A., & Graber, K. C. (2014). Sixth-grade physical education: An acculturation of bullying and fear. *Research Quarterly for Exercise and Sport, 85*(3), 398–408.

Oh, Y. J., Zhang, J., Fang, M.-L., & Fukuoka, Y. (2021). A systematic review of artificial intelligence chatbots for promoting physical activity, healthy diet, and weight loss. *International Journal of Behavioral Nutrition and Physical Activity, 18*(1), 1–25.

Orrow, G., Kinmonth, A. L., Sanderson, S., & Sutton, S. (2012). Effectiveness of physical activity promotion based in primary care: Systematic review and meta-analysis of randomised controlled trials. *British Medical Journal, 344,* e1389.

Pabayo, R., Belsky, J., Gauvin, L., & Curtis, S. (2011). Do area characteristics predict change in moderate-to-vigorous physical activity from ages 11 to 15 years? *Social Science and Medicine, 72*(3), 430–438.

Prochnow, T., Delgado, H., Patterson, M. S., & Meyer, M. R. U. (2020). Social network analysis in child and adolescent physical activity research: A systematic literature review. *Journal of Physical Activity and Health, 17*(2), 250–260. https://doi.org/10.1123/jpah.2019-0350

Pulido, R., Banks, C., Ragan, K., Pang, D., Blake, J. J., & McKyer, E. L. (2019). The impact of school bullying on physical activity in overweight youth: Exploring race and ethnic differences. *Journal of School Health, 89*(4), 319–327. https://doi.org/10.1111/josh.12740

Rafaeli, E., Cranford, J. A., Green, A. S., Shrout, P. E., & Bolger, N. (2008). The good and bad of relationships: How social hindrance and social support affect relationship feelings in daily life. *Personality and Social Psychology Bulletin, 34*(12), 1703–1718.

Ravenek, M. J., & Schneider, M. A. (2009). Social support for physical activity and perceptions of control in early Parkinson's disease. *Disability and Rehabilitation, 31*(23), 1925–1936. https://doi.org/10.1080/09638280902850261

Rhodes, R. E., Baranova, M., Christian, H., & Westgarth, C. (2020). Increasing physical activity by four legs rather than two: Systematic review of dog-facilitated physical activity interventions. *British Journal of Sports Medicine, 54*(20), 1202–1207. https://doi.org/10.1136/bjsports-2019-101156

Rhodes, R. E., Guerrero, M. D., Vanderloo, L. M., Barbeau, K., Birken, C. S., Chaput, J. P., Faulkner, G., Janssen, I., Madigan, S., Mâsse, L. C., McHugh, T-L., Perdew, M., Stone, K., Shelley, J., Spinks, N., Tamminen, K. A., Tomasone, J. R., Ward, H., Welsh, F., & Tremblay, M. S. (2020). Development of a consensus statement on the role of the family in the physical activity, sedentary, and sleep behaviours of children and youth. *International Journal *of Behavioral Nutrition and Physical Activity, 17*(1), 1–31. https://doi.org/10.1186/s12966-020-00973-0

Rhodes, R. E., Spence, J. C., Berry, T., Faulkner, G., Latimer-Cheung, A. E., O'Reilly, N., Tremblay, M. S., & Vanderloo, L. (2019). Parental support of the Canadian 24-hour movement guidelines for children and youth: Prevalence and correlates. *BioMed Central Public Health, 19*(1), 1–12.

Rich, E., & Mansfield, L. (2019). Fat and physical activity: Understanding and challenging weight stigma - Special Issue of Fat Studies: An Interdisciplinary Journal of Body Weight and Society. *Fat Studies, 8*(2), 99–109. https://doi.org/10.1080/21604851.2019.1552823

Roman, C. G., & Taylor, C. J. (2013). A multilevel assessment of school climate, bullying victimization, and physical activity. *Journal of School Health, 83*(6), 400–407.

Russell, D., & Cutrona, C. (1984, August). The provisions of social relationships and adaptation to stress. Paper presented at the annual meeting of the American Psychological Association. Toronto, Ontario, Canada.

Sarason, B. R., Pierce, G. R., & Sarason, I. G., (1990). Social support: The sense of acceptance and the role of relationships. In B. R. Sarason, I. G. Sarason, & G. R. Pierce (Eds.), *Social support: An interactional view* (pp. 97–128). New York, NY: Wiley.

Sarason, B. R., Pierce, G. R., Shearin, E. N., Sarason, I. G., Waltz, J. A., & Poppe, L. (1991). Perceived social support and working models of self and actual others. *Journal of Personality and Social Psychology, 60*(2), 273.

Sarason, I. G., Levine, H. M., Basham, R. B., & Sarason, B. R. (1983). Assessing social support: The Social Support Questionnaire. *Journal of Personality and Social Psychology, 44*(1), 127.

Sarason, I. G., Mankowski, E. S., Peterson, A. V. Jr., & Dinh, K. T. (1992). Adolescents' reasons for smoking. *Journal of School Health, 62*(5), 185–190.

Sarason, I. G., Sarason, B. R., & Pierce, G. R. (1992). Three contexts of social support. In H. O. F. Veiel & U. Baumann (Eds.), *The meaning and measurement of social support* (pp. 143–154). New York, NY: Hemisphere Publishing.

Sattler, K. M., Deane, F. P., Tapsell, L., & Kelly, P. J. (2018). Gender differences in the relationship of weight-based stigmatisation with motivation to exercise and physical activity in overweight individuals. *Health Psychology Open, 5*(1), 2055102918759691. https://doi.org/10.1177/2055102918759691

Sawka, K. J., McCormack, G. R., Nettel-Aguirre, A., Hawe, P., & Doyle-Baker, P. K. (2013). Friendship networks and physical activity and sedentary behavior among youth: A systematized review. *International Journal of Behavioral Nutrition and Physical Activity, 10*(1), 1–9.

Sbarra, D. A., Law, R. W., & Portley, R. M. (2011). Divorce and death: A meta-analysis and research agenda for clinical, social, and health psychology. *Perspectives on Psychological Science, 6*(5), 454–474.

Scarapicchia, T. M. F., Amireault, S., Faulkner, G., & Sabiston, C. M. (2017). Social support and physical activity participation among healthy adults: A systematic review of prospective studies. *International Review of Sport and Exercise Psychology, 10*(1), 50–83. https://doi.org/10.1080/1750984X.2016.1183222

Shirazipour, C. H., Evans, M. B., Leo, J., Lithopoulos, A., Martin Ginis, K. A., & Latimer-Cheung, A. E. (2020). Program conditions that foster quality physical activity participation experiences for people with a physical disability: A systematic review. *Disability and Rehabilitation, 42*(2), 147–155. https://doi.org/10.1080/09638288.2018.1494215

Short, C. E., Hayman, M., Rebar, A. L., Gunn, K. M., De Cocker, K., Duncan, M. J., Turnbull, D., Dollman, J., van Uffelen, J. G. Z., & Vandelanotte, C. (2016). Physical activity recommendations from general practitioners in Australia. Results from a national survey. *Australian and New Zealand Journal of Public Health, 40*(1), 83–90. https://doi.org/10.1111/1753-6405.12455

Smith-Ray, R. L., Mama, S., Reese-Smith, J. Y., Estabrooks, P. A., & Lee, R. E. (2012). Improving participation rates for women of color in health research: The role of group cohesion. *Prevention Science, 13*(1), 27–35.

Springer, A. E., Kelder, S. H., & Hoelschler, D. M. (2006). Social support, physical activity, and sedentary behavior among 6th-grade girls: A cross-sectional study. *International Journal of Behavioral Nutrition and Physical Activity, 3*(1), 1–10.

Stephenson, A., McDonough, S. M., Murphy, M. H., Nugent, C. D., & Mair, J. L. (2017). Using computer, mobile and wearable technology enhanced interventions to reduce sedentary behaviour: A systematic review and meta-analysis. *International Journal of Behavioral Nutrition and Physical Activity, 14*(1), 105–121. https://doi.org/10.1186/s12966-017-0561-4

Stevens, M., Rees, T., Coffee, P., Haslam, S. A., Steffens, N. K., & Polman, R. (2018). Leaders promote attendance in sport and exercise sessions by fostering social identity. *Scandinavian Journal of Medicine & Science in Sports, 28*(9), 2100–2108. https://doi.org/10.1111/sms.13217

Sylaska, K. M., & Edwards, K. M. (2014). Disclosure of intimate partner violence to informal social support network members: A review of the literature. *Trauma, Violence, & Abuse, 15*(1), 3–21.

Tandon, P. S., Zhou, C., Sallis, J. F., Cain, K. L., Frank, L. D., & Saelens, B. E. (2012). Home environment relationships with children's physical activity, sedentary time, and screen time by socio economic status. *International Journal of Behavioral Nutrition and Physical Activity, 9*(1), 1–9. https://doi.org/10.1186/1479-5868-9-88

Tay, L., Tan, K., Diener, E., & Gonzalez, E. (2013). Social relations, health behaviors, and health outcomes: A survey and synthesis. *Applied Psychology, Health and Well-Being, 5*(1), 28–78.

Vancampfort, D., Damme, T. V., Firth, J., Hallgren, M., Smith, L., Stubbs, B., Rosenbaum, S., & Koyanagi, A. (2019). Correlates of leisure-time sedentary behavior among 181,793 adolescents aged 12–15 years from 66 low- and middle-income countries. *Public Library Of Science ONE, 14*(11), e0224339. https://doi.org/10.1371/journal.pone.0224339

Vancampfort, D., Stubbs, B., Lara, E., Vandenbulcke, M., Swinnen, N., & Koyanagi, A. (2019). Correlates of sedentary behavior in middle-aged and old age people with mild cognitive impairment: A multinational study. *International Psychogeriatrics, 31*(4), 579–589. https://doi.org/10.1017/S1041610218001163

Vancampfort, D., Stubbs, B., Mugisha, J., Firth, J., Schuch, F. B., & Koyanagi, A. (2018). Correlates of sedentary behavior in 2,375 people with depression from 6 low- and middle-income countries. *Journal of Affective Disorders, 234*, 97–104. https://doi.org/10.1016/j.jad.2018.02.088

Vancampfort, D., Stubbs, B., Smith, L., Gardner, B., Herring, M. P., Firth, J., & Koyanagi, A. (2019). Correlates of sedentary behavior among community-dwelling adults with anxiety in six low- and middle-income countries. *Psychiatry Research, 273*, 501–508. https://doi.org/10.1016/j.psychres.2019.01.064

Vaux, A. (1988). *Social support: Theory, research, and intervention.* New York, NY: Praeger.

Vaux, A. (1992). Assessment of social support. In H. O. F. Veiel & U. Baumann (Eds.), *The meaning and measurement of social support* (pp. 193–216). New York, NY: Hemisphere Publishing.

Weiss, R. S. (1974). The provisions of social relationships. In Z. Rubin (Ed.), *Doing unto others* (pp. 17–26). Englewood Cliffs, NJ: Prentice-Hall.

Yang, C. H., Maher, J. P., & Conroy, D. E. (2015). Implementation of behavior change techniques in mobile applications for physical activity. *American Journal of Preventive Medicine, 48*(4), 452–455.

Yao, C. A., Rhodes, R. E. (2015). Parental correlates in child and adolescent physical activity: A meta-analysis. *International Journal of Behavioral Nutrition and Physical Activity, 12*(1), 1–38. https://doi.org/10.1186/s12966-015-0163-y

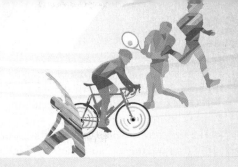

CHAPTER 4

Physical Environment

LEARNING OBJECTIVES

After completing this chapter, you will be able to:

- Outline the importance of the physical and built environment on physical activity and sedentary behaviors.
- Describe how modernization has influenced levels of physical activity and sedentary behavior.
- Describe the influence of the environment on travel patterns.
- Describe environmental prompts that increase physical activity.
- Differentiate between perceived and actual access to physical activity resources.
- Describe the socioecological model applied to physical activity and sedentary behavior.
- Outline physical environmental correlates of physical activity and sedentary behavior.

Introduction

In George Orwell's classic novel *1984*, a dark picture of a futuristic society in fear of the ever-present, watchful eye of the enigmatic dictator called Big Brother is described (Orwell, 1949). In *1984*, members of the "Outer Party" were awakened with a whistle every morning at the same time. Three minutes after the sound of the whistle, a fitness instructor would appear on the telescreen. Outer Party members did not think about having time for exercise, they did not consider if they had the confidence to complete the exercise, nor did they have intentions regarding the frequency, duration, intensity, or type of physical activity. They simply did their morning exercises. Why? Because their environment was structured so that each day they would do what was called the "physical jerks." No questions, no options. And, if they did attempt to miss the exercise

sessions, they would be quickly chastised and brought back into behavioral conformity. Unlike the dismal exercise adherence we have in most countries, in Big Brother's world there were no exercise adherence problems—only 100% prevalence, 100% maintenance.

So, did Orwell find the answer to promoting the initiation and maintenance of physical activity? Is it a plausible model for current society? Definitely not. However, some components of Big Brother's world are appealing. For example, in his world there are no motivational problems associated with being physically active. What is clear is that one's environment has the potential to be related to behavioral outcomes. In this chapter, we focus on factors within one's physical environment that may be related to either increased or diminished levels of physical activity and sedentary behavior. The **physical environment** includes all of your indoor

75

and outdoor surroundings. Thus, the physical environment includes both designed and natural infrastructures. Designed infrastructures include houses, stores, fitness facilities, and recreational parks. In comparison, examples of natural infrastructures include oceans, lakes, and mountains.

The **built environment** is part of the physical environment, but it refers to only the designed, human-made surroundings. The built environment ranges in scale from infrastructures for walking and cycling, availability of public transit, **street connectivity**, housing density, parks, **green spaces** (i.e., an area of grass, trees, or other vegetation set apart for recreational purposes), and **land use mix** (i.e., diversity or variety of land uses such as residential, commercial, industrial, and agricultural). For example, a diverse land use mix is associated with shorter travel distances between places of interest and activities (Sallis et al., 2020).

Examining the effect of the physical environment on people's physical activity and sedentary behavior is a more recent area of inquiry in comparison to individual and social factors. However, the physical environment represents an intense area of study since 2000, accounting for about 30% of all psychology of physical activity research (Rhodes & Nasuti, 2011). When reviewing the literature examining the impact of physical environmental factors on physical activity participation, a pattern of research emerges. Based on this pattern of research, the following components

of the physical environment and its relationship to physical activity and sedentary behavior are addressed in this chapter: **modernization**, travel, climate/seasonal variations, **point-of-choice prompts**, and environmental correlates of physical activity and sedentary behavior. To better understand how the physical environment affects our physical activity behavior, let's first take a closer look at how the environment influences young children's ability to delay gratification.

Influences of the Physical Environment on Delayed Gratification

Delayed gratification is the ability to reject immediately available smaller rewards in favor of later larger rewards. For example, can you forgo buying those jeans to save money to buy a car in the next year? People's ability to delay gratification has been linked to many positive outcomes, including academic success, physical health, psychological health, and social competence (Drobetz, Maercker, & Forstmeier, 2012; Moffitt et al., 2011).

For the purposes of this chapter, a functional starting point is with Walter Mischel and his colleagues' research regarding delayed gratification in 4-year-old children (for a review, see Mischel, Shoda, & Rodriguez, 1989). Using primarily laboratory research techniques, the typical protocol involved children being shown toys, marshmallows, and candies. The researcher then explained to the children that they can either have the treat or play with the toy immediately or have additional treats or toys if they wait a few minutes until the researcher returns to the room. In other words, the child could eat the one marshmallow right away or wait 20 minutes for two marshmallows. The researcher would then leave the room and return in 20 minutes. As expected, the children, on average, were not very successful in delaying their gratification. Most would quickly play with the toys or eat the candies. Only about one-third of the children could wait until the researcher returned (Mischel et al., 1989).

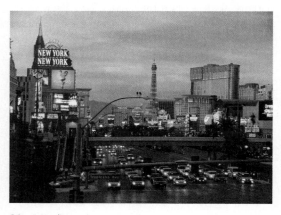

© Steve Hoskinson/Shutterstock.

A longitudinal study of these children found that a child's ability to delay gratification for a longer period of time as a preschooler was associated with important outcomes, such as adolescent academic strength, social competence, and the ability to handle stress as an adult. In some children, it was also associated with higher Scholastic Aptitude Test (SAT) scores and decreased likelihood of illegal drug use in adulthood (Ayduk et al., 2000).

CRITICAL THINKING ACTIVITY 4-1

How successful are you at delaying gratification? How has this affected your overall health?

A number of potential explanations were offered why some children could wait and others could not resist the temptation. It was hypothesized that some children have the skills necessary to wait for gratification. Potentially, these skills could be taught to children, or the temptation of early consumption could be removed from the child's environment. In subsequent studies, Mischel and his colleagues (1989) examined different strategies that could help the child become more successful. Using the typical protocol, the children were assigned to one of three possible environments. In Condition 1, the children were asked to wait while the candy was in plain view on the table. In Condition 2, the children were asked to wait while the candy was in plain view on the table, but they had been taught to cope by thinking about fun thoughts while waiting for the researcher to return. In Condition 3, the children were asked to wait while the candy was on the table but under a cover. In other words, in Condition 3 the physical environment was changed.

As expected, the children in Condition 1 typically ate the candy and could not delay gratification. In Condition 2, the children were more successful than those who were not taught the coping strategy from Condition 1; that is, the children who had been taught to cope by thinking about fun thoughts (Condition 2) were more successful than those who were not taught the coping strategy (Condition 1). However, for Condition 3, where the physical environment was changed (i.e., the candy was covered), the children were also more successful in waiting for their reward (Mischel et al., 1989). Based on these findings, it appears that changing the physical environment can change children's ability to delay their gratification—changing their physical environment changed their behavior.

Interestingly, Mischel and his colleagues assessed whether the 4-year-olds' performance on the delayed gratification task would predict their body mass index (BMI) 30 years later. As part of a longitudinal study, a subset (n = 164) of the children were followed up on about 30 years later and were asked to self-report their height and weight. The researchers found that children who had a longer delay of gratification at age 4 also had a lower BMI 30 years later (Schlam, Wilson, Shoda, Mischel, & Ayduk, 2013). Potentially identifying children with greater difficulty in delaying gratification could help detect children at risk of becoming either overweight or obese.

How does this relate to physical activity and sedentary behavior? Dzewaltowski and his colleagues (Dzewaltowski, Johnston, Estabrooks, & Johannes, 2000) suggested the following: First, like waiting for a second candy, the benefits of physical activity participation are sometimes more distal than the acute benefits of sedentary behavior. Second, like waiting for candy, physical activity often requires coping skills to complete. Take, for example, an individual who plans to exercise after work. Before he goes to exercise, he decides to stop at home. While at home, he turns on the television and finds an entertaining program and in the end does not exercise. It can be concluded based on what we know from Mischel and his colleagues' study that if the television option was removed from the environment, then the individual might not have been tempted and would have followed through on his exercise plans. So, when an environment is risky (i.e., there is a candy waiting to be eaten or a television show waiting to be watched), it is important to ensure that individuals have appropriate coping skills.

However, when the environment is supportive (i.e., no candy, accessible physical activity options), even those people without appropriate coping skills can be successful (Dzewaltowski et al., 2000). In short, it is the physical environment that changed the children's behavior regardless of the skills they possessed. Does this generalize to physical activity and sedentary behavior? That is, by having a physical environment that makes it easy to be active and stand, will people be more active and stand more? Let's now see what the research says about the role that our physical environment has on our physical activity and sedentary behaviors.

Modernization of the Physical Environment: A Comparison of Two Cultures

Modernization refers to the transformation from a rural and agrarian society to an urban and industrial society. To take a look at the effects of modernization of our physical environment on physical activity levels, we can examine the following two very different cultures: (1) the Inuit, who have experienced rapid modernization, and (2) the **Old Order Amish**, who have resisted modernization. Comparing and contrasting these two cultures has enabled researchers to examine the effects of modernization (or resistance to modernization) on health and physical activity.

The Case of the Inuit

In a landmark series of studies, Andris Rode and Roy Shephard (1993, 1994) examined the effects of a rapidly changing physical environment on the Inuit people living in Igloolik, which is located in the remote northern Canadian territory of Nanavut. Igloolik has a **polar climate**; 9 months of the year the average temperature is below freezing. Historically, the people of Igloolik lived a hunting and trapping lifestyle that required high levels of daily physical activity. However, in the latter half of the 20th century, the people of Igloolik went through a rapid period of acculturation to a sedentary lifestyle. In essence, their hunter-gatherer lifestyle quickly shifted to a more mechanized Western lifestyle.

As shown in **Figure 4-1**, the people of Igloolik experienced dramatic changes in their physical environment from 1970 to 1990, with significant increases in the ratio of snowmobiles, boats, cars, and all-terrain vehicles to households. Instead of walking, the Inuit could now take a sedentary form of transportation. As well, their outdoor activities declined and were often replaced by sedentary indoor activities such as watching television. Did this dramatic and rapid change in their physical environment affect their health? Yes!

Using a longitudinal study design, Rode and Shephard examined various health outcomes of a sample of Igloolik adults (age range = 20 to 60 years) with surveys and testing that they administered in 1970, 1980, and 1990. In 1970, much of the population continued traditional hunting and fishing activities, and physical activity levels were high. One of the primary indicators of decreased physical activity was the sum of skinfolds, which assesses the amount of subcutaneous body fat. A higher number on this assessment is related to increased adiposity. The 40- to 49-year-old Inuit people assessed in 1970 had a relatively low sum of skinfolds (16.3 mm for men and 21 mm for women). Individuals in the same age category in 1990 had scores four times that of their predecessors (46.9 mm for

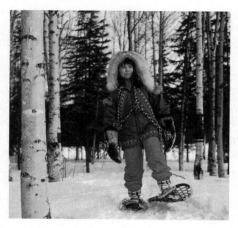

© Chris Arend/Design Pics Inc/Alamy Stock Photo.

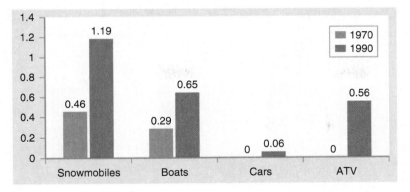

Figure 4-1 Ratio of Vehicles to Households.

Data from Rode, A., & Shephard, R. J. (1994). Physiological consequences of acculturation: A 20-year study of fitness in an Inuit community. *European Journal of Applied Physiology and Occupational Physiology, 69,* 516–524.

men and 85.4 mm for women; see **Figure 4-2**). Similarly, significant decreases in aerobic power via a step test were found from 1970 to 1990 (see **Figure 4-3**). The researchers concluded that changes in the Inuit's physical environment were responsible for the dramatic reduction of lifestyle physical activity and rise in sedentary behavior, particularly through the use of snowmobiles in place of walking through deep snow.

The Case of the Old Order Amish

Another method to assess the impact of modernization on physical activity is to examine the Old Order Amish because their lifestyle, in contrast to the Inuit, has not changed much in the last 150 years (Bassett, Schneider, & Huntington, 2004). The Old Order Amish believe in separation from the outside world and a simplistic lifestyle. In their clothing, lifestyle, and religion, the Amish people emphasize humility, nonviolence, and traditional values rather than advancement and technology. They do not drive automobiles, use electrical appliances, or employ other modern conveniences such as dishwashers and washing machines.

They have elected to keep most types of modern technology out of their lives, to live close to the land, and to maintain strong family and community ties. Labor-intensive farming remains the main occupation, whereby the Amish men still

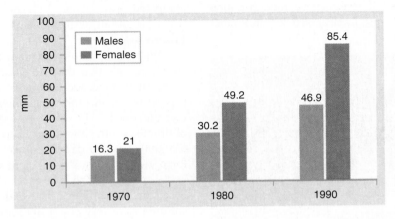

Figure 4-2 Sum of Skinfolds (adults aged 40 to 49 years).

Data from Rode, A., & Shephard, R. J. (1994). Physiological consequences of acculturation: A 20-year study of fitness in an Inuit community. *European Journal of Applied Physiology and Occupational Physiology, 69,* 516–524.

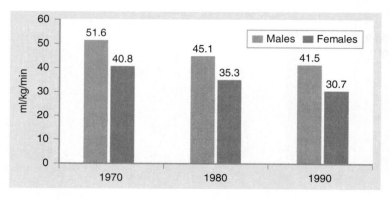

Figure 4-3 Changes in Aerobic Power Over a 20-Year Period.

Data from Rode, A., & Shephard, R. J. (1994). Physiological consequences of acculturation: A 20-year study of fitness in an Inuit community. *European Journal of Applied Physiology and Occupational Physiology, 69*, 516–524.

till the soil with horses. The Amish people tend to either walk or use horse-drawn carriages for transportation. The Amish women do most of the childcare, cooking, and cleaning. The children are educated in their own schools, and formal education ends after the eighth grade. In short, the Old Order Amish have resisted modernization. Has this resistance to modernization had an effect on their physical activity and sedentary behavior levels? From the standpoint of energy expenditure, the Amish people's lifestyle might resemble that of rural residents in North America in the mid-to-late 1800s.

In a series of studies, David Bassett and his colleagues (2004, 2007; Eslinger et al., 2010; Tremblay, Eslinger, Copeland, Barnes, & Bassett, 2008) examined if resistance to modernization had any effect on physical activity and other health parameters of Old Order Amish children and adults. In one study, the children (aged 6 to 18 years) wore a pedometer for a week and their height and weight were assessed to compute their BMI. The main findings were that the Amish children had higher levels of physical activity (as determined by their pedometer step count), lower rates of sedentary time, and lower rates of overweight and obesity compared to youth living in modern societies.

More specifically, obesity was rare in the Amish children. Only 1.4% of the Amish youth were classified as obese based on their BMI, compared to about 8% of Canadian and American youth at the time the study was conducted. As well, only 7% of Amish youth were overweight, compared with about 25% of Canadian and American youth at the time of the study (see **Figure 4-4**).

With regard to physical activity, **Figure 4-5** clearly reveals that the Old Order Amish children, on average, took significantly more steps than children in other industrialized countries (age range = 5 to 12 years). As a reasonable rule of thumb, youth should accumulate a minimum of 9,000 steps per day. Of course, more is better for optimal health (Adams, Johnson, & Tudor-Locke, 2013; Tudor-Locke et al., 2011a, 2011b). Based on these values, the Old Order Amish children were very physically active. In fact, the Old Order Amish children took about 5,000 to 6,000 more steps per day than North American

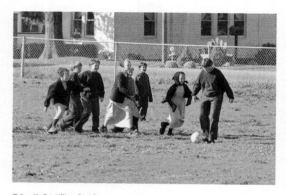

© Ilene MacDonald/Alamy Stock Photo.

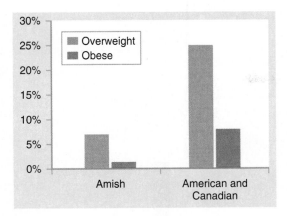

Figure 4-4 Percent of Amish Children with Overweight and Obesity Compared with Their American and Canadian Counterparts.

Data from Bassett, D. R. Jr., Tremblay, M. S., Esliger, D. W., Copeland, J. L., Barnes, J. D., & Huntington, G. E. (2007). Physical activity and body mass index of children in an Old Order Amish community. *Medicine and Science in Sports and Exercise, 39*, 410–415.

children, and they had significantly lower obesity rates.

Of importance, Old Order Amish youth had higher levels of physical activity than children living in industrialized societies, despite less participation in competitive sports, no formal exercise classes, and no physical education classes. Old Order Amish children accumulated steps in a variety of ways throughout the day. For example, they walked to school regardless of the weather, and they performed activity-intense farm and household chores such as feeding and tending to farm animals, harvesting crops, sweeping, cleaning floors on their hands and knees, as well as laundry, meal preparation, and childcare activities. Despite the lack of formal physical education classes, the schoolchildren are given two recesses and a 1-hour lunch each school day, in which most of this time is spent engaged in active play.

Similar results were obtained with Old Order Amish adults, with Amish men accumulating an average of 18,425 steps per day and Amish women accumulating an average of 14,196 steps per day (see **Figure 4-6**). These Amish adult daily step values are about two-thirds higher than estimates from other epidemiological pedometer-assessed step values in other American adult populations (Bassett, Wyatt, Thompson, Peters, & Hill, 2010).

As well, only 4% of the Amish adults were obese. Of interest, there was no evidence of an age-related decline in physical activity between 6 to 60 years of age for the Old Order Amish. In contrast, American adults take only one-half as many steps as elementary school children in the United States (6,000 vs. 12,000 steps/day; Tudor-Locke et al., 2004). The study of a culture that has resisted modern technology can help us understand the impact of modern technology on

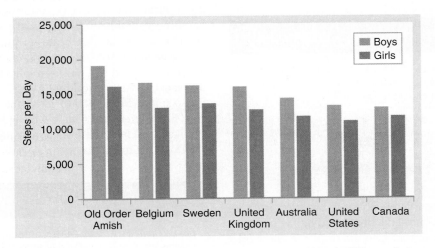

Figure 4-5 Average Number of Steps per Day in Elementary School Children in Different Cultures.

Data from Bassett, D. R. Jr., Pucher, J., Buehler, R., Thompson, D. L., & Crouter, S. E. (2008). Walking, cycling, and obesity rates in Europe, North America, and Australia. *Journal of Physical Activity and Health, 5*, 795–814.

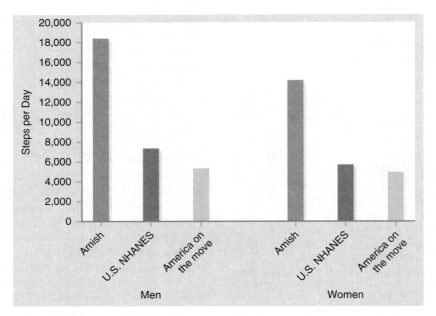

Figure 4-6 Comparison of Daily Step Counts Between Old Order Amish Adults and Contemporary U.S. Adults from the "America on the Move" Epidemiological Study.

Note: The average number of steps per day taken by Amish men and women were 18,425 steps per day and 14,196 steps per day, respectively. These values are considerably higher than recent estimates for contemporary U.S. adults.

Data from Bassett, D. R. Jr., Schneider, P. L., & Huntington, G. E. (2004). Physical activity in an Old Order Amish community. *Medicine and Science in Sports and Exercise, 36*, 79–85.

people's physical activity and weight status. In short, by examining a culture that refrains from using automobiles, modern labor-saving devices, and screen entertainment, it is possible to estimate how these advances have impacted our lives.

CRITICAL THINKING ACTIVITY 4-2

Can you think of other societies that have gone through rapid periods of modernization? How has this affected their health?

Travel Patterns

Youth Travel Patterns

Active travel is an approach to transportation that focuses on physical activities, such as walking, biking, and skateboarding, as opposed to automobile travel, to get to places like work, school, shops, and parks. Active travel is an important way for youth to get physical activity.

School-age children who travel to school by active means accumulate more physical activity and are more physically fit that those who travel by passive means, such as car and bus (Ostergaard, Kolle, Steene-Johannssen, Anderssen, & Anderson, 2013; Pizarro et al., 2013). Unfortunately, there has been a dramatic decline in the number of children who walk, skateboard, or bike to school or engage in active leisure activities in many parts of the world, and this has been ongoing for over 30 years (see Active Healthy Kids Canada, 2013). For example, from 1969 to 1990, the percentage of U.S. children and youth who either walked or biked to school fell from almost 48% to 13% (McDonald, Brown, Marchetti, & Pedroso, 2011).

CRITICAL THINKING ACTIVITY 4-3

Did you walk or bike to elementary school? How did this affect your level of daily physical activity as a youth?

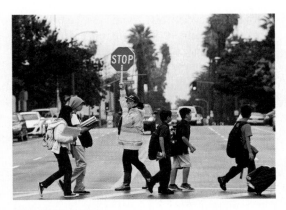

© Rappensuncle/iStock/Getty Images.

The distance from a child's home to school is a strong indicator of active travel. Early research in this area found that children living within a quarter mile of their school were 14 times more likely to walk to school than children living greater than 1 mile away from their school (McDonald et al., 2011). Unfortunately, many students face long trips not possible by active means. The likelihood of children walking or biking to school is positively associated with shorter trips, self-reporting as male, higher land use mix (i.e., retail, recreation, and residential spaces), low-density traffic, and presence of street trees (Su et al., 2013). The community and neighborhood environment can facilitate active transportation to school and other nearby locations through the presence of neighborhood schools, sidewalks, bike lanes, and traffic-calming mechanisms such as crosswalks and traffic signals.

In a systematic review of 52 studies, Schoeppe and colleagues (Schoeppe, Duncan, Badland, Oliver, & Curtis, 2013) examined children and youth's (aged 3–18 years) independent mobility and active travel with regard to physical activity, sedentary behavior, and weight status. Independent mobility is defined as the freedom to travel around either their own neighborhood or city without adult supervision (Tranter & Whitelegg, 1994). Thus, independent mobility could be for the purposes of either play or travel to places such as school, leisure facilities, parks, and friends' houses. The researchers found that most studies focused on active travel to and/or from school,

and that these studies found a positive association with physical activity. In other words, children and youth who walked to school engaged in more physical activity than those who were driven to school. The same relationship was detected for active travel to leisure-related places and independent mobility with physical activity. A more recent systematic review found that parents with concerns about street connectivity and distance cited lower active transport behavior among their children (Aranda-Balboa et al., 2020), suggesting that the built environment was a critical factor for active transport within the family.

Unfortunately, few studies have examined whether a correlation exists between active travel to school and self-reported screen time or objectively measured sedentary behavior. The researchers concluded that children who have the freedom to play outdoors and travel actively without adult supervision accumulate more physical activity than those who do not.

In addition to built environment factors, many parents will site safety as a main reason for restricting the independent mobility of their children (Stone et al., 2014). In an attempt to bring clarity to this issue, Datar and colleagues (Datar, Nicosia, Shier, 2013) examined the relationship between parent-perceived neighborhood safety and children's physical activity, sedentary behavior, body mass, and obesity status using 9 years of longitudinal data (1999 to 2007) on a cohort of about 19,000 American kindergartners. The children's height and weight measurements and

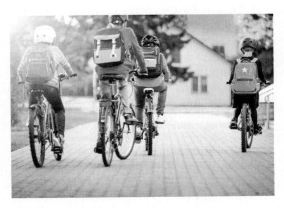

© LeManna/Shutterstock.

parent perceptions of neighborhood safety were assessed when the children were in kindergarten and in the first, third, fifth, and eighth grades. Dependent variables included age- and gender-specific BMI percentile, obesity status, and parent- or child-reported weekly physical activity and television watching. The researchers found that children whose parents perceived their neighborhoods as unsafe watched more television and participated in less physical activity. No significant association, however, was found between parent-perceived neighborhood safety and children's BMI. A recent systematic review on the correlates of parental support of child physical activity also echoed this finding (Rhodes et al., 2020); those parents who perceived environmental safety concerns for physical activity, were less likely to support their children in physical activity than parents who did not share these concerns.

CRITICAL THINKING ACTIVITY 4-4

What types of interventions can be developed to get children and youth to walk or bike to school more?

Travel in Different Countries

An example of the relationship between physical activity and one's environment can be found in the travel patterns of people from different countries. Bassett and his colleagues (Bassett, Pucher, Buehler, Thompson, & Crouter, 2008) conducted an international examination of the relationship between active transportation (defined as the percentage of trips taken by walking, bicycling, and public transit) and obesity rates in Europe, North America, and Australia. They found that countries with the highest levels of active transportation generally had the lowest obesity rates.

They found that Europeans walked and biked significantly more than Americans. For example, in 2000, Europeans walked 382 kilometers per person, compared to 140 kilometers per person for Americans. As another example, also in 2000,

Europeans bicycled 188 kilometers, compared to Americans biking 40 kilometers per person. The researchers concluded that walking and bicycling are far more common in European countries than in the United States, Australia, and Canada, and that active transportation is inversely related to obesity in these countries.

D'Haese and colleagues (2015) explored how the physical environment was associated with active transportation among children across North America, Europe, and Australia through a review of 65 papers. The authors found that active transportation to school (walking or cycling) was positively associated with walkability, but not in any other context (such as leisure time active transport). General safety and traffic safety were associated with active transportation to school in North America and Australia but not associated with active transportation to school in Europe. There is a need for studies conducted in Asia, Africa and South-America to further explore regional differences.

Active travel can also help adults meet the recommended levels of physical activity. Buehler and colleagues (Buehler, Pucher, Merom, & Bauman, 2011) conducted a longitudinal study to examine the proportion of walking and cycling trips in Germany and the United States. They found that Germans walk and cycle significantly more than Americans (see **Table 4-1**). The researchers concluded that the high prevalence of active travel in Germany shows that daily walking and cycling can help a large proportion of the population meet recommended physical activity levels.

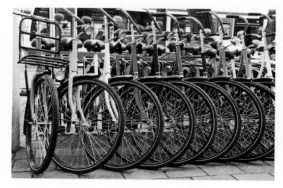

© Vitaly Titov/Shutterstock.

Table 4-1 Comparison of Active Travel in the United States and Germany

	United States		Germany	
	2001/2002	2008/2009	2001/2002	2008/2009
Note: Between 2001/2002 and 2008/2009, the proportion of "any walking" was stable in the United States (18.5%) but increased in Germany from 36.5% to 42.3%. The proportion of "any cycling" in the United States remained at 1.8% but increased in Germany from 12.1% to 14.1%. In 2008/2009, the proportion of "30 minutes of walking and cycling" in Germany was 21.2% and 7.8%, respectively, compared to 7.7% and 1.0% in the United States.				
Any walking	18.5%	18.5%	36.5%	42.3%
Any cycling	1.8%	1.8%	12.1%	14.1%
30 minutes of walking a day		7.7%		21.2%
30 minutes of cycling a day		1.0%		7.8%

Data from Buehler, R., Pucher, J., Merom, D., & Bauman, A. (2011). Active travel in Germany and the U.S.: Contributions of daily walking and cycling to physical activity. *American Journal of Preventive Medicine, 41,* 241–250.

People who engage in active travel also have a lower mortality rate. In other words, it appears that people who engage in active travel live longer than those who either drive or take other sedentary forms of travel. For example, Andersen, Schnohr, Schroll, and Hein (2000) observed that cycling to work decreased mortality rates by 40% among Danish men and women. Similarly, a multifaceted cycling demonstration project in Odense, Denmark, reported a 20% increase in cycling levels from 1996 to 2002 and a 5-month increase in life expectancy for men (Pucher et al., 2010). In fact, some evidence suggests that active travel may even have a positive effect on diabetes prevention (Saunders, Green, Petticrew, Steinbach, & Roberts, 2013).

While much research has been conducted on children and working-age adults and active transport, there is also good evidence for the role the built environment plays in promoting this form of physical activity for older adults. Cerin et al. (2017) conducted a review of 42 studies on active transportation and older adults (aged ≥ 65 years). They found considerable evidence of positive associations with total walking for transport and residential density/urbanisation, walkability, street connectivity, overall access to destinations/services, land use mix, pedestrian-friendly features. They also showed that littering, vandalism, and decay were negatively related to total walking for transport.

Case Study: Undergraduate Student Active Transport

College life involves many potential opportunities for being physically active through active transport, including travel to and from campus as well as between buildings as one moves from class to class. Based on this premise, Wilson and colleagues (2020) explored the contribution of active transport to physical activity among college students by surveying a sample of 3,714 students enrolled in general health and wellness courses at a large university in the northeast of the United States. The results showed that active transport physical activity influenced a significant proportion of the volume of physical activity that contributed to meeting public health guidelines (of 150 min of moderate or vigorous intensity physical activity per week). Women, in particular, were more likely to have their active transportation contribute to meeting public health guidelines. The findings reinforce the importance of facilitating and promoting active transport for health benefits among college students.

Seasonal Variation

A **season** is a division of the year marked by changes in weather, ecology, and hours of daylight. Very hot and humid temperatures, very cold and dry temperatures, high rainfall, strong winds, and snow may reduce the likelihood of people being physically active. Although the meteorological factors associated with the seasons cannot be changed, our ability to identify specific seasons that are associated with low physical activity behavior and high sedentary behavior is important for promotion efforts.

When researchers design studies that focus on physical activity, they typically take great care to assess physical activity at a consistent time of the year across study groups. For example, if an intervention study that targeted increased physical activity completed the baseline measure in the middle of a cold winter and then completed the post assessment in the temperate weather of the spring, chances are that the group would show increased physical activity. This practice highlights the recognition in the scientific community that physical activity varies based upon seasonal changes.

Research reveals a relationship between weather and physical activity that is associated with seasonal changes in temperature. For example, in Australia, where the climate is temperate, only swimming varies with the seasons, while every other form of physical activity remains unchanged (Stephens & Caspersen, 1994). In contrast, data collected from Canada and Scotland show wide variations in physical activity across the seasons. For example, walking and cycling are highest in the months of June, July, and August and lowest during November, December, January, and February in these two countries (Stephens & Caspersen, 1994).

Carly Rich and her colleagues (Rich, Griffiths, & Dezateux, 2012) reviewed 16 studies examining seasonal variation in sedentary behavior and physical activity in children aged 2 to 18 years. They only included studies that used accelerometer-determined sedentary behavior and physical activity. Accelerometers are considered the gold standard method to assess physical activity in young populations because self-report or parent proxy reports may overestimate physical activity levels of children. The researchers found seasonal variation in physical activity, particularly for children living in the United Kingdom. Not surprisingly, physical activity levels were highest in the summer and lowest in the winter. The study findings were inconclusive for sedentary behavior, possibly due to the low number of studies examining this relationship. A more recent review and meta-analysis by Zheng and colleagues (2021) of 26 studies showed that higher temperatures were again associated with more moderate-to-vigorous physical activity, while lower temperature and heavily rainfall was associated with longer sedentary behavior time. Increasing opportunities for physical activity during poor weather, in particular during winter, may mitigate declines in physical activity.

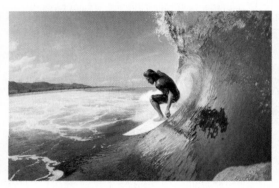

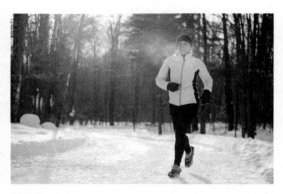

A study conducted by Anna Goodman and her colleagues (2014) found that hours of daylight is related to physical activity in children. They examined data of 23,188 children ages 5 to 16 years old from nine different countries. Of this large dataset, 439 of these children were further examined because they contributed data both immediately before and after the clocks changed (i.e., daylight saving time). Typically, users of daylight-saving time adjust clocks forward 1 hour near the start of spring and then adjust them backward 1 hour in the fall. Although the total number of daylight hours in the day is fixed, putting the clocks forward in the spring shifts daylight hours from the very early morning to the evening.

Goodman and her colleagues (2014) then examined the correlation between the time of sunset and physical activity levels measured by accelerometers. The date of accelerometer data collection was matched to time of sunset and to weather characteristics such as daily precipitation, humidity, wind speed, and temperature. Adjusting for child characteristics (i.e., age and gender) and weather covariates, they found that longer evening daylight was independently related with a small increase in daily physical activity. In other words, a later hour of sunset (i.e., extended evening daylight) was associated with increased daily activity across the full range of time of sunset, and this association was only partly attenuated after adjusting for the weather covariates.

The researchers concluded that their study findings provide evidence that evening daylight plays a causal role in increasing physical activity in the late afternoon and early evening—a time that is important for children's outdoor physical activity. In fact, the researchers calculated that if this proposal would be in effect, British children would have 200 extra waking daylight hours per year. In turn, this would increase the average time children could engage in moderate to vigorous physical activity from 33 to 35 minutes daily. In short, introducing additional daylight hours may positively increase children's evening outdoor play.

There has also been an increase in research on the impact that climate change across the planet may have on physical activity. For example, Obradovich and Fowler (2017) used data on reported participation in recreational physical activity from nearly 2 million US adults, coupled with daily meteorological data. The results showed that both cold and hot temperatures, as well as precipitation days, reduce physical activity, as noted in prior research. The researchers then used 21 climate models to project the possible physical activity effects of future climatic changes by 2050 and 2099. Their results indicated that physical activity may increase most during the winter in northern states and decline during the summer in southern states. Relatedly, Bernard et al. (2021) conducted a narrative synthesis of 74 research papers on physical activity and air pollution, extreme weather conditions, greenhouse gas emissions, and natural disasters. Results indicated a consistent negative effect of air pollution, extreme temperatures and natural disasters on physical activity participation, particularly for adults with chronic diseases, higher body mass index, and the elderly. Climate change is likely to impact physical activity on a worldwide scale.

CRITICAL THINKING ACTIVITY 4-5

Do you think that **daylight saving time** affects your physical activity level?

While considerable research on weather has been explored with children and youth, those rainy days can also affect adults and sometimes prompt us in choosing to curl-up with a movie or a good book instead of a long evening walk. Not surprisingly, the effect of seasonal variations also affects older adults. For example, Aspvik and colleagues (2018) showed that older adults had a higher physical activity level in warmer than in colder months, and this was particularly dependent on the participant's fitness level, environmental precipitation, and gender. In warmer months, increasing precipitation negatively influenced physical activity in both unfit females and males. In colder months, increasing precipitation positively influenced physical activity for physically fit males, but not for females and unfit males. Finally, there is also evidence that owning a dog can affect seasonal variations in outdoor physical activity. Wharf-Higgins and colleagues (2011), in an observational study of park use across multiple seasons in Western Canada, showed that moderate and vigorous physical activity was prevalent in parks during warmer weather among non-dog owners, while dog walking was consistent in parks year-round and regardless of the weather condition. Clearly, the dog needs a walk, rain or shine!

Point-of-Choice Environmental Prompts

Stair climbing is an activity that can easily be integrated into everyday life and has positive health effects. Point-of-choice prompts (or point-of-decision prompts) are informational or motivational signs and messages near stairs and elevators/escalators aimed at increased stair climbing. Kelly Brownell and his colleagues (Brownell, Stunkard, & Albaum, 1980; Study 1) provided the seminal study on the potential impact of one's physical environment on physical activity levels. Their paper outlined the impact of a simple environmental manipulation intended to increase stair use at a shopping mall, a train station, and a bus terminal. In each setting, the stairs and escalator were side by side. Prior to the intervention, the research team documented the naturally occurring activity patterns of individuals confronted with the option of using a set of stairs or an escalator. To ensure that the recorded use rates were reliable, each site was visited on two occasions and stair use was monitored at peak times (i.e., 11 a.m. to 1 p.m. at the mall, 7:30 a.m. to 9:30 a.m. at the train station, and 3:30 p.m. to 5:30 p.m. at the bus terminal). In the initial observations, only about 5% of the people used the stairs.

The environmental manipulation introduced was a simple sign placed at the stairs/escalator choice point. The sign—which was 3 × 3 ½ feet in size—depicted a lethargic heavy heart riding up the escalator and a healthy slim heart climbing the stairs (see **Figure 4-7**). Over 45,600 observations were made during the baseline and intervention phases of the study. Following the intervention, the percentage of people using the stairs increased to about 16% (Brownell et al., 1980). These results not only demonstrate the usefulness of this paradigm, but also suggest the strength of simple, inexpensive public health interventions to increase people's physical activity.

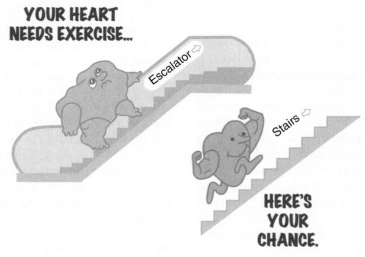

Figure 4-7 The Point-of-Choice Prompt to Encourage Stair Use.

Brownell, K. D., Stunkard, A. J., & Albaum, J. M. (1980). Evaluation and modification of exercise patterns in the natural environment. *American Journal of Psychiatry, 137,* 1540–1545.

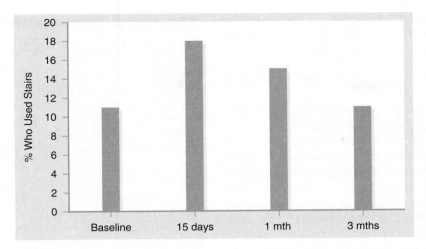

Figure 4-8 Percentage of People Who Used the Stairs During the Intervention and Follow-up.

Data from Brownell, K. D., Stunkard, A. J., & Albaum, J. M. (1980). Evaluation and modification of exercise patterns in the natural environment. *American Journal of Psychiatry, 137,* 1540–1545.

Interestingly, Brownell and his colleagues found that the impact of the intervention was different for Caucasians and African Americans. Although there were no baseline differences between the groups, African Americans were less likely to use the stairs following the intervention. Furthermore, although men and women differed in their stair use at baseline (7% and 5%, respectively), both increased at the same rate following the intervention (15% and 13%, respectively). Perhaps the most important finding of the study was that the percentage of individuals with obesity who used the stairs (1.5%) quadrupled (6.7%) during the intervention phase (Brownell et al., 1980).

In a second study, Brownell and his associates (1980; Study 2) examined the lasting impact of their environmental intervention on stair use. To do so, they collected baseline data for a week to determine the typical frequency of stair use at a commuter train station. This time the sign was placed by the set of stairs and escalator for 2 weeks. Average stair use increased from 11% to over 18% during the 2-week intervention period. The sign was then removed and follow-up assessments were conducted to examine how long the change would last. After 1 month without the sign, people's stair use had decreased to about 15%; after 3 months,

people's stair use had returned to baseline levels (see **Figure 4-8**).

A study conducted in Scotland used a similar point-of-choice design. Using a subway in Glasgow, the researchers placed a sign that read "Stay healthy, save time, use the stairs" in close proximity to a set of stairs that was adjacent to an escalator (Blamey, Mutrie, & Aitchison, 1995). Just as in the Brownell studies, stair use increased when the prompt was present. In fact, stair use nearly doubled for men (from 12% to 22%) and almost tripled for women (from 5% to 14%). This study design has been replicated in several other areas (e.g., shopping malls) and countries (Boen, Maurissen, & Opdenacker, 2010).

Systematic reviews of multiple studies on the effectiveness of point-of-choice prompts and similar choice architecture have now generally shown the same results as these early findings (Bellicha et al., 2015; Landais et al., 2020; Nocon et al., 2010). For example, Landais and colleagues (2020) reviewed 88 studies where prompts were included at a point of decision to engage in physical activity or sedentary behavior in the workplace or community. Of these 88 studies, 68% reported an effect of choice prompts on behavior. In an interesting study design, Rhian Evans and his colleagues (2012) experimentally examined if point-of-choice prompts could reduce sitting time at work. They examined if point-of-choice prompting software placed on people's computer was able to reduce long uninterrupted sedentary periods and total sedentary time at work. People were randomized to either an education group (n = 14) or a point-of-choice prompting group (n = 14). The education group received a brief education session on the importance of reducing long sitting periods at work; the point-of-choice group received the same education along with prompting software on their personal computers that reminded them to stand up every 30 minutes. Sitting time was then measured objectively using an activity monitor for 5 workdays at baseline and 5 workdays during the intervention. The number and time spent sitting in events longer than 30 minutes in duration were the main outcome measures.

At baseline, the participants spent almost 6 hours (76%) of their time at work sitting. Of that time, 3.3 hours a day was spent sitting in 3.7 events that lasted longer than 30 minutes. During the intervention, compared with baseline, the point-of-choice prompt group reduced the number and duration of sitting events that were greater than 30 minutes. However, there was no significant difference in total sitting time between groups. The researchers concluded that point-of-choice prompting software on work computers recommending taking a break from sitting plus education is superior to education alone in reducing long, uninterrupted sedentary periods at work.

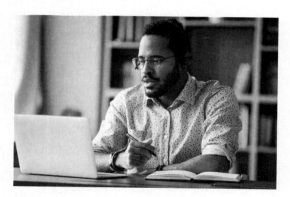

© fizkes/Shutterstock.

Physical Environment Correlates

Despite the continued efforts of health professionals and agencies to encourage people to participate in physical activity, many people are not active enough to achieve optimal health benefits. To develop effective health policies and interventions aimed at increasing people's physical activity levels and reducing their sedentary behaviors, the main correlates and determinants of these behaviors need to be understood. While individual characteristics (e.g., age, gender, and ethnicity) and social characteristics (e.g., parents, peers, teammates) are important correlates of our physical activity and sedentary behavior, so, too, are aspects of the physical environment.

Several reviews have been undertaken in an attempt to examine the physical environmental correlates of physical activity and to a lesser extent, sedentary behavior (e.g., Barnett et al., 2017; Biddle, Petrolini, & Pearson, 2014; Carlin et al., 2017; Kärmeniemi et al., 2018; Kaushal & Rhodes, 2014; Laxer & Janssen, 2013; McGrath et al, 2015; van Loon, Frank, Nettlefold, & Naylor, 2014). A major criticism of this research is the reliance on self-reported and non-validated assessments of both physical activity and sedentary behavior and the physical environment, as well as a focus on cross-sectional designs. Before strong conclusions can be drawn regarding physical environment correlates of physical activity, better quality research is still needed in this emerging area of study.

However, with that being said, the existing research is consistent with associations between our physical environment and both our physical activity and sedentary behaviors, with larger associations typically found for the perceived versus the actual environment and for self-reported versus objective measures. Of importance, the magnitude of the effect tends to be small, yet these associations often include a breadth of environmental variables, such as walkability, residential density, urbanization, street connectivity, access to/availability of destinations and services, infrastructure and streetscape, and safety. See **Table 4-2**

Table 4-2 Summary of Built Environment Correlates of Physical Activity

Correlate	Relationship to Physical Activity
Cul-de-sacs	Positive
Park space	Positive
Neighborhood walkability (e.g., sidewalks)	Positive
Commercial density	Positive
Residential density	Positive
Distance to school	Negative with youth PA
Recreation sites	Negative with youth PA
Low speed limits	Lower speed limits related to greater PA
Land use mix	Positive
Aesthetics (e.g., greenery, cleanliness)	Positive
Personal safety (e.g., graffiti, incivilities)	Positive
Violence	Negative

walking, cycling, and public transportation was associated with increased overall physical activity, although the effects are small and sometimes inconsistent. The findings provide some support for the creation of infrastructure that facilitates physical activity. Research of this kind with a focus on sedentary behavior is still needed before conclusions can be drawn (Stappers et al., 2019).

For people who live in cities, urban sprawl is negatively associated with physical activity and health. **Urban sprawl** (also known as suburban sprawl) represents the expansion of auto-oriented, low-density development. In other words, it is the spreading of urban development, such as houses and shopping centers on undeveloped land near a city. Characteristics of urban sprawl include increased distances between homes and destinations, lower population densities, and disconnected street patterns.

Another physical environmental correlate of physical activity is pollution. Jennifer Roberts and her colleagues (Roberts, Voss, & Knight, 2014) found that increased community level air pollution is associated with reduced exercise, particularly among normal weight individuals. Not surprisingly, air pollution is often perceived as a barrier to physical activity in urban areas. Researchers from the University of Copenhagen, however, found that the beneficial effects of physical activity are more important for our health than the negative effects of air pollution, as it relates to the risk of premature mortality; that is, the benefits of activity outweigh the harmful effects of air pollution (Andersen et al., 2015).

for a summary of the built environment correlates of physical activity and sedentary behavior.

Some of the most compelling research for the directionality of the built environment on physical activity and sedentary behavior comes from natural experiments or location changes. Natural experiments involve situations where parks, trails, bike lanes and walkways have been constructed and researchers have been present to monitor behavior before and after these environmental changes. Location change studies offer situations where cohorts of people move to new cities or locations with different environments and researchers assess changes to physical activity and sedentary behavior practices. Kärmeniemi and colleagues (2018) reviewed 21 cohort studies and 30 natural experiments of how these types of environmental changes may impact physical activity. The researchers found that more accessibility and infrastructure for

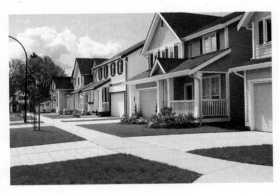

© Hannamariah/Shutterstock.

Despite the adverse effects of air pollution on health, air pollution should be not perceived as a barrier to exercise in urban areas. The researchers concluded that even for those living in the most polluted areas, it is healthier to run, walk, or cycle to work rather than remain inactive.

Perceptions of one's environment compared to the actual environment can be quite different. You may perceive a walking path to be quite safe while your friends may not. Or you may perceive that there are many gyms close to your house while your neighbors may not. In many cases, personal perceptions are a stronger determinant of behavior than the actual environment. However, there are a number of objective environmental criteria that could influence behavior. We know that awareness of positive environmental attributes for physical activity is important. Studies have shown that people who do not perceive their environment as safe or walkable, even when objective

data show otherwise, are less likely to engage in physical activity (Khoosari et al., 2014; Loh et al., 2020). Thus, environmental interventions must make changes to the actual environment and target changes in perceptions of that environment to enable behavior change.

The importance of perceptions of the built environment in behavior demonstrates an interplay between the individual, the environment, and the behavior. Socioecological models posit that behavior is influenced by multiple factors ranging from higher-level policy and built environment to individual motivations, demographic, and biological factors (Stokols, 1996). This has also been the guiding framework for physical activity and sedentary behavior when understanding relationships with the physical environment (Owen et al., 2011; Bornstein & Davis, 2014) (**Figure 4-9**).

In this framework, the influence of the built environment on behavior may be indirect through

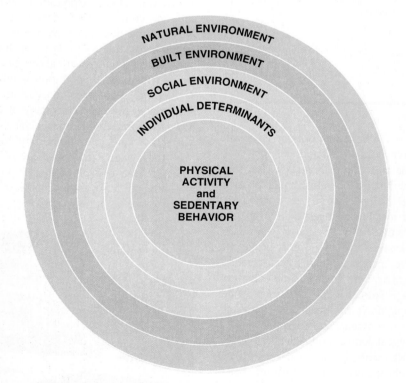

Figure 4-9 Socioecological model and physical activity.

Adapted from Bornstein, D. B. & Davis, W. K. (2014). The Transportation Profession's Role in Improving Public Health, *ITE Journal, 84*, 19–24. https://www.researchgate.net/publication/264347123_The_Transportation_Profession %27s_Role_in_Improving_Public_Health individual-level perceptions or direct and independent of individual perceptions (Spence and Lee, 2003). The framework also suggests there may be interactions across multiple levels of influence on behavior (Emmons, 2000).

These different relationships between the physical environment and individual perceptions were tested in two reviews by Rhodes and colleagues (Rhodes, Saelens, & Sauvage-Mar, 2018; Rhodes, Zhang, & Zhang, 2020). In their review of 46 studies comparing the direct and indirect relationships of the built environment on physical activity, the authors found evidence that environmental infrastructure that was accessible and convenient was related to total physical activity through self-efficacy and perceived control (see Chapter 14). In terms of active travel specifically, environmental infrastructure that was accessible and convenient had an indirect route through individual habits (see chapter 17). They found no evidence that the built environment had a direct association with physical activity after controlling for these individual-level factors. In the review of 22 studies investigating interactions between the built environment and individual perceptions, Rhodes et al. found that access to recreation predicted leisure-time physical activity only when people had positive intentions to engage in physical activity. They also found that people who enjoyed physical activity less were more likely to be active when the built environment was more aesthetically pleasing (e.g., attractive sights). The results highlight the need for coordinated interventions of individual and environmental change. Research on the physical environment, individual perceptions, and sedentary behavior is still needed in order to uncover how these factors are linked.

Home Environment Correlates

It is important to examine if the home environment (also known as the microenvironment) is correlated to exercise and sedentary behavior, especially for young children who have limited independent mobility (Kausal et al., 2014; Maitland, Stratton, Foster, Braham, & Rosenberg,

2013). Considering the substantial amount of time children spend at home, there has been little investigation of how the home physical environment either constrains or supports children's physical activity and sedentary behavior.

Two reviews of the literature examining the home physical environment on children's physical activity and sedentary behavior have shed some light on this important research area (Kausal & Rhodes, 2014; Maitland et al., 2013). The number of televisions in a home is positively correlated with sedentary behaviors. Interventions that change the home environment by introducing television-limiting devices are effective in reducing sedentary behavior in children. These interventions include such things as television-locking devices, curriculums on media awareness to reduce television watching, setting media use goals, and television-monitoring devices.

In general, home physical activity equipment is unrelated to physical activity behavior, and an inverse relationship exists between physical activity equipment and sedentary behavior. The size of the exercise equipment, however, appears to matter, because large exercise equipment, such

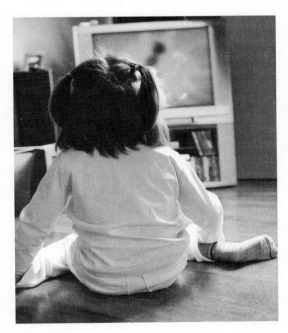

© Pressmaster/Shutterstock.

Table 4-3 Summary of the Home Environment Correlates of Physical Activity

Correlate	Relationship
Media equipment in the home	Positively associated with children's sedentary behavior Inconsistent results for physical activity
Media equipment in the child's bedroom	Positively associated with children's sedentary behavior
Yard space	Positively associated with physical activity
Physical activity equipment	Small positive association with physical activity Inverse relationship with sedentary behavior

as treadmills and prominent exergaming materials (e.g., exergaming bike, dance mats), are more effective than smaller, **peripheral** devices for increasing physical activity levels. A peripheral is a device that is connected, but it is not an integral part of an activity. It expands capabilities, but it does not form part of the core activity environment architecture.

Socioeconomic status moderates the effects of the home environment on physical activity. For example, children from lower-income households have greater media access in their bedrooms and have more daily screen time compared to children from higher-income households. As well, children from lower-income households have less access to portable play equipment (e.g., bikes, jump ropes) compared to higher-income children (Tandon et al., 2012). **Table 4-3** summarizes the home environment correlates of physical activity.

Summary

George Orwell (1949) described the fictional world of Big Brother where behavior was simply a reaction to environmental cues and stimulants.

More scientifically, Walter Mischel and his associates (1989) showed that one's environment has the potential to be related to behavioral outcomes. It was concluded that when an environment is supportive, both individuals with and without appropriate coping skills could be successful.

To examine the generalizability of Mischel's findings, this chapter examined the relationship between the physical environment and physical activity and sedentary behavior.

As common sense might predict, weather changes are related to either increased or decreased physical activity. Brownell and associates' (1980) seminal study on the impact of a simple sign to promote the use of stairs rather than escalators provides good support for point-of-choice (i.e., stairs or escalator) environmental influences on physical activity. However, the translation of those findings to more distal physical activity participation within a fitness facility is mixed. Due to the relative infancy of the field, a clear consensus on how best to change environments to promote activity is ongoing. Some research suggests that the relationship may be influenced by factors such as age, cognitions, and habit.

Vignette: Clayton

I played sports in high school and lifted weights in college. But when I graduated from business school, I went into finance, got married, and quickly became a dad, so my involvement in physical activity all but vanished. I jokingly competed with two work buddies over whose waistband was expanding the fastest.

A few of my colleagues would get up at unreasonably early hours to hit the gym. But most of the fellow junior analysts I worked with came down on the side of preferring a bit more sleep before work hours—not to mention drinks and dinners whenever the bulk of us clocked out.

My health wasn't the only thing I was not paying attention to. I was pretty absentminded when it came to my home life. My wife wasn't happy with my long hours at work. Nor did she approve of my drinking habits. I loved my kids, but I could tell they felt I wasn't there for them as strongly as she was. I kept arguing that I should get cut a bit more slack since I was bringing home most of our income. But I see now that my reasoning was not just selfish but misguided.

She filed for divorce shortly after our youngest son's third birthday. The stress of dealing with lawyers, the tumult and adjustment of moving into my own studio apartment in midtown Manhattan, and the radical shift in my mood resulted in my putting on even more weight and using more alcohol.

It was only when my habits started affecting my work that I considered making some health-related changes. I was told during an annual physical that I had high blood pressure, high cholesterol, and at risk of an imminent heart attack if I didn't alter my habits as soon as possible. When my boss pulled me aside and said he was worried about how my unraveling was impacting the morale of our company, the reality of all I was doing to myself truly hit.

I took 10 days off work, per my boss's recommendation. I booked appointments with a nutritionist and trainer who had each been recommended by one of my college friends. I held out on the mental health component for some time because I was, to be honest, ashamed of needing emotional help of any kind—or admitting I had issues that couldn't be solved with the perfect algorithm on a spreadsheet. But once I returned to work I tentatively started seeing a psychiatrist, who specialized not only in prescribing the right drugs but also in counseling.

I'd say the transition away from whole boxes of pizza, chugged six packs of beer, and the insidious comfort of my couch and television was quite possibly one of the hardest behavioral adjustments I ever made. I'd put it on par with the actual divorce itself. So ensconced had I become in my own self-destructive routine that I wasn't even aware of how insurmountable it would be to wriggle out of it until I actually tried.

My wife and kids ended up coming over one weekend to help me get my place into shape. She and I were on talking terms and, though there would always be some level of tension and resentment between us, she did care enough about me to ensure I wouldn't fall through any cracks. Together, we single-handedly discarded all junk food in the apartment as well as all beer, liquor, and wine (despite my pleading with her to not throw out the top-shelf stuff). Seeing an obvious look of worry in my kids' young faces made me keep at it. It wasn't about doing this just for myself, it was about doing this, also, for my family.

As part of my plan with my personal trainer, I started walking to and from work. I used to take cabs, even though my new apartment was only about 15 blocks from the office. Another change: taking the stairs. I've been at it for about 2 months now and I can make it up about 12 flights before I have to take the elevator the rest of the way up to the 35th floor where my office is. (When I started I could barely do one flight.) My goal by the end of the year is to be able to make it the whole way.

I consider myself lucky to live in such a walkable environment as New York City. It's not as hard as I thought to squeeze more activity into my day. And with access to my company's gym, I can—if time permits—lift weights during those rare extended breaks from work.

A big shift in how much I work out is keeping a pair of sneakers and having several days' worth of gym clothes at my office. If I had to go home to change I'd honestly stay parked on the couch watching television.

What's been the best outcome of my new effort to be healthy is the quality time I now spend with my boys. My coworkers also have kids and they don't give me slack for leaving work early every other Friday to take the boys out for dinner. And while I have yet to spend a Saturday or Sunday without my Blackberry attached to my

hip, I'm able to at least run around Central Park with them as they learn to bike ride.

I'm hoping the fact that I can keep up with them might work in my favor as I soon try to get back into the dating world.

Key Terms

active travel An approach to travel that focuses on physical activities, such as walking and cycling, as opposed to car travel, to get to work, school, and other destinations.

built environment The part of the physical environment that includes the human-made surroundings that provide the setting for human activity.

daylight saving time Adjustment of the time to achieve longer evening daylight, especially in summer, by setting the clocks an hour ahead of the standard time.

delayed gratification The ability to reject immediately available smaller rewards in favor of later larger rewards.

green space An area of grass, trees, or other vegetation set apart for recreational or aesthetic purposes in an otherwise urban environment.

land use mix The diversity or variety of land uses, such as residential, commercial, industrial, and agricultural.

modernization The transformation of a society from rural and agrarian to an urban and industrial one.

Old Order Amish Religious community that emphasizes humility, nonviolence, and traditional values rather than advancement and technology.

peripheral A device that is connected to a host architecture but is not an integral part.

physical environment The part of the environment that includes all of a person's indoor and outdoor surroundings, both those that have been designed (e.g., neighborhoods and parks) and those that occur naturally (e.g., oceans and mountains).

point-of-choice prompt Informational or motivational signs near where alternative behavioral options are available and where decisions to act are likely.

polar climate Climate characterized by a lack of warm summers. Every month a polar climate has an average temperature of less than 10°C (50°F).

season A division of the year marked by changes in weather, ecology, and hours of daylight.

street connectivity How often streets or roadways intersect.

urban sprawl The expansion of auto-oriented, low-density development outside of city centers. Also known as suburban sprawl.

Review Questions

1. What is the physical environment? What is the built environment? Provide examples of each.

2. Define *delayed gratification*. How is delayed gratification related to participation in physical activity?

3. Define *modernization*. Compare and contrast the Inuit and the Old Order Amish to highlight the effects of modernization (or resistance to modernization) on health and physical activity.

4. Define *active travel*. How is travel related to our physical activity behaviors?

5. How does climate affect our physical activity levels?

6. What are point-of-choice prompts and how do they affect people's behavior with regard to physical activity?

7. Describe some physical environment correlates of physical activity behavior.

Applying the Concepts

1. How did the built environment in which Clayton lived and worked influence his exercise behavior?
2. What changes did Clayton make to his environment (and the way he interacted

with it) to increase the likelihood that he would engage in healthy behaviors, such as exercise and dietary changes?

References

Active Healthy Kids Canada. (2013). Are we driving our kids to unhealthy habits? Retrieved from http://dvqdas9jty7g6 .cloudfront.net/reportcard2013/AHKC-Summary-2013 .pdf

Adams, M. A., Johnson, W. D., & Tudor-Locke, C. (2013). Steps/day translation of the moderate-to-vigorous physical activity guideline for children and adolescents. *International Journal of Behavioral Nutrition and Physical Activity, 10*(49). https://doi.org/10.1186/1479-5868-10-49

Andersen, L. B., Schnohr, P., Schroll, M., & Hein, H. O. (2000). All-cause mortality associated with physical activity during leisure time, work, sports, and cycling to work. *Archives of Internal Medicine, 160*(11), 1621–1628.

Aranda-Balboa, M. J., Huertas-Delgado, F. J., Herrador-Colmenero, M., Cardon, G., & Chillo, P. (2020). Parental barriers to active transport to school: a systematic review. *International Journal of Public Health, 65*(1), 87–98.

Aspvik, N. P., Viken, H., Ingebrigtsen, J. E., Zisko, N., Mehus, I., & Wisløff, U. (2018). Do weather changes influence physical activity level among older adults? – The Generation 100 study. The *Public Library of Science One, 13*(70), e0199463.

Ayduk, O., Mendoza-Denton, R., Mischel, W., Downey, G., Peake, P. K., & Rodriguez M. (2000). Regulating the interpersonal self: Strategic self-regulation for coping with rejection sensitivity. *Journal of Personality and Social Psychology, 79*(5), 776–792.

Barnett, D. W., Barnett, A., Nathan, A., Van Cauwenberg, J., & Cerin, E. (2017). Built environmental correlates of older adults' total physical activity and walking: A systematic review and meta-analysis. *International Journal of Behavioral Nutrition and Physical Activity, 14*(1), 103.

Bassett, D. R. Jr., Pucher, J., Buehler, R., Thompson, D. L., & Crouter, S. E. (2008). Walking, cycling, and obesity rates in Europe, North America, and Australia. *Journal of Physical Activity and Health, 5*(6), 795–814.

Bassett, D. R. Jr., Schneider, P. L., & Huntington, G. E. (2004). Physical activity in an Old Order Amish community. *Medicine and Science in Sports & Exercise, 36*(1), 79–85.

Bassett, D. R. Jr., Tremblay, M. S., Esliger, D. W., Copeland, J. L., Barnes, J. D., & Huntington, G. E. (2007). Physical activity and body mass index of children in an Old Order Amish community. *Medicine and Science in Sports and Exercise, 39*(3), 410–415.

Bassett, D. R., Wyatt, H. R., Thompson, H., Peters, J. C., & Hill, J. O. (2010). Pedometer-measured physical activity and health behaviors in U.S. adults. *Medicine and Science in Sport and Exercise, 42*(10), 1819–1825.

Bellicha, A., Kieusseian, A., Fontvieille, A. M., Tataranni, A., Charreire, H., & Oppert, J. M. (2015). Stair-use interventions in worksites and public settings—A systematic review of effectiveness and external validity. *Preventive Medicine, 70*, 3–13.

Bernard, P., Chevance, G., Kingsbury, C., Baillot, A., Romain, A. J., Molinier, V., & Dancause, K. N. (2021). Climate change, physical activity and sport: A systematic review. *Sports Medicine, 51*(5), 1041–1059.

Biddle, S. J., Petrolini, I., & Pearson, N. (2014). Interventions designed to reduce sedentary behaviours in young people: A review of reviews. *British Journal of Sports Medicine, 48*(3), 182–186.

Blamey, A., Mutrie, N., & Aitchison, T. (1995). Health promotion by encouraged use of stairs. *The British Medical Journal, 311*(7000), 289–290.

Boen, F., Maurissen, K., & Opdenacker, J. (2010). A simple health sign increases stair use in a shopping mall and two train stations in Flanders, Belgium. *Health Promotion International, 25*(2), 183–191.

Bornstein, D. B. & Davis, W. K. (2014). The Transportation Profession's Role in Improving Public Health, *ITE Journal, 84*, 19–24. https://www.researchgate.net/publication /264347123_The_Transportation_Profession%27s_Role _in_Improving_Public_Health

Brownell, K. D., Stunkard, A. J., & Albaum, J. M. (1980). Evaluation and modification of exercise patterns in the natural environment. *The American Journal of Psychiatry, 137*(12), 1540–1545.

Buehler, R., Pucher, J., Merom, D., & Bauman, A. (2011). Active travel in Germany and the U.S.: Contributions of daily walking and cycling to physical activity. *American Journal of Preventive Medicine, 41*(3), 241–250.

Carlin, A., Perchoux, C., Puggina, A., Aleksovska, K., Buck, C., Burns, C., Cardon, G., Chantal, S., Ciarapica, D., Condello, G., Coppinger, T., Cortis, C., D'Haese, S., De Craemer, M., Di Blasio, A., Hansen, S., Iacoviello, L., Issartel, J., Izzicupo, P., Jaeschke, L., Kanning, M., Kennedy, A., Lakerveld, J., Ling, F. C. M., Luzak, A., Napolitano, G., Nazare, J. A., Pischon, T., Polito, A., Sannella, A., Schulz, H., Sohun, R., Steinbrecher, A.,

Schlicht, W., Ricciardi, W., MacDonncha, C., Capranica, L., & Boccia, S. (2017). A life course examination of the physical environmental determinants of physical activity behaviour: A "Determinants of Diet and Physical Activity" (DEDIPAC) umbrella systematic literature review. *The Public Library of Science One, 12*(8), e0182083.

Cerin, E., Nathan, A., van Cauwenberg, J., Barnett, D. W., & Barnett, A. (2017). The neighbourhood physical environment and active travel in older adults: A systematic review and meta-analysis. *International Journal of Behavioral Nurtrition and Physical Activity, 14*(1), 1–23.

Datar, A., Nicosia, N., & Shier, V. (2013). Parent perceptions of neighborhood safety and children's physical activity, sedentary behavior, and obesity: Evidence from a national longitudinal study. *American Journal of Epidemiology, 177*(10), 1065–1073.

D'Haese, S., Vanwolleghem, G., Hinckson, E., De Bourdeaudhuij, I., Deforche, B., Van Dyck, D., & Cardon, G. (2015). Cross-continental comparison of the association between the physical environment and active transportation in children: A systematic review. *International Journal of Behavioral Nurtrition and Physical Activity, 12*(1), 1–14.

Drobetz, R., Maercker, A., & Forstmeier, S. (2012). Delay of gratification in old age: Assessment, age-related effects, and clinical implications. *Aging Clinical and Experimental Research, 24*(1), 6–14.

Dzewaltowski, D. A., Johnston, J. A., Estabrooks, P. A., & Johannes, E. (2000, October). *Health Places.* Paper presented at the Governors Conference on the Prevention of Child Abuse and Neglect. Topeka, KS.

Emmons, K. Health behaviors in a social context. In: Berkman L, Kawachi I, editors. *Social Epidemiology, 137.* Oxford: Oxford University Press; 2000. p. 242–66.

Eslinger, D. W., Tremblay, M. S., Copeland, J. L., Barnes, J. D., Huntington, G. E., & Bassett, D. R. Jr. (2010). Physical activity profile of Old Order Amish, Mennonite, and contemporary children. *Medicine and Science in Sports and Exercise, 42,* 296–303.

Evans, R. E., Fawole, H. O., Sheriff, S. A., Dall, P. M., Grant, P. M., & Ryan, C. G. (2012). Point-of-choice prompts to reduce sitting time at work: A randomized trial. *American Journal of Preventive Medicine, 43*(3), 293–297.

Eyler, A. A., Baker, E., Cromer, L., King, A. C., Brownson, R. C., & Donatelle, R. J. (1998). Physical activity and minority women: A qualitative study. *Health Education & Behavior, 25*(5), 640–652.

Goodman, A., Page, A. S., Cooper, A. R., & International Children's Accelerometry Database (ICAD) Collaborators. (2014). Daylight saving time as a potential public health intervention: An observational study of evening daylight and objectively measured physical activity among 23,000 children from 9 countries. *International Journal of Behavioral Nutritional and Physical Activity, 11*(1), 1–9. https://doi.org/10.1186/1479-5868-11-84

Karmeniemi, M., Lankila, T., Ikaheimo, T., Koivumaa-Honkanen, H., & Korpelainen, R. (2018). The built environment as a determinant of physical activity: A systematic review of longitudinal studies and natural experiments. *Annals of Behavioral Medicine, 52*(3), 239–251.

Kaushal, N., & Rhodes, R. E. (2014). The home physical environment and its impact of physical activity and sedentary behavior: A systematic review. *Preventive Medicine, 67,* 221–237.

Kottyan, G., Kottyan, L., Edwards, N. M., & Unaka, N. I. (2014). Assessment of active play, inactivity, and perceived barriers in an inner city neighborhood. *Journal of Community Health, 39*(3), 538–544.

Landais, L. L., Damman, O. C., Schoonmade, L. J., Timmermans, D. R. M., Verhagen, E. A. L. M., & Jelsma, J. G. M. (2020). Choice architecture interventions to change physical activity and sedentary behavior: A systematic review of effects on intention, behavior and health outcomes during and after intervention. *International Journal of Behavioral Nutrition and Physical Activity, 17*(1), 1–37.

Laxer, R. E., & Janssen, I. (2013). The proportion of youths' physical inactivity attributable to neighbourhood built environment features. *International Journal of Health Geographics,* Jun 18;*12*(1), 1–13: https://doi.org/10.1186/1476-072X-12-31

Maitland, C., Stratton, G., Foster, S., Braham, R., & Rosenberg, M. (2013). A place for play? The influence of the home physical environment on children's physical activity and sedentary behaviour. *International Journal of Behavioral Nutrition and Physical Activity, 10*(1), 1–21. https://doi.org/10.1186/1479-5868-10-99

McDonald, N. C., Brown, A. L., Marchetti, L. M., & Pedroso, M. S. (2011). U.S. school travel, 2009: An assessment of trends. *American Journal of Preventive Medicine, 41*(2), 146–151.

McGrath, L. J., Hopkins, W. G., & Hinckson, E. A. (2015). Associations of objectively measured built-environment attributes with youth moderate–vigorous physical activity: A systematic review and meta-analysis. *Sports Medicine, 45*(6), 841–865.

Mischel, W., Shoda, Y., & Rodriguez, M. L. (1989). Delay of gratification in children. *Science, 244*(4907), 933–938.

Moffitt, T. E., Arseneault, l., Belsky, D., Dickson, N., Hancox, R. J., Harrington, H., Houts, R., Poulton, R., Roberts, B. W., Ross, S., Sears, M. R., Murray Thomson, W., & Caspi, A. (2011). A gradient of childhood self-control predicts health, wealth, and public safety. *Proceedings of the National Academy of Sciences of the United States of America, 108*(7), 2693–2698.

Obradovich, N., & Fowler, J. H. (2017). Climate change may alter human physical activity patterns. *Nature Human Behaviour, 1*(5), 1–7.

Orwell, G. (1949). *1984.* San Diego, CA: Harcourt, Brace, Jovanovich.

Ostergaard, L., Kolle, E., Steene-Johannessen, J., Anderssen, S. A., & Andersen, L. B. (2013). Cross- sectional analysis of the association between mode of school transportation and physical fitness in children and adolescents. *International Journal of Behavioral Nutrition and Physical Activity, 10*(19). https://doi.org/10.1186/1479-5868-10-91

Owen, N., Sugiyama, T., Eakin, E. E., Gardiner, P. A., Tremblay, M. S., & Sallis, J. F. (2011). Adults' sedentary behavior-determinants and interventions. *American Journal of Preventive Medicine, 41*(2), 189–196.

Pizarro, A. N., Ribeiro, J. C., Marques, E. A., Mota, J., & Santos, M. P. (2013). Is walking to school associated with improved metabolic health? *International Journal of Behavioral Nutrition and Physical Activity, 10*(1). https://doi.org/10.1186/1479-5868-10-12

Pucher, J., Buehler, R., Bassett, D. R., & Dannenbert, A. L. (2010). Walking and cycling to health: A comparative analysis of city, state, and international data. *American Journal of Public Health, 100*(10), 1986–1992.

Rhodes, R. E., & Nasuti, G. (2011). Trends and changes in research on the psychology of physical activity across 20 years: A quantitative analysis of 10 journals. *Preventive Medicine, 53*(1-2), 17–23.

Rhodes, R. E., Perdew, M., & Malli, S. (2020). Correlates of parental support of child and youth physical activity: A systematic review. *International Journal of Behavioral Medicine, 27*(6), 636–646.

Rhodes, R. E., Saelens, B. E., & Sauvage-Mar, C. (2018). Understanding physical activity through interactions between the built environment and social cognition: A systematic review. *Sports Medicine, 48*(8), 1893–1912.

Rhodes, R. E., Zhang, R., & Zhang, C. Q. (2020). Direct and indirect relationships between the built environment and individual-level perceptions of physical activity: A systematic review. *Annals of Behavioral Medicine, 54*(7), 495–509.

Rich, C., Griffiths, L. J., & Dezateux, C. (2012). Seasonal variation in accelerometer-determined sedentary behaviour and physical activity in children: A review. *International Journal of Behavioral Nutritional and Physical Activity, 9*(49). https://doi.org/10.1186/1479-5868-9-49

Rode, A., & Shephard, R. J. (1993). Acculturation and loss of fitness in the Inuit: The preventive role of active leisure. *Arctic Medical Research, 52*(3), 107–112.

Rode, A., & Shephard, R. J. (1994). Physiological consequences of acculturation: A 20-year study of fitness in an Inuit community. *European Journal of Applied Physiology and Occupational Physiology, 69*(6), 516–524.

Sallis, J. F., Cerin, E., Kerr, J., Adams, M. A., Sugiyama, T., Christiansen, L. B., . . . , & Owen, N. (2020). Built environment, physical activity, and obesity: Findings from the International Physical Activity and Environment Network (IPEN) adult study. *Annual Review of Public Health, 41*, 119–139.

Saunders, L. E., Green, J. M., Petticrew, M. P., Steinbach, R., & Roberts, H. (2013). What are the health benefits of active travel? A systematic review of trials and cohort studies. *PLoS One, 8*(8), e69912.

Schlam, T. R., Wilson, N. L., Shoda, Y., Mischel, W., & Ayduk, O. (2013). Preschoolers' delay of gratification predicts their body mass 30 years later. *The Journal of Pediatrics, 162*(1), 90–93.

Schoeppe, S., Duncan, M. J., Badland, H., Oliver, M., & Curtis, C. (2013). Association of children's independent mobility and active travel with physical activity, sedentary behavior, and weight status: A systematic review. *Journal of Science and Medicine in Sport, 16*(4), 312–319.

Spence, J. C., & Lee, R. E. (2003). Toward a comprehensive model of physical activity. *Psychology of Sport and Exercise, 4*(1), 7–24.

Stappers, N. E. H., Van Kann, D. H. H., Ettema, D., De Vries, N. K., & Kremers, S. P. J. (2018). The effect of infrastructural changes in the built environment on physical activity, active transportation and sedentary behavior—A systematic review. *Health & Place, 53*, 135–149.

Stephens, T., & Caspersen, C. J. (1994). The demography of physical activity. In C. Bouchard & R. J. Shepard (Eds.), *Physical activity, fitness, and health: International proceedings and consensus statement* (pp. 204–213). Champaign, IL: Human Kinetics.

Stokols D.(1996). Translating social ecological theory into guidelines for community health promotion. *American Journal of Health Promotion, 10*(4), 282–298.

Stone, M. R., Faulkner, G. E., Mitra, R., & Buliung, R. N. (2014). The freedom to explore: Examining the influence of independent mobility on weekday, weekend and after-school physical activity behaviour in children living in urban and inner-suburban neighbourhoods of varying socioeconomic status. *International Journal of Behavioral Nutrition and Physical Activity, 11*(1), 1–11.

Su, J. G., Jerrett, M., McConnell, R., Berhane, K., Dunton, G., Shankardass, K., Reynolds, K., Chang, R., & Wolch, J. (2013). Factors influencing whether children walk to school. *Health & Place, 22*, 153–161. https://doi.org/10.1016/j.healthplace.2013.03.011. Epub 2013 Apr 17.

Tandon, P. S., Zhou, C., Sallis, J. F., Cain, K. L., Frank, L. D., & Saelens, B. E. (2012). Home environment relationships with children's physical activity, sedentary time, and screen time by socioeconomic status. *International Journal of Behavioral Nutritional and Physical Activity, 9*(1), 1–9. https://doi.org/10.1186/1479-5868-9-88

Tranter, P., & Whitelegg, J. (1994). Children's travel behaviour in Canberra: Car-dependent lifestyles in a low density city. *Journal of Transport Geography, 2*(4), 265–273.

Tremblay, M. S., Esliger, D. W., Copeland, J. L., Barnes, J. D., & Bassett, D. R. (2008). Moving forward by looking back: Lessons learned from long-lost lifestyles. *Applied Physiology, Nutrition, and Metabolism, 33*(4), 836–842.

Tudor-Locke, C., Craig, C. L., Beets, M. W., Belton, S., Cardon, G. M., Duncan, S., Hatano, Y., Lubans, D. R., Olds, T. S., Raustorp, A., Rowe, D. A., Spence, J. C., Tanaka, S., & Blair, S. N. (2011). How many steps/day are enough? For children and adolescents. *International Journal of Behavioral Nutrition and Physical Activity, 8*(1), 1–14. https://doi.org/10.1186/1479-5868-8-78

Tudor-Locke, C., Craig, C. L., Brown, W. J., Clemes, S. A., De Cocker, K., Giles-Corti, B., Hatano, Y., Inoue, S., Matsudo,

S. M., Mutrie, N., Oppert, J-M., Rowe, D. A., Schmidt, M. D., Schofield, G. M., Spence, J. C., Teixeira, P. J., Tully, M. A., & Blair, S. N. (2011). How many steps/day are enough? For adults. *International Journal of Behavioral Nutritional and Physical Activity, 8*(1), 1–17. https://doi.org/10.1186/1479-5868-8-79

Tudor-Locke, C., Ham, S. A., Macera, C. A., Ainsworth, B. E., Kirkland, K. A., Reis, J. P., & Kimsey, C. D. (2004). Descriptive epidemiology of pedometer-determined physical activity. *Medicine and Science in Sports and Exercise, 36*(9), 1567–1573.

Van Loon, J., Frank, L. D., Nettlefold, L., & Naylor, P. J. (2014). Youth physical activity and the neighbourhood environment: Examining correlates and the role of neighbourhood definition. *Social Science & Medicine, 104*, 107–115.

Wharf Higgins, S. J., Temple, V. A., & Rhodes, R. E. (2011). Unleashing physical activity: An observational study of park use, dog walking and physical activity. *Journal of Physical Activity and Health, 8*(6), 766–774.

Wilson, O. W. A., Elliott, L. D., Duffey, M., Papalia, Z., & Bopp, M. (2020). The contribution of active travel to meeting physical activity recommendations among college students. *Journal of Transport & Health, 18*, 100890.

Zheng, C., Feng, J., Huang, W. Y., & Heung-Sang Wong, S. (2021). Associations between weather conditions and physical activity and sedentary time in children and adolescents: A systematic review and meta-analysis. *Health & Place, 69*, 102546.

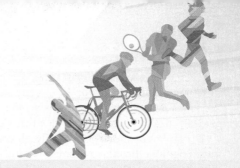

CHAPTER 5

Digital Environment

LEARNING OBJECTIVES

After completing this chapter, you will be able to:

- Describe digital health and digital literacy.
- Identify individual correlates of digital health use pertaining to physical activity.
- Understand the effectiveness of digital health interventions on physical activity.
- Understand the effectiveness of digital health interventions on sedentary behavior.

Introduction

Chapters 3 and 4 highlighted the roles that the social and physical environment play in physical activity and sedentary behavior, and in the 20th century this may have been encompassing of the key environments that represent the background to health behavior psychology. In fact, group interventions, environment promotion campaigns, and individual behavior change counselling represented the main implementation avenues for intervention before 2010 (Rhodes & Nasuti, 2011). However, now firmly in the 21st century, we would be remiss to not include a chapter on the role of the digital environment in explaining and changing physical activity and sedentary behavior.

The need to understand the role of the digital environment in health behaviors like physical activity and sedentary behavior stems from the near ubiquitous role that technology features into our work and leisure. **Digital health** is defined as the general use of information and communication technologies for health (World Health Organization, 2016). Internet and smartphone use has grown exponentially in the last decade to a point where >90% of the population in high income countries and >50% of those in medium income countries have regular access to these technologies (Roser et al., 2019). This high prevalence opens up the possibility for these increasingly prevalent technological tools to improve health behaviors (Widmer et al., 2015). Conversely, the rise in technology-based platforms can also facilitate poor health through increased sedentary behavior; in fact, screen-time is one of the most prevalent forms of sedentary behavior (Tremblay et al., 2017). The COVID-19 pandemic has further accentuated our use of technology, which has both driven a large desire to use digital health for physical activity (Parker et al., 2021; Wilke et al., 2020), yet also fortified our reliance on screen-based sedentary behaviors (Moore et al., 2020; Stockwell et al., 2021).

The depth of application of digital health is vast, encompassing health behavior tracking (e.g., smoking, dietary assessment and monitoring), health behavior interventions (e.g., text messaging, internet interventions, serious games), health outcomes and processes (e.g., CVD risk factor monitoring, daily glucose readings, cognitive health assessments), and patient-care decision making (e.g., zoom-based health care, video counselling). The breadth of digital health is also impressive, ranging from cardiovascular disease (Widmer et al., 2015) and cancer control (Roberts et al., 2017) to family and adolescent behavioral interventions (Rose et al., 2017) or worksite health promotion (Howarth et al., 2018). As one might expect, the change in this scientific literature is also rapid, mimicking the speed of the technological age and making it difficult to keep reviews of various digital health domains timely and relevant. In this chapter, we will overview the demographic correlates of digital health, followed by physical activity and sedentary behavior as it pertains to web-based internet interventions (eHealth), mobile health (**mHealth**) and movement trackers, gaming, and social media.

Use of Digital Health Applications

While technology like smartphones and the internet is almost ubiquitous in contemporary society, it is still critical to understand whether people are using digital health technologies for health-related matters. Contemporary evidence suggests that about one-third of smartphone owners use health-related applications. For example, over 90% of Canadians own smartphones (Statistics Canada, 2020), and spend almost three hours per day using apps (Briggs, 2018). Still, the most popular apps are for games and social networking; approximately 30% of app downloads are health-related (Sydow, 2021). A similar finding was reported recently from an adult population sample in Hong Kong, where 97% reported using mobile devices (Xie et al., 2018). Despite this near majority use of mobile phones, health app use comprised a much smaller subset of the sample. Xie et al. (2018) found that 32% used healthy living apps, 13% used health tracking (e.g., vital signs, measuring health), 11% used their phone for medical reminders, 7% used their phone to seek out health information, and <2% used their phone for telehealth. These findings tell us that many people who have access to digital health are not using it at present.

Correlates of Digital Health Use

Based on this information about the variation in digital health use, it is critical to understand the profiles of those who use digital health compared with those who do not. This information can assist to better target digital health interventions to current users. More importantly, understanding the correlates of digital health use can help identify underserved groups who may need assistance in accessing and applying digital health technologies to improve their health.

Table 5-1 outlines the collation of results of several surveys on the correlates of various aspects of digital health use among adults, using large samples from Australia, the United States, Denmark, and Hong Kong (Boakye et al., 2018; Holt et al., 2019; Nikoloudakis et al., 2018; Xie et al., 2018).

The results of these surveys showed that women clearly use digital health technology more than men, although this is a well-established finding for all health information/services seeking behaviors and thus not specific to digital health (Boakye et al., 2018). Those using digital health were also likely to have a higher income, be White compared to Black (in the U.S.), use social media more, not smoke, and report less sedentary behavior than those not using digital health. There were some mixed findings across these international surveys. For example, more formal education and younger adulthood (compared to other age groups) were associated with digital health use in Australia and the United States, but there was no association between education or age and digital health use in China or

Table 5-1 Correlates of Digital Health Use among Adults

Correlate	Finding
Demographics	
Gender	Women are more likely to use digital health than men
Income	People with higher incomes are more likely to use digital health than those with lower incomes
Education	Mixed Results
Age	Mixed Results
Occupation	No Association
Marital Status	Mixed Results
Geographic Location	No Association
Race	White people are more likely to use digital health than Black people
Health Indicators	
Health Status	No Association
Comorbidities	Mixed Results
Body Mass Index	No Association
Technology-Related Aspects	
Social Media Users	More likely to use digital health than those who do not use social media
Digital Health Literacy	People with more digital health literacy are more likely to use digital health than people with less digital health literacy
Health Behaviors	
Smoking Status	Non-smokers are more likely to use digital health than smokers
Physical Activity	Mixed Results
Healthy Eating	No Association
Drinking Alcohol	No Association
Sedentary Behavior	Those who engage in more sedentary behavior are less likely to use digital health than those who engage in less sedentary behavior

Data from Boakye, E. A., Mohammed, K. A., Geneus, C. J., Tobo, B. B., Wirth, L. S., Yang, L., & Osazuwa-Peters, N. (2018). Correlates of health information seeking between adults diagnosed with and without cancer. *PLoS One*, 13, e0196446; Holt, K. A., Karnoe, A., Overgaard, D., Nielsen, S. E., Kayser, L., Røder, M. E., & From, G. (2019). Differences in the level of electronic health literacy between users and nonusers of digital health services: An exploratory survey of a group of medical outpatients. Interactive *Journal of Medical Research, 8*(2), e8423. Nikoloudakis, I. A., Vandelanotte, C., Rebar, A. L., Schoeppe, S., Alley, S., Duncan, M. J., & Short, C. E. (2018). Examining the correlates of online health information–seeking behavior among men compared with women. *American Journal of Men's Health, 12*, 1358–1367. Xie, Z., Nacioglu, A., & Or, C. (2018). Prevalence, demographic correlates, and perceived impacts of mobile health app use amongst Chinese adults: Cross-sectional survey study. *JMIR: mHealth and uHealth, 6*, e103.

Europe. The results underscore that there may be some cultural differences in digital health use. Interestingly, there are also several demographic variables that seem unrelated to digital health use, including occupation, health status and body mass index, healthy eating, or drinking alcohol. Whether physical activity is related to general digital health use is unclear at present, with a large survey of Australian adults showing no relationship (Nikoloudakis et al., 2018), yet a population sample of adults in the United States shows that digital health use favors those who are physically active (Boakye et al., 2018).

Digital Health Literacy and Technology Use

Many of the correlates noted in Table 5-1 are relatively unchangeable in terms of health behaviors and conditions that represent the intended outcomes of digital health interventions. By contrast, one construct with growing recognition as an antecedent of digital health use is **eHealth literacy** (or digital health literacy), which is defined as the users' competence to engage with digital health services (Norman & Skinner, 2006). This construct is a more specified version of health literacy, which is the ability to gain access to, understand, and use information to promote and maintain good health (Nutbeam, 2000).

Many studies have supported the association between eHealth literacy and digital health use (Choi & DiNitto, 2013; Holt et al., 2019; Lepore et al., 2019; Vajaean & Baban, 2015). For example, Lepore and colleagues (2019) examined how eHealth literacy affected the participation of internet-based peer support groups for cancer survivors, which is a scalable digital health approach to addressing their information and support needs. The results showed that cancer survivors with lower eHealth literacy were more likely to report difficulties using the internet support groups, and this resulted in greater distress before and after online chats during the intervention and post-intervention. Holt et al. (2019) showed a similar relationship between

eHealth literacy and use of government online patient health services. In fact, eHealth literacy was the only predictor of use for these patient services even when considering demographic and background health indicators of the participants in the study. The results underscore the potential importance of promoting eHealth literacy to increase digital health use.

User Engagement and Digital Health

Adherence and retention to any health behavior intervention is always critical in order to understand whether the components of the intervention are effective. In face-to-face environments and social groups, attention may be easier to attain than the digital health environment. Digital health interventions are often implemented and followed by the user, at their own pace, and without any social commitment. For example, if you are training in a gym, you may have a workout partner or a coach who will notice if you are absent. This creates a sense of social commitment. If you have downloaded an app or visited a health website for physical activity tips, you are often reliant on yourself for that ongoing commitment to engage with the material.

Recent statistics found that over two-thirds of those in North America who download a behaviour change app only use it once (Byrnes, 2019). Even among those who continue beyond the initial trial, there is a significant lack of persistent engagement. Several studies have found that adherence to such apps dropped under 50% within 1-2 months (Choi et al., 2016; Hassandra et al., 2017; Serrano et al., 2017). Thus, digital health intervention designers are often very concerned with user engagement because it is exceedingly difficult to evaluate whether an intervention to change physical activity or reduce sedentary behavior has utility if people will not even engage with the material to begin with. Engagement in digital health technology is a function of many things, including content, usability, visual design, and overall product quality

(Baumel & Kane, 2018). In the sections below, we review how effective internet interventions, mobile health (mHealth), gaming, and social media have been with maintaining engagement and subsequently changing physical activity and sedentary behavior.

Because user engagement is so important to the success of digital health behavior interventions, frameworks are needed to develop the intervention with a strong focus on the user experience. Use of these types of frameworks are very common in all human-computer interaction design; however, Mummah and colleagues (2016) developed a framework specific for digital interventions to change health behavior. Their framework is called IDEAS (Integrate, Design, Assess, Share). It highlights the critical importance of integrating (I) the insights of target users and the application of behavioral theory (see Chapters 14–17) in designing digital health interventions right from the start of development. Creators of the intervention are then recommended to use iterative design (DE) approaches with target user feedback. This involves building prototypes and working through all of the applications of the digital health intervention with behavioral scientists and target users. After a prototype (or minimal viable product) has been produced, Mummah and colleagues recommend that pilot and feasibility testing (for usability of the product) followed by efficacy testing (for effectiveness in behavior change) be conducted for rigorous assessment (A). Finally, the product findings should be shared (S) with researchers, developers, and industry partners to help advance understanding and continue with its refinement (see **Figure 5-1**).

Internet Interventions

Most of the first digital health interventions designed to change physical activity and reduce sedentary behavior were web browser or email-based approaches. This is because access to the internet has had a high prevalence for over 20 years, resulting in 66% of the world's population and 94% of North America currently having access (Internet usage statistics, 2022). Thus, health behavior interventions delivered over the internet have high reach, flexibility, and low cost. Several reviews have appraised the effectiveness of internet-based interventions for changing physical activity (Beleigoli et al., 2019; Davies et al., 2012; Hou et al., 2014; Jahangiry et al., 2017; Joseph et al., 2014; Rose et al., 2017). Internet interventions focused on reducing sedentary behavior have seen far less attention than those targeting physical activity, so a full understanding of their effectiveness is not yet available. There is some irony, of course, in sitting at a computer to receive an intervention designed to prevent sitting; yet, preliminary findings with adolescents suggest that interventions to reduce sedentary behavior through web-based approaches may hold some utility and warrant further research (Rose et al., 2017).

For physical activity, one of the earliest reviews and meta-analyses of internet interventions was from Davies and colleagues (2012), who showed an effect size of $d = .14$ among 34 studies, favoring the internet intervention over control groups. A review conducted a few years later (Joseph et al., 2014), this time of 72 studies, showed that 61% of studies reported increases in physical activity from the internet intervention.

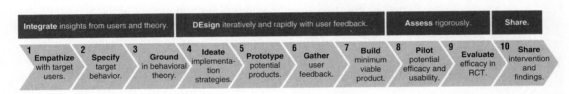

Figure 5-1 The IDEAS framework for digital interventions to change health behavior.

Mummah, S. A., Robinson, T. N., King, A. C., Gardner, C. D., & Sutton, S. (2016). IDEAS (Integrate, Design, Assess, and Share): A framework and toolkit of strategies for the development of more effective digital interventions to change health behavior. *Journal of Medical Internet Research, 18*(12), e5927. Retrieved from https://doi.org/10.2196/jmir.5927

These mixed results have continued in more recent reviews of internet interventions on physical activity (Beleigoli et al., 2019; Jahangiry et al., 2017; Rose et al., 2017).

The generally mixed findings have prompted an exploration into moderators of the effectiveness of physical activity interventions. Jahangiry and colleagues (2017) showed that younger people (< 45 years of age) compared to older people, short term assessments of physical activity (<6 weeks) compared to longer intervention assessment times, more active participants at baseline compared to inactive participants, and higher quality studies were more likely to show increased physical activity outcomes. Most recently, Smith and Liu (2020) explored whether engagement in the internet intervention material affected the success of physical activity behavior change. The researchers found that usage metrics (number of logins, login frequency, and usage of online tools) were related to the physical activity outcomes. This suggests, as noted above, that the design of the intervention to bring participants back to it and its content are critical to the overall success in behavior change.

Because the usage of materials in the intervention is important to physical activity, some reviews have reported on the most common content found in internet interventions. Davies et al. (2012) showed that inclusion of educational material on the benefits of physical activity and how to build self-efficacy was linked to increased effectiveness. In line with this finding, many internet interventions have been based on theories with strong educational and self-efficacy building materials such as social cognitive theory (see Chapter 14), the health belief model (see Chapter 15), and the transtheoretical model of behavior change (see Chapter 16) (Hou et al., 2014). Duff and colleagues (2017) explored the specific behavior change techniques typically found in internet interventions for populations with cardiovascular disease. They found that content about the health consequences from regular physical (in)activity (78%), how to set physical activity goals (74%), advice on how to self-monitor progress (48%) and information about creating social support for physical activity (48%) were the most common aspects of the interventions.

In summary, physical activity interventions using web-based browsers and email have been well-studied. A similar focus of these types of interventions on sedentary behavior has seen less attention. In general, internet interventions show small increases in physical activity, particularly among younger and middle-aged adults over the short term, but the engagement with the internet intervention material, such as educational content, is important to this success. Innovative ways to maintain engagement throughout the intervention may be paramount.

Mobile Health Technology and Wearables

Mobile phones have been used in text messaging health interventions for over two decades and this form of intervention helped to develop the term *mHealth* as a name for mobile phone based health promotion (Khan et al., 2017). Text messaging interventions have shown general support for making small changes in physical activity (Vandelanotte et al., 2016); however, a more contemporary focus in mHealth has been with smartphone app technology, often in conjunction with movement trackers. This development in the expansion of mHealth technology has been equally supported by research.

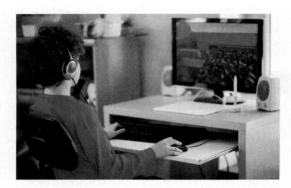

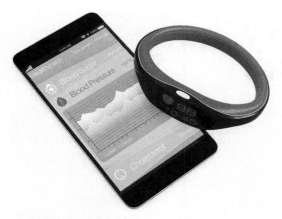

© Chesky_W/iStock/Getty Iamges Plus/Getty Images.

For example, a review of mHealth technology studies by Müller and colleagues (2018) showed that research publications on mHealth and physical activity or sedentary behavior have increased at a rate of 26% per year since 2000! Most of these papers have studied physical activity and have been focused on what the authors refer to as Generation 2 technologies (e.g., smartphones, wearables), while Generation 1 (e.g., text messages) research has decreased. In this section, we give an overview of this research on both smartphones and their often-associated companion wearable movement trackers in physical activity and sedentary behavior.

The high volume of research that has focused on mHealth and physical activity in the last 10 years has enabled the production of several reviews and meta-analyses to inform us about whether this technology is useful in promotion. In one of the highest quality reviews, Mönninghoff and colleagues (2021) assessed 117 studies, collectively featuring 21,118 participants, to examine whether mHealth interventions promoted four categories of physical activity (walking, moderate-to-vigorous physical activity, energy expenditure and total physical activity), and whether there were any conditions that improved or impaired the success of these interventions. The authors found mHealth interventions increased physical activity across all four of these categories (see **Table 5-2**).

Of particular note, however, the most effective behavior change was through increased walking (SMD = 0.46), with a smaller effect on moderate-to-vigorous intensity physical activity (SMD = 0.28). These results may reflect that step count is used as a feedback metric for most mHealth applications, which corresponds perfectly with walking. Among the small number of studies that included longer follow-up measurement periods, the authors found that both the walking and moderate-to-vigorous intensity physical activity changes were sustained. This is very promising, as it suggests that mHealth may be maintainable, which is often not the case in other forms of physical activity intervention (McEwan et al., 2022).

Table 5-2 **Effect Sizes of mHealth Interventions by Different Classifications of Physical Activity as Reported in Mönninghoff et al. 2021**

Physical Activity Category	# of Studies	Effect Size (standardized mean difference)	95% Confidence interval
Walking	77	0.46	0.36 to 0.55
MVPA	62	0.28	0.21 to 0.35
Total Physical Activity	33	0.34	0.20 to 0.47
Energy Expenditure	5	0.44	0.13 to 0.75

Note: MVPA = moderate to vigorous intensity physical activity.

Data from Mönninghoff, A., Kramer, J. N., Hess, A. J., Ismailova, K., Teepe, G. W., Tudor Car, L. T., Müller-Riemenschneider, F., Kowatsch, T. (2021). Long-term effectiveness of mHealth physical activity interventions: Systematic review and meta-analysis of randomized controlled trials. *Journal of Medical Internet Research, 23*, e26699.

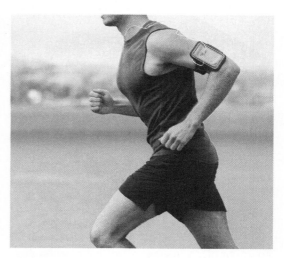

© Maridav/Shutterstock.

While the findings of mHealth studies have been promising, some of these results may be a result of weaker study designs and biases in measurement. For example, Mönninghoff and colleagues (2021) highlighted that many of the studies in their review (80%) had study designs with considerable bias. Relatedly, Romeo and colleagues (2019) conducted a systematic review and meta-analysis aimed to determine the effectiveness of smartphone apps for increasing only objectively measured physical activity in adults. As we have highlighted previously in Chapter 1, self-reported physical activity may be prone to measurement error and recall bias, so objective assessments of physical activity are helpful to improve the accuracy of research findings. The authors identified six studies that met their criteria and concluded that physical activity apps produced a non-significant increase in behavior, and that studies with higher objective physical activity results were more likely to be over short time-periods rather than longer time periods. Studies of mHealth technologies with adolescents and children have also been less convincing (Böhm et al., 2019). These results show that caution still needs to be taken when appraising app-based interventions, and the findings may change over time as experiments with mHealth become more rigorous.

Considerable research in mHealth has focused on physical activity, yet there is less evidence to appraise the effectiveness of these interventions in decreasing sedentary behavior. Still, some early reviews suggest that mHealth may be effective in some cases. Direito and colleagues (2017) reviewed five studies on the effect of mHealth interventions on sedentary behavior and showed a small overall reduction (SMD = -0.26). Buckingham et al. (2019) reviewed 10 studies that examined mHealth interventions to change sedentary behavior in the workplace and showed that four

of these studies reported reductions. At present, there are too few studies to reach a conclusion of the effectiveness of mHealth interventions in reducing sedentary behavior.

In research using mHealth, it is often difficult to separate smartphone apps from trackers because they are so interconnected. However, some research has focused specifically on the effectiveness of movement trackers for producing changes in physical activity. This is important research because movement trackers, such as those produced by Fitbit, Apple Watch, and Garmin represent an enormous business. Wearables are the number one selling fitness product and collectively represent a multi-billion dollar business (The Global Health and Fitness Association, 2020). Thus, the establishment of their effectiveness for changing behavior is important information to guide consumers. Reviews of interventions using wearables have generally shown support for increasing physical activity. For example, Gal and colleagues (2018) reviewed 18 randomized controlled trials featuring wearables and showed a meaningful increase in physical activity in minutes per day (SMD = 0.43) and an increase in daily step count (SMD = 0.51). Importantly, they found that removing biased studies improved the intervention effects. More recently, Brickwood et al. (2019) reviewed 28 trials with wearables and also showed a significant increase in daily step count (SMD = 0.24), moderate and vigorous physical activity (SMD = 0.27), and energy expenditure (SMD = 0.28), yet a non-significant decrease in sedentary behavior (SMD 0.20). It should be noted that these results are all from studies with adults. Limited research on the effect of wearables on physical activity and sedentary behavior has been conducted with children and adolescents, yet the results have not been as convincing (Böhm et al., 2019).

Behavior Change Content in mHealth Interventions

As noted earlier in this chapter, engagement with digital health content is essential in order to produce effective interventions. Thus, a full understanding of the content of mHealth physical activity interventions is needed. Several reviews have detailed the most common behavior change techniques in mHealth interventions for physical activity and sedentary behavior (Buckingham et al., 2019; Direito et al., 2017; Eckerstorfer et al., 2018). Frequently employed intervention content included the key components of control theory (See Chapter 16), such as goal setting, self-monitoring of behavior, feedback on behavior, and prompts/cues. For anyone who has used a physical activity tracker, none of this content will be particularly surprising. Setting step (or other categories of physical activity) goals, monitoring progress, and receiving prompts and cues with feedback are the main functions of these products.

Other common content for mHealth interventions in this review included social support or social comparison, instructions on how to perform the behavior, information about health consequences, and adding objects to the environment. Diereito and colleagues (2017) point out that while these techniques are used in >50% of mHealth research, they represent a small number of possible behavior change techniques, as outlined in Michie et. al.'s (2013) behavior change technique taxonomy.

While most reviews of behavior change techniques in mHealth have just detailed the content, Eckerstorfer et al. (2018) examined which of these behavior change techniques correlated with physical activity change. They found that mHealth interventions that included behavioral goals and self-monitoring each led to more intervention success. By contrast, content with general health information, plans involving where and when, and instructions on how to be active were not associated with greater intervention success. Taken together, the results support the general inclusion of goal setting and self-monitoring in mHealth interventions, yet there is still considerable room for innovation and application of various behavior change techniques.

Exergames

One of the emergent areas of research in physical activity and technology is the combination of video games and movement-based skills. These forms of games are often called active video games or **exergames**, where gameplay requires the player to move in order to interact with the avatar on screen. Videogames have received negative attention with their links to prolonged sedentary behaviour and maladaptive psychological and scholarly outcomes (Carson et al., 2016), but exergames appear to be one way to increase human movement behavior without altering the type of activity itself (Spence et al., 2017). The video game industry has tremendous global reach. Videogames represent a 85+ billion dollar annual industry (Statista.com, 2021), which is more than the gross domestic product of many countries! Video games are no longer an activity purely for young males either: for over a decade, the average age of players in the U.S. is > 30, and nearly half of game players are women (Entertainment Software Association, 2009). Games are played using traditional consoles, virtual reality (VR), and smartphones.

In terms of exergames, they have also shown enormous popularity since the time they hit the marketplace at the turn of the century. For example, the Nintendo Wii sold close to 100 million units (Nintendo Co. Ltd., 2012) and Microsoft Kinect was the fastest selling consumer electronics device of all time (BBC News, 2011). Pokemon

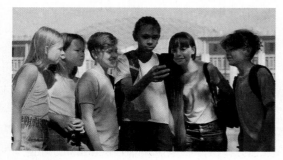

Go, an augmented reality game on smartphones, debuted to a massive success in 2016. Since that time, virtual reality (VR) exergames on platforms such as Occulus have also seen a large consumer interest. This demonstrates the enormous reach of diverse forms of exergames into households. Research on exergames has typically attempted to answer two questions: 1) Do exergames provide public health benefits? 2) Do exergames affect behavioural adherence?

Health Benefits of Exergames

Exergames are a relatively new physical activity, so it is important to classify their typical energy expenditure, similar to our compendium of other activities (Ainsworth et al., 2011). Perhaps the most important question in this type of research is whether exergames can meet the intensity guidelines for public health, which are in the moderate to vigorous intensity category (World Health Organization, 2020). To examine this research question, several early reviews have been conducted on various exergames and the energy expenditure required in a bout of play (Barnett et al., 2011; Biddiss & Irwin, 2010; Mark et al., 2008; Peng et al., 2012; Primack et al., 2012). All the reviews concluded that exergames have a lot of variability in the energy expenditure required to play, and many are in the moderate to lower intensity range (Kari, 2017). For example, the meta-analysis results conducted for this research question by Barnett and colleagues (2011) showed that the average

energy expenditure was 3.1 METs, which is the low-end of moderate intensity activity. The researchers found that age and gender did not explain the differences in expenditure, so it can be attributed to the actual games played. Games attached to cycle ergometers and exergames that involve dancing or boxing are among the highest energy expenditure for exergames. Warburton and colleagues also showed that exergames produce higher energy expenditure at lower rates of perceived exertion than ordinary activity, suggesting people may work harder but not perceive the extra effort (Warburton et al., 2009). Overall, it appears that some exergames can provide doses of physical activity at health enhancing MVPA intensity, but most of these games would be classified in the light intensity range of physical activity and thus contribute to lessening sedentary behavior (Kari, 2017).

Recently, Viana et al. (2021) examined the effects of exergames on muscle strength across 47 studies. Their meta-analyses showed no significant differences between exergames and non-exercise control groups in heathy/unhealthy middle-aged/older adults. However, exergames provided a greater increase in strength outcomes among individuals with clinical conditions when compared to usual care interventions. The results highlight that the health benefits of exergames may be more profound for older adults, those with clinical conditions, or for rehabilitation purposes. This has been supported in several reviews of the literature (Andrade et al., 2019; Kappen et al., 2019; Qian et al., 2020).

More recent reviews have also shown evidence that the bout of activity provided by exergames may be sufficient to improve aspects of mental health. For example, Li and colleagues (2016) engaged in a systematic review and meta-analysis of nine studies to discover the overall effect size of exergames on treating depressive symptoms. They found a significant effect size of $g = -0.21$, showing that playing exergames had a small but meaningful effect on relieving depressive symptoms. In a more recent review, Zeng et al. (2018) explored the effect of virtual reality exergaming on mental

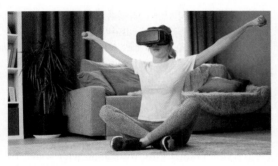

© MYDAYcontent/Shutterstock.

health across five studies. The majority of these studies reported significant improvements in anxiety- and depression-related measures following VR exercise, including reduced tiredness and tension, in addition to increased energy and enjoyment.

Exergames and Activity Adherence

Exergames are relatively unique among physical activities because they were designed to be fun enough for families to purchase. This provides the possibility for the activities to be reinforcing enough to promote continued physical activity. Results, however, are mixed on whether exergames can improve adherence when compared to other physical activities (Peng et al., 2012). For example, in a series of studies with exercise bikes that were augmented with video game technology, Rhodes and colleagues (Mark & Rhodes, 2013; Rhodes, Beauchamp, et al., 2018; Rhodes et al., 2017; Rhodes, Kaos, et al., 2018) showed that the exergame bike had a high initial frequency of use, but this effect began to wane after the first week and dropped off in use quite precipitously thereafter unless new weekly gaming content was provided (Kaos et al., 2018). This effect where initial use and interest wanes over time seems common among the early exergame studies (Barnett et al., 2011). Newer exergames, such as those with virtual reality enhancements, may hold more utility for long term adherence (Ng et al., 2019). Further, the proposed mechanism for why exergames

might result in better adherence compared to traditional physical activities has been supported. In multiple relevant studies, exergames were associated with more fun and enjoyment compared to the traditional activities (Kari, 2017; Mark & Rhodes, 2013; Rhodes et al., 2019; Rhodes et al., 2009).

Research on exergames remains relatively untapped at present due to several challenges. One issue in this line of research is the slow process of research when paired with the speed of the videogame industry. Most of our knowledge of exergames is on platforms and games that are now gone from the marketplace. Researchers are finding it difficult to keep up with this pace. Second, exergaming research that attempts to foster maintenance is needed to demonstrate that the initial high participation rates can be sustained. There may be several reasons for the diminishing effect of exergames in the early research trials that mimic the same issues around engagement with all digital health interventions (e.g., technical glitches, professional design, uninteresting narratives and design).

In addition, one of the faulty assumptions in exergame research may be that videogames generally sustain playing behaviour and therefore exergames should show continued adherence without decline. Videogames, similar to these exergame results noted above, show decline in playing frequency as games become familiar and the novelty wears (Koster, 2004). To sustain videogame play, manufacturers continually develop new games and new editions of the same games. The videogame marketplace is well-timed so that new games are constantly made available to satiate the needs of gamers who have completed or become bored of their older games. It would stand to reason that exergames would require the same approach as ordinary video games for behavioural maintenance (Kaos et al., 2018).

Finally, a source of variability in exergames is the necessary trade-off that designers make when blending quality exercise and gaming. Exergames, which are "exercise first," may not appeal to the same players as those which are a "games first" design. Exergame design will undoubtedly continue to improve, and after 20 years in our marketplace and society, this research domain is also poised to continue to grow, diversify, and develop.

Social Media

More than half of the world now uses social media (> 80% in North America), such as Facebook, WhatsApp, YouTube, Twitter and Instagram, and spends an average of two and a half hours per day on these platforms (Chaffey, 2021). Furthermore, the adoption of social media is still in a growth phase with nearly 500 million new users annually. Thus, social media is positioned as a powerful medium to potentially reach and influence physical activity and sedentary behaviors (see **Figure 5-2**).

The advances in social media make it difficult to address all the potential behavior change techniques possible on social media platforms, which include but are not limited to social support and comparison, health information, and behavioral instruction. Research on social media as an intervention to promote physical activity is in its early phases. Still, there are some reviews that help to provide an initial assessment of its

utility. In one of the earliest reviews, Williams and colleagues (2014) assessed 12 intervention trials examining the use of social media to promote physical activity. In these studies, participants were mainly middle-aged Caucasian women of mid-to-high socioeconomic status. There were also a variety of interventions, comparison groups and outcomes that made the assessment challenging, yet the authors concluded that changes in physical activity were not significantly different in the social media condition to the control condition ($d = 0.13$).

A few years later, Ann et al. (2017) reviewed 22 studies regarding the effectiveness of social media-based interventions about weight-related behaviors, including physical activity and sedentary behavior. The majority (n = 17) used Facebook, followed by Twitter (n = 4) and Instagram (n = 1). The 12 studies that assessed physical activity showed no effect on energy expenditure, total physical activity, and light, moderate, vigorous, and moderate-to-vigorous physical activity. The one study that assessed sedentary behavior also showed no effect from the social media intervention (Joseph et al., 2015). The authors, however, did report a significant

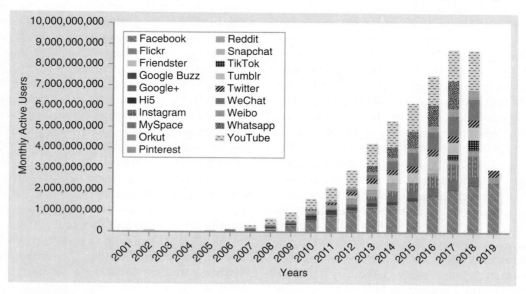

Figure 5-2 Rate of number of people using social media platforms from 2004 to 2019.

overall effect on step count resulting from social media interventions.

The most recent and comprehensive review on social media and physical activity was conducted by Goodyear and colleagues (2021). This review sought to update the evidence since the prior research review by Williams and colleagues in 2014. The authors found that most of the new studies have featured young female adults (aged 18–35) attending university, with Facebook being the predominant form of social media intervention, followed by a handful of studies using Twitter, Reddit, WeChat, and Instagram. Facebook groups and the accessibility of information and interaction were the main characteristics of these social media interventions. These more recent studies were also more likely to include metrics of engagement to characterize the success of the intervention. Metrics of engagement varied, and included participation in social media groups, hours spent on social media, and the frequency of views, posts, comments, and likes. The authors reported that average engagement in the intervention was high (between 50% and 100%) and time on social media for the intervention ranged from one to two hours per week when this was reported. Despite this generally high engagement, the effectiveness in changing physical activity was mixed. Specifically, only 4 of the 10 physical activity studies showed significant behavior change.

Social media use has also expanded considerably during the COVID-19 pandemic (Chaffey, 2021) and this has also been apparent in physical activity-related social media (Goodyear, Boardley, et al., 2021). For example, Parker and colleagues (2021) surveyed a large sample of Australians to explore the use of digital exercise platforms during the first lockdown (April and May 2020). They found that digital platform use was diverse and included social media services for exercise (e.g., YouTube, Instagram, and Facebook). Overall, 39.5% of adults reported using these platforms for physical activity. Rhodes et al. (2020) showed that those people who moved from face-to-face exercise programming to online exercise videos (e.g., on YouTube) reported they were more likely to stay active during the early phase of the lockdowns. However, while the use of YouTube exercise programming videos was initially high, the continued use of this medium may not have lasted. Sui et al. (2022) showed that ten of the most highly frequented exercise YouTube channels decreased views and likes significantly across the first months of the pandemic, and these declines were often after the first week.

Taken together, social media holds the promise of reaching and influencing physical activity and sedentary behaviors across diverse members of society. Current research, however, has tended to focus on select groups (young adult women) and the results of this research have been mixed in terms of whether social media can change physical activity. Too little research have been conducted on sedentary behavior at present to fully understand whether the results are similar to physical activity. One of the reasons for this mixed effect on behavior may be the types of behavior change techniques that social media can typically confer (e.g., social support, information about health consequences) compared to mHealth apps or web-based interventions that often include self-monitoring, personalized feedback, and goal setting related behavior change techniques. These latter behavior change techniques are often considered the most powerful elements of interventions (Knittle et al., 2018; McEwan et al., 2019). Future research that explores different aspects of social media that correspond with the most effective behavior change approaches may yield more effective interventions.

CRITICAL THINKING ACTIVITY 5-2

Do you think your social media use influences your sedentary behavior or physical activity? If so, how? If not, why not?

One interesting area of study related to social media and digital health generally is the application of artificial intelligence chatbots, or conversational agents. These approaches have been used to change physical activity and sedentary behavior, with 5 of 7 intervention studies showing positive behavior change effects (Oh et al., 2021).

Conversational Agents and Physical Activity Behavior

A review of 20 studies that used conversational agents to change physical activity was conducted by Luo et al. (2021), and here are some highlights of the review findings:

- There was a moderate level of evidence that people would engage with and benefit from conversational agents.
- A lot of people tended to drop-out of these interventions regularly.
- It is unknown whether the effects of conversational agents on changing physical activity lead to long-term behavior change.
- Some people reported concerns, including safety, privacy, and that the conversational agents felt unnatural.

CRITICAL THINKING ACTIVITY 5-3

How does it make you feel when you interact with a chat-bot or conversational agent? Do you think it could be useful to help people get social support to change their behavior?

Summary

Technology like smartphones and the internet is ubiquitous in our lifestyles, so it is important to understand how digital health technology affects our physical activity and sedentary behaviors. Screen-time is an often-used marker of sedentary behavior itself and therefore, a reduction of technology use, particularly leisure-time screen use, is recommended in public health messaging (Ross et al., 2020). However, the role of web-based, mHealth, exergames, and social media programming as interventions designed to reduce sedentary behavior and/or increase physical activity is a dynamic and burgeoning domain of research. Women clearly use digital health technology more than men, and there are other noteworthy demographic correlates (income, ethnicity, education, selected health behavior profiles), yet eHealth literacy may be the most critical correlate of those who use digital health technology compared to those who are less likely. Thus far, research evidence supports small physical activity changes from web-based interventions, although these approaches seem most effective for younger adults and short-term changes to physical activity. Early-phase research has also supported the effectiveness of mHealth technologies such as apps and trackers in making changes in physical activity, though ongoing engagement in the digital health intervention material is challenging and directly linked to success. Exergames (including smartphone-based, console-based, and VR) have also shown some success, particularly in the short term, for promoting physical activity but they also have steep drop-offs in use. These games are often associated with light intensity physical activity, so many exergames are better considered as an intervention for reducing sedentary behavior rather than increasing moderate-to-vigorous intensity physical activity. Finally, social media interventions are the least studied form of digital health interventions for physical activity and sedentary behavior, and their effectiveness is mixed at present. Continued advancements in digital health intervention quality and application will certainly change our understanding of how technology can be used for increasing physical activity and reducing sedentary behavior.

Vignette: Deshaun

As part of our Exercise Psychology class, I had to keep track of the time I spent on my phone and computer last week. You wouldn't believe the amount of time I spent in front of screens. It's interesting though, because I'm really active still. There's this idea that screen time is bad because it means you're sitting, slouching, and not moving. But that's not how I roll. I'm always on the move. I play basketball and I use my phone while I'm waiting off the court. I use my phone while I'm walking to class. Even when I use my computer or watch TV, I'm usually doing different things too. I'm not a guy who sits for hours with a backache staring at my screen.

My professor presents a lot of studies that link "screen time" to bad outcomes, like poor mental health and more inactivity, but I think that's outdated. It may be that decades ago, screen time meant you were locked into a stationary office chair or a couch. But now, with all the innovation going on about virtual and augmented reality, that can't be true anymore.

You wouldn't believe this, but I brought up my points about screens not necessarily meaning being sedentary to my exercise psychology professor and she thought it was a good point! She got so excited thinking about it that we've decided to do a study on it together. I start working with her after class next week to figure out what we'll do.

Just got back from meeting with my professor about that study. The study plan is not fully developed yet, but the basic idea is that we'll track whether people are moving, sitting, standing, or lying down while using their screens and come up with how much of screen-time is actually spent being sedentary. We'll look for differences in this between people too, because she thinks office workers will probably be more sedentary while using a screen compared to students – I'm not sure about that yet. The best thing about this whole study is that we can collect the data without asking participants to self-report questions– after they give us permission, of course. We'll be sticking a posture and movement monitor on them and then access their device usage data from their phones and computers. Can't wait to see what happens–and to show the field that screen time doesn't equal being lazy!

Key Terms

digital health The general use of information and communication technologies for health.
eHealth literacy The users' competence needed to engage with digital health services; digital health literacy.

exergames Video games in which gameplay requires the player to move in order to interact with the avatar on screen.
mHealth Health promotion using mobile phones as the primary mechanism.

Review Questions

1. Define e-Health literacy. How is e-Health literacy related to digital health?
2. What are exergames? Are they effective in promoting physical activity?
3. Are digital health physical activity interventions effective? If so, what seems to be the most effective?
4. What is user engagement? Is user engagement related to physical activity? If so, how?
5. Are wearables associated with improvements in physical activity? What behavior change techniques do wearables typically use to change behavior?
6. Have digital health interventions been effective at reducing sedentary behavior? What is the research so far?

Applying the Concepts

1. How did Deshaun's e-Health literacy affect their appraisal of the professor's definition of sedentary behavior?
2. How will Deshaun use digital health information to evaluate the study they plan to perform?

References

Ainsworth, B. E., Haskell, W. L., Herrmann, S. D., Meckes, N., Bassett, D. R., Tudor-Locke, C., Greer, J. L., Vezina, J., Whitt-Glover, M. C. & Leon, A. S. (2011). 2011 Compendium of physical activities. *Medicine & Science in Sports & Exercise, 43*(8), 1575–1581.

An, R., Ji, M., & Zhang, M. S. (2017). Effectiveness of social media-based interventions on weight-related behaviors and body weight status: Review and meta-analysis. *American Journal of Health Behavior, 41*(6), 670–682.

Andrade, A., Correia, C. K., & Coimbra, D. R. (2019). The psychological effects of exergames for children and adolescents with obesity: A systematic review and meta-analysis. *Cyberpsychology, Behavior, and Social Networking, 22*(11), 724–735.

Barnett, A., Cerin, E., & Baranowski, T. (2011). Active video games for youth: A systematic review. *Journal of Physical Activity and Health, 8*(5), 724–737.

Baumel, A., & Kane, J. M. (2018). Examining predictors of real-world user engagement with self-guided eHealth interventions: Analysis of mobile apps and websites using a novel dataset. *Journal of Medical Internet Research, 20*(12), e11491.

BBC News. (2011). Microsoft Kinect 'fastest-selling device on record'. Retrieved March 10, 2011, from http://www.bbc.co.uk/news/business-12697975

Beleigoli, A. M., Andrade, A. Q., Cançado, A. G., Paulo, M. N., Diniz, M. D. F. H?., & Ribeiro, A. L. (2019). Web-based digital health interventions for weight loss and lifestyle habit changes in overweight and obese adults: Systematic review and meta-analysis. *Journal of Medical Internet Research, 21*(1), e9609.

Biddiss, E., & Irwin, J. (2010). Active video games to promote physical activity in children and youth: A systematic review. *Archives of Pediatric and Adolescent Medicine, 164*(7), 664–672.

Boakye, E. A., Mohammed, K. A., Geneus, C. J., Tobo, B. B., Wirth, L. S., Yang, L., & Osazuwa-Peters, N. (2018). Correlates of health information seeking between adults diagnosed with and without cancer. *The Public Library of Science One, 13*(5), e0196446.

Böhm, B., Karwiese, S. D., Böhm, H., & Oberhoffer, R. (2019). Effects of mobile health including wearable activity trackers to increase physical activity outcomes among healthy children and adolescents: Systematic review. *Journal of Medical Internet Research: mHealth and uHealth, 7*(4), e8298.

Brickwood, K. J., Watson, G., O'Brien, J., & Williams, A. D. (2019). Consumer-based wearable activity trackers increase physical activity participation: Systematic review and meta-analysis. *Journal of Medical Internet Research mHealth and uHealth, 7*(4), e11819.

Briggs, P. (2018). *Canada Mobile Time Spent and Ad Spending 2018: How Consumers and Advertisers Are Using Search, Social, Messaging and Gaming.* Insider Intelligence. Accessed October 18, 2022. https://www.insiderintelligence.com/content/canada-mobile-time-spent-and-ad-spending-2018

Buckingham, S. A., Williams, A. J., Morrissey, K., Price, L., & Harrison, J. (2019). Mobile health interventions to promote physical activity and reduce sedentary behaviour in the workplace: A systematic review. *Digital Health, 5*, 1–50.

Byrnes, N. (2019). Mobile technologies could revolutionize health care if it can overcome challenges. *MIT Technology. Review.* Retrieved 18 Dec 2019, from https://www.technologyreview.com/s/529031/mobile-healths-growing-pains

Carson, V., Hunter, S., Kuzik, N., Gray, C. E., Poitras, V. J., Chaput, J. P., Saunders, T. J., Katzmarzyk, P. T., Okely, A. D., Gorber, S. C., Kho, M. E., Sampson, M., Lee, H., & Tremblay, M. S. (2016). Systematic review of sedentary behaviour and health indicators in school-aged children and youth: an update. *Applied Physiology, Nutrition, and Metabolism, 41*(6), S240–S265.

Chaffey, D. (2021). Global social media statistics research summary 2022. *Smart Insights.* https://www.smartinsights.com/social-media-marketing/social-media-strategy/new-global-social-media-research/#:~:text=More%20than%20half%20of%20the,social%20media%20is%202h%2027m.

Choi, J., Lee, J., & Vittinghoff, E. (2016). mHealth physical activity intervention: A randomized pilot study in physically inactive pregnant women. *Maternal Child Health Journal, 20*(5), 1091–1101.

Choi, N. G., & DiNitto, D. M. (2013). The digital divide among low-income homebound older adults: Internet use patterns, eHealth literacy, and attitudes toward computer/internet use. *Journal of Medical Internet Research, 15*(5), e2645.

Davies, C. A., Spence, J. C., Vandelanotte, C., Caperchione, C. M., & Mummery, W. K. (2012). Meta-analysis of internet-delivered interventions to increase physical activity levels. *International Journal of Behavioral Nutrition and Physical Activity, 9*(1), 52.

Direito, A., Carraça, E., & Rawstorn, J. (2017). mHealth technologies to influence physical activity and sedentary behaviors: Behavior change techniques, systematic review and meta-analysis of randomized controlled trials. *Annals of Behavioral Medicine, 51*(2), 226–239.

Duff, O. M., Walsh, D. M. J., Furlong, B. A., O'Connor, N. E., Moran, K. A., & Woods, C. B. (2017). Behavior change techniques in physical activity eHealth interventions for people with cardiovascular disease: Systematic review. *Journal of Medical Internet Research, 19*(8), e7782.

Eckerstorfer, L. V., Tanzer, N. K., Vogrincic-Haselbacher, C., Kedia, G., Brohmer, H., Dinslaken, I., & Corcoran, K. (2018). Key elements of mHealth interventions to successfully increase physical activity: Meta-regression. *Journal of Medical Internet Regression mHealth and uHealth, 6*(11), e10076.

Entertainment Software Association. (2009). Industry facts. Retrieved June 3, from http://www.theesa.com/facts/index.asp

Gal, R., May, A. M., van Overmeeren, E. J., Simons, M., & Monninkhof, E. M. (2018). The effect of physical activity interventions comprising wearables and smartphone applications on physical activity: A systematic review and meta-analysis. *Sports Medicine - Open, 4*(1), 1–15.

Goodyear, V. A., Boardley, I., Chiou, S. Y., Fenton, A. A. M., Makopoulou, K., Stathi, A., Wallis, G. A., Veldhuijzen van Zanten, J. J. C. S., & Thompson, J. L. (2021). Social media use informing behaviours related to physical activity, diet and quality of life during COVID-19: A mixed methods study. *BioMed Central Public Health, 21*(1), 1–14.

Goodyear, V. A., Wood, G., Skinner, B., & Thompson, J. L. (2021). The effect of social media interventions on physical activity and dietary behaviours in young people and adults: A systematic review. *International Journal of Behavioral Nurtrition and Physical Activity, 18*(1), 1–18.

Hassandra, M., Lintunen, T., & Hagger, M. S. (2017). An mHealth app for supporting quitters to manage cigarette cravings with short bouts of physical activity: A randomized pilot feasibility and acceptability study. *Journal of Medical Internet Research, 5*(5), 6252.

Holt, K. A., Karnoe, A., Overgaard, D., Nielsen, S. E., Kayser, L., Røder, M. E., & From, G. (2019). Differences in the level of electronic health literacy between users and nonusers of digital health services: An exploratory survey of a group of medical outpatients. *Interactive Journal of Medical Research, 8*(2), e8423.

Hou, S. I., Charlery, S. A. R., & Roberson, K. (2014). Systematic literature review of Internet interventions across health behaviors. *Health Psychology and Behavioral Medicine: an Open Access Journal, 2*(1), 455–481.

Howarth, A., Quesada, J., Silva, J., Judycki, S., & Mills, P. R. (2018). The impact of digital health interventions on health-related outcomes in the workplace: A systematic review. *Digital Health, 4*, 1–18.

Internet usage statistics. (2022). *Internet world stats: Usage and population statistics.* https://www.internetworldstats.com/stats.htm

Jahangiry, L., Farhangi, M. A., Shab-Bidar, S., Rezaei, F., & Pashaei, T. (2017). Web-based physical activity interventions: A systematic review and meta-analysis of randomized controlled trials. *Public Health, 152*, 36–46.

Joseph, R. P., Durant, N. H., Benitez, T. J., & Pekmezi, D. W. (2014). Internet-based physical activity interventions. *American Journal of Lifestyle Medicine, 8*(1), 42–67.

Joseph, R. P., Keller, C., Adams, M. A., & Ainsworth, B. E. (2015). Print versus a culturally-relevant Facebook and text message delivered intervention to promote physical activity in African American women: A randomized pilot trial. *BioMed Central Women's Health, 15*(1), 1–18.

Kaos, M. D., Beauchamp, M. R., Bursick, S., Latimer-Cheung, A. E., Hernandez, H., Warburton, D. E., Yao, C., Ye, Z.,

Graham, T. C., & Rhodes, R. E. (2018). Efficacy of online multi-player versus single-player exergames on adherence behaviours among children: A nonrandomized control trial. *Annals of Behavioral Medicine, 20*, 1–12.

Kappen, D. L., Mirza-Babaei, P., & Nacke, L. E. (2019). Older adults' physical activity and exergames: A systematic review. *International Journal of Human–Computer Interaction, 35*(2), 140–167.

Kari, T. (2017). Promoting physical activity and fitness with exergames: Updated systematic review of systematic reviews. In B. Dubbels (Ed.), *Transforming Gaming and Computer Simulation Technologies across Industries* (pp. 225–245). IGI Global.

Khan, N., Marvel, F. A., Wang, J., & Martin, S. S. (2017). Digital health technologies to promote lifestyle change and adherence. *Current Treatment Options Cardiovascular Medicine, 19*(8), 1–12.

Knittle, K., Nurmi, J., Crutzen, R., Hankonen, N., Beattie, M., & Dombrowski, S. U. (2018). How can interventions increase motivation for physical activity? A systematic review and meta-analysis. *Health Psychology Review, 12*(3), 211–230.

Koster, R. (2004). *A Theory of Fun for Game Design.* Paraglyph Press.

Lepore, S. J., Rincon, M. A., Buzaglo, J. S., Golant, M., Lieberman, M. A., Bass, S. B., & Chambers, S. (2019). Digital literacy linked to engagement and psychological benefits among breast cancer survivors in Internet-based peer support groups. *European Journal of Cancer Care, 28*(4), e13134.

Li, J., Theng, Y. L., & Foo, S. (2016). Effect of exergames on depression: A systematic review and meta-analysis. *Cyberpsychology, Behavior, and Social Networking, 19*(1), 34–42.

Luo, T. C., Aguilera, A., Lyles, C. R., & Figueroa, C. A. (2021). Promoting physical activity through conversational agents: Mixed methods systematic review. *Journal of Medical Internet Research, 23*(9), e25486.

Mark, R., & Rhodes, R. E. (2013). Testing the effectiveness of exercise videogame bikes among families in the home-setting: A pilot study. *Journal of Physical Activity and Health, 10*(2), 211–221.

Mark, R., Rhodes, R. E., Warburton, D. E. R., & Bredin, S. S. G. (2008). Interactive video games and physical activity: A review of literature and future directions. *Health &Fitness Journal of Canada, 1*(1), 14–24.

McEwan, D., Kouvousis, C., Ray, C., Wyrough, A., Beauchamp, M. R., & Rhodes, R. E. (2019). Examining the active ingredients of physical activity interventions underpinned by theory versus no stated theory: A meta-analysis. *Health Psychology Review, 13*(1), 1–17. https://doi.org/10.1080/17437199.2018.1547120

McEwan, D., Rhodes, R. E., & Beauchamp, M. (2022). What happens when the party is over? Sustaining physical activity behaviors after intervention cessation. *Behavioral Medicine, 48*(1), 1–9.

Michie, S., Richardson, M., Johnston, M., Abraham, C., Francis, J., Hardeman, W., Eccles, M. P., Cane, J., & Wood, C. E. (2013). The behavior change technique taxonomy (v1) of 93 hierarchically clustered techniques: Building an international consensus for the reporting of behavior change interventions. *Annals of Behavioral Medicine, 46*(1), 81–95. AU:The reference I found on Google Scholar was different.

Mönninghoff, A., Kramer, J. N., Hess, A. J., Ismailova, K., Teepe, G. W., Tudor Car, L. T., Müller-Riemenschneider, F., & Kowatsch, T. (2021). Long-term effectiveness of mhealth physical activity interventions: Systematic review and meta-analysis of randomized controlled trials. *Journal of Medical Internet Research, 23*(4), e26699.

Moore, S. A., Faulkner, G., Rhodes, R. E., Brussoni, M., Chulak-Bozzer, T., Ferguson, L. J., Mitra, L. J., Mitra, R., O'Reilly, N., Spence, J. C., Vanderloo, L. M., & Tremblay, M. S. (2020). Impact of the COVID-19 virus outbreak on movement and play behaviours of Canadian children and youth: A national survey. *International Journal of Behavioral Nutrition and Physical Activity, 17*(1), 1–11.

Müller, A. M., Maher, C. A., Vandelanotte, C., Hingle, M., Middelweerd, A., Lopez, M. L., DeSmet, A., Short, C. E., Nathan, N., Hutchesson, M. J., Poppe, L., Woods, C. B., Williams, S. L., & Wark, P. A. (2018). Physical activity, sedentary behavior, and diet-related eHealth and mHealth research: Bibliometric analysis. *Journal of Medical Internet Research, 20*(4), e8954.

Mummah, S. A., Robinson, T. N., King, A. C., Gardner, C. D., & Sutton, S. (2016). IDEAS (Integrate, Design, Assess, and Share): A framework and toolkit of strategies for the development of more effective digital interventions to change health behavior. *Journal of Medical Internet Research, 18*(12): e5927. https://doi.org/10.2196/jmir.5927

Ng, Y. L., Ma, F., Ho, F. K., Ip, P., & Fu, K. W. (2019). Effectiveness of virtual and augmented reality-enhanced exercise on physical activity, psychological outcomes, and physical performance: A systematic review and meta-analysis of randomized controlled trials. *Computers in Human Behavior, 99*, 278–291.

Nikoloudakis, I. A., Vandelanotte, C., Rebar, A. L., Schoeppe, S., Alley, S., Duncan, M. J., & Short, C. E. (2018). Examining the correlates of online health information–seeking behavior among men compared with women. *American Journal of Men's Health, 12*(5), 1358–1367.

Nintendo Co. Ltd. (2012). Consolidated Sales Transition by Region. http://www.nintendo.co.jp/ir/library/historical_data/pdf/consolidated_sales_e1206.pdf

Norman, C. D., & Skinner, H. A. (2006). eHEALS: The eHealth literacy scale. *Journal of Medical Internet Research, 8*(4), e507.

Nutbeam, D. (2000). Advancing health literacy: A global challenge for the 21st century. *Health Promotion International, 15*(3), 183–184.

Oh, Y. J., Zhang, J., Fang, M.-L., & Fukuoka, Y. (2021). A systematic review of artificial intelligence chatbots for promoting physical activity, healthy diet, and weight loss. *International Journal of Behavioral Nutrition and Physical Activity, 18*(1), 1–25.

Parker, K., Uddin, R., Ridgers, N. D., Brown, H., Veitch, J., Salmon, J., Timperio, A., Sahlqvist, S., Cassar, S., Toffoletti, K., Maddison, R., & Arundell, L. (2021). The use of digital platforms for adults' and adolescents' physical activity during the COVID-19 pandemic (our life at home): Survey study. *Journal of Medical Internet Research, 23*(2), e23389.

Peng, W., Crouse, J. C., & Lin, J. H. (2012). Using active video games for physical activity promotion: A systematic review of the current state of research. *Health Education and Behavior, 40*(2), 171–192. https://doi.org/DOI: 10.1177/1090198112444956

Primack, B. A., Carroll, M. V., McNamara, M., Klem, M. L., King, B., Rich, M., Chan, C. W., & Nayak, S. (2012). Role of video games in improving health-related outcomes: A systematic review. *American Journal of Preventitive Medicine, 42*(6), 630–638.

Qian, J., McDonough, D. J., & Gao, Z. (2020). The effectiveness of virtual reality exercise on individual's physiological, psychological and rehabilitative outcomes: A systematic review. *International Journal of Environmental Research and Public Health, 17*(11), 4133.

Rhodes, R. E., Beauchamp, M., Blanchard, C. M., Bredin, S. S. D., Warburton, D. E. R., & Maddison, R. (2018). Use of in-home stationary cycling equipment among parents in a family-based randomized trial intervention. *Journal of Science and Medicine in Sport, 21*(10), 1050–1056.

Rhodes, R. E., Beauchamp, M. R., Blanchard, C. M., Bredin, S. S. D., Warburton, D. E. R., & Maddison, R. (2019). Predictors of stationary cycling exergame use among inactive children in the family home. *Psychology of Sport and Exercise, 41*, 181–190.

Rhodes, R. E., Blanchard, C. M., Beauchamp, M. R., Bredin, S. S. D., Maddison, R., & Warburton, D. E. R. (2017). Stationary cycling exergame use among inactive children in the family home: A randomized trial. *Journal of Behavioral Medicine, 40*(6), 978–988.

Rhodes, R. E., Kaos, M. D., Beauchamp, M. R., Bursick, S. K., Latimer-Cheung, A. E., Hernandez, H., Warburton, D. E., Ye, Z., & Nicholas Graham, T. C. N. (2018). Effects of home-based exergaming on child social cognition and subsequent prediction of behavior. *Scandinavian Journal of Medicine and Science in Sports, 28*(10), 2234–2242.

Rhodes, R. E., Liu, S., Lithopoulos, A., Zhang, C. Q., & Garcia-Barrera, M. A. (2020). Correlates of perceived physical activity transitions during the COVID-19 pandemic among a sample of Canadian adults. *Applied Psychology: Health and Well-Being, 12*(4), 1157–1182. https://doi.org/10.1111/aphw.12236

Rhodes, R. E., & Nasuti, G. (2011). Trends and changes in research on the psychology of physical activity across 20 years: A quantitative analysis of 10 journals. *Preventive Medicine, 53*(1-2), 17–23.

Rhodes, R. E., Warburton, D. E. R., & Bredin, S. S. (2009). Predicting the effect of interactive video bikes on exercise adherence: An efficacy trial. *Psychology, Health & Medicine, 14*(6), 631–641.

Roberts, A. L., Fisher, A., Smith, L., Heinrich, M., & Potts, H. W. W. (2017). Digital health behaviour change interventions targeting physical activity and diet in cancer survivors: A systematic review and meta-analysis. *Journal of Cancer Survivorship, 11*(6), 704–719.

Romeo, A., Edney, S., Plotnikoff, R., Curtis, R., Ryan, J., Sanders, I., Crozier, A., & Maher, C. (2019). Can smartphone apps increase physical activity? Systematic review and meta-analysis. *Jornal of Medical Internet Research, 21*(3), e12053.

Rose, T., Barker, M., Jacob, C. M., Morrison, L., Lawrence, W., Strömmer, S., Vogel, C., Woods-Townsend, K., Farrell, D., Inskip, H., & Baird, J. (2017). A systematic review of digital interventions for improving the diet and physical activity behaviors of adolescents. *Journal of Adolescent Health, 61*(6), 669–677.

Roser, M., Ritchie, H., & Ortiz-Ospina, E. (2019). *Internet.* Ourworldindata.org. Retrieved March 10 from https://ourworldindata.org/internet

Ross, R., Chaput, J., Giangregorio, L., Janssen, I., Saunders, T. J., Kho, M. E., Poitras, V. J., Tomasone, J. R., El-Kotob, R., McLaughlin, E. C., Duggan, M., Carrier, J., Carson, V., Chastin, S. F., Latimer-Cheung, A. E., Chulak-Bozzer, T., Faulkner, G., Flood, S. M., Gazendam, M. K., Healy, G. N., Katzmarzyk, P. T., Kennedy, W., Lane, K. N., Lorbergs, A., McLaren, K., Marr, S., Powell, K. E., Rhodes, R. E., Ross-White, A., Welsh, F., Willumsen, J., & Tremblay, M. S. (2020). Canadian 24-hour movement guidelines for adults aged 18–64 years and adults aged 65 years or older: An integration of physical activity, sedentary behaviour, and sleep. *Applied Physiology, Nutrition, and Metabolism, 45*(10), S57–S102. https://doi.org/10.1139/apnm-2020-0467

Serrano, K. J., Coa, K. I., & Yu, M. (2017). Characterizing user engagement with health app data: A data mining approach. *Transl Behav Med 7*(2), 277–785.

Smith, N., & Liu, S. (2020). A systematic review of the dose-response relationship between usage and outcomes of online physical activity weight-loss interventions. *Internet Interventions, 22*, 100344.

Spence, J. C., Rhodes, R. E., & Carson, V. (2017). Challenging the dual-hinge approach to intervening on sedentary behavior. *American Journal of Preventive Medicine, 52*(3), 403–406.

Statista.com. (2021). *Video game industry - Statistics & facts.* https://www.statista.com/topics/868/video-games/#dossier Keyfigures

Statistics Canada. (2020). Smartphone use and smartphone habits by gender and age group. https://doi.org/10.25318/2210011501-eng

Stockwell, S., Trott, M., Tully, M., Shin, J., Barnett, Y., Butler, L., McDermot, D., Schuch, F., & Smith, L. (2021). Changes in physical activity and sedentary behaviours from before to during the COVID-19 pandemic lockdown: A systematic review. *British Medical Journal Open Sport & Exercise Medicine, 7*(1), e000960.

Sui, W., Rush, J., & Rhodes, R. E. (2022). Engagement with online fitness videos on YouTube and Instagram during the COVID-19 pandemic: A longitudinal study. *Journal of Medical Internet Research: Formative Research.*

Sydow, L. (2021). Pumped up: Health and fitness app downloads rose 30% in a landmark year for mobile wellness. *App Annie.* https://www.appannie.com/en/insights/market-data/health-fitness-downloads-rose-30-percent/

The Global Health and Fitness Association. (2020). Wearables continue to transform the fitness industry. https://www.ihrsa.org/improve-your-club/wearables-continue-to-transform-the-fitness-industry/

Tremblay, M. S., Aubert, S., Barnes, J. D., Saunders, T. J., Carson, V., Latimer-Cheung, A. E., Chastin, S. F., Altenburg, T. M., & Chinapaw, M. J. M. (2017). Sedentary behavior research network (SBRN) – Terminology consensus project process and outcome. *International Journal of Behavioral Nutrition and Physical Activity, 14*(1),1–17.

Vajaean, C. C., & Baban, A. (2015). Emotional and behavioral consequences of online health information seeking: The role of eHealth literacy. *Cognition, Brain, Behavior, 19*(4), 327–345.

Vandelanotte, C., Muller, A. M., Short, C. E., Hingle, M., Nathan, N., Williams, S. L., Lopez, M. L., Parekh, S., & Maher, C. A. (2016). Past, present, and future of eHealth and mHealth research to improve physical activity and dietary behaviors. *Journal of Nutrition Education and Behavior, 48*(3), 219–228.

Viana, R. B., de Oliveira, V. N., Dankel, S. J., Loenneke, J. P., Abe, T., da Silva, W. F., & de Lira, C. A. B. (2021). The effects of exergames on muscle strength: A systematic review and meta-analysis. *Scandanavian Journal of Medicine & Science in Sport, 31*(8), 1592–1611.

Warburton, D. E. R., Sarkany, D., Johnson, M., Rhodes, R. E., Whitford, W., Esch, B. T. A., & Bredin, S. S. D. (2009). Metabolic requirements of interactive video game cycling. *Medicine+ Science in Sports+ Exercise, 41*(4), 920–926.

Widmer, R. J., Collins, N. M., Collins, C. S., West, C. P., Lerman, L. O., & Lerman, A. (2015). Digital health interventions for the prevention of cardiovascular disease: A systematic review and meta-analysis. *Mayo Clinic Proceedings, 90*(4), 469–480.

Wilke, J., Mohr, L., Tenforde, A. S., Edouard, P., Fossati, C., Gonzalez-Gross, M., & Yuki, G. (2020). Restrictercise! Preferences regarding digital home training programs during confinements associated with the COVID-19 pandemic. *International Journal of Environment Research and Public Health, 17*(18). https://doi.org/10.3390/ijerph17186515

Williams, G., Hamm, M. P., Shulhan, J., Vandermeer, B., & Hartling, L. (2014). Social media interventions for diet and exercise behaviours: A systematic review and meta-analysis of randomised controlled trials. *British Medical Journal Open, 4*(2), e003926.

World Health Organization. (2016). Monitoring and evaluating digital health interventions: A practical guide to conducting research and assessment. http://www.who.int/reproductivehealth/publications/mhealth/

World Health Organization. (2020). Physical Activity. https://www.who.int/news-room/fact-sheets/detail/physical-activity

Xie, Z., Nacioglu, A., & Or, C. (2018). Prevalence, demographic correlates, and perceived impacts of mobile health app use amongst Chinese adults: Cross-sectional survey study. *Journal of Medical Internet Research: mHealth and uHealth,* 6(4), e9002.

Zeng, N., Pope, Z., Lee, J. E., & Gao, Z. (2018). Virtual reality exercise for anxiety and depression: A preliminary review of current research in an emerging field. *Journal of Clinical Medicine,* 7(3), 42.

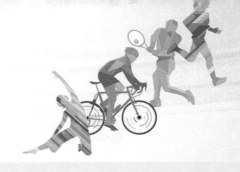

Psychological Health Effects of Exercise and Sedentary Behavior

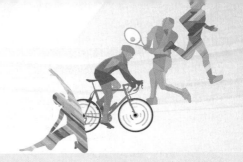

CHAPTER 6

Health-Related Quality of Life and Positive Psychology

LEARNING OBJECTIVES

After completing this chapter, you will be able to:

- Distinguish among quality of life, standard of living, and health-related quality of life.
- Measure your health-related quality of life using assessment tools.
- Understand how physical activity and sedentary behavior affect health-related quality of life in a variety of populations.
- Define positive psychology and happiness.
- Explain how exercise and sedentary behavior are related to our happiness levels.
- Describe how exercise affects feeling states.

Introduction

Historically, researchers focused on how physical activity could reduce negative mood states and psychological disorders such as anxiety and depression. This line of research found that exercise is a viable intervention to reduce these negative mood states and disorders in both healthy and clinical populations. The flip side to this line of inquiry is the following question: Can exercise improve positive mood states, such as happiness, vigor, energy, and enthusiasm, and overall quality of life?

Like many people, Martin Luther King Jr. believed that quality of life is very important, as evidenced in his following quote: "The quality,

not the longevity, of one's life is what is important." (n.d.). In other words, it is the quality of one's life, not the quantity of life, that needs to be fostered. Interestingly, increase people's quality of life and their quantity of life will also increase (Leaf et al., 2021).

The purpose of this chapter is to examine how physical activity and sedentary behavior affect people's **health-related quality of life (HRQoL)** and **positive psychology** (e.g., happiness and flourishing). First, we will define and determine how HRQoL is measured, and then we will examine the effects of physical activity and sedentary behavior on HRQoL in a variety of special populations (e.g., cancer patients, diabetics, and older adults). Finally, we will define positive psychology and examine its relationship to our quality of life, in particular the relationship between happiness and positive feeling states with physical activity and sedentary behavior.

Health-Related Quality of Life

Quality of life is a broad multidimensional term that assesses people's perceived quality of their daily life. In other words, quality of life is a subjective evaluation of both positive and negative aspects of people's general well-being and their ability to function on daily tasks. Although many different conceptualizations of quality of life exist, the World Health Organization (WHO) envisions quality of life as a broad concept consisting of the following six domains: physical health, psychological health, independence, social relationships, spirituality, and the environment (WHO, 2012; see **Figure 6-1**). **Table 6-1** provides a description of each of these domains.

Factors that play a role in people's quality of life vary according to personal preferences, but they often include financial security, job satisfaction, family life, health, and safety. For example, financial decisions usually involve a tradeoff whereby quality of life is either decreased by

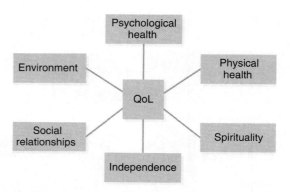

Figure 6-1 WHO Quality of Life.

Data from World Health Organization. (2012). WHOQOL. Measuring quality of life. Retrieved October 26, 2022, from https://www.who.int/tools/whoqol

saving money or increased by spending money. A person may buy that new car she has been eyeing, or she may decide to not buy the car and save her money to purchase a house in the future instead of continuing to rent an apartment. As well, sickness and pandemics, such as COVID-19, have negative impacts on people's quality of life (Nobari et al., 2021).

Commuting to work provides another good example of something that can affect people's quality of life. Many people save money on housing by living further away from work. However, living farther from work requires a longer

Table 6-1 World Health Organization Multidimensional Quality of Life Model

Domain	Quality of Life Example
1. Physical health	Energy, fatigue, pain, discomfort, sleep, and rest
2. Psychological health	Body image and appearance, negative feelings, positive feelings, self-esteem, thinking, learning, memory, and concentration
3. Independence	Mobility, activities of daily living, dependence on medicinal substances medical aids, and work capacity
4. Social relationships	Personal relationships, social support, and sexual activity
5. Environment	Financial resources, freedom, physical safety and security, health and social care, home environment, and recreation opportunities
6. Spirituality	Religion, personal beliefs

Data from World Health Organization. (2012). WHOQOL. Measuring quality of life. Retrieved October 26, 2022, from https://www.who.int/tools/whoqol

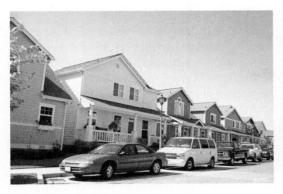

© Ligonography/iStock/Getty Images Plus/Getty Images.

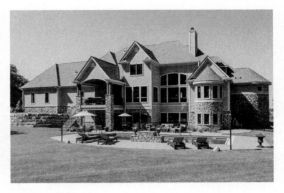

© Tim Abramowitz/E+/Getty Images.

commute (usually both in distance and time) to the office. The extra time spent traveling reduces the available time that the commuter will have with family, friends, and doing leisure activities, but it offers more affordable housing and suburban amenities. In popular job centers, such as major urban areas like New York City, London, Hong Kong, and Tokyo, it is not uncommon for people to spend 2 hours commuting one way to live in more affordable and larger housing in the suburbs. Some people consider this tradeoff worthwhile for their quality of life, whereas others choose to maximize their quality of life by spending more money on housing to live closer to work. In short, perceptions of quality of life vary greatly from person to person.

CRITICAL THINKING ACTIVITY 6-1

What is more important to your quality of life? To live close to work or to live in the suburbs?

The terms quality of life and standard of living are often incorrectly used interchangeably. **Standard of living** refers to levels of wealth, comfort, and material goods. Although standard of living is often measured by a person's income, it can include many other factors, such as quality and availability of employment, class disparity, poverty rate, quality and affordability of housing, inflation rate, number of days off for holidays

per year, affordable (or free) access to quality healthcare, quality and availability of education, life expectancy, incidence of disease, cost of goods and services, economic and political stability, political and religious freedom, environmental quality, climate, and safety. In comparison, quality of life is related to how people feel about their lives and themselves. A person can have a very high standard of living, as measured by having a high-income level, yet have a low quality of life. Or a person can have a low standard of living and a high quality of life.

The application of quality of life to the impact of diseases and treatments on people's lives has given rise to a field of research called health-related quality of life (HRQoL). This field assesses how people's quality of life affects their physical, social, and mental health. Most people would agree that either increasing or maintaining health improves overall quality of life. Not surprisingly, people with chronic diseases (e.g., diabetes, cancer, stroke, arthritis, and hypertension) tend to have lower HRQoL than healthy people.

Measuring Health-Related Quality of Life

HRQOL-14 Measure

Many assessment tools exist to measure HRQoL. A popular HRQoL assessment is the Centers for Disease Control and Prevention's (CDC) HRQOL-14 Measure. The HRQOL-14 measure has been used since 1993 in epidemiological studies to assess behavioral risk factors for health in the United States. This measure has three modules. The Healthy Days Core Module includes four core questions (see **Table 6-2**). These questions are useful at the national level to identify health disparities and track population trends. For example, almost 16% of Americans report that they have either fair or poor health (question 1 of the Healthy Days Core Module; Zack, 2013). Certain groups are more at-risk for poor HRQoL. For example, women, older adults, individuals with obesity, minority racial/ethnic groups, those with less education, those who speak another language besides English at home, and those with a disability have higher percentages of fair or poor health and report more physically and mentally unhealthy days than their peers (Zack, 2013; Zack, Moriarty, Stroup, Ford, & Mokdad, 2004).

With regard to age, a negative linear relationship with HRQoL is evidenced, with 9% of adults ages 18 to 24 years reporting either fair or poor health, compared to 30% of adults aged 75 or older. As well, a positive relationship exists between education level and overall health, with 37% of people with less than a high school education reporting either fair or poor health, compared to 7% of people who have graduated college. For weight status, 38% of people who are overweight or obese report either fair or poor health, compared to 11% of normal weight individuals (National Center for Chronic Disease Prevention and Health Promotion, 2011). In short, demographic variables (such as age, weight status, and education) are related to people's HRQoL.

The Activity Limitations Module contains five questions that assess physical, mental, or emotional problems or limitations a person may have in his or her daily life (see **Table 6-3**). Finally, the Healthy Days Symptoms Module contains five questions that assess a person's recent pain, depression, anxiety, sleeplessness, vitality and the cause, duration, and severity of a current activity limitation an individual may have had in his or her life during the past 30 days (see **Table 6-4**).

CRITICAL THINKING ACTIVITY 6-2

Complete the Healthy Days Core Module. What does this tell you about your HRQoL? What can you do to improve your HRQoL?

Table 6-2 **CDC HRQOL-14: Healthy Days Core Module**

1. Would you say that in general your health is (circle one):

   Excellent   Very Good   Good   Fair   Poor

2. Now thinking about your PHYSICAL HEALTH, which includes physical illness and injury, how many days during the past 30 days was your physical health NOT good?

   _____ Number of Days

3. Now thinking about your MENTAL HEALTH, which includes stress, depression, and problems with emotions, how many days during the past 30 days was your mental health NOT good?

   _____ Number of Days

4. During the past 30 days, how many days did POOR PHYSICAL OR MENTAL HEALTH keep you from doing your usual activities, such as self-care, work, or recreation?

   _____ Number of Days

Centers for Disease Control and Prevention. National Center for Chronic Disease Prevention and Health Promotion. Division of Population Health. Retrieved from https://www.cdc.gov/hrqol/hrqol14_measure.htm. Reference to specific commercial products, manufacturers, companies, or trademarks does not constitute its endorsement or recommendation by the U.S. Government, Department of Health and Human Services, or Centers for Disease Control and Prevention.

Table 6-3 CDC HRQOL-14: Activity Limitations Module

These next questions are about physical, mental, or emotional problems or limitations you may have in your daily life.

1. Are you LIMITED in any way in any activities because of any impairment or health problem?

   YES or NO

2. What is the MAJOR impairment or health problem that limits your activities?
   a. Arthritis/rheumatism
   b. Back or neck problem
   c. Fractures, bone/joint injury
   d. Walking problem
   e. Lung/breathing problem
   f. Hearing problem
   g. Eye/vision problem
   h. Heart problem
   i. Stroke problem
   j. Hypertension/high blood pressure
   k. Diabetes
   l. Cancer
   m. Depression/anxiety/emotional problem
   n. Other impairment/problem

3. For HOW LONG have your activities been limited because of your major impairment or health problem?
   a. Days
   b. Weeks
   c. Months
   d. Years

4. Because of any impairment or health problem, do you need the help of other persons with your PERSONAL CARE needs, such as eating, bathing, dressing, or getting around the house?
   a. Yes
   b. No

5. Because of any impairment or health problem, do you need the help of other persons in handling your ROUTINE needs, such as everyday household chores, doing necessary business, shopping, or getting around for other purposes?
   a. Yes
   b. No

Centers for Disease Control and Prevention. National Center for Chronic Disease Prevention and Health Promotion. Division of Population Health. Retrieved from https://www.cdc.gov/hrqol/hrqol14_measure.htm. Reference to specific commercial products, manufacturers, companies, or trademarks does not constitute its endorsement or recommendation by the U.S. Government, Department of Health and Human Services, or Centers for Disease Control and Prevention.

Table 6-4 CDC HRQOL-14: Healthy Days Core Module

Please indicate the number of days that represent your response to each item.	# of Days
During the past 30 days, how many days did PAIN make it hard for you to do your usual activities, such as self-care, work, or recreation?	
During the past 30 days, how many days have you felt SAD, BLUE, or DEPRESSED?	
During the past 30 days, how many days have you felt WORRIED, TENSE, or ANXIOUS?	
During the past 30 days, how many days have you felt you did NOT get ENOUGH REST or SLEEP?	
During the past 30 days, how many days have you felt VERY HEALTHY and FULL OF ENERGY?	

Centers for Disease Control and Prevention. National Center for Chronic Disease Prevention and Health Promotion. Division of Population Health. Retrieved from https://www.cdc.gov/hrqol/hrqol14_measure.htm. Reference to specific commercial products, manufacturers, companies, or trademarks does not constitute its endorsement or recommendation by the U.S. Government, Department of Health and Human Services, or Centers for Disease Control and Prevention.

Health-Related Quality of Life, Exercise, and Sedentary Behavior

General Population

Physical activity is positively associated with higher HRQoL across the lifespan (Gopinath, Hardy, Baur, Burlutsky, & Mitchell, 2012; Luncheon & Zack, 2011). In other words, physical activity enhances people's HRQoL from childhood, to adulthood, and into older adulthood (Marker, Steele, & Nose, 2018; Sivaramakrishnan et al., 2019). For example, data obtained from the Healthy Days Core Module of the CDC HRQOL-14 reveals that physical activity is positively related to HRQoL. With regard to exercise, 11.3% of active people report to be in either fair or poor health, compared to 30.2% of inactive people (National Center for Chronic Disease Prevention and Health Promotion, 2011).

Nonactive people also report poorer physical and mental health than active individuals. For example, nonactive people report that of the past 30 days their physical health was not good for an average of 6.6 days, compared with 2.6 days for active people. Similarly, nonactive people report of the past 30 days that their mental health was not good for 5.1 days, compared to 3.0 for active people. Finally, nonactive people report that of the past 30 days their poor physical or mental health kept them from doing their usual activities (e.g., self-care, work, or recreation activities) for an average of 4.6 days, compared to 1.5 days for active individuals (see **Figure 6-2**).

Whereas physical activity positively influences HRQoL, obesity negatively influences HRQoL. But which has more of an impact on HRQoL, physical activity or weight status? Herman, Hopman, Vanderkerhof, and Rosenberg (2012) attempted to answer this question using a cross-sectional sample of 110,986 adults who completed measures of their HRQoL and activity levels. The researchers found that inactive individuals had a greater likelihood of worse health and activity limitation due to either illness or injury at all body mass index (BMI) levels. Conversely, in active individuals, being underweight, overweight, or obese had little effect on health and activity limitation due to illness or injury. The researchers concluded that when examining BMI and physical activity in combination, physical activity is the more important correlate of HRQoL, regardless of weight status. This reinforces the importance of physical activity to health outcomes over and above the benefits related to either weight loss or maintenance.

How does sedentary behavior affect HRQoL? People who spend more time engaged in sedentary behaviors such as television viewing, computer and video game use, and reading have lower HRQoL than their less sedentary counterparts (Boberska et al., 2018; Gopinath et al., 2012). Researchers found an inverse association between screen time and quality of life in university students (Lavados-Romo, Andrade-Mayorga, Morales, Muñoz, & Balboa-Castillo, 2021; Whitaker et al., 2022).

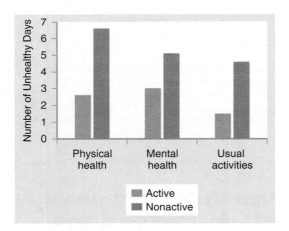

Figure 6-2 Leisure-Time Physical Activity and Health-Related Quality of Life Responses to the Healthy Days Core Module.
Note: Healthy Days Core Module (Questions 2–4) 2. Now thinking about your physical health, which includes physical illness and injury, for how many days during the past 30 days was your physical health not good? 3. Now thinking about your mental health, which includes stress, depression, and problems with emotions, for how many days during the past 30 days was your mental health not good? 4. During the past 30 days, for about how many days did poor physical or mental health keep you from doing your usual activities, such as self-care, work, or recreation?

Data from National Center for Chronic Disease Prevention and Health Promotion. (2011). HRQOL tables and maps. Retrieved March 7, 2014, from http://www.cdc.gov/hrqol/data.htm

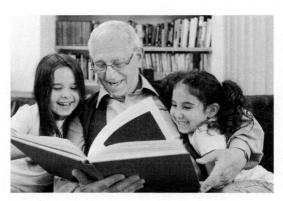

© Noam Armonn/Shutterstock.

Students with a longer screen exposure time had a lower quality of life, specifically in the domains of social relationships and psychological health, regardless of sex, physical activity level, or socioeconomic level.

Health-Related Quality of Life and Physical Activity in Special Populations

In general, people who engage in physical activity tend to have better HRQoL compared with sedentary people. For example, college students with higher levels of sport and physical activity have more positive HRQoL compared to less active students (Snedden et al., 2019). In comparison, people with chronic diseases such as diabetes, hypertension, asthma, heart disease, and stroke tend to have lower HRQoL than people without these chronic diseases. Thus, it is important to examine ways to increase the HRQoL of these special populations. Common types of interventions to improve HRQoL are behavioral interventions, medication, education, and surgery.

Physical activity is another intervention that may improve the HRQoL of people with chronic diseases. In general, physical activity improves HRQoL in people with chronic diseases and conditions such as cancer, chronic pain, kidney disease, osteoporotic vertebral fracture, intermittent claudication, and multiple sclerosis (Anjos et al., 2022; Reina-Gutiérrez et al., 2022; Soares-Miranda, et al., 2021). For example, Latimer-Cheung and colleagues (2013) found that among those with mild to moderate disability from multiple sclerosis, exercise training was effective for improving aerobic capacity and muscular strength, as well as HRQoL. In this section, we will discuss how physical activity and sedentary behavior affect the HRQoL of people suffering with leading causes of death such as diabetes and cancer. As well, we will examine HRQoL and physical activity in older adults, which is a population at increased risk for both physical inactivity and sedentary behavior and lower levels of HRQoL than younger populations.

Cancer Populations

Cancer is a broad group of diseases involving unregulated cell growth. Cancer can affect any part of the body, and its defining feature is the rapid creation of abnormal cells that grow beyond their usual boundaries. These unregulated cells can then invade adjoining parts of the body and spread to other organs. The causes of cancer are diverse, complex, and only partially understood. About 30% of cancer deaths are directly related to the following five risk factors: (1) high BMI, (2) low fruit and vegetable intake, (3) lack of physical activity, (4) tobacco use, and (5) alcohol use.

Worldwide, an estimated 19.3 million new cancer cases and almost 10.0 million cancer deaths occurred in 2020 (Sung et al., 2021).

The most common forms of this disease are lung cancer, stomach cancer, liver cancer, colorectal cancer, and breast cancer. Prevalence and incidence rates of cancer are rising largely due to the fact that people are living longer and lifestyle changes resulting in increased obesity and inactivity.

A **cancer survivor** is a person with cancer who is still living. The number of cancer survivors in the United States increased from 3 million in 1971 to 16.9 million in 2019. The number of cancer survivors is projected to increase to 22.2 million by 2030. Many people with cancer live a long time after diagnosis. Cancer survivors face many physical and emotional challenges throughout their treatment and recovery, including persistent and profound adverse effects on

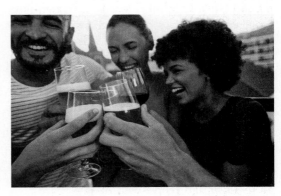

© Pixdeluxe/E+/Getty Images.

their HRQoL. Because HRQoL is an important determinant of cancer survivorship, it is important to examine methods to increase HRQoL, both during and after the end of active treatment. Research reveals that physical activity can improve HRQoL in cancer survivors during active treatment (Mishra et al., 2012a).

What are the effects of physical activity on cancer survivors who have finished cancer treatment? Fuller and his colleagues (2018) reviewed this area of research, and they found that physical activity had a positive impact on HRQoL. They concluded that physical activity has an important role in helping to manage physical function, mental health, general well-being, and quality of life in people undergoing and recovering from cancer and the side effects of treatment. As well, a review found that physical activity is an effective intervention for improving the quality of life of breast cancer patients; with yoga being the most recommended type of exercise (Mokhatri-Hesari & Montazeri, 2020). The benefits to HRQoL are sufficient for the recommendation that cancer survivors follow the current physical activity guidelines, with specific exercise program adaptations based on disease and treatment-related adverse events.

While physical activity is beneficial in improving HRQoL among cancer survivors, sedentary behavior has a detrimental effect (Yan et al., 2021). That is, with cancer survivors, a positive relationship exists between moderate to vigorous physical activity and HRQoL. In contrast, a negative relationship exists between sedentary behavior and HRQoL. In other words, increased time spent exercising was associated with improved HRQoL while increased time in sedentary behavior was associated with poorer HRQoL among cancer survivors. Thus, it is important to displace sedentary behavior with exercise to improve the quality of life.

Diabetic Populations

Diabetes refers to a group of diseases that affect how the body uses blood glucose (also known as blood sugar). People with diabetes have high blood sugar, meaning that they have too much glucose in their blood, which can lead to serious health issues. Worldwide, as of 2019, diabetes affects 463 million adults (aged 20 to 79 years), and it is the eighth leading cause of death. The number of people with diabetes is expected to rise to 700 million by 2045 (IDF Diabetes Atlas, Ninth edition, 2021). Understanding how to prevent and treat diabetes is a major public health concern because of its high prevalence and serious negative side effects.

Low levels of HRQoL are associated with increased mortality in people with diabetes. Chia-Lin Li and colleagues (2013) found that increased mortality risk was associated with reduced HRQoL in diabetic patients who reported no physical activity, indicating that engaging in physical activity may improve survival in diabetic patients who have poor quality of life. As well, a positive relationship exists between physical activity levels and HRQoL, in particular physical health, in diabetic patients (Imayama, Plotnikoff, Courneya, & Johnson, 2011; Thiel et al., 2017).

Older Adults

Older adults are typically defined as persons 60 years of age and older. The world population is rapidly aging. Between 2000 and 2050, the proportion of the world's population aged 60 years and older will double from about 11% to 22%. The absolute number of people aged 60 years and older is expected to increase from 605 million to

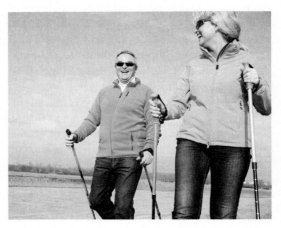

© Paul/F1online/Getty Images.

2 billion over the same period (WHO, 2014). As we become more of an aged society, understanding how HRQoL later in life can be maintained or improved by exercising is an important public health question. Literature reviews in older adults have found strong evidence for the beneficial effects of physical activity for HRQoL among this special population (Marquez, Aguiñaga, Vásquez, Conroy, Erickson, et al. 2020; Sivaramakrishnan et al., 2019).

What about sedentary behavior and HRQoL in older adults? Using a prospective cohort design, Balboa-Castillo and his colleagues (Balboa-Castillo, Leon-Munoz, Rodriguez-Artalejo, & Guallar-Castillon, 2011) examined if both sedentary behavior and physical activity were associated with HRQoL in older adults. Participants self-reported their physical activity behavior, sedentary behavior (i.e., number of hours sitting per week), and HRQoL by using the SF-36. The data were collected on a large representative sample of older adults living in Spain over a 9-year period. The researchers found a positive relationship between exercise behavior and the HRQoL dimensions of physical functioning, physical role, bodily pain, social functioning, vitality, emotional role, and mental health. They also found that the number of sitting hours showed a gradual and inverse relationship with most of the SF-36 scales. In short, more physical activity and less sitting were independently associated with better long-term HRQoL in older adults. What happens if sedentary behavior is replaced with physical activity that is of equal duration on HRQoL of older adults? Japanese researchers examined this research question in 287 older Japanese adults (aged 65–84 years). They found that replacing sedentary behaviors with moderate to vigorous physical activity resulted in better physical HRQoL in these older adults (Yasunaga et al., 2018).

In general, increased levels of physical activity and decreased levels of sedentary behavior are related to improving HRQoL in both healthy and diseased populations. As the number of people with chronic diseases increases, further understanding of the dose–response effects of both physical activity and sedentary behavior on HRQoL is needed.

CRITICAL THINKING ACTIVITY 6-3

What effect do you think sedentary behavior has on adolescents' HRQoL? Provide research from other populations to justify your response.

Positive Psychology

Psychology traditionally has focused on mental illness (e.g., personality disorders, anxiety disorders, and depressive disorders) or other psychological problems (e.g., nonclinical depression and anxiety symptoms) and how to treat these issues. Positive psychology, by contrast, is a relatively new field that focuses on how to help people prosper and lead healthy, happy lives (Seligman, Steen, Park, & Peterson, 2005). Positive psychology was founded on the following three ideas that people want to: (1) lead meaningful and fulfilling lives, (2) foster what is best within themselves, and (3) enhance their experiences of love, work, and play. Positive psychology has the following three central concerns of: (1) positive emotions, (2) positive individual traits, and (3) positive institutions (see **Table 6-5** for a description of these concerns).

Of importance, before we begin to examine this literature, definitional clarity among the terms affect, mood, and emotion is needed (Stevens et al., 2020). Affect is a generic term that covers a broad range of feelings that people can experience. It is an umbrella concept that encompasses both people's emotions and moods (Ekkekakis, 2008, 2013). Emotions are intense feelings that are either directed at a specific person or event. Examples of emotions are reacting with anger immediately when another driver cuts you off, being nervous right before you give a presentation, or being happy when you receive a compliment.

Moods are feelings that tend to be less intense than emotions, and they usually are not directed at either a person or an event. In other words, moods differ from emotions in that they are less specific, less intense, and less likely to be triggered by either a particular person or event.

Table 6-5 Central Concerns of Positive Psychology

Concern	Description of Research Focus
Positive emotions	Study of contentment with the past, happiness in the present, and hope for the future
Positive individual	Study of strengths and virtues (e.g., capacity for love and work, courage, compassion, resilience, creativity, curiosity, integrity, self-knowledge, moderation, self-control, and wisdom)
Positive institutions	Study of the meaning and purpose as well as the strengths that foster better communities, such as justice, responsibility, civility, parenting, nurturance, work ethic, leadership, teamwork, purpose, and tolerance

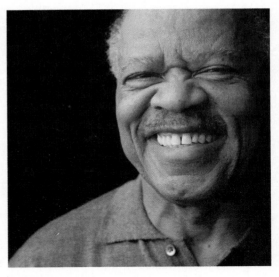

© Ryan McVay/Lifesize/Thinkstock.

For example, if someone is rude to you, you may feel angry right away. That intense feeling of anger usually comes and goes quickly, even in a matter of seconds. In comparison, when you are in a good mood, you can feel good for several hours. See **Figure 6-3** for a graphical distinction among emotions, moods, and affect.

Relationship among affect, mood, and emotion

Affect

Emotions

Moods

Figure 6-3 Relationship Among Affect, Mood, and Emotion.

Positive Psychology, Physical Activity, and Sedentary Behavior

Not surprisingly, most of the scientific research in the psychology of physical activity and sedentary behavior has focused on the impact of these behaviors on negative psychological states, such as depression and anxiety (see Chapters 10 and 11 for the information). More recently, researchers have also studied the effects of physical activity and sedentary behavior on feeling states, such as happiness, vigor, energy, and tranquility (Rodriguez-Ayllon et al., 2019). In this section, we will examine how various positive psychology concepts are related to both physical activity and sedentary behavior.

Can exercise give you more energy? It might seem counterintuitive that expending energy through exercise would increase feelings of energy and reduce feelings of fatigue. When a person is tired, the last thing they want to do is exercise. However, regular low-intensity exercise may help boost energy levels in people suffering from fatigue.

Tim Puetz and his colleagues (Puetz, Flowers, & O'Connor, 2008) studied whether exercise can be used to treat fatigue in a laboratory study. The participants were 36 young adults who were not regular exercisers and who also complained of persistent fatigue. People who reported fatigue due to serious medical conditions, such as those with chronic fatigue syndrome, were excluded from the study. One group of fatigued adults was randomized to a prescribed 20 minutes of moderate-intensity aerobic exercise three times a week for 6 weeks. The second group of adults engaged in low-intensity aerobic exercise for the same time period. A third group, the control group, did not exercise.

The participants in the exercise conditions exercised on bikes in the laboratory because this enabled the researchers to control their exertion levels. The low-intensity exercise was equivalent to a leisurely, easy walk. The more intense exercise was similar to a fast-paced uphill walk. Vigor and fatigue mood states were obtained at the beginning of the third exercise session each week for 6 weeks.

Both of the exercise groups had about a 20% increase in energy levels by the end of the study, compared to the control group. Interestingly, the low-intensity group reported a 65% drop in feelings of fatigue, compared to a 49% drop in the moderate-intensity biking group. The researchers concluded that for people with low activity levels, lower-intensity exercise may be the most effective way to reduce fatigue because a moderate-intensity exercise regime may be too intense for their fitness level.

Meta-analyses provide further confirmation that physical activity increases people's feelings of energy and reduces their feelings of fatigue in both healthy populations and populations enrolled in cardiac rehabilitation programs (Puetz, Beasman, & O'Connor, 2006; Puetz, O'Connor, & Dishman, 2006). Thus, lacing up your running shoes and doing some physical activity may provide that burst of energy you are looking for. Let's take a closer look at these meta-analyses.

Puetz, Beasman, and O'Connor (2006) conducted a meta-analysis to examine the effects of chronic exercise on feelings of energy and fatigue in 70 randomized controlled trials that enrolled a total of 6,807 participants. They found that

chronic exercise increased feelings of energy and lessened feelings of fatigue compared with control conditions (mean ES = .37). In a second meta-analysis, Puetz, O'Connor, and Dishman (2006) found that this positive energy-enhancing effect of exercise was also evidenced in people enrolled in cardiac rehabilitation exercise programs. In their review of 36 studies consisting of a total of 4,765 participants, they found that exercise improved feelings of energy and decreased fatigue for this special population.

In another meta-analysis, Justy Reed and Deniz Ones (2006) examined the effects of acute aerobic exercise on positive affect. They reviewed 158 studies with a total sample size of 13,101 participants. They found that exercisers had higher positive affect levels compared with inactive controls. They also noted that the positive effects of physical activity on affect lasted for at least 30 minutes after exercise before returning to baseline levels.

Most of the studies integrated into these meta-analyses refer to either specific exercise programs or to physical activity that is planned and structured. These studies generally do not refer to unstructured daily activities, such as walking or gardening. Thus, researchers have attempted to measure the association between physical activity and mood in everyday life. Understanding this association and the manner in which exercise contributes to enhanced positive feelings in everyday life may help to answer whether people can manage their mood through their lifestyle physical activities.

An interesting research technique called ecological momentary assessment enables researchers to comprehensively examine the association between daily mood and physical activity because the data are assessed in real time when the assumed effect of exercise on mood happens. Ecological momentary assessment refers to a category of methods that involve the collection of real-time data about current states (e.g., mood, activity) in the natural environment repeatedly over time. This technique reduces recall bias because the data are recorded when events occur and enables researchers to obtain data that have higher

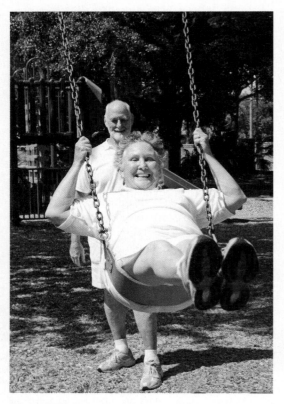

© iStockphoto/Thinkstock.

diurnal variations in mood, they found that feeling states were significantly better after exercise.

In another study, Martina Kanning and Wolfgang Schlicht (2010) examined the relationship between daily activities and mood in healthy people during their everyday life. They had 13 participants complete a standardized diary and report their mood (i.e., valence, energetic arousal, and calmness) over a 10-week period, resulting in 1,860 measurement points. They found that the participants felt more content (valence), awake (energetic arousal), and calm (calmness) after being physically active (e.g., walking and gardening) compared to when they were inactive. They also found that the positive mood–physical activity relationship was affected by the individual baseline mood level, with the greatest effect seen when the participants' mood was depressed.

CRITICAL THINKING ACTIVITY 6-4

What would you tell someone who says they do not exercise because they are too tired? Is this a valid excuse for not engaging in exercise?

ecological validity compared with data collected in the laboratory. In addition, multiple assessments of mood from each participant allow for higher-power analyses. In short, ecological momentary assessment provides a strong external validity of within-subject variations in physical activity and mood (Degroote, DeSmet, De Bourdeaudhuij, Van Dyck, & Crombez, 2020).

A review of the ecological momentary assessment studies found that being in nature and physical activity relates to better well-being and happiness (de Vries, Bart, Baselmans, & Meike Bartels, 2021). In one study Heather Hausenblas and her colleagues (Hausenblas, Gauvin, Symons Down, & Duley, 2008) analyzed the effects of abstinence from regular exercise on feeling states with ecological momentary assessment. Participants were deprived of their scheduled exercise on 3 days and maintained their regular exercise routine on 3 other days. After controlling for

A main area of inquiry in positive psychology is how to help people become happier. **Happiness** is a state of mind or a feeling characterized by contentment, love, satisfaction, pleasure, or joy, and it is a fundamental human goal. Research in this rapidly growing field often studies what makes people happy and how they can lead fulfilling and satisfying lives. Emerging evidence indicates that happiness also influences health. Conversely, unhappiness (i.e., not being cheerful, joyful, or glad) is related to mental and physical problems, such as depression, cardiovascular disease, lower immune response, and a shorter lifespan (Chida & Steptoe, 2008; Zhang et al., 2022). Positive psychology interventions are designed to enhance positive feelings, positive cognitions, and/or positive behaviors, as opposed to interventions aimed at reducing symptoms, problems, or disorders (Bolier et al., 2013).

Chida and Steptoe (2008) conducted a meta-analysis to examine the relationship between positive psychological well-being and physical health in both healthy and diseased populations (N = 70 studies). They found that both positive affect (e.g., emotional well-being, positive mood, joy, happiness, vigor, energy) and positive trait-like dispositions (e.g., life satisfaction, hopefulness, optimism, sense of humor) were associated with reduced mortality in healthy and diseased populations. Interestingly, the protective effects of positive psychological well-being were independent of negative affect. The authors concluded that positive psychological well-being has a favorable effect on survival in a variety of populations.

Are people who exercise and stand happier? It appears that people who exercise are happier than people who are inactive or sedentary in both the short and the long term (Matheson, 2014; Richards et al., 2015). A survey of 12,492 university students from 24 countries found that higher sedentary behavior was associated with poorer life satisfaction and lower happiness (Pengpid & Peltzer, 2019). In addition, moderate and high physical activity was related to higher life satisfaction, greater happiness, and better perceived health. Wang and colleagues (2012) conducted a longitudinal study to examine the association between changes in leisure-time physical activity and happiness. The participants were 17,276 randomly selected Canadians older than 12 years of age. People who reported clinical depression or the use of antidepressants at baseline or follow-up were excluded from the study. As well, people who reported preexisting unhappiness at baseline were also excluded from the study. To assess happiness, participants answered the following question: "Would you describe yourself as being usually _____" by selecting one of the following predefined responses of: "happy and interested in life," "somewhat happy," "somewhat unhappy," "unhappy with little interest in life," and "so unhappy that life is not worthwhile." The researchers combined "happy and interested in life" with "somewhat happy" responses into an overall "happy" category and combined the remaining responses as "unhappy."

Happy participants were classified as physically active or inactive at baseline and then followed up to examine whether they became unhappy. The researchers found that people who exercised were less likely to be unhappy after 2 years and 4 years. In contrast, people who were inactive over time were more than twice as likely to be unhappy as those who remained active. Compared with those who became active, inactive participants who remained inactive were also more likely to become unhappy. As well, people who went from active to inactive were more likely to become unhappy. In short, exercise is associated with maintaining happiness and avoiding unhappiness in the long term.

Satisfaction with life is related to peoples' physical and mental health and is a key determinant of happiness throughout the lifespan. Physical activity is related to enhanced satisfaction with life in a variety of populations, including college students (An et al., 2020). In other words, people report greater satisfaction with life on days when they are more active. What is the relationship between satisfaction with life and sedentary behavior? Jaclyn Maher and her colleagues (Maher, Doerksen, Elavsky, & Conroy, 2014) examined whether physical activity and sedentary behavior were related to satisfaction with life in college students. They selected college students because satisfaction with life appears to worsen more during young adulthood (18 to 25 years) than any other time in the adult lifespan. Thus, college students represent a high-risk group for decreased satisfaction with life. Using an ecological momentary assessment design, they had 128 college students wear an accelerometer to objectively measure physical activity and sedentary behavior for 14 days.

The participants were also asked to complete self-report assessments of their physical activity, sedentary behavior, and satisfaction with life at the end of each day. To assess satisfaction with life, the study used the following single item: "I was satisfied with my life today." The students rated this item on a visual analogue scale ranging from 0 ("strongly disagree") to 100 ("strongly agree"). They found that the students' daily satisfaction with life was related to greater amounts of physical activity and lower amounts of sedentary behavior. In other words, increasing daily physical activity and reducing daily sedentary behavior were associated with increased satisfaction with life in college students.

Smartphones are central to college students' lives, keeping them constantly connected with friends, family, and the Internet. Emerging research is revealing that high cell phone use has negative health outcomes. For example, cell phone use is related to lower cardiorespiratory fitness and more sedentary behavior in college students (Lepp, Jacob, Barkley, & Karpinski, 2014). In another study, Andrew Lepp and his colleagues (2013) found that cell phone use is negatively related to grade point average (GPA) and happiness and positively related to anxiety in college students. In other words, high-frequency cell phone users tended to have lower GPAs, higher anxiety, and lower satisfaction with life (happiness) relative to their peers who used their cell phones less often. These results suggest that students should reduce their cell phone use so that it does not negatively affect their academic performance, mental and physical health, and overall well-being or happiness.

A measure used to assess positive feeling states (including happiness) is the Exercise-Induced Feeling Inventory (Gauvin & Rejeski, 1993). This inventory is a 12-item multidimensional inventory consisting of four 3-item subscales: positive engagement, revitalization, tranquility, and physical exhaustion. Participants are asked to rate the extent to which they are currently experiencing each of the 12 items on a scale ranging from 0 ("do not feel") to 4 ("feel very strongly"). See **Table 6-6** for information on these items. Researchers have found that people report improved positive feelings immediately following exercise compared to their pre-exercise scores (Bryan, Pinto Zipp, & Parasher, 2012; Rendi, Szabo, Szabo, Velenczei, & Kovacs, 2008; Szabo & Abraham, 2013). This positive mood–inducing effect is seen for a variety of exercise types (e.g., aerobic or weight training), exercise levels (regular exercisers, sedentary people), and age groups (young adults and older adults). That is, immediately following exercise, people typically report increased positive engagement, revitalization, and tranquility with decreased physical exhaustion.

Although most of the research reveals that exercise induces positive feelings, there are some

CRITICAL THINKING ACTIVITY 6-5

Does your cell phone use have a positive or negative affect on your exercise behavior?

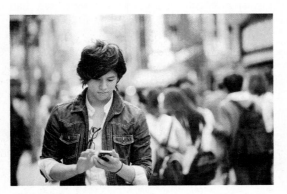

© Johnny Greig/E+/Getty Images.

Table 6-6 Items from the Exercise-Induced Feeling Scale

Subscale	Items
Positive engagement	Enthusiastic Happy Upbeat
Revitalization	Refreshed Energetic Revived
Tranquility	Calm Relaxed Peaceful
Physical exhaustion	Fatigued Tired Worn-out

Gauvin, L., & Rejeski, W. J. (1993). The Exercise-Induced Feeling Inventory: Development and initial validation. *Journal of Sport and Exercise Psychology, 15,* 403–423.

exceptions to this "rule." The positive feeling state effect following exercise is not evidenced in all populations and exercise environments. For example, Brian Focht and his colleagues (Focht, Gauvin, & Rejeski, 2004) found that older, obese adults with knee osteoarthritis did not exhibit improvements in feeling states that are often observed following acute exercise in younger, more physically active populations. In another study, Brian Focht and Heather Hausenblas (2006) found that women with high social physique anxiety only had improvements in their positive feeling states when they exercised alone in a private environment. When these women with high social physique anxiety exercised in a public environment (i.e., co-ed gym), they did not experience improvements in their mood. The researchers hypothesized that for women with high social physique anxiety, exercising in a public co-ed gym is anxiety provoking. This finding suggests that women with body image concerns may have better adherence to home-based or private exercise compared to gym-based exercise programs.

As another example, outdoor exercise tends to result in better improvements in mood and feeling states compared to indoor exercise. Researchers from Canada found that postmenopausal women reported better affective responses to exercise and exercise adherence during outdoor exercise compared to indoor exercise (Lacharite-Lemieux, Brunelle, & Dionne, 2015). In a 12-week trial, the researchers randomized 23 healthy postmenopausal women (age range = 52 to 69 years) to either an outdoor training or an indoor training exercise program. Each participant exercised three times a week for 1-hour durations of both aerobic and resistance training. After the 12 weeks of exercise, the researchers found that the outdoor exercise group had greater improvements in exercise-induced feelings, affect, and depressive symptoms compared to the indoor exercise group. As well, adherence was significantly higher in those who participated in the outdoor exercise program compared to those who participated in the indoor exercise program.

Furthermore, Matthew Fraser and his colleagues (2019) examined the effects of two different types of green exercise – walking and golfing – on participants feeling states. They found that participants who walked outside improved in all four subscales of the Exercise-Induced Feeling Inventory, whereas the participants who golfed showed no significant improvements. Based on the findings, distinct differences were evidenced in the perception of the environment. The golf participants noted natural elements as obstacles to effective performance, whereas the walking participants found that natural stimuli as evoking positive feelings. The researchers concluded that the benefits of green exercise may be reduced when greater levels of directed attention towards the activity are exhibited during green exercise, as with an activity such as golf.

Summary

In this chapter, we examined how physical activity and sedentary behavior affects people's positive mood and health-related quality of life (HRQoL) in a variety of populations. In general, exercise improves people's HRQoL and sedentary behavior decreases people's HRQoL. As well, both acute and chronic bouts of exercise improve our positive mood states. In other words, people who exercise report that they are happier and have more energy than their sedentary counterparts. More research is needed in this emerging field of inquiry.

Vignette: Beverly

I received a devastating diagnosis of cancer shortly after my 34th birthday. My husband and I had begun putting aside money for a second child, and our first was about to turn 6. My husband was the first person who noticed a lump in my left breast. And because my paternal grandmother died of cancer before I was born, I didn't waste any time seeking medical attention.

An ultrasound by the end of the week produced inconclusive but concerning results. So I immediately underwent a biopsy. The 4 days I had to wait for the results were agonizing. I barely slept, ate, or remained emotionally present at the elementary school I then worked at as an English teacher. About 30 days after hearing the confirmation that I had stage 2A breast cancer, I began treatment.

In my case, this meant a mastectomy in order to forgo radiation and an immediate reconstruction. It took me about 3 weeks to fully recover my strength and feel comfortable enough to come off the pain killers I'd been put on. And about the only exercise I could do was to walk slowly around our house while performing the basic arm movements a physical therapist showed me the morning after my surgery.

I continued to work with a physical therapist for months after I was able to return to work. After I was cleared for exercise by my doctor, I went on to work with a personal trainer, who helped me rebuild my upper body strength with a simple weight training regimen and elastic band routine I could do at home. The trainer also helped me find a cardiovascular program appropriate for my energy levels, schedule, and preferred pace of movement. Eventually, she introduced me to cycling.

My husband, a former football player in college, had outfitted our home with a weight rack and treadmill. And once I expressed to him my desire to take charge of my health by making physical activity a regular part of my life, he agreed to join me at a cycling studio that offered daily classes.

It was important to me to impart to my son how important mommy's new routine was now that she was out of the hospital. At first, he was sad that I'd go to the gym after work on most days of the week rather than bring him to baseball or soccer practice. But once I convinced him that my going to the gym was a way for me to stay home for good—and be around to be his mommy for longer—he eventually got the message. In fact, he even started asking me over for dinners, "Mommy, did you do your exercise today?"

Cancer, to me, was a horrifying experience. I've been in remission for 2 years now, but I'm still worried I might not be in the clear. I was diagnosed relatively young, which increases my odds that I could have a reoccurrence. Hence why it's so crucial for me to have not just a means of keeping my body in its healthiest form ever, but also finding activities that keep me feeling empowered and in control of my life.

I derive immense joy from being a mother and a wife and teaching English at the magnet school I now work at, but few things compare to the feeling I get when I reach that 15-mile mark on my bike or when I round the final bend of a 3-mile jog around my neighborhood, make it through 10 pushups without touching my knees on the floor, or reach the peak of the mountain my husband and son hike up with me on some weekends without feeling winded.

I would never in a million years have asked to be diagnosed with cancer. It's a traumatic experience for anyone, and its imprint will always linger in my life, as well as on the lives of everyone who has known and loved me. But that it galvanized me to take charge of my health and be more aware of my body—not to mention the time I have here on earth and its meaning—has indeed been a blessing (albeit a very unexpected, hidden, and conflicting one).

I can honestly say that at 36 I feel healthier than I've ever felt in my life. I have more energy. I enjoy my days more. And I come home from my workouts with more of me to share with the family I deeply and truly love. I will, of course, have to adjust my workout schedule slightly over the next year, because my husband and I are, at long last, finally expecting that second child.

Key Terms

cancer A broad group of diseases characterized by unregulated cell growth.

cancer survivor A person with cancer of any type who is still living.

diabetes A group of diseases that affect how the body uses blood glucose.

happiness A state of mind or a feeling characterized by contentment, love, satisfaction, pleasure, or joy.

health-related quality of life (HRQoL) An assessment of how an individual's quality of life affects their physical, mental, and social health.

positive psychology The study of happiness and how people can become happier and more fulfilled.

quality of life A broad, multidimensional term that encompasses a person's perceived quality of his or her daily life.

standard of living Refers to the level of wealth, comfort, material goods, and necessities available to a certain socioeconomic class in a certain geographic area.

Review Questions

1. Define the terms "quality of life" and "standard of living". How do these two terms differ? Provide examples.
2. Describe the domains of the World Health Organization's conceptualization of quality of life.
3. Define health-related quality of life.
4. The CDC's Healthy Days Core Module items are useful at the national level to identify health disparities and track population trends. Based on the results of surveys using the module, which groups are more at risk for poor HRQoL?
5. What is ecological momentary assessment? Describe an ecological momentary assessment study and its main findings.
6. What is positive psychology? How is positive psychology related to physical activity and sedentary behavior?

Applying the Concepts

1. What HRQoL domains did Beverly's adoption of physical activity help her improve?
2. How did Beverly's standard of living contribute to her overall quality of life, despite having and being in remission from cancer?

References

An, H-Y., Chen, W., Wang, C. W., Yang, H-F., Huang, W-T., et al. (2020). The relationships between physical activity and life satisfaction and happiness among young, middle-aged, and older adults. *International Journal of Environmental Research and Public Health, 17*(13), 4817. https://doi.org/10.3390/ijerph17134817

Anjos, J. M., Neto, M. G., Dos Santos, F., de Oliveira Almeida, K., Bocchi, E. A. et al. (2022). The impact of high-intensity interval training on functioning and health-related quality of life In post-stroke patients: A systematic review with meta-analysis. *Clinical Rehabilitation, 36,* 726–739. https://doi.org/10.1177/02692155221087082

Balboa-Castillo, T., Leon-Munoz, L. M., Rodriquez-Artalejo, F., & Guallar-Castillon, P. (2011). Longitudinal association of physical activity and sedentary behavior during leisure time with health-related quality of life in community-dwelling older adults. *Health and Quality of Life Outcomes, 9*(1), 1–10.

Boberska, M., Szczuka, Z., Kruk, M., Knoll, N., Keller, J., et al. (2018). Sedentary behaviours and health-related quality of life. A systematic review and meta-analysis. *Health Psychology Review, 12*(2), 195–210. https://doi.org/10.1080/17437199.2017.1396191

Bolier, L., Haverman, M., Westerhof, G. J., Riper, H., Smit, F., & Bohlmeijer, E. (2013). Positive psychology interventions: A meta-analysis of randomized controlled studies. *BioMed Central Public Health, 13*(1), 1–20.

Bryan, S., Pinto Zipp, G., & Parasher, R. (2012). The effects of yoga on psychosocial variables and exercise adherence: A randomized, controlled pilot study. *Alternative Therapies in Health & Medicine, 18*(5), 50–59.

Chida, Y., & Steptoe, A. (2008). Positive psychological well-being and mortality: A quantitative review of prospective observational studies. *Psychosomatic Medicine, 70*(7), 741–756.

Degroote, L., DeSmet, A., De Bourdeaudhuij, I., Van Dyck, D., & Crombez, G. (2020). Content validity and methodological considerations in ecological momentary assessment studies on physical activity and sedentary behaviour: A systematic review. *International Journal of Behavioral Nutrition and Physical Activity,* 17(1), 1–13. https://doi.org/10.1186/s12966-020-00932-9

de Vries, L. P., Baselmans, B., & Bartels, M. (2021). Smartphone-based ecological momentary assessment of well-being: A systematic review and recommendations for future studies. *Journal of Happiness Studies, 22*(5), 2361–2408. https://doi.org/10.1007/s10902-020-00324-7

Ekkekakis, P. (2008). Affect, mood, and emotion (Chapter 28). In G. Tenenbaum, R. C. Eklund, & A. Kamata (eds) *Measurement in sport and exercise psychology* (pp. 321–332). Human Kinetics.

Ekkekakis, P. (2013). *The measurement of affect, mood, and emotion.* Cambridge University Press.

Focht, B. C., Gauvin, L., & Rejeski, W. J. (2004). The contribution of daily experiences and acute exercise to fluctuations in daily feeling states among older, obese adults with knee osteoarthritis. *Journal of Behavioral Medicine, 27*(2), 101–121.

Focht, B. C., & Hausenblas, H. A. (2006). Exercising in public and private environments: Effects on feeling states in women with social physique anxiety. *Journal of Applied Biobehavioral Research, 11*(3–4), 147–165.

Fraser, M., Munoz, S-A., & MacRury, S. (2019). Does the mode of exercise influence the benefits obtained by green exercise? *International Journal of Environmental Research and Public Health, 20,* 3004. https://doi.org/10.3390/ijerph16163004

Fuller, J. T., Hartland, M. C., Maloney, L. T., & Davison, K. (2018). Therapeutic effects of aerobic and resistance exercises for cancer survivors: A systematic review of meta-analyses of clinical trials. *British Journal of Sports Medicine, 52*(20):1311. https://doi.org/10.1136/bjsports-2017-098285

Gauvin, L., & Rejeski, W. J. (1993). The exercise-induced feeling inventory: Development and initial validation. *Journal of Sport & Exercise Psychology, 15*(4), 403–423.

Hausenblas, H. A., Gauvin, L., Symons Downs, D., & Duley, A. R. (2008). Effects of abstinence from habitual involvement in regular exercise on feeling states: An ecological momentary assessment study. *British Journal of Health Psychology, 13*(2), 237–255.

Herman, K. M., Hopman, W. M., Vanderkerkhof, E. G., & Rosenberg, M. W. (2012). Physical activity, body mass index, and health-related quality of life in Canadian adults. *Medicine and Science in Sports and Exercise, 44*(4), 625–636.

Imayama, I., Plotnikoff, R. C., Courneya, K. S., & Johnson, J. A. (2011). Determinants of quality of life in adults with type 1 and type 2 diabetes. *Health and Quality of Life Outcomes, 9*(1), 1–9. https://doi.org/10.1186/1477-7525-9-115

International Diabetes Foundation. (2021). Diabetes atlas. Retrieved April 13, 2014, from https://diabetesatlas.org/

Kanning, M., & Schlicht, W. (2010). Be active and become happy: An ecological momentary assessment of physical activity and mood. *Journal of Sport and Exercise Psychology, 32*(2), 253–261.

Lacharite-Lemieux, M., Brunelle, J. P., & Dionne, I. J. (2015). Adherence to exercise and affective responses: Comparison between outdoor and indoor training. *Menopause, 22*(7), 731–740.

Latimer-Cheung, A. E., Pilutti, L. A., Hicks, A. L., Martin Ginis, K. A., Fenuta, A. M., MacKibbon, K. A., & Motl, R. W. (2013). Effects of exercise training on fitness, mobility, fatigue, and health-related quality of life among adults with multiple sclerosis: A systematic review to inform guideline development. *Archives of Physical Medicine and Rehabilitation, 94*(9), 1800–1823.

Lavados-Romo, P., Andrade-Mayorga, O., Morales, G., Muñoz, S., & Balboa-Castillo, T. (2021). Association of screen time and physical activity with health-related quality of life in college students. *Journal of the American College of Health,* 1–6. https://doi.org/10.1080/07448481.2021.1942006

Leaf, D. E., Tysinger, B., Goldman, D. P., & Lakdawalla, D. N. (2021). Predicting quantity and quality of life with the Future Elderly Model. *Health Economics, 30* (Suppl 1): 52–79. https://doi.org/10.1002/hec.4169

Lepp, A., Barkley, J. E., Sanders, G. J., Rebold, M., & Gates, P. (2013). The relationship between cell phone use, physical and sedentary activity, and cardiorespiratory fitness in a sample of U.S. college students. *International Journal of Behavioral Nutrition and Physical Activity, 10*(1), 1–9. https://doi.org/10.1186/1479-5868-10-79

Lepp, A., Jacob E., Barkley, A., & Karpinski, C. (2014). The relationship between cell phone use, academic performance, anxiety, and satisfaction with life in college students. *Computers in Human Behavior, 31,* 343–350. https://doi.org/10.1016/j.chb.2013.10.049

Li, C., Chang, H-Y., Hsu, C-C., Lu, J. & Fang, H-L. (2013). Joint predictability of health-related quality of life and leisure time physical activity on mortality risk in people with diabetes. *BioMed Central Public Health, 13*(1), 1–10.

Luncheon, C., & Zack, M. (2011). Peer Reviewed: Health-related quality of life and the physical activity levels of middle-age women, California Health Interview Survey, 2005. *Preventing Chronic Disease, 8*(2), A36.

Maher, J. P., Doerksen, S. E., Elavsky, S., & Conroy, D. E. (2014). Daily satisfaction with life is regulated by both physical activity and sedentary behavior. *Journal of Sport and Exercise Psychology, 36*(2), 166–178.

Maher, J. P., Doerksen, S. E., Elavsky, S., Hyde, A. L., Pincus, A. L., Ram, N., & Conroy, D. E. (2013). A daily analysis of physical activity and satisfaction with life in emerging adults. *Health Psychology, 32*(6), 647–656.

Marker, A. M., Steele, R. G., & Nose, A. E. (2018). Physical activity and health-related quality of life in children and adolescents: A systematic review and meta-analysis. *Health Psychology, 37*(10), 893–903. https://doi.org/10.1037/hea0000653

Marquez, D. X., Aguiñaga, S., Vásquez, P. M., Conroy, D. E., Erickson, K. I., et al. A systematic review of physical activity and quality of life and well-being (2020). *Translational Behavioral Medicine, 10*(5), 1098–1109. https://doi.org/10.1093/tbm/ibz198

Martin Luther King, Jr. (n.d.). BrainyQuote.com. Retrieved September 13, 2015, from BrainyQuote.com. http://www.brainyquote.com/quotes/quotes/m/martinluth297515.html

Matheson, G. (2014). Changing level of physical activity and changing degree of happiness. *Clinical Journal of Sport Medicine, 24*(2), 162–163.

Mishra, S I., Scherer, R. W., Geigle, P. M., Berlanstein, D. R., Topaloglu, O., Gotay, C. C., & Snyder, C. (2012a). Exercise interventions on health-related quality of life for cancer survivors. *Cochrane Database Systematic Reviews*, (8). https://doi.org/10.1002/14651858.CD007566.pub2

Mishra, S. I., Scherer, R. W., Snyder, C., Geigle, P. M., Berlanstein, D. R., & Topaloglu, O. (2012b). Exercise interventions on health-related quality of life for people with cancer during active treatment. *Cochrane Database Systematic Reviews*, (8). https://doi.org/10.1002/14651858.CD008465.pub2

National Center for Chronic Disease Prevention and Health Promotion. (2011). HRQOL tables and maps. Retrieved March 7, 2014, from https://www.cdc.gov/hrqol/index.htm

Mokhatri-Hesari, P., & Montazeri, A. (2020). Health-related quality of life in breast cancer patients: Review of reviews from 2008 to 2018. *Health and Quality of Life Outcomes, 18*(1), 1–26. https://doi.org/10.1186/s12955-020-01591-x

Nobari, H., Fashi, M., Eskandari, A., Villafaina, S., Murillo-Garcia, A., & Pérez-Gómez, J. (2021). Effect of COVID-19 on health-related quality of life in adolescents and children: A systematic review. *International Journal of Environmental Research and Public Health, 18*(9), 4563.

Pengpid, S., & Peltzer, K. (2019). Sedentary behaviour, physical activity and life satisfaction, happiness and perceived health status in university students from 24 countries. *International Journal of Environmental Research and Public Health, 16*(12), 2084. https://doi.org/10.3390/ijerph16122084

Puetz, T. W., Beasman, K. M., & O'Connor, P. J. (2006). The effect of cardiac rehabilitation exercise programs on feelings of energy and fatigue: A meta-analysis of research from 1945 to 2005. *European Journal of Cardiovascular Prevention and Rehabilitation, 13*(6), 886–893.

Puetz, T. W., Flowers, S. S., & O'Connor, P. J. (2008). A randomized controlled trial of the effect of aerobic exercise training on feelings of energy and fatigue in sedentary young adults with persistent fatigue. *Psychotherapy and Psychosomatics, 77*(3), 167–174.

Puetz, T. W., O'Connor, P. J., & Dishman, R. K. (2006b). Effects of chronic exercise on feelings of energy and fatigue: A quantitative synthesis. *Psychological Bulletin, 132*(6), 866–876.

Reina-Gutiérrez, S., Cavero-Redondo, I., Martínez-Vizcaíno, V., Núñez de Arenas-Arroyo, S., López-Muñoz, P., Álvarez-Bueno, C., Guzmán-Pavón, M. J., & Torres-Costoso, A. (2022). The type of exercise most beneficial for quality of life in people with multiple sclerosis: A network meta-analysis. *Annals of Physical and Rehabilitation Medicine, 65*(3):101578. https://doi.org/10.1016/j.rehab.2021.101578. Epub 2021 Nov 22.

Rendi, M., Szabo, A., Szabo, T., Velenczei, A., & Kovacs, A. (2008). Acute psychological benefits of aerobic exercise: A field study into the effects of exercise characteristics. *Psychology, Health& Medicine, 13*(2), 180–184.

Richards, J., Jiang, X., Kelly, P., Chau, J., Bauman, A., & Ding, D. (2015). Don't worry, be happy: Cross-sectional associations between physical activity and happiness in 15 European countries. *BioMed Central Public Health, 15*(1), 1–8. https://doi.org/10.1186/s12889-015-1391-4

Rodriguez-Ayllon, M., Cadenas-Sánchez, C., Estévez-López, F., Muñoz, N. E., Mora-Gonzalez, J. et al. (2019). Role of physical activity and sedentary behavior in the mental health of preschoolers, children and adolescents: A systematic review and meta-analysis. *Sports Medicine, 49*(9), 1383–1410. https://doi.org/10.1007/s40279-019-01099-5

Seligman, M. E., Steen, T. A., Park, N., & Peterson, C. (2005). Positive psychology progress: Empirical validation of interventions. *The American Psychologist, 60*(5), 410–421.

Sivaramakrishnan, D., Fitzsimons, C., Kelly, P., Ludwig, K., Mutrie, N., Saunders, D. H., & Baker, G. (2019). The effects of yoga compared to active and inactive controls on physical function and health related quality of life in older adults- systematic review and meta-analysis of randomised controlled trials. *International Journal of Behavioral Nutrition and Physical Activity, 16*(1), 1–22. https://doi.org/10.1186/s12966-019-0789-2

Snedden, T. R., Scerpella, J., Kliethermes, S. A., Norman, R. S., Blyholder, L., et al. (2019). Sport and physical activity level impacts health-related quality of life among collegiate students, *American Journal of Health Promotion, 33*(5): 675–682. https://doi.org/10.1177/0890117118817715

Soares-Miranda, L., Lucia, A., Silva, M., Peixoto, A., Ramalho, R., Correia da Silva, P., et al. (2021). Physical fitness and health-related quality of life in patients with colorectal cancer. *International Journal of Sports Medicine, 42*(10), 924–929. https://doi.org/10.1055/a-1342-7347

Stevens, C. J., Baldwin, A. S., Bryan, A. D., Conner, M., Rhodes, R. E., & Williams, D. M. (2020). Affective determinants of physical activity: A conceptual framework and narrative review. *Frontiers in Psychology, 11*(568331), 1–19.

Sung, H., Ferlay, J., Siegel, R. L., Laversanne, M., Soerjomataram, I., Jemal, A., & Bray, F. (2021). Global cancer statistics 2020: GLOBOCAN estimates of incidence and mortality worldwide for 36 cancers in 185 countries. *CA: Cancer Journal for Clinicians, 71*(3), 209–249. https://doi.org/10 .3322/caac.21660

Szabo, A., & Abraham, J. (2013). The psychological benefits of recreational running: A field study. *Psychology, Health, & Medicine, 18*(3), 251–261.

Thiel, D. M., Sayah, F. A., Vallance, J. K., Johnson, S. T. & Johnson, J. A. (2017). Association between physical activity and health-related quality of life in adults with type 2 diabetes. *Canadian Journal of Diabetes, 41*(1), 58–63. https://doi.org/10.1016/j.jcjd.2016.07.004

Wang, F., Orpanan, H. M., Morrison, H., de Groh, M., Dai, S., & Luo, W. (2012). Long-term association between leisure-time physical activity and changes in happiness: Analysis of the Prospective National Population Health Survey. *American Journal of Epidemiology, 176*(2), 1095–1100.

Whitaker, K. M., Jones, M. A., Wallace, M. K., Catov, J., & Gibbs, B. B. (2022). Associations of objectively measured physical activity and sedentary time with pregnancy-specific health-related quality of life. *Midwifery, 104,* 103202. https://doi.org/10.1016/j.midw.2021.103202

World Health Organization. (2012). WHOQOL. Measuring quality of life. Retrieved October 26, 2022, from https:// www.who.int/tools/whoqol

World Health Organization. (2012). GLOBOCAN 2012: Estimated cancer incidence, mortality, and prevalence worldwide in 2012. Retrieved April 8, 2014, from http:// globocan.iarc.fr/Pages/fact_ sheets_cancer.aspx

World Health Organization. (2014). *Ageing.* Retrieved April 16, 2014, from http://www.who.int/ageing/en/

Yan, R., Che, B., Lv, B., Wu, P., Lu, X., Zhang, X., et al. (2021). The association between physical activity, sedentary time and health-related quality of life in cancer survivors. *Health and Quality Life Outcomes, 19*(1), 1–12. https://doi .org/10.1186/s12955-020-01575-x

Yasunaga, A., Shibata, A., Ishii, K., Inoue, S., Sugiyama, T., et al., (2018). Replacing sedentary time with physical activity: Effects on health-related quality of life in older Japanese adults. *Health and Quality of Life Outcomes, 16*(1), 1–5. https://doi.org/10.1186/s12955-018-1067-8

Zack, M. M. (2013). Health-related quality of life—United States, 2006 and 2010. *Morbidity and Mortality Weekly Report, 62*(Suppl 3), 105–111.

Zack, M. M., Moriarty, D. G., Stroup, D. F., Ford, E. S., & Mokdad, A. H. (2004). Worsening trends in adult health-related quality of life and self-rated health-United States, 1993–2001. *Public Health Reports, 119*(5), 493–506.

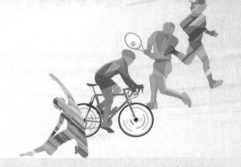

CHAPTER 7

Personality Traits

LEARNING OBJECTIVES

After completing this chapter, you will be able to:

- Describe the history of trait psychology and the main personality traits used to understand human behavior.
- Discuss the research that has applied the five-factor and three-factor models of personality to physical activity and sedentary behavior.
- Discuss the advantages and limitations of using personality traits to customize interventions to increase physical activity.

Introduction

Have you ever tried to characterize yourself or another person in terms of a general disposition? Do you consider yourself sociable or upbeat? Have you ever suggested that someone is a kind or gentle person? Are there other times where you have suggested that someone is generally mean-spirited or selfish? If you have made these characterizations, then you may be operating on the underlying assumption that people behave in stable and enduring patterns of behavior, thoughts, and feelings. You are describing **personality trait** psychology. In this chapter, we will outline the history of trait psychology, overview the structure of the most popular personality models, discuss the relationship between personality and physical activity and sedentary behavior, and conclude with the contemporary evidence for how personality may be used in physical activity interventions.

Personality theory has a rich history, tracing back to Hippocrates' treatise "On the Nature of Man" (460 BC), which proposed that individual differences in emotions and behavior were based on four bodily humours: sanguine, phlegmatic, choleric, and melancholic (Stelmack & Stalikas, 1991). While the theory lost favor as science advanced, the basic foundations that: 1) typologies can be observed from a person's emotions and behavior, and 2) these typologies are linked to physiology are still critical to personality theory. Personality research was the source of several spirited debates over the 20th century (Digman, 1990; McCrae & Costa, 1995; Wiggins, 1997). Early 20th century personality theory (Jung, 1923; Sheldon & Stevens, 1942) reiterated the notion of somatotypes (i.e., the idea that body types determined personality), although this was also eventually refuted (e.g., Hammond, 1957; Lerner, 1969; Slaughter, 1970). Debates in the second half of the 20th century focused on whether people are influenced by the situation and not individual personality differences (Mischel, 1968) and whether personality traits are actually mechanisms/causes of behavior

(Costa & McCrae, 2009). Some scientists believe that personality is a reflection of a person's neurology or physiology and is thus controlled by a person's genes. They refer to personality traits as being genotypic. By contrast, others suggest that personality merely describes behavior, and thus refer to personality traits as being phenotypic. They do not describe how the behavior is caused.

In the last 30 years; however, personality researchers have amassed a considerable body of evidence to support the importance of personality traits as mechanisms of behavior. This research has provided evidence that personality is structured similarly across over 50 cultures (Costa & McCrae, 2009; McCrae et al., 2000), can be inherited through your genetics (Jang et al., 1996; Riemann et al., 1997), has high stability across time with a predictable life-course trajectory (Roberts et al., 2006), are related to childhood temperament (Rothbart et al., 2000, Rothbart, 2007), and does not relate strongly to parental rearing style (Costa & McCrae, 2009; McCrae et al., 2000).

CRITICAL THINKING ACTIVITY 7-1

Although personality is considered unchangeable and consistent, it is thought to stabilize in early adulthood and show some minor variability across adult life (Costa & McCrae, 2009). Think of your own personality: have you changed in sociability, conscientiousness, or openness since the beginning of high school? What changed? What stayed consistent?

In the past, there has been a lack of agreement over the basic definition of personality. In this chapter, we use the definition provided by the American Psychological Association that *personality* is defined as "individual differences in characteristic patterns of thinking, feeling and behaving" (American Psychological Association, 2020). Overall, personality traits represent enduring and consistent individual differences across the lifespan (McCrae et al., 2000; Roberts, Walton, & Viechtbauer, 2006). Many researchers further theorize that personality has an evolutionary/biological/genetic basis (Gray, 1991;

Zuckerman, 2005) but that the expression of a trait is still culturally and environmentally conditioned (Eysenck, 1970; Funder, 2001; McCrae et al., 2000). For example, a student with high **extraversion** may choose to socialize a lot more with friends in their free time than a student lower on extraversion, but both individuals will choose not to talk during class because this is a cultural standard of respect for one's teacher and fellow students. This has direct implications for how personality integrates with social, cognitive, and environmental models to explain physical activity, and we will discuss this later in the chapter.

Structure of Personality

Another major area of debate and active scholarship over the last 80 years has been on the creation of working models of personality. Researchers have asked and attempted to answer questions like: How many personality traits do we have? Which traits are the most important? How do traits relate to each other? The person who started this process—the proverbial grandfather of all personality trait research—was Gordon Allport. Allport (1937) surmised that the best way to start answering these questions was through the use of language. This was based on the premise that all important human feelings, characteristics, and behaviors would be present in our language. Basically, if something was important, he assumed we would have created a word for it. His assumption became known as the fundamental lexical

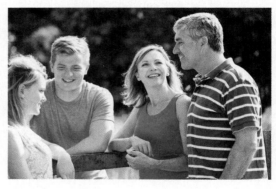

© Monkey Business Images/Shutterstock.

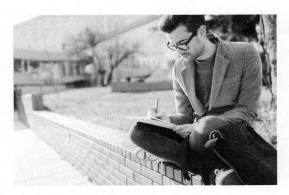

© Supersizer/iStock/Getty Images Plus/Getty Images.

hypothesis. Allport and his colleagues identified 18,000 potential human traits by looking up these descriptions in English dictionaries (Allport & Odbert, 1936).

Of course, 18,000 traits do not make for a very parsimonious theory of personality! Certainly, some of these words are synonyms for each other, and other words may be representative of a collection of other words. In order to make sense of all of these potential descriptors, researchers began to reduce these data with the use of analytical techniques called factor analysis (Guilford & Guilford, 1934). Factor analysis reduces data to common elements. With the use of factor analysis and careful scrutiny of the English terms, Raymond Cattell (1947) identified 16 traits that he felt characterized the larger collection of traits. This 16PF (i.e., personality factors) became the dominant trait framework of the 1950s and 1960s. These traits include warmth, reasoning, emotional stability, dominance, liveliness, rule-consciousness, social boldness, sensitivity, vigilance, abstractness, privateness, apprehension, openness to change, self-reliance, perfectionism, and tension. Cattell also developed 5 *supertraits* that encompass these 16 more specific traits. These included extraversion, anxiety, tough-mindedness, independence, and self-control.

Taking the supertrait approach to understanding personality, Eysenck developed his theory with two factors: (1) extraversion-introversion (i.e., the tendency to be sociable, assertive, energetic, seek excitement, and experience positive affect) and (2) neuroticism-emotional stability (i.e., the

tendency to be emotionally unstable, anxious, self-conscious, and vulnerable) (Eysenck & Eysenck, 1963). More than his predecessors, Eysenck also theorized that personality traits had a biological and genetic basis. He suggested that extraversion and **neuroticism** could be linked to biological systems and brain chemistry. He later added a third trait called **psychoticism** (i.e., risk taking, impulsiveness, irresponsibility, manipulativeness, sensation-seeking, tough-mindedness, non-pragmatism) to his model (Eysenck, 1970). This model serves as one of the dominant frameworks of personality to the present day.

Still, during the mid-20th century, personality trait psychology suffered from an abundance of investigator-created traits and independent research agendas (Digman, 1990). Because of this, it was difficult for research to advance with any common theoretical model. A move toward a common trait taxonomy has helped bridge this gap. The most popular personality model at present is a five-factor taxonomy (see **Table 7-1**).

This model suggests that neuroticism (i.e., the tendency to be emotionally unstable, anxious, self-conscious, and vulnerable); extraversion (i.e., the tendency to be sociable, assertive, energetic, seek excitement, and experience positive affect); **openness to experience/ intellect** (i.e., the tendency to be perceptive, creative, reflective, and appreciate fantasy and

CRITICAL THINKING ACTIVITY 7-2

For some people, all of the subtrait descriptions explain them very well. For example, some extraverts are active, social, positive, and adventurous. Other people may express one particular facet more than others. For example, someone may be super orderly but not score as high on self-discipline, although both are facet traits of conscientiousness. The difference highlights why some researchers prefer the specific facet traits to understand people, whereas others prefer the more general supertraits. Look at the descriptors for each of the five factors. Is there one facet that best describes you, or do they all describe you about the same?

Table 7-1 **Primary Factor Descriptions for the Five Factor Model of Personality**

Characteristic tendencies of individuals scoring on the high or low end of each bipolar dimension of the Big Five personality factors.

Trait Dimension		Characteristic Tendencies
Extraversion	(+) Extravert	Sociable; assertive; energetic; excitement seeking; affectionate; talkative; friendly; warm; spontaneous; active; propensity towards positive affect.
	(−) Introvert	Reclusive; reserved; aloof; quiet; inhibited; passive; cold; propensity toward negative affect under conditions of high stimulation.
Neuroticism	(+) Neurotic	Emotionally reactive/unstable; anxious; self-conscious; vulnerable; high-strung; worrying; insecure.
	(−) Emotionally stable	Calm; emotionally stable; secure; relaxed; self-satisfied; comfortable; unperturbed.
Conscientiousness	(+) Conscientious	Orderly; dutiful; self-disciplined; achievement oriented; reliable; persevering; hardworking; punctual; neat; careful; well-organized.
	(−) Undirected	Disorganized; negligent; undependable; poor time management/planning skills; lacking self-discipline.
Openness	(+) Open-minded	Reflective; perceptive; creative; welcoming; unconventional; non-traditional; intellectual; original; imaginative; daring; complex; independent; broad interests.
	(−) Closed-minded	Simple; pragmatic; conforming; traditional; unadventurous; "down to earth"; conventional; uncreative; narrow interests.
Agreeableness	(+) Agreeable	Lighthearted; easy going; cooperative; kind; optimistic; altruistic; trustworthy; generous; soft-hearted; forgiving; sympathetic; acquiescent; selfless; good-natured; lenient; trusting.
	(−) Antagonistic	Ruthless; vengeful; callous; selfish; irritable; critical; suspicious; argumentative; cynical; competitive.

Wilson, K.E. & Rhodes, R.E. (2021). Personality and physical activity. In Z. Zenko & L. Jones (Eds.), Essentials of exercise and sport psychology: An open access textbook (pp. 114–149). *Society for the Transparency, Openness, and Replication in Kinesiology.*

aesthetics); **agreeableness** (i.e., tendency to be kind, cooperative, altruistic, trustworthy, and generous); and **conscientiousness** (i.e., the tendency to be ordered, dutiful, self-disciplined, and achievement oriented) are the basic factors of personality structure.

Similar to the work of both Cattell and Eysenck, these common-factor taxonomies are thought to represent the basic building blocks of personality, and subsequently cause the expression of more specific subtraits (Costa & McCrae, 2009). Thus, individuals high in extraversion may express this higher-order trait through excitement seeking, sociability, a positive outlook, and energetic activity.

Mixtures of these five factors of personality may also produce traits of interest. For example, type A behavior (Jenkins, 1976) may be a combination of high extraversion, high neuroticism, low agreeableness, and high conscientiousness. Although it is important to continue with a higher-order supertrait understanding of personality and behavior, these facets or specific traits may help define the relationship between personality and specific behaviors such as physical activity (Costa & McCrae, 1992). The greater specificity provided by these facet traits allows for a more precise understanding of personality relationships with an outcome variable; indeed, it is this higher level of specificity and its applied value in understanding traits and behavior that defines the facet approach (Costa & McCrae, 1995). In the next section, we review the research conducted on both supertraits and their more specific facet traits and physical activity.

Personality and Physical Activity

Although several pathways for how personality interacts with health have been postulated, the main focus in this chapter is the evidence that personality traits influence physical activity through a health behavior model (Wiebe & Smith, 1997). This position suggests that the principal impact of personality on health-oriented behaviors is through the quality of one's health practices. More specifically, personality is hypothesized to affect social cognitions (e.g., perceptions, attitudes, norms, self-efficacy) toward a behavior, which, in turn, influence the health behavior itself (Ajzen, 1991; Bogg, Voss, Wood, & Roberts, 2008; McCrae & Costa, 1995; Rhodes, 2006; Wilson, 2019). We overview the evidence for this chain of personality to social cognition to physical activity later in the chapter; still, the first consideration should be whether there is any evidence for a physically active personality.

Research on personality and physical activity has spanned over 50 years. While early work considered sport performance and the potential impact of physical activity on personality (Eysenck, Nias, & Cox, 1982), more recent approaches have focused on physical activity and the health behavior model. In 2006, Rhodes and Smith reviewed and systematically appraised the relationship between personality and physical activity for Eysenck's (1970) three-factor model, the five-factor model, and Cattel's (1947) 16 personality factors among 35 samples. More recent meta-analyses extend these findings. Wilson and Dishman (2015) conducted a meta-analysis of 64 studies on the application of the five factor model and physical activity, and Sutin and colleagues (2016) conducted a more selected meta-analysis of 16 population samples. The results of these meta-analyses of the five-factor model can be found in **Figure 7-1**.

Rhodes and Smith (2006) found small positive associations between extraversion ($r = 0.23$), conscientiousness ($r = 0.20$) and physical activity and a small negative relationship with neuroticism ($r = -0.11$). The findings identified no meaningful association between agreeableness and openness to experience and physical activity. Rhodes and Smith (2006) further concluded that age, sex, and study design did not appear to affect the overall results of these analyses, but they did suggest that European studies had a lower correlation between extraversion and physical activity compared to North American studies.

The more recent Wilson and Dishman (2015) and Sutin and colleagues (2016) meta-analyses found generally similar outcomes to the earlier Rhodes and Smith (2006) study. Both of the more recent meta-analyses found positive associations between extraversion (both $r = 0.11$) and conscientiousness (both $r = 0.10$) and physical activity and negative associations with neuroticism (both $r = -0.07$). Overall, these reviews lead to the conclusion that physical activity has a reliable, yet small positive association with extraversion and conscientiousness. Neuroticism has a negative relationship with physical activity, but the association may not be practically relevant. Study design characteristics were formally

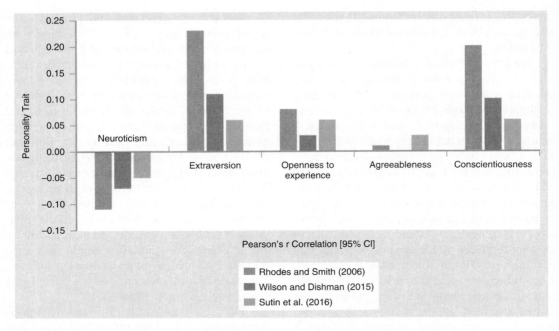

Figure 7-1 Relationship Between the Five-Factor Model and Personality.

Data from Rhodes, R. E., & Smith, N. E. I. (2006). Personality correlates of physical activity: A review and meta-analysis. *British Journal of Sports Medicine, 40,* 958–965. Wilson, K. E., & Dishman, R. K. (2015). Personality and physical activity: A systematic review and meta-analysis. *Personality and Individual Differences, 72,* 230–242. Sutin, A. R., Stephan, Y., Luchetti, M., Artese, A., Oshio, A., & Terracciano, A. (2016). The five-factor model of personality and physical inactivity: A meta-analysis of 16 samples. *Journal of Research in Personality, 63,* 22–28.

examined as moderators of the effects in the Wilson and Dishman (2015) meta-analysis. While nearly all of the deviations were not in a meaningful effect size range (Cohen, 1992), the findings with extraversion also corroborated the prior review by Rhodes and Smith (2006) showing larger correlations in samples from North American compared to samples from Europe. The evidence also suggests that personality and physical activity relationships are not dependent on specific demographic characteristics but there may be some differences by the type of physical activity and geographic region.

When taken together, it appears that neuroticism, extraversion, and conscientiousness are the most reliable, yet small, correlates of physical activity. Extraversion concerns the differences in preference for social interaction and lively activity (Eysenck, 1970; McCrae & Costa, 1995). The seeking out of physical activity behaviors appears a logical extension for people high in this trait, whereas the disinterest in physical activity

seems likely for those low in extraversion (Eysenck et al., 1982). Individuals high in neuroticism represent those people with less emotional stability and more distress, anxiety, and depression than those with lower neuroticism.

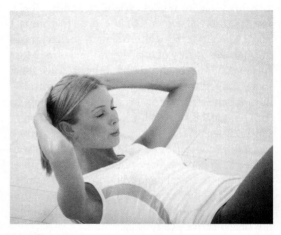

© Goodluz/Shutterstock.

Avoidance of physical activity or cancellation of physical activity plans is a logical extension of this trait. The relationship between conscientiousness and health behaviors more generally also has been established (Booth-Kewley & Vickers, 1994; O'Connor, Conner, Jones, McMillan, & Ferguson, 2009). In fact, Bogg and Roberts (2013) emphasize conscientiousness as an important epidemiological factor that protects against mortality. High scores on conscientiousness represent a purposeful, self-disciplined individual (Digman, 1990; McCrae & Costa, 1995), suggesting that this factor may be important in terms of adherence behavior. The predisposition to maintain physical activity behavior appears to be logical for individuals who possess higher conscientiousness than their low conscientiousness counterparts and partly underpin one's self-control over impulsive decision-making (Mao et al., 2018).

Personality and Physical Activity Preferences

Physical activity is a complex concept and cannot be captured comprehensively with any one measurement method because different physical activities are characterized with different skill requirements and energy expenditures (Ainsworth et al., 2011; Pate et al., 1995). It may be that the relationship between personality traits and physical activity are best understood by different types or characterizations of physical activity. With this in mind, Rhodes and Smith (2006) and Wilson and Dishman (2015) also examined specific physical activity characteristics and personality. Specifically, Rhodes and Smith noted that strenuous and moderate-intensity modalities of physical activity may be associated with personality factors of neuroticism, extraversion, and conscientiousness more than lower-intensity activities. This possibility was formally examined and corroborated in the Wilson and Dishman (2015) meta-analysis. They showed that extraversion and physical activity were intensity dependent, where the relationship with physical activity was larger

for moderate-to-vigorous physical activity (r = .13) than for mild-to-moderate physical activity (r = .04). This effect was exemplified in a specific study of participation in different physical activities conducted by Howard, Cunningham, and Rechnitzer (1987). The authors found that high-extraversion individuals were more likely to engage in swimming, aerobic conditioning, dancing, and tennis. By contrast, less extraverted individuals were more inclined to engage in gardening and home improvement, while no differences were identified for walking, jogging, golf, and cycling. A more recent study replicated and extended these results, and showed there was no relationship between neuroticism, extraversion, or conscientiousness and leisure-time walking (Rhodes, Courneya, Blanchard, & Plotnikoff, 2007). One might expect, based on these findings, that extraversion predicts participation in higher intensity activities, such as those endorsed in national physical activity recommendations (U.S. Department of Health and Human Services, 2018, World Health Organization, 2020), highlighting the potential importance that those with higher introversion may be at risk and require intensified physical activity promotion considerations.

Wilson and Dishman (2015) also showed that the association between conscientiousness and how physical activity was measured mattered. Conscientiousness was linked more to the frequency of activity (r = .21) than quantity (r = .06) or volume (r = .07). (Wilson & Dishman, 2015). It may be that the propensity to plan and be dutiful in high conscientiousness individuals is linked more to the number of times physical activity is scheduled and not the behavior itself.

A recent meta-analysis of 39 studies also highlighted significant positive relationships between extraversion, facet traits impulsivity and sensation seeking, with participation in high-risk sports like skydiving, mountain climbing, surfing, or hang-gliding, among others (McEwan, Boudreau, Curran, & Rhodes, 2019). Participation in these types of activities was also negatively associated with neuroticism. One of the earliest examinations in this area was a study on

Preferences for Exercise and Personality

Courneya & Hellsten (1998) conducted a study with undergraduate students to explore how personality traits relate to physical activity preferences. Those who preferred moderate-to-vigorous physical activity scored low on neuroticism. Not surprisingly, extraversion was related to preferences for exercising with others (e.g., group or supervised exercise) rather than alone. Those reporting an openness to experience had several preferences, including outdoor activity (rather than home or gym), recreational activity (rather than competitive), unsupervised exercise, and spontaneous (rather than scheduled) activity. Interestingly, those who scored higher for agreeableness preferred aerobics to weight-training (Courneya & Hellsten, 1998). Finally, conscientiousness was associated with a preference for scheduled activity and high intensity, rather than moderate intensity exercise. These findings show that personality traits may affect many different preferences for physical activities and assist practitioners in suggesting activities that are more likely to match a client's personality to help with sustaining adherence.

skydiving, where Hymbaugh and Garrett (1974) reported higher levels of sensation seeking scores for skydivers compared to a normative control group. It is possible that individuals with strong sensation seeking, which involves a willingness to take physical risks for the attainment of novel, varied, and intense sensations/experiences (Zuckerman, 2005), seek high risk physical activities as a logical extension of this desire. Neuroticism is characterized by feelings such as worry, fear, and anxiety (Costa & McCrae, 1995), so its seems sensible that individuals who are inclined toward neuroticism would be less likely to participate in high risk sports. McEwan et al. did not show a relationship between high-risk sports and conscientiousness and agreeableness, which is interesting. While it may be tempting to label high-risk sport participants as reckless and disagreeable, participants are no more reckless,

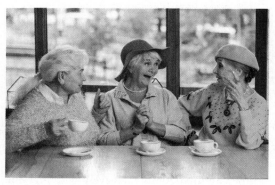

© DenisProduction.com/Shutterstock.

non-conformist, or angry than individuals who do not partake in such activities.

Lower-Order Traits

As mentioned earlier in the chapter, the super-traits featured in the five-and three-factor models are very useful for understanding the basic building blocks of personality structure, but more specific underlying traits may describe exercise behavior and physical activity better. Rhodes and Pfaeffli (2012) reviewed the evidence among 29 peer-reviewed studies and 42 samples for several of these more specific traits and their relationship with physical activity.

One of the most popular traits applied to health behavior is type A personality. **Type A personality** gained popularity from its association with coronary heart disease (Jenkins, 1976).

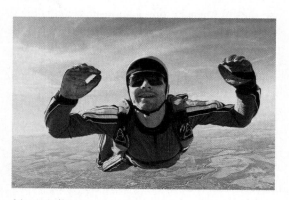

© Germanskydiver/Shutterstock.

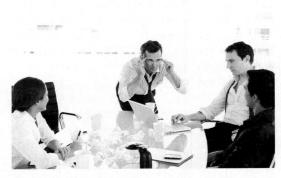

© AIMSTOCK/iStock/Getty Images Plus/Getty Images.

It is marked by a blend of competitiveness and hostility with agitated behavior and continual movement patterns; thus, physical activity could conceivably be a natural extension of type A individuals. Rhodes and Pfaeffli reviewed six studies that appraised the relationship between type A personality and physical activity. Overall, five of the six studies showed some significant positive association between type A personality and physical activity in the small to medium effect size range.

Another trait that has received some research attention in the physical activity domain is optimism. Dispositional optimism is defined as generalized expectations of positive outcomes. It stands to reason that individuals with high optimism would conceivably hold higher regard for the positive health benefits of physical activity, and perhaps participate more than their more pessimistic (or less optimistic) counterparts. Rhodes and Pfaeffli (2012), however, found no support for optimism as a correlate.

Extraversion's **activity trait** represents a disposition toward a fast lifestyle and being high energy, fast talking, and keeping busy, as opposed to a more laissez-faire disposition. These properties could conceivably make regular physical activity a behavior of choice given its energy demands. Rhodes and Pfaeffli's (2012) literature review identified six studies that have applied the activity trait of extraversion with physical activity. In all cases, the activity trait showed a medium to large effect-size correlation with behavior ($r = 0.24$ to $r = 0.52$). More compelling, the three direct tests that compared the predictive capacity of activity against the supertrait of extraversion showed the superiority of the activity trait. Overall, the results suggest that extraversion's activity trait is a reliable and strong predictor of physical activity. The authors speculated that extraversion's activity trait makes regular physical activity a natural behavior of choice given its energy demands (Rhodes & Pfaeffli, 2012).

Extraversion's sociability facet trait is often considered its cornerstone (Costa & McCrae, 1995). People high in sociability prefer the company of others and gravitate to social situations with people. The social component that accompanies many physical activities could therefore make for a logical outlet among highly sociable people. To this end, sociability had been assessed for its relationship with physical activity in six studies (Rhodes & Pfaeffli, 2012). Only two of these studies supported a relationship between sociability and physical activity, suggesting that it may not be a reliable correlate.

Complementary to the examination of extraversion's facet traits, conscientiousness's facet of **industriousness-ambition** has also received attention in four studies (Rhodes & Pfaeffli, 2012). The trait comprises aspects of achievement-striving and self-discipline, and a natural extension of this type of disposition could be regular exercise given its challenge, impact on health and appearance, and self-regulatory barriers. Three of the four studies found a significant relationship between this trait and behavior, suggesting that it may be the critical link between conscientiousness and physical activity. Despite this association, Rhodes and Pfaeffli (2012) noted that the industriousness-ambition and physical activity relationship does not seem to hold once extraversion's activity facet is controlled for in multivariate analyses. Thus, many aspects of conscientiousness and industriousness—ambition related to physical activity are most likely accounted for by the activity trait.

Since the review by Rhodes and Pfaeffli (2012), some research has investigated people with "distressed"or **type D personalities**, which reflect tendencies to experience higher levels of negative affect and social inhibition (Denollet, 1998). Those with high type D personalities were found to participate in significantly less physical activity than non-type D personalities (Borkoles, Polman, & Levy, 2010). In addition, the facet trait of **grit** (i.e., the tendency to persevere and be passionate about long-term goals) was found to correlate with adherence to a moderate and high intensity exercise (Reed, Pritschet, & Cutton, 2013). Similar to grit, Gerber et al. (2012) found that mental toughness was associated with meeting physical activity guidelines for adolescents.

How Does Personality Affect Physical Activity?

Personality theorists and social psychologists generally agree that behavioral action is unlikely to arise directly from personality (Ajzen, 1991; Bandura, 1998; Eysenck, 1970; McCrae & Costa, 1995; McCrae et al., 2000; Rhodes, 2006). Instead, personality is thought to influence behavioral perceptions, expectations, and cognitions. The theory of planned behavior (TPB; Ajzen, 1991) (see Chapter 14 for more information on the Theory of Planned Behavior) has been the leading model to test this assumption in the physical activity domain, with 16 such studies (Davies, Mummery, & Steele, 2010; McEachan, Sutton, & Myers, 2010; Rhodes & Pfaeffli, 2012). The relationship between personality and the

TPB is specific. According to Ajzen (1991), personality should affect behavior through the constructs of attitude, subjective norm, and perceived behavioral control. Thus, TPB should mediate personality and physical activity relations. However, this was only supported in three of the 16 studies. Overall, the results suggest that the TPB may not always fully mediate personality.

One of the reasons for the mixed results of the TPB as a mediator of personality, may be explained by dual-process theories (Deutsch & Strack, 2006), which propose that behavior is the result of a combination of planned "cold" operations and more impulsive "hot" drives. Social cognitive approaches such as theory of planned behavior incorporate the "cold" operations well, but generally neglect the "hot" component such as affect (Stevens et al., 2020; Rhodes & Kates, 2015; see Chapter 17). It is plausible that the relationship between extraversion and impulsivity, or extraversion and the affective response to heightened arousal, for example, partially influences physical activity behavior beyond the observed relationships between extraversion and social cognitive constructs (Rhodes & Wilson, 2020). The research is too limited to explore this possibility at present, so it remains an area of future study.

Another way that personality may affect behavior is by interacting with physical activity motivation. A recent review of factors that interact with the intention–behavior relationship found convincing evidence that conscientiousness may alter this relationship (Rhodes, Cox, & Sayar, 2022). The basic premise for this finding is that people who are more conscientious are more likely to act on their good intentions than their less conscientious counterparts. It may be that the disposition toward achievement keeps high-conscientiousness individuals from slipping in their original physical activity plans (see **Figure 7-2**). Some evidence suggests that extraversion may interact with intention (Rhodes et al., 2022). The theory behind this proposed relationship is that individuals high on extraversion may facilitate their intentions by gravitating toward more active

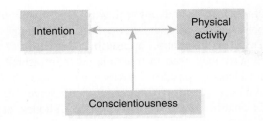

Figure 7-2 Personality as a Moderator of Physical Activity Intention.

environments than do more introverted individuals; however, the evidence for this association is more mixed than conscientiousness.

Personality is conceived as having an evolutionary basis, so the question of whether there is genetic overlap between personality and physical activity is also of keen interest. Heritability of physical activity ranges from 48 to 71% (de Moor & de Geus, 2012; Stubbe et al., 2006), and heritability of the five-factor model personality traits ranges from 41 to 61% (Jang, Livesley, & Vernon, 1996; Riemann, Angleitner, & Strelau, 1997; Vukasovic & Bratko, 2015). With such large heritability among these aspects, there is certainly the potential for an overlap between the heritability of physical activity and that of personality, and early investigations support such genetic links between personality traits and physical activity. For example, in a sample of adolescent and young adult Croatian twin pairs, 100% of the correlation between physical activity and extraversion and nearly 100% of the association between physical activity and neuroticism was accounted for by genetic overlap, after controlling for age and sex (Butkovic, Vukasovic Hlupic, & Bratko, 2017). Longitudinal sampling of 10,105 twins surveyed from 1991 to 2009 indicated that the association between neuroticism and physical activity was observed to be the result of a shared genetic source (de Moor & de Geus, 2018). By contrast, this same study found the association between extraversion and physical activity was partly due to shared genes, but also partly due to the impact of extraversion on physical activity (e.g., higher levels of extraversion predisposing individuals to more frequent opportunities for

physical activity). The genetic association between extraversion and physical activity was also found in a sample of adolescent and young adult twins (Schutte, Nederend, Bartels, & de Geus, 2019). This cutting-edge early research suggests a common genetic etiology between physical activity and key personality traits.

Longitudinal Associations Between Physical Activity and Personality

Most of the research that has been conducted on physical activity and personality involves cross-sectional research or short longitudinal surveys (e.g., less than 1 month). These studies provide us with only a snapshot that personality and physical activity are related to each other, and we often infer from theory that the relationship is most likely representing how personality affects behavior. A few studies have examined the interconnected relationship between personality and physical activity across extended periods of time, which helps us better understand the direction of the relationship. Overall, longitudinal evidence indicates that relationships between personality and physical activity are quite stable across the lifespan (Rhodes & Wilson, 2020). For example, a population-based study using the Netherlands Twin Registry collected data every two years from 1991 to 2002 and demonstrated that regular exercisers were significantly more extroverted and generally more emotionally stable (low neuroticism) than non-exercisers across age categories from early adolescence (10–15 yrs.) to old age (>60 yrs.) (de Moor et al., 2006).

Repeated longitudinal measurement also provides the opportunity to explore differences between people and within the same person over time. For example, Mõttus et al. (2017) showed that while extraversion and conscientiousness predict between-person physical activity, neuroticism predicts changes in physical activity withinpeople over time. The differences may help us understand how to promote physical activity. Given that extraversion and conscientiousness only showed up as between-person differences, these study findings suggest that it may be worth targeting physical activity promotion efforts differently for people with high or low extraversion and conscientiousness. Whereas, because neuroticism was found to change in accordance with physical activity behavior, it may be that interventions could target change in physical activity behavior *through* efforts to reduce neuroticism. However, until more experimental work is done, we can't be sure if a change in neuroticism would lead to physical activity or if changes in physical activity drive future reductions in neuroticism.

Related to this point above, evidence is also increasing to suggest that while personality does appear to influence physical activity as theorized (Kern, Reynolds, & Friedman, 2010), there are some cases where longstanding physical activity may affect personality (Stephan, Boiché, Canada, & Terracciano, 2014; Stephan, Sutin, Luchetti, Bosselut, & Terracciano, 2018; Stephan, Sutin, et al., 2014). This supports a hypothesis that personality and physical activity relations are bidirectional. For example, a recent longitudinal study showed that lower physical activity was associated with declines in conscientiousness, openness, extraversion, and agreeableness over the course of 20 years, although the effect sizes were very small and may not be practically meaningful (Stephan et al., 2018). Though the existing longitudinal research is interesting , the hypothesis of bi-directionality has mixed support, highlighting the need for further investigation (Allen, Magee, Vella, & Laborde, 2017).

Personality and Intervention

One of the struggles as a health educator interested in promoting physical activity is what to do with personality traits. Based on their enduring and stable nature, it seems like a difficult enterprise to plan an intervention to change a person's personality! Personality traits have been shown to change, particularly in adolescence, but change among adults generally unfolds very slowly across the life cycle (McCrae et al., 2000). Unlike self-efficacy or attitudes, a strong correlation

of personality and physical activity represents a potential obstacle and not a target for change. Thus, the promotion approach taken with personality may need to resemble other intractable correlates of physical activity, such as age, disability, or gender (Coulter, Mallett, Singer, & Gucciardi, 2016; Ferguson, 2013; Rhodes & Boudreau, 2017; Wilson et al., 2019). For example, the negative correlation of physical activity and advancing age does not signal an intervention to reverse time! Instead, health promoters need to consider age and target effective interventions for older adults. Similarly, introverts or less conscientious individuals may need targeted interventions to help them increase physical activity despite a natural inclination to be less active.

Some evidence suggests that individual differences in extraversion and neuroticism may impact how effective different promotional strategies are for influencing behavior change. For example, preliminary research suggests that personality traits may interact with promotional message content to affect how that content is processed (Wilson & Estabrooks, 2020). Messages about physical activity that were presented in a gain-framed format (i.e. listing the benefits of physical activity) were perceived more positively by university undergraduate students who scored high for those with a profile of high extraversion and low neuroticism (called approach motivation). By contrast, loss-framed messages (i.e. listing the costs of being physically inactive) were perceived more negatively by people who scored high for avoidance motivation (high neuroticism and low extraversion). In another example, extraverts and those high in neuroticism increased physical activity in response to a mobile app intervention under a condition of social comparison, but not peer pressure (Lepri, Staiano, Shmueli, Pianesi, & Pentland, 2016). Not all interventions, however, have shown results dependent on personality traits. For example, Kahlin et al. (2016) found no evidence that personality moderated the success of a school-based intervention among inactive female adolescents. By contrast, Zaitsu et al. (2015) showed evidence that older adults who were more neurotic and introverted than their counterparts participated more in an exergame intervention. It is therefore possible that the type of physical activity intervention would need to be *tailored* (i.e., matched) based on the extraversion/neuroticism profile of the respondent for effectiveness, yet the mixed results show that a continuation of this research is needed to fully understand the conditions.

The proposal for personality-matched interventions to assist with the well-established relationship between conscientiousness and physical activity also has appeal, but the research on this approach is very limited at present. Rhodes and Matheson (2008) examined whether a planning intervention among low-conscientiousness individuals could help improve physical activity over a control group of undergraduate students. The effects were null, but it may have been from an ineffective intervention, as most of the participants reported that they did not even complete the planning worksheet. More recently, a planning intervention had a significant impact on the translation of intention for physical activity into successful performance of the behavior in a clinical sample of people undergoing cardiac rehabilitation, but only for those with high levels of conscientiousness (Lippke, Pomp, & Fleig, 2018). This underscores the importance of identifying methods to assist individuals with low levels of conscientiousness in following through on behavioral intentions. Similarly, Why and colleagues (Why, Huang, & Sandhu, 2010) examined the effects of a walking intervention and found that messages were more effective in increasing walking behavior among conscientious individuals than their less conscientious counterparts. The results here underscore that personality traits may need to be targeted to help less conscientious individuals.

CRITICAL THINKING ACTIVITY 7-4

If personality is enduring and immutable, how can one use it to promote physical activity intervention? What might you do to screen and promote physical activity for those low on extraversion and conscientiousness?

Personality and Sedentary Behavior

Given the newer focus on sedentary behavior and health, it is not surprising that far less is known about the association between personality traits and sitting, TV watching, video game play, and computer use than for moderate and vigorous physical activity. Nonetheless, it stands to reason that some of the associations between physical activity and personality may be reversed in sedentary behavior. In support of this supposition, a meta-analysis of 23 cross-sectional studies and three longitudinal studies by Allen et al. (2017) showed a small positive correlation between neuroticism and sedentary behavior (r = .08) and a small negative correlation between conscientiousness and sedentary behavior (r = -.08). Another meta-analysis by Sutin et al. (2016) showed similar findings. Specifically, higher values in neuroticism were associated with sedentary behavior, while higher values in conscientiousness were associated with less sedentary behaviors.

Specific analyses in Allen et al. (2017) helped to show that the type of sedentary behavior also affected the findings. In particular, a positive correlation between extraversion and the use of social media was shown, but this was not identified with video gaming. Neuroticism was also associated with the use of social media, but not with more general use of the internet or computing. Some of these results are correspondent with personality theory. One might expect that while the high-energy extravert may seek out activity, the introvert may be motivated to stay home and watch screens from the relative quiet of one's home. Thus, an extravert's use of social media is higher than an introvert, yet they strongly reject that TV can replace socialization as a viable pastime (Weaver, 2003). Sedentary behaviors may also represent a safe and easy behavior for neurotics who tend to be high in anxiety, depressive tendencies, and self-reproach. Overall, the associated evidence on personality and sedentary behavior is still in its infancy. Continued work in this is needed to support our understanding of how personality relates to sedentary behaviors, and

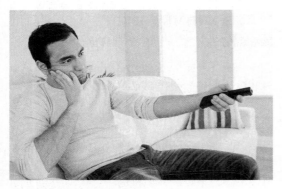

© Wavebreakmedia Ltd/Getty Images Plus/Getty Images.

whether any of these findings hold promotional utility to help decrease sedentary behavior.

Summary

Personality trait psychology has a rich and spirited history, but contemporary research has supported the premise that people have enduring and stable individual differences in how they express thoughts, feelings, and actions. Personality traits are typically organized by supertraits, and then more specific facet traits that are a consequence of the supertrait. The most popular personality supertrait model is the five-factor model composed of neuroticism, extraversion, openness to experience, agreeableness, and conscientiousness.

A series of reviews have identified extraversion, neuroticism, and conscientiousness as the key supertraits related to physical activity. A subsequent review of the more specific traits suggested that extraversion's trait of activity/adventurousness and conscientiousness's trait of achievement striving/ambition may be the critical components that are related to physical activity. Type A personality, which includes components of both the activity and achievement-striving traits (as well as hostility), has also been shown as a reliable predictor of physical activity. These traits are hypothesized to affect a behavior such as physical activity through social cognitive constructs such as attitudes, norms, and self-efficacy. For example, your level of extraversion may affect your perceptions of confidence, your appraisal of how much fun it may be to perform a physical activity, the assessment of whether physical activity is beneficial, or your feeling/shyness about how others will perceive you doing physical activity. Personality may also affect the success of holding to positive physical activity intentions. Research has been quite convincing in demonstrating that people low on conscientiousness have more difficulty holding to their initial physical activity intentions than those who are high on conscientiousness.

Sedentary behaviors also have personality correlates that tend to be the opposite of physical activity, such as low extraversion and high neuroticism. Still, the type of sedentary behavior appears to have slightly different trait makeups, and research in this area is ongoing.

The findings suggest that understanding "at risk" personalities may be important when creating interventions. Interventions that consider a person's introversion, for example, and that target physical activity behaviors accordingly (e.g., home based, solo or with one friend, low intensity) may have utility. This topic has not yet received much attention from researchers. Future research is needed to examine this personality-matching strategy.

Vignette: Lauren

There is no way you'll ever get me to go to a gym unless it's a few months before a wedding or a summer event where I need to wear a swimsuit. Even then, I need to be screamed at by a personal trainer or fitness instructor to actually break a sweat.

I hate working out. I always have. I use the excuse that my bone structure doesn't allow me to move as fluidly as some of my friends who are more sports and activity oriented. But that's a lie I came up with in high school in a failed attempt to get an exemption from P.E. class. The truth is, I'm just not a fan of exercise.

I was the younger sister of two very active older brothers—both of whom went on to play sports in college. And I was intimidated by their involvement in athletics. I far preferred to camp out in my room (or on the sidelines of their games) and read than attempt to keep up with them. In this regard, I took after my mother—who was perfectly content staying at home to garden while my father went rock climbing, hiking, and biking with my brothers.

I wouldn't exactly call myself lazy. I have a lot on my plate between work, a 9 year old and a 6 year old at home, and a mother who is exhibiting the early stages of Alzheimer's and isn't adjusting well to her new senior living establishment. On many occasions, I've made plans to hit a yoga, spin, or Zumba class with a friend of mine. But at the last minute, I end up canceling, often because I get anxious about how much time the class will take out of my day and I feel guilty because I think I should be doing other things.

I'm also incredibly wary about my interest in planning my workouts. To be frank, I'm just not much of a planner. I prefer to be spontaneous. I know I should be more active—especially because I sit at a desk all day for work and commute to and from it via car. But there's nothing that makes me excited about forcing myself to move.

My husband is a different story entirely. He wakes up around 5:30 each morning to go for a bike ride before heading to work. After work he does yoga, while I come home to cook, clean around the house, and (if there's time) catch an episode of one of my favorite television shows after we put the kids to bed.

He's tried for about 5 years now to get me to bike with him. But I'm not interested. I've fallen

off. I don't like the dirt that accumulates on my calves. (I can barely stand the mud his shoes are covered in when he gets home from an extended ride. I make him remove his socks and shoes and wipe his legs and feet off before he even thinks of entering our house—but that's another story.)

We have been incredibly fortunate between my job and his to afford to outfit our basement with a home gym. It's nothing impressive. But we've managed to squeeze in a stationary bike, a treadmill, a squat rack, and a full rack of free weights. And for Christmas this past year, my husband bought me a series of way too many sessions with a personal trainer who comes to our apartment twice a week to walk me through a basic weight-training regimen. I've been following this program somewhat against my will for several months now, and I enjoy the changes I'm seeing in my body. But I wish I could just achieve them through diet alone.

I've been diagnosed in the past with generalized anxiety disorder. And my husband has, on more than one occasion, suggested I may be a bit of a hypochondriac. (Again, here, I take after my mother.) I know about the health benefits of physical activity. I'm reminded of them ad nauseam by the personal trainer I work with and by my husband. But for me to stick with any program is just too much to deal with on top of everything I do at work and home.

My being active is completely dependent on the fitness professional who comes to my house two times a week and barks orders at me no matter how much I protest. I'm not sure how long this new weight program will even last. (I could quit tomorrow, were it not for the slight relief seeing myself in the mirror affords me from my anxiety over aging.) But I guess one does what one has to in order to remain healthy.

Key Terms

activity trait A disposition toward a fast lifestyle. Individuals with this trait are high energy, fast talking, and tend to keep busy.
agreeableness Tendency to be kind, cooperative, altruistic, trustworthy, and generous.

conscientiousness Tendency to be ordered, dutiful, self-disciplined, and achievement oriented.
extraversion Tendency to be sociable, assertive, energetic, seek excitement, and experience positive affect.

grit The tendency to persevere and be passionate about long-term goals.

industriousness-ambition Tendency toward achievement-striving and self-discipline.

neuroticism Tendency to be emotionally unstable, anxious, self-conscious, and vulnerable.

openness to experience/intellect Tendency to be perceptive, creative, and reflective, and to appreciate fantasy and aesthetics.

personality traits Enduring and consistent individual-level differences in tendencies to show consistent patterns of thoughts, feelings, and actions.

psychoticism Tendency toward risk taking, impulsiveness, irresponsibility, manipulativeness, sensation-seeking, tough-mindedness, and nonpragmatism.

type A personality Personality type characterized by a blend of competitiveness and hostility with agitated behavior and continual movement patterns.

type D personality Personality type that experiences distress in the form of higher levels of negative affect and social inhibition.

Review Questions

1. Describe how personality traits are structured.
2. What are the five supertraits in the five-factor model?
3. What supertraits have been linked with physical activity?
4. What traits may determine whether good physical activity intentions translate into behavior?
5. Describe the current evidence for lower-order personality traits and physical activity. What key specific traits may be important?

Applying the Concepts

1. What personality factors might account for Lauren's lack of enthusiasm for and commitment to fitness?
2. What personality traits might account for the enthusiasm and regularity with which Lauren's husband exercises?

References

Ajzen, I. (1991). The theory of planned behavior. *Organizational Behavior and Human Decision Processes, 50*(2), 179–211.

Allport, G. W. (1937). *Personality*. New York, NY: Henry Holt.

Allport, G. W., & Odbert, H. S. (1936). Trait names: A psycholexical study. *Psychological Monographs, 47*(1), i.

Allen, M. S., Walter, E. E., & McDermott, M. S. (2017). Personality and sedentary behavior: A systematic review and meta-analysis. *Health Psychology, 36*(3), 255–263.

Allen, M. S., Magee, C. A., Vella, S. A., & Laborde, S. (2017). Bidirectional associations between personality and physical activity in adulthood. *Health Psychology, 36*(4), 332–336.

Ainsworth, B. E., Haskell, W. L., Herrmann, S. D., Meckes, N., Bassett, D. R., Tudor-Locke, C., . . . Leon, A. S. (2011). 2011 Compendium of Physical Activities: A second update of codes and MET values. *Medicine & Science in Sports & Exercise, 43*(8), 1575–1581.

American Psychological Association. (2020). Personality. Retrieved from www.apa.org/topics/personality/

Bandura, A. (1998). Health promotion from the perspective of social cognitive theory. *Psychology and Health, 13*(4), 623–649.

Bogg, T., & Roberts, B. W. (2013). The case for conscientiousness: Evidence and implications for a personality trait marker of health and longevity. *Annals of Behavioral Medicine, 45*(3), 278–288. doi: 10.1007/s12160-012-9454-6

Bogg, T., Voss, M. W., Wood, D., & Roberts, B. W. (2008). A hierarchical investigation of personality and behavior: Examining neo-socioanalytic models of health-related outcomes. *Journal of Research in Personality, 42*(1), 183–207.

Booth-Kewley, S., & Vickers Jr, R. R. (1994). Associations between major domains of personality and health behavior. *Journal of Personality, 62*(3), 281–298.

Borkoles, E., Polman, R., & Levy, A. (2010). Type-D personality and body image in men: The role of exercise status. *Body Image, 7*(1), 39–45.

Butkovic, A., Vukasovic Hlupic, T., & Bratko, D. (2017). Physical activity and personality: A behaviour genetic analysis. *Psychology of Sport and Exercise, 30*, 128–134.

Cattell, R. B. (1947). Confirmation and clarification of primary personality factors. *Psychometrica, 12*(3), 197–220.

Cohen, J. (1992). Quantitative methods in psychology: A power primer. In *Psychological Bulletin*.

Costa, P. T., & McCrae, R. R. (2009). The five factor model and the NEO Inventories. In J. N. Butcher (Ed.), *Oxford Handbook of Personality Assessment*. Oxford University Press.

Costa, P. T., & McCrae, R. R. (1992). Revised NEO Personality Inventory (NEO-PI-R) and NEO Five-Factor Inventory (NEO-FFI) Professional Manual. Odessa, FL: Psychological Assessment Resources.

Costa Jr, P. T., & McCrae, R. R. (1995). Domains and facets: Hierarchical personality assessment using the Revised NEO Personality Inventory. *Journal of Personality Assessment, 64*(1), 21–50.

Coulter, T. J., Mallett, C. J., Singer, J. A., & Gucciardi, D. F. (2016). Personality in sport and exercise psychology: Integrating a whole person perspective. *International Journal of Sport and Exercise Psychology, 14*(1), 23–41.

Courneya, K. S., & Hellsten, L. A. (1998). Personality correlates of exercise behavior, motives, barriers and preferences: An application of the five-factor model. *Personality and Individual Differences, 24*(5), 625–633.

Davies, C. A., Mummery, W. K., & Steele, R. M. (2010). The relationship between personality, theory of planned behaviour, and physical activity in individuals with type II diabetes. *British Journal of Sports Medicine, 44*(13), 979–984.

De Moor, M., Beem, A. L., Stubbe, J. H., Boomsma, D. I., & De Geus, E. J. C. (2006). Regular exercise, anxiety, depression and personality: A population-based study. *Preventive Medicine, 42*(4), 273–279. doi: 10.1016/j.ypmed.2005.12.002

De Moor, M., & De Geus, E. (2018). Causality in the associations between exercise, personality, and mental health. In H. Budde & M. Wegner (Eds.), *The Exercise Effect on Mental Health* (pp. 67–99). CRC Press.

Denollet, J. (1998). Personality and risk of cancer in men with coronary heart disease. *Psychological Medicine, 28*(4), 991–995.

Deutsch, R., & Strack, F. (2006). Duality models in social psychology: From dual processes to interacting systems. *Psychological Inquiry, 17*(3), 166–172.

Digman, J. M. (1990). Personality structure: Emergence of the five-factor model. *Annual Review of Psychology, 41*(1), 417–440.

Eysenck, H. J. (1970). *The structure of human personality*. (3rd ed.). London: Methuen.

Eysenck, H. J., & Eysenck, S. B. J. (1963). *Manual for the Eysenck Personality Inventory*. San Diego, CA: Educational and Industrial Testing Service.

Eysenck, H. J., Nias, D. K. B., & Cox, D. N. (1982). Sport and personality. *Advances in Behavior Research and Therapy, 4*(1), 1–56.

Ferguson, E. (2013). Personality is of central concern to understand health: Towards a theoretical model for health psychology. *Health Psychology Review, 7*(sup1), S32–S70.

Funder, D. C. (2001). Personality. *Annual Review of Psychology, 52*, 197–221.

Gerber, M., Kalak, N., Lemola, S., Clough, P. J., Puhse, U., Elliot, C., . . . & Brand, S. (2012). Adolescents' exercise and physical activity are associated with mental toughness. *Mental Health and Physical Activity, 5*(1), 35–42.

Gray, J. A. (1991). The neuropsychology of temperament. In J. Strelau & A. Angleitner (Eds.), Guilford, J. P., & Guilford, R. B. (1934). An analysis of the factors in a typical test of introversion-extroversion. *Journal of Abnormal and Social Psychology, 28*(4), 377–399.

Hammond, W. (1957). The status of physical types. *Human biology, 29*(3), 223–241.

Hymbaugh, K., & Garrett, N. D. (1974). Sensation seeking among skydivers. *Perceptual and Motor Skills, 38*, 118.

Jang, K. L., Livesley, W. J., & Vernon, P. A. (1996). Heritability of the big five personality dimensions and their facets: A twin study. *Journal of Personality, 64*(3), 577–591.

Jenkins, C. D. (1976). Recent evidence supporting psychologic and social risk factors for coronary disease. *New England Journal of Medicine, 294*(19), 1033–1038.

Jung, C. G. (1923). *Psychological types: Or, the psychology of individuation*. Paul, Trench, Trubner.

Kahlin, Y., Werner, S., Edman, G., Raustorp, A., & Alricsson, M. (2016). Physical self-esteem and personality traits in Swedish physically inactive female high school students: An intervention study. *International Journal of Adolescent Medicine and Health, 28*(4), 363–372.

Kern, M. L., Reynolds, C. A., & Friedman, H. S. (2010). Predictors of physical activity patterns across adulthood: A growth curve analysis. *Personality and Social Psychology Bulletin, 36*(8), 1058–1072.

Lepri, B., Staiano, J., Shmueli, E., Pianesi, F., & Pentland, A. (2016). The role of personality in shaping social networks and mediating behavioral change. *User-Modeling and User Adaptation Interaction, 26*(2), 14–175.

Lerner, R. M. (1969). The development of stereotyped expectancies of body build-behavior relations. *Child Development*, 137–141.

Lippke, S., Pomp, S., & Fleig, L. (2018). Rehabilitants' conscientiousness as a moderator of the intention–planning-behavior chain. *Rehabilitation Psychology, 63*(3), 460–467.

Mao, T., Pan, W., Zhu, Y., Yang, J., Dong, Q., & Zhou, G. (2018). Self-control mediates the relationship between personality trait and impulsivity. *Personality and Individual Differences, 129*, 70–75.

McCrae, R. R., & Costa Jr, P. T. (1995). Trait explanations in personality psychology. *European Journal of Personality, 9*(4), 231–252.

McCrae, R. R., Costa Jr, P. T., Ostendorf, F., Angleitner, A., Hrebickova, M., Avia, M. D., . . . Smith, P. B. (2000). Nature over nurture: Temperament, personality, and life-span development. *Journal of Personality and Social Psychology, 78*(1), 173–186.

McEwan, D., Boudreau, P., Curran, T., & Rhodes, R. E. (2019). Personality traits of high-risk sport participants: A meta-analysis. *Journal of Research in Personality, 79*, 83–93.

McEachan, R., Sutton, S., & Myers, L. (2010). Mediation of personality influences on physical activity within the theory of planned behavior. *Journal of Health Psychology, 15*(8), 1170–1180.

Mischel, W. (1968). *Personality and assessment.* New York, NY: John Wiley & Sons.

Mõttus, R., Epskamp, S., & Francis, A. (2017). Within-and between individual variability of personality characteristics and physical exercise. *Journal of Research in Personality, 69*, 139–148.

O'Connor, D. B., Conner, M., Jones, F., McMillan, B., & Ferguson, E. (2009). Exploring the benefits of conscientiousness: An investigation of the role of daily stressors and health behaviors. *Annals of Behavioral Medicine, 37*(2), 184–196.

Pate, R. R., Pratt, M., Blair, S., Haskell, W. L., Macera, C. A., & Bouchard, C. . . . & Wilmore, J. H. (1995). Physical activity and public health: A recommendation from the Centers of Disease Control and Prevention and the American College of Sports Medicine. *Journal of the American Medical Association, 273*(5), 402–407.

Reed, J., Pritschet, B. L., & Cutton, D. M. (2013). Grit, conscientiousness, and the transtheoretical model of change for exercise behavior. *Journal of Health Psychology, 18*(5), 612–619.

Rhodes, R. E. (2006). The built-in environment: The role of personality with physical activity. *Exercise and Sport Sciences Reviews, 34*(2), 83–88.

Rhodes, R. E., & Matheson, D. H. (2008). Does personality moderate the effect of implementation intentions on physical activity? *Annals of Behavioral Medicine, 35*, S209.

Rhodes, R. E., & Pfaeffli, L. A. (2012). Personality and physical activity. In E. O. Acevedo (Ed.), *The Oxford handbook of exercise psychology* (pp. 195–223). New York, NY: Oxford University Press.

Rhodes, R. E., & Smith, N. E. I. (2006). Personality correlates of physical activity: A review and meta-analysis. *British Journal of Sports Medicine, 40*(12), 958–965.

Rhodes, R., & Boudreau, P. (2017). Physical activity and personality traits. In *Oxford Research Encyclopedia of Psychology* (pp. 1–20). Oxford Press. https://doi.org/10.1093/acrefore/9780190236557.013.210

Rhodes, R. E., Courneya, K. S., Blanchard, C. M., & Plotnikoff, R. C. (2007). Prediction of leisure-time walking: An integration of social cognitive, perceived environmental, and personality factors. *International Journal of Behavioral Nutrition and Physical Activity, 4*(1), 1–11.

Rhodes, R. E., & Kates, A. (2015). Can the affective response to exercise predict future motives and physical activity behavior? A systematic review of published evidence. *Annals of Behavioral Medicine, 49*(5), 715–731.

Rhodes, R. E., Cox, A., & Sayar, R. (2022). What predicts the physical activity intention-behavior gap? A systematic review. *Annals of Behavioral Medicine, 56*(1), 1–20.

Rhodes, R. E., & Wilson, K. E. (2020). Personality and physical activity. In D. Hackfort & R. J. Schinke (Eds.), *The Routledge International Encyclopedia of Sport and Exercise Psychology* (pp. 413–425). Taylor and Francis.

Riemann, R., Angleitner, A., & Strelau, J. (1997). Genetic and environmental influences on personality: A study of twins reared together using the self- and peer report NEO-FFI scales. *Journal of Personality, 65*(3), 449–475.

Rothbart, M. K. (2007). Temperament, development, and personality. *Current Directions in Psychological Science, 16*(4), 207–212.

Roberts, B. W., Walton, K. E., & Viechtbauer, W. (2006). Patterns of mean-level change in personality traits across the life course: A meta-analysis of longitudinal studies. *Psychological Bulletin, 132*(1), 1–25.

Schutte, N. M., Nederend, I., Bartels, M., & de Geus, E. J. (2019). A twin study on the correlates of voluntary exercise behavior in adolescence. *Psychology of Sport and Exercise, 40*, 99–109.

Sheldon, W. H., & Stevens, S. S. (1942). The varieties of temperament; a psychology of constitutional differences.

Slaughter, M. (1970). An Analysis of the relationship between somatotype and personality traits of college women. *Research Quarterly. American Association for Health, Physical Education and Recreation, 41*(4), 569–575. doi: 10.1080/10671188.1970.10615017

Stelmack, R. M., & Stalikas, A. (1991). Galen and the humour theory of temperament. *Personality and Individual Differences, 12*(3), 255–263. http://dx.doi.org/10.1016/0191-8869(91)90111-N

Stephan, Y., Boiché, J., Canada, B., & Terracciano, A. (2014). Association of personality with physical, social, and mental activities across the lifespan: Findings from US and French samples. *British Journal of Psychology, 105*(4), 564–580.

Stephan, Y., Sutin, A. R., & Terracciano, A. (2014). Physical activity and personality development across adulthood and old age: Evidence from two longitudinal studies. *Journal of Research in Personality, 49*, 1–7.

Stephan, Y., Sutin, A. R., Luchetti, M., Bosselut, G., & Terracciano, A. (2018). Physical activity and personality development over twenty years: Evidence from three longitudinal samples. *Journal of Research in Personality, 73*, 173–179.

Stevens, C. J., Baldwin, A. S., Bryan, A. D., Conner, M., Rhodes, R. E., & Williams, D. M. (2020). Affective determinants of physical activity: A conceptual framework and narrative review. *Frontiers in Psychology, 11*,(568331), 1–19.

Stubbe, J. H., Boomsma, D. I., Vink, J. M., Cornes, B. K., Martin, N. G., Skytthe, A.,. . . & de Geus, E. J. (2006). Genetic influences on exercise participation in 37, 051 twin pairs from seven countries. *Public Library of Science One, 1*(1), e22.

Sutin, A. R., Stephan, Y., Luchetti, M., Artese, A., Oshio, A., & Terracciano, A. (2016). The five-factor model of personality and physical inactivity: A meta-analysis of 16 samples. *Journal of Research in Personality, 63*, 22–28.

U.S. Department of Health and Human Services. (2018). *Physical Activity Guidelines for Americans* (2nd ed.). US Department of Health and Human Services.

Vukasovic, T., & Bratko, D. (2015). Heritability of personality: A meta- analysis of behavior genetic studies. *Psychological Bulletin, 141*(4), 769–785.

Why, Y. P., Huang, R. Z., & Sandhu, P. K. (2010). Affective messages increase leisure walking only among conscientious individuals. *Personality and Individual Differences, 48*(6), 752–756.

Wiebe, D. J., & Smith, T. W. (1997). Personality and health: Progress and problems in psychosomatics. In R. Hogan, J. Johnson & S. Briggs (Eds.), *Handbook of Personality Psychology*. San Diego, CA: Academic Press.

Wiggins, J. S. (1997). In defense of traits. In R. Hogan, J. A. Johnson, & S. R. Briggs (Eds.), *Handbook of personality psychology* (pp. 95–115). San Diego, CA: Academic Press.

Wilson, K. (2019). Personality and physical activity. In M. H. Anshel & S. J. Petruzzello (Eds.), *APA's Handbook of Sport and Exercise Psychology* (2, 219–239): American Psychological Association.

Wilson, K. E., & Dishman, R. K. (2015). Personality and physical activity: A systematic review and meta-analysis. *Personality and Individual Differences, 72*, 230–242.

Wilson, K., & Estabrooks, P. A. (2020). Physical activity promotion message perceptions biased by motivational dispositions. *Appl Psychol Health Well Being*. doi: 10.1111 /aphw.12199

World Health Organization. (2020). Physical activity. https:// www.who.int/news-room/fact-sheets/detail/physical -activity

Zaitsu, K., Nishimura, Y., Matsuguma, H., & Higuchi, S. (2015). Association between extraversion and exercise performance among elderly persons receiving a videogame intervention. *Games for Health Journal, 4*(5), 375–380.

Zuckerman, M. (2005). *Psychobiology of personality* (2nd ed.). Cambridge, England: Cambridge University Press.

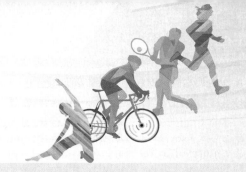

CHAPTER 8

Cognition

LEARNING OBJECTIVES

After completing this chapter, you will be able to:

- Describe the general anatomy of the brain.
- Explain cognition and different aspects of it.
- Describe the state of evidence on physical activity and sedentary behavior with cognition across the lifespan.
- Understand whether physical activity and sedentary behavior play roles in the prevention and treatment of attention-deficit/hyperactivity disorder and cognitive impairment.

Introduction

People will often report that they think better or have less brain fog after they work out. Parents, guardians, and teachers often report that their children and students can focus better and are less disruptive following recess and physical education. These anecdotes suggest that physical activity may have a positive effect on our cognitive abilities. This chapter will discuss what cognition is and the science behind how physical activity and sedentary behavior affect our cognitive ability. But before we begin to examine this literature, let's take a closer look at the brain.

The Brain

You may have heard our brain described as the command center or engine. In a lot of ways, those descriptions aren't far off. This amazing organ is responsible for how we feel, how we behave, what we think, and how our feelings, thoughts, and actions interact with one another. The human brain weighs about 1,400 grams, or roughly 3 pounds. It is thought to consist of about 100 billion individual neurons, and it has a texture similar to firm jelly. Despite its small size, the brain is the control center of our nervous system, the storage vault for our memories, and the source of our feelings. The brain is often referred to as the most complex structure in the universe.

Without a brain, we would not be able to think, move, speak, or even breathe. Like any complex machine or computer, the brain contains many parts, each of which has subparts, which themselves have subparts, all the way down to 100 billion or so neurons. Let's consider the brain's general structure and functions so that we can better understand the impact that physical activity and sedentary behavior have on it.

People Are Not Right-Brained or Left-Brained

The brain has two nearly symmetrical halves or **brain hemispheres**, split down the middle and connected by the **corpus callosum**, connective flat neural fibers that relay information from one hemisphere to the other. Although the hemispheres look similar, there are important features that distinguish one from the other (Sherman, 2019). It varies from person to person, but for most people, the left hemisphere is slightly larger than the right hemisphere. The hemispheres also function differently. The left hemisphere tends to be more associated with language use and comprehension, although notably, this is reversed for some people. For others, language dominance is equally spread across both hemispheres. The right hemisphere tends to be more dominant in control of **spatial-visual processes**. This is how we sense the interrelations of things in space around us (e.g., navigating where we are going, representing a concept through drawing). But again, the brain hemisphere in which these processes are controlled varies from person-to-person. It is theorized that the left and right hemispheres of the human brain have specialized functioning, evolving from features originating more than 500 million years ago. Our early ancestors' left hemisphere was specialized for control of well-established patterns of behavior under familiar circumstances, while the right hemisphere was primarily accountable for emotional arousal responses and responding to unexpected threats or challenges (MacNeilage et al., 2009).

Given the historical research and evolutionary origins into differences between the brain hemispheres, it is not surprising that people started theorizing that differences in how people act and think may be explained simply by which hemisphere they are using. Because simple stories are easier to sell, this idea that people are left-brained or right-brained spread rapidly through media and popular books. However, it has been debunked many times. The truth is that pretty much nothing happens in isolation in one part of the brain. It is just not that simple. Even language, which tends to be thought of as one of the functions most segmented to a single hemisphere, requires both sides of the brain working together. Rather, the large majority of human functioning occurs as a result of active networks that spread across large areas of both sides of the brain. So, going forward in this chapter, we will describe functioning in certain brain areas, but just keep in mind that it usually isn't as clear-cut as that. Certain brain areas may be more dominant than others for certain processes, but functioning involves more areas of the brain than one, and even the area that is most dominant for certain functions varies from person-to-person.

Brain Anatomy and Functioning

The three main parts of the brain are the cerebrum, brainstem, and cerebellum (see **Figure 8-1**). The biggest part of the brain is the cerebrum, or cortex, and it fills up most of the skull. The cerebrum makes up about 80% of the brain's weight. The cerebral cortex is divided into four sections: the frontal lobe, parietal lobe, occipital lobe, and temporal lobe (see **Table 8-1**). Brain anatomical, clinical, and neuroimaging data have provided important insights

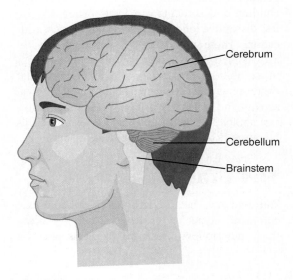

Figure 8-1 Major Parts of the Brain.

Table 8-1 **Functions of the Four Lobes of the Cerebrum**

Lobe	Functioning Associated with the Lobe
Frontal	Reasoning, planning, parts of speech, movement, emotions, and problem solving
Parietal	Movement, orientation, recognition, and perception of stimuli
Occipital	Visual processing
Temporal	Perception and recognition of auditory stimuli, memory, and speech

into the types of activities that each part of the brain is most associated with. The cerebrum is considered the main driver behind memory, problem solving, thinking, and feeling. This part of the brain also largely controls movement.

Lying at the back of the brain is the cerebellum, which is also known as the little brain. The cerebellum functions include maintaining balance and coordinating voluntary muscle movement. However, it is also important for visuospatial functioning, learning and memory, language, and problem solving. Damage to the cerebellum results in tremors, abnormal posture, and a loss of muscle tone. Attention-deficit/hyperactivity disorder, autism spectrum disorders, and schizophrenia are associated with cerebellar activity (O'Halloran et al., 2012).

The brainstem sits beneath the cerebrum and in front of the cerebellum. This structure is responsible for basic vital life functions such as breathing, digesting food and circulating blood. In other words, it is responsible for the non-thinking actions, and it oversees all the functions your body needs to stay alive.

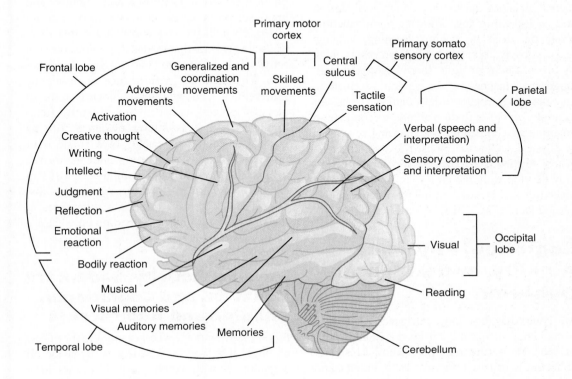

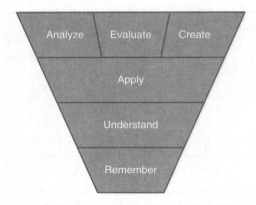

Figure 8-2 Example of a Bloom's Cognitive Taxonomy.

What Is Cognition?

Historically, the term **cognition** comes from the Latin verb *cognōscere*, meaning "to know," "to conceptualize," or "to recognize." Today, cognition represents a wide group of mental processes that reflect a person's knowledge or awareness. These mental processes interact in a hierarchical fashion and include thinking, knowing, remembering, reasoning, decision making, learning, judging, and problem solving. Mental processes high in the hierarchy include those associated with language, imagination, perception, evaluation, and planning. Higher-order cognitive tasks, for example, would include planning to compete in an ironman competition or choosing to engage in physical activity as opposed to watching television. **Figure 8-2** represents a common taxonomy developed by Bloom for classifying learning objectives that is based on higher-order cognitive tasks (Bloom et al., 2013).

Cognition, Physical Activity, and Sedentary Behavior

An issue that has long intrigued researchers is contained in the dictum by the Roman poet, Juvenal: 'Mens sana in corpore sano.' This Latin aphorism is usually translated as "a sound mind in a sound body" or "a healthy mind in a healthy body." The intended meaning here is that only a healthy body can support a healthy mind, so we should strive to keep our bodies in top condition. However, is this aphorism supported by science?

Hundreds, if not thousands, of studies have been carried out to determine if there is a relationship between physical activity and the brain; that is, whether acute and chronic physical activity influence cognitive functioning. A burgeoning body of literature is also evolving suggesting sedentary behavior may reduce cognitive functioning, especially being sedentary for long periods of time. Researchers have used a variety of different types of cognitive functioning tasks (e.g., memory, mathematical ability, verbal ability, reasoning, creativity, academic achievement, mental age, intelligence quotient, reaction time, and perception) to examine these important research questions.

To inform the 2018 Health and Human Services Physical Activity Guidelines for Americans, an umbrella review was conducted investigating physical activity interventions and cognitive and brain outcomes across all ages (Erickson et al., 2019). Overall, the review concluded that there was solid evidence that moderate-vigorous physical activity led to improvements in cognitive function. This includes performance on academic achievement and neuropsychological tests of memory, processing speed, and executive functioning. There was strong evidence for the immediate cognitive benefits of a single bout of physical activity, and strong evidence for the benefits of physical activity to reduce risks of cognitive impairments such as Alzheimer's disease. There were also important differences in the strength of evidence depending on what age groups were being studied.

Physical Activity, Sedentary Behavior, and Cognition in Children and Adolescents

A good starting point when examining the effects of physical activity and sedentary behavior on cognition is with youth. Several reviews have found that both acute and chronic physical activity positively influences brain health and cognition in children (Chaddock, Pontifex, Hillman, & Kramer, 2011; Hillman, Kamijo, & Scudder, 2011; Mahar, 2011). For example, Fedewa and Ahn (2011) undertook a meta-analysis of 59 studies examining the effects of physical activity on cognitive performance of school-age children between the ages of 3–18 years. They found that being physically active has a small benefit on children's achievement (ES = 0.28), with aerobic exercise having the greatest effect.

Donnelly and colleagues (2016) built on these findings by reviewing the evidence of physical activity and fitness on cognitive functioning and academic achievement in children aged 5–13 year old. They found 64 studies that investigated physical activity or fitness and cognitive functioning and 73 others that investigated physical activity or fitness and academic achievement. Overall, the results showed that fitness, single bouts of physical activity, and physical activity interventions improve children's cognitive functioning. The results of physical activity or fitness and academic achievement was less certain, with some evidence suggesting more activity was associated with better academic achievement, but the lack of randomized controlled trials on the topic resulted in inconclusive findings. Overall, Erickson's et al. umbrella review declared a moderate strength of evidence for the benefits of physical activity on cognitive functioning for children aged 6–13 years and insufficient evidence for those aged 14–18 years (Erickson et al., 2019).

In school-age children and youth aged 5–17 years, watching TV for more than 2 hours per day was associated with increased body mass index (BMI), decreased fitness, lower self-esteem and pro-social behaviors (emotional stability, sensitive, outgoing, self-controlled), and decreased academic achievement (school performance, grade point average; Tremblay et al., 2011).

Notably, the evidence of physical activity and cognitive functioning in infants and children younger than 6 years old is insufficient and too limited to make firm conclusions (Erickson

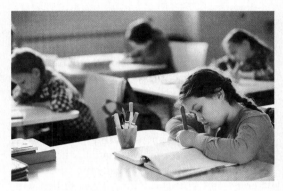

© Mediaphotos/Getty Images.

et al., 2019). There are two reviews that show preliminary evidence that physical activity may be associated with better cognitive functioning (Carson et al., 2016; Zeng et al., 2017). Carson et al. (2016) reviewed all study design types looking at physical activity and cognitive functioning in children younger than 5 years old. They found seven studies with a total of 414 participants from five countries, including two observational and five experimental studies. Physical activity showed enhancement effects for about 65% of the assessed cognitive functioning outcomes. Most studies (six of the seven) were rated as having a high risk of bias. Zeng et al. (2017) reviewed only randomized controlled trials and found that of five randomized controlled trials reviewed, four found that physical activity enhancements lead to increased cognitive functioning. Importantly, the included trials in that review had broadly defined cognitive functioning outcomes that included academic achievement, cognitive learning, language, concentration, attention, memory, and intelligence. Given the low number of eligible trials and the broad conceptualization of cognition, strong conclusions about physical activity and cognition from these reviews cannot be made. Rather, there are calls for more rigorous studies.

A review considering 37 studies (31 observational, six experimental) of cognition and sedentary behavior representing more than 14,000 children younger than 5 years from nine countries found that sedentary behavior was associated with lower cognitive development outcomes (Carson et al., 2015). However, the findings also highlighted that the activity being engaged in (e.g., reading vs. watching TV) likely differentially impacts cognition. Evidence is also building for the context-specificity of the link between sedentary behavior and cognition for children older than 5 years (Aggio et al., 2016; Carson et al., 2017; Haapala et al., 2014). Not surprisingly, time spent sitting while doing academic work seems associated with higher scores on cognitive or academic outcomes; whereas time spent watching TV is linked with lower scores.

Classroom-Based Physical Activity

Given the strong evidence of the immediate benefits of physical activity on cognitive function, it may seem logical to consider physical education classes as the target for increasing physical activity of schoolchildren. There are several reasons why this may not be the case. First, time allocated to physical education has steadily declined in most high-income nations. For example, less than half of American high school students attend physical education classes at least once weekly, and one in four children aged 6–17 years participated in 60 minutes of physical activity every day (Centers for Disease Control and Prevention, 2020a). Second, there is also a decline in recess, which is an opportunity for students to obtain unstructured physical activity. In fact, it is estimated that only 57% of school districts require regularly scheduled recess for elementary school children (Lee et al., 2007). Third, coupled with the decline in physical education classes is the fact that children often get limited physical activity, with only 40% of time spent in physical education classes engaged in moderate-vigorous physical activity (Hollis et al., 2017). Finally, the current emphasis on end-of-grade testing can cause decreased opportunities during school for students to be physically active by inadvertently pressuring administrators and teachers to spend more sedentary time in the classroom and less time in physical education in an effort to improve standardized testing scores.

If physical activity is to be increased in elementary schools, venues other than physical education need to be developed and evaluated. An alternative to physical education for increased physical activity is the regular classroom where students spend most of their time. Indeed, children are easily accessible in school settings because they spend a large portion of their day at school. In many countries, children spend about 6–8 hours a day at school. Thus, a practical, although challenging, solution is to promote classroom-based physical activity (Donnelly & Lambourne, 2011). Classroom-based physical activity is either linked to an established curriculum or it's coupled with the teachers' existing lessons. Thus, the physical activity is integrated with the academic lesson and does not take time away from the curriculum.

One such classroom-based program is the Physical Activity Across the Curriculum (PAAC). This program is guided by the association among physical activity, fitness, fatness, and academic achievement; it provides a unique opportunity to improve both health (e.g., fitness levels) and cognitive achievement of children during school. PAAC lessons can be used in a variety of academic areas, including math, language arts, geography, history, spelling, science, and health. An example of a math lesson might consist of students hopping and skipping across the room and counting their own "laps," as well as adding or multiplying laps of groups of children (i.e., 6 children × 6 laps each = 36). Geometry might be taught by having students form different shapes, such as squares or triangles, while either walking or skipping. Geography can be taught by having children run to the appropriate area designated for one of the directions (i.e., north, south, east, west). For example, if the teacher calls the state of Florida, students would run or skip to the south space. A floor mat with letters printed on it could be used to teach spelling; the children spell out words by hopping onto the letters. The scope of physically active lessons is almost limitless.

The conceptual framework for PAAC includes no additional teacher preparation time, uses existing academic lessons, has no additional costs, and incorporates activities that are fun for both students and teachers. Additionally, PAAC promotes the concept that physical activity can occur at many times and places without the need to report to a special place (such as a gym or track) and to change into gym clothes. Specifically, PAAC promotes 90 minutes a week of moderate to vigorous physically active academic lessons that last about 10 minutes each. The lessons are delivered intermittently throughout the school day. Lessons are mostly delivered in the classroom but can also be delivered in alternate school sites, such as hallways and outdoors.

Donnelly and his colleagues (2009, 2017) conducted a 3-year cluster randomized controlled trial in elementary schools. This is a unique trial in which groups of subjects, in this case schools (as opposed to individual participants), are randomized. The point of this trial was to compare changes in fitness and fatness surrounding changes in academic achievement in schools that either received PAAC or schools that served as controls. The participants were children in grades two and three initially and progressed to grades four and five. The authors found that the overall change in BMI for PAAC schools compared to control schools was not significantly different. However, the change in BMI from baseline to 3 years was significantly influenced by exposure to PAAC; that is, as minutes of PAAC exposure increased, the change in BMI decreased. More specifically, schools with 75 minutes or more of PAAC a week showed significantly smaller increases in BMI at 3 years compared to schools with fewer than 75 minutes of PAAC each week.

A secondary outcome examined was daily physical activity that was measured by accelerometers. The researchers found that children in the PAAC schools had significantly greater levels of physical activity during the school day (by 12%) and on the weekends (by 17%) compared to children in the control schools. Children in PAAC schools also had a 27% greater level of moderate to vigorous physical activity compared to children in the control schools. Another secondary outcome assessed by the researchers was academic achievement. Academic achievement was measured with the Wechsler Individual Achievement Test-Second Edition (Wechsler, 2005) by a third party. This test assesses the academic achievement of children in the following four areas: reading, math, oral language, and writing. There was no significant difference in academic achievement from PAAC, suggesting the activity program neither diminished nor improved academic achievement (Donnelly et al., 2017).

CRITICAL THINKING ACTIVITY 8-1

Excluding recess and physical education classes, how could you increase physical activity for children while they are at school?

Other research examining the impact of physically active academic instruction is promising (see Singh, Uijtdewilligen, Twick, van Mechelen, & Chinapaw, 2012) and supports the findings of Donnelly and Lambourne (2011). For example, a review by Mahar (2011) revealed that students who participated in classroom-based physical activities that incorporated academic concepts had better attention-to-task than control students. As well, a review by the Centers for Disease Control and Prevention (2010) found that interventions that combined physical activity and academic lessons resulted in students having improvements in on-task behavior, word recognition, and spatial, reading, and math aptitude. In summary, the literature strongly supports the relationship between physical activity, cognition, and academic performance in youth. There is no scientific evidence to support the argument that increasing the time allotted to physical activity during the school day results in decreased academic performance.

In short, schools may be able to address several health issues in conjunction with improving academic performance by delivering academic lessons using physical activity in the classroom (Donnelly & Lambourne, 2011).

Attention Deficit Hyperactivity Disorder

Attention Deficit Hyperactivity Disorder (ADHD) is one of the most common childhood disorders and can continue through adolescence and into adulthood. 6.1 million (9.4%) of children in America have been diagnosed with ADHD, with boys almost twice as likely as girls to be diagnosed (Centers for Disease Control and Prevention, 2020b). Some evidence suggests that transgender individuals are more likely than boys or girls to be diagnosed with ADHD (Dawson et al., 2017). Symptoms include difficulty staying focused and paying attention, difficulty controlling behavior, and/or hyperactivity. These symptoms can make it difficult for a child with ADHD to succeed in school, get along with other children or adults, or finish tasks at home.

Brain imaging studies have revealed that in a youth with ADHD, the brain matures in a normal pattern but is delayed, on average, by about 3 years (Shaw et al., 2007). The delay is most pronounced in brain regions involved in thinking, paying attention, and planning. Inattention, hyperactivity, and impulsivity are the main behaviors of ADHD. It is normal for all children to be inattentive, hyperactive, or impulsive sometimes, but for children with ADHD, these behaviors are more severe, intense, and frequent. To be diagnosed with this disorder, a child must show a pattern of inattention and/or hyperactive impulsivity that interferes with functioning or development (American Psychiatric Association, 2013). Symptoms of ADHD are separated into two main categories: inattention and hyperactive impulsivity. See **Table 8-2** for a description of the diagnosable symptoms. To be diagnosed, several symptoms would be present before the age of 12 years, present in multiple settings (not just school), and cause interference in daily life. Also, it must be ruled out that the symptoms are not better explained by other mental disorders, such as mood disorders or anxiety disorders (See Chapters 10 and 11). In adulthood, symptoms can present a bit differently. For example, hyperactivity may be more recognizable as restlessness.

Table 8-2 Symptoms of Attention Deficient Hyperactivity Disorder

Inattention: Observe six or more symptoms of inattention for children up to age 16 years, or 5 or more for adolescents aged 17 years and older and adults; symptoms of inattention have been present for at least 6 months, and they are inappropriate for developmental level.

- Often fails to give close attention to details or makes careless mistakes in schoolwork, at work, or with other activities.

- Often has trouble holding attention on tasks or play activities.

- Often does not seem to listen when spoken to directly.

- Often does not follow through on instructions and fails to finish schoolwork, chores, or duties in the workplace (e.g., loses focus, side-tracked).

- Often has trouble organizing tasks and activities.

- Often avoids, dislikes, or is reluctant to do tasks that require mental effort over a long period of time (such as schoolwork or homework).

- Often loses things necessary for tasks and activities (e.g., school materials, pencils, books, tools, wallets, keys, paperwork, eyeglasses, mobile telephones).

- Is often easily distracted.

- Is often forgetful in daily activities.

Hyperactivity and Impulsivity: Observe six or more symptoms of hyperactivity-impulsivity for children up to age 16 years, or 5 or more for adolescents aged 17 years and older and adults; symptoms of hyperactivity-impulsivity have been present for at least 6 months to an extent that is disruptive and inappropriate for the person's developmental level.

- Often fidgets with or taps hands or feet, or squirms in seat.

- Often leaves seat in situations when remaining seated is expected.

- Often runs about or climbs in situations where it is not appropriate (adolescents or adults may be limited to feeling restless).

- Often unable to play or take part in leisure activities quietly.

- Is often "on the go" acting as if "driven by a motor."

- Often talks excessively.

- Often blurts out an answer before a question has been completed.

- Often has trouble waiting their turn.

- Often interrupts or intrudes on others (e.g., butts into conversations or games).

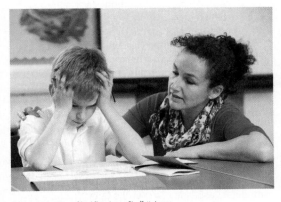

© Monkeybusinessimages/iStock/Getty Images Plus/Getty Images.

Approximately 75% of children with ADHD are receiving some type of treatment (Centers for Disease Control and Prevention, 2020b). The main treatment for ADHD is drug therapy, which uses psychostimulants to help increase attention and focus through enhancing dopamine regulation in the frontal lobe and striatum (Vaidya et al., 1998). There are some who do not respond fully to medication or experience unwanted side effects (Toomey et al., 2012). Most people being treated for ADHD are taking medication, while less than half are receiving behavioral treatment such as social skills training or cognitive behavioral therapy. Evidence suggests behavioral treatment can be effective for persistent reduction and management of symptoms. For example, a review of treatments of ADHD in adults compared cognitive behavioral therapy treatment to relaxation and education treatments. The review showed cognitive behavioral therapy reduces both clinically and self-assessed ADHD symptoms more than two times that of relaxation and education (Safren et al., 2010). Treatments can relieve many symptoms of ADHD, but there is currently no cure for the disorder. With treatment, most people with ADHD can be successful in school, work, and social situations and lead productive lives. Evidence is building showing that physical activity can help children and adults with ADHD mitigate symptoms (Gapin et al., 2011).

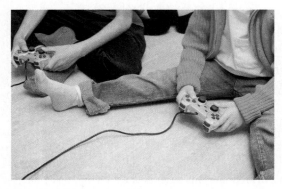

© JupiterImages/Creatas/Getty Images.

For example, a review of intervention studies of physical activity and ADHD in children and adolescents reviewed 16 studies and found that short bouts of physical activity (20–30 minutes) results in improved processing speed, working memory, planning and problem solving in children and adolescents with ADHD (Suarez-Manzano et al., 2018). The same review also found that regular engagement in physical activity of at least 30 minutes of physical activity on 3 or more days/week for at least 5 consecutive weeks led to further advancements in attention, inhibition, emotional control, behavior and motor control in children and adolescents with ADHD.

CRITICAL THINKING ACTIVITY 8-2

Why do you think physical activity can mitigate ADHD symptoms?

The verdict is still out in terms of whether reducing sedentary behavior can help alleviate ADHD symptoms. That some ADHD symptoms manifest as a lack of prolonged sedentary behavior (e.g., not being able to stay seated) complicates the scientific investigation because it blurs the line between symptoms (being able to stay seated) and treatment (reduction of sitting time). Not surprisingly, children who were less sedentary at age 7 were found to have more ADHD symptoms at age 14 (Brandt et al., 2021).

Interestingly though, observational evidence suggests that screentime is associated with more ADHD symptoms in adolescents; whereas non-screentime sedentary behavior is not associated with ADHD symptoms (Suchert et al., 2017). Overall, the field of investigation into cognition, ADHD, and sedentary behavior is underdeveloped. There remains a lot to understand about how movement and ADHD are connected, but there seems to be sufficient evidence to suggest that physical activity can reduce cognitive symptoms of ADHD in children.

CRITICAL THINKING ACTIVITY 8-3

For you to be more active while studying and learning, what would need to change? Think about change at levels, including students, lecturers, learning resources, and university systems.

Distance Education, Physical Activity, and Sedentary Behavior

When considering in-classroom, face-to-face learning environments, evidence tends to support that physical activity is beneficial for learning outcomes. However, nowadays, a lot of us are doing our education remotely online. Researchers from the Netherlands were interested to see how physical activity and sedentary behavior impacted distance education outcomes (Gijselaers et al., 2016).

What they did: Physical activity and sedentary behavior of 1,110 adult distance education students were self-reported and then tested whether they were associated with study progress (the number of successfully passed modules) assessed 14 months later.

What they found: Physical activity was not associated with study progress, but sedentary behavior was. People who were more sedentary tended to have passed more modules, or progress further in their study.

So, what does this mean?: Should we encourage people to be more sedentary so they will do better in study? The researchers don't think so. Maybe instead, the system should change so that study and learning are not necessarily sedentary activities.

Adult Populations

Overall, there is insufficient evidence to rule on whether physical activity or sedentary behavior impacts cognition in young and middle aged adults (aged 18–50 years) (Erickson et al., 2019). It is not that there is evidence to suggest the effects of physical activity or sedentary behavior on cognition may or may not be present, but rather it is that researchers have tended to focus on either children or older adults; there is a dearth of evidence into the general, healthy adult population.

There have been reviews of the effects of physical activity on cognition in adults of all ages (including older adults) and this line of research supports that physical activity is beneficial for cognition both acutely and chronically. Smith and his colleagues (2010) conducted a large meta-analysis of randomized controlled trials examining the association between aerobic exercise training on cognition of adults. They reviewed 29 studies with data from 2,049 adults aged 18 or older. The studies reviewed had to incorporate aerobic exercise for at least one month, have supervised exercise training, and have incorporated a non-aerobic-exercise control group. They found that adults who were randomly assigned to receive aerobic exercise training had modest improvements in attention, processing speed, executive function, and memory compared to the control participants who did not receive exercise training. **Processing speed** refers to the speed at which the brain processes information. Faster processing speed means more efficient thinking and learning. **Executive functioning** is the cognitive process that regulates the ability to organize thoughts and activities, prioritize tasks, manage time efficiently, and make decisions. They found that aerobic exercise did not appear to benefit working memory (i.e., short-term memory). Smith et al. (2010) also found via moderator analyses that studies using combined aerobic exercise and strength training interventions improved attention, processing speed, and working memory to a greater extent than aerobic exercise alone.

A systematic review of thirteen studies that investigated the effects on cognition of intervention programs aimed at reducing at-work sedentary time reported that nine found nonsignificant results, two studies found that the interventions enhanced cognitive outcomes, and another two found that the interventions led to decrements in cognitive outcomes (Magnon et al., 2018). These mixed findings lead to the conclusion that there is insufficient evidence that reducing sedentary behavior at work impacts cognition.

Older Adult Populations

With age, physical and cognitive functioning decline. It is well-established that as we age, both the structure and function of our brain changes. These changes are associated with decreased cognitive function. For example, as we age, our reaction time becomes slower, our memory is not as good, and we may have a more difficult time making decisions. We know that physical activity is beneficial for healthy aging, and it may also help maintain good cognitive functioning in older adults. A great deal of research has examined the relationship between physical activity and cognitive functioning in older adults, and some evidence suggests there is also a connection between cognition and sedentary behavior.

Most of the research done on physical activity and cognition has been done in older adult samples, which has resulted in a moderate level of evidence suggesting that both acute and long-term physical activity improve cognition (Erickson et al., 2019). There is a bit of mixed evidence on whether aerobic exercise, resistance training, or a combination of both provides the greatest benefits for cognition, but findings are favorable regardless of which type of activity is being engaged in. Notably, there seems to be a difference in genders of the effects of physical activity on cognition. Effects seem to be greater for studies with samples made up of more women than men. These conclusions about the state of evidence come from many meta-analyses and systematic reviews—a few of which, we'll cover now.

Northey et al. (2018) reviewed 39 randomized controlled trials of exercise interventions of community-dwelling older adults aged 50 years and up. Findings revealed that the exercise interventions enhanced cognition by an effect size of 0.29, with interventions of aerobic exercise, resistance training, combined training, and tai chi all showing significant effects. Further analysis suggests that durations of 45 minutes to 1 hour per session of at least moderate intensity were associated with the largest effects.

Ogawa and colleagues (2016) conducted a systematic review of the effects of **exergaming** interventions on cognition in older adults. Seven studies were reviewed, and the findings suggest that exergaming is beneficial for cognition. Notably though, there was insufficient evidence to determine whether exergaming had added benefits to cognition beyond physical activity that is not technology-driven. Because studies did not control for dose or intensity of physical activity, this question remains unanswered.

Although there is not a large enough body of evidence to make firm conclusions about the impact of sedentary behavior on cognition in older adults, there are some studies that provide preliminary evidence about whether there is an effect. Some evidence suggests that TV watching is associated with poorer cognition later in life (Hamer & Stamatakis, 2014). Some evidence shows cross-sectional associations of more sedentary behavior with poorer cognition (Falck, Landry, et al., 2017; Vance et al., 2005). Edwards and Loprinzi (2017) analyzed data from more than 2,000 older adults aged 60–85 years and found that people who engaged in more than 5 hours/day of sedentary behavior had poorer cognition than those who engaged in less sedentary behavior. However, when accounting for people's physical activity, the link between sedentary behavior and cognition washed out, meaning that it may be that physical activity could buffer from some of the potential deleterious effects of sedentary behavior on cognition. Importantly though, the evidence is still preliminary. We cannot be certain that this buffering effect is real until more investigation has been done on the topic. Next, we'll consider how physical activity and sedentary behavior prevent and treat cognitive impairment, including dementia.

CRITICAL THINKING ACTIVITY 8-4

How does physical activity affect cognitive abilities across the lifespan?

Physical Activity, Sedentary Behavior, and Cognitive Impairment

Cognitive Impairment, Dementia, and Alzheimer's Disease

Mild cognitive impairment is an intermediate stage between the expected cognitive decline of normal aging and the more pronounced decline of dementia. It involves problems with memory, language, thinking, and judgment that are greater than typical age-related changes. A person with mild cognitive impairment may be aware that their memory or mental function has slipped, and family and close friends may also notice a change. However, these changes are not generally severe enough to interfere with the person's day-to-day life and usual activities.

Mild cognitive impairment increases a person's risk of later developing dementia, including Alzheimer's disease, especially when the person's main difficulty is with memory. **Dementia** (which literally means "madness from the mind") is a serious loss of global cognitive ability in a previously unimpaired person, beyond what might be expected from normal aging. Although dementia is far more common in older adults, it can occur before the age of 65, in which case it is termed **early onset dementia**. Dementia is not a single disease, but rather a nonspecific illness syndrome (i.e., set of signs and symptoms). It can affect memory, attention, language, and problem solving. It is normally required to be present for at least 6 months to be diagnosed. Especially in the later stages of the condition, affected persons may be disoriented in time (not knowing what day of the week, day of the month, or even what year it is), in place (not knowing where they are), and in person (not knowing who they or others around them are). Dementia, though often treatable to some degree, is usually due to causes that are progressive and incurable.

There are many specific types and causes of dementia, often showing slightly different symptoms. One of the most common forms of dementia is **Alzheimer's disease**, a neurodegenerative disease characterized by a progressive deterioration of higher cognitive functioning in the areas of memory, problem solving, and thinking. **Table 8-3** lists potential signs of Alzheimer's disease.

Physical Activity and Sedentary Behavior in Preventing Cognitive Impairment

Determining the effects of physical activity and sedentary behavior for people at risk for dementia is very important. Can increasing physical activity or reducing sedentary behavior be used as treatments for dementia? Can increasing movement improve cognitive function in those at risk for dementia? Within this chapter section, we will consider the state of the evidence for these questions.

There is strong evidence that physical activity improves cognition in people with dementia and moderate evidence that physical activity reduces risks of dementia and cognitive impairment, including Alzheimer's disease (Erickson et al., 2019). For example, Beckett and colleagues (2015) reviewed prospective studies that investigated

Table 8-3 Signs of Alzheimer's Disease

Sign	Example
Recent memory loss	Asking the same question repeatedly, forgetting about already asking it.
Difficulty completing familiar tasks	Making a drink or cooking a meal but forgetting and leaving it.
Problems communicating	Difficulty with language by forgetting simple words or using the wrong ones.
Disorientation	Getting lost on a previously familiar street close to home and forgetting how they got there or would get home again.
Poor judgment	Forgetting all about the child they are watching and just leaving the house for the day.
Problems with abstract thinking	Difficulty with money and finances.
Misplacing things	Putting items in the wrong places and forgetting about doing this.
Mood changes	Swinging quickly through a set of moods.
Personality changes	Becoming irritable, suspicious, or fearful.
Loss of initiative	Showing less interest in starting something or going somewhere.

Data from American Academy of Family Physicians. (2001). The signs of dementia (patient information). *American Family Physician, 63,* 717–718.

whether physical activity prevented Alzheimer's disease in individuals 65 years or older. Review findings from 10 studies representing 20,326 participants showed that 1,358 participants were prospectively diagnosed with Alzheimer's disease (a rate of 6.7%), and older adults who were more physically active were less likely to be diagnosed than those who were less physically active, with a risk ratio of 0.61. The researchers concluded that given the limited treatment options, greater emphasis should be paid to primary prevention through physical activity among individuals at high risk of Alzheimer's disease, such as those with a strong genetic and family history.

A meta-analysis by Sofi and colleagues (2011) sought to examine the association between physical activity and cognitive decline in participants. Their review included 15 prospective cohort studies with 30,331 participants without dementia (aged 35 and older) who were followed for a period of 1–12 years. Of the 30,331 followed, the researchers found that 3,003 of the participants had developed cognitive decline. Of importance, physically active people at baseline had a significantly reduced rate of developing cognitive decline during the follow-up period. In fact, highly physically active people had a 38% reduced risk of cognitive decline compared to inactive people. Furthermore, even low to moderate intensity physical activity had a protective effect against cognitive impairment, reducing the risk of cognitive decline by 35%. The authors concluded that all levels of physical activity may protect against the occurrence of cognitive decline.

There is also some empirical evidence to suggest that sedentary behavior plays a role in risks of cognitive impairment. A study of more than 30,000 people older than 50 years found that being sedentary for more than 8 hours/day was associated with 1.56 times higher odds for mild cognitive impairment than those who were sedentary for less than eight hours/day (Vancampfort et al., 2018). Overall, though, the evidence is mixed. One systematic review of the association between sedentary behavior and cognition in adults older than 40 years found that there was insufficient evidence to determine whether

sedentary behavior impacts future risks of dementia (Falck, Davis, et al., 2017). However, another more recent review and meta-analysis with no age restrictions found that sedentary behavior was significantly associated with increased risk of dementia to a risk ratio of 1.30 (Yan et al., 2020).

Physical Activity and Sedentary Behavior in Improving Cognition in People with Cognitive Impairment

There is little evidence to determine whether reductions in sedentary behavior are valuable for cognition of people with cognitive impairment. Some preliminary studies suggest there may be potential benefits (Dillon & Prapavessis, 2020), but the evidence is inconclusive. There is, however, moderate evidence that physical activity improves cognition in those with dementia (Erickson et al., 2019). Many reviews have led to this conclusive state of the evidence, including one which reviewed 130 studies of older adults with dementia that investigated 133 different cognitive outcomes assessed using 267 different assessment tools (Gonçalves et al., 2018). An important finding of this review was that, although cognitive gains were valued, the most sought-after outcome for these patients and their caregivers was enjoyment. This highlights that intervention developers must always consider how to engage people within physical activity programs and enhance enjoyment, amidst focusing on enhancing cognitive benefits of the activities. To provide more insight into the process of intervention development, let's zoom in on a specific intervention program.

German researchers examined the effects of a home-based physical activity program on clinical symptoms, functional abilities, and caregiver burden in patients with Alzheimer's disease (Holthoff et al., 2015). Using a randomized controlled trial design involving 30 patients (mean age 72 years old) with Alzheimer's disease and their caregivers were allocated to either a home-based 12-week

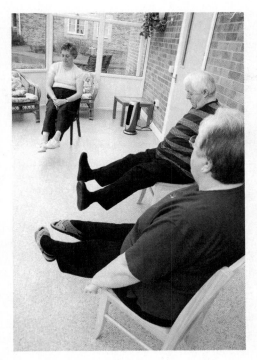

© Lucianne Pashley/Age fotostock/Alamy Stock Photo.

physical activity intervention group or the usual care group. The intervention changed between passive, motor-assisted, or active-resistive leg training and changes in direction on a movement trainer using a chair. Participants were required to train 3 times a week for 30 minutes at a self-selected time with at least 1 day without training in between 2 training days.

The researchers found that the control group experienced decreases in activities of daily living performance at weeks 12 and 24, whereas daily activity living performance of patients in the intervention group remained stable. Analyses of executive function and language ability revealed that patients in the intervention group improved during the intervention and returned to initial performance at week 12, whereas the controls revealed continuous worsening. Analyses of reaction time, hand-eye quickness, and attention revealed improvement only in the intervention group. Caregiver burden remained stable in the intervention group but worsened in the control group (see **Figure 8-3**).

Holthoff and colleagues (2015) concluded that physical activity in a home-based setting might be an effective and intrinsically motivating way to promote physical activity training in Alzheimer's patients and regulate caregiver burden.

Mechanism of Effect

Most of the research examining the mechanisms of how physical activity or sedentary behavior affects brain function has been undertaken with animal models. Based on these studies, there are several potential mechanisms that have been investigated, which are described in **Table 8-4** (Voss et al., 2014). Much of the observed changes in the brain involve **neurogenesis** (i.e., new nerve cell generation), **neurotransmitters** (i.e., chemical substances that transmit nerve impulses across a synapse, the tiny communication gap between the neurons in the brain), and vascular adaptations, such as the formation of new blood vessels (van Praag, 2009). In fact, van Praag (2009) stated that animal research reveals

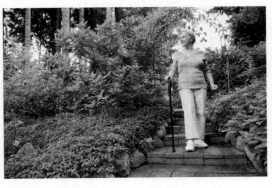

© Fancy/Veer/Corbis/Getty Images.

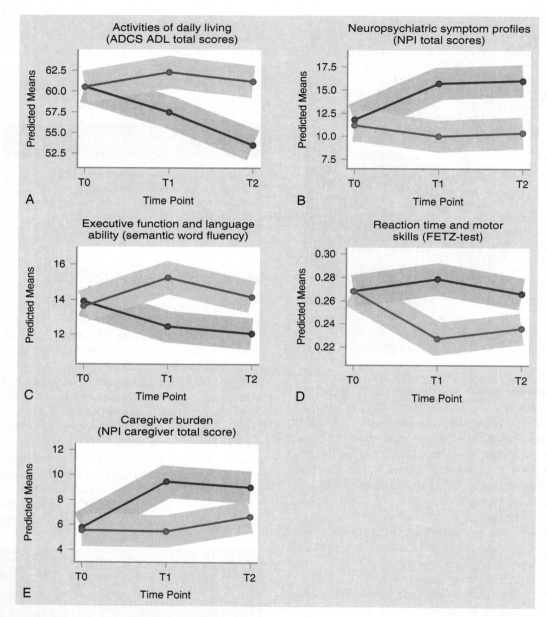

Figure 8-3 Effects of Physical Activity on Clinical Performance.
This figure shows the effects of physical activity on the patients when compared to the control group for the 3 time points (T0, baseline; T1, 3 months later or after completion of the intervention; and T2, 3 month follow-up). Activities of daily living (ADCS ADL total scores): Patients in the control group experienced significant decreases in their performance over 12 weeks and at the 3 month follow-up, whereas patients in the intervention group remained stable during the study period and follow up (a). Neuropsychiatric symptom profiles (NPI total scores): Controls suffered a considerable increase in behavioral changes over 24 weeks, whereas patients in the intervention group remained stable over 24 weeks (b). Executive function and language ability: Patients in the intervention group improved during the intervention period and returned to initial performance after completion but without revealing the continuous worsening over 24 weeks demonstrated in the controls (c). Reaction time, hand-eye quickness, and attention (FETZ-test or Ruler Drop Test): Only patients in the intervention group improved their performance during the study period (d). Caregiver burden (NPI): Burden increased in the control group during the first 3 months whereas caregiver burden remained stable in the intervention group during the study period (e).

Holthoff, V. A., Marschner, K., Scharf, M., Steding, J., Meyer, S., Koch, T., & Donix, M. (2015). Effects of physical activity training in patients with Alzheimer's dementia: Results of a pilot RCT study. *PLoS ONE, 10*(4): e0121478. https://doi.org/10.1371/journal.pone.0121478

Table 8-4 Description of The Neurophysiological Mechanisms Likely Explaining Why Physical Activity and Sedentary Behavior impact Cognition

Mechanism	Description	How is it Relevant to Cognition?	Physical Activity/ Sedentary Behavior
Neurogenesis	The birth of new neurons	Neurogenesis in the hippo-campus is associated with gains in learning and memory processes.	Some evidence suggests physical activity enhances neurogenesis and sedentary behavior reduces neurogenesis.
Synaptic Plasticity	Strengthening efficiency in the junctions between neurons that allows them to share information	Learning and storing of memo-ries are directly reliant on synaptic plasticity.	Physical activity facilitates synaptic plasticity and sedentary behavior may suppress it.
Growth Factors	Proteins that stimulate tissue growth	Growth factors such as Brain-Derived Neurotrophic Factor regulate and enhance the survival and maturation of new neurons.	Growth factor modulation is enhanced by physical activity and decreased by sedentary behavior.
Cerebrovascular Remodeling	Alterations in the structure and functioning of the brain	Structural changes or functional adaptations can enhance the strong connection between neurons and the cerebrovascular system that is essential for cognition.	Cerebrovascular remodeling has been shown to be a response to physical activity, but it is unclear if sedentary behavior leads to cerebrovascular remodeling.
Neuroendocrine Functioning	The process by which cells make hormones in response to mes-sages from the nervous system	Neuroendocrine functioning is crucial for problem solving and the body's response to stress.	Physical activity activates enhancement of neuroendocrine functioning, whereas sedentary behavior leads to poorer neuroendocrine functioning.
Inflammation	Inflammatory responses to oxidative stress	Inflammation is associated with higher likelihood of dementia and poorer cognition.	Physical activity leads to adaptive anti-inflammatory responses to stress, and early evidence sug-gests sedentary behavior may lead to more inflammatory stress responses.
Brain Volume	Brain volume loss is a marker of neurodegeneration.	Brain volume declines naturally with ageing and is associated with declines in cognitive outcomes.	Physical activity can forestall age-related declines in brain volume; it is unknown whether sedentary behavior impacts brain volume.

(continues)

Table 8-4 Description of The Neurophysiological Mechanisms Likely Explaining Why Physical Activity and Sedentary Behavior impact Cognition   *(continued)*

Mechanism	Description	How is it Relevant to Cognition?	Physical Activity/ Sedentary Behavior
Higher-Level Brain Function	Monitoring changes in blood-oxygenation can demonstrate differences of the functional capacity of the prefrontal cortex.	Higher-level brain function illustrates efficiency of top-down attention control and decreased response conflict.	Physical activity enhances higher-level brain functioning; it is unknown if sedentary behavior is associated with higher-level brain function.

Data from Voss, M. W., Carr, L. J., Clark, R., & Weng, T. (2014). Revenge of the "sit" II: Does lifestyle impact neuronal and cognitive health through distinct mechanisms associated with sedentary behavior and physical activity? *Mental Health and Physical Activity, 7*(1), 9–24. https://doi.org/10.1016/j.mhpa.2014.01.001

that physical activity is the strongest neurogenic stimulus. Much of this neurogenesis occurs in the hippocampus of the brain, which is an important area for learning and memory. Hillman and his colleagues (2008) stated that this hippocampus cell proliferation is the most consistently observed effect from physical activity and that it can occur at all stages of life.

Preliminary research is also revealing that physical activity can lead to changes in the brain, making it more plastic (i.e., its ability to change physically, functionally, and chemically), and improving memory and motor skill coordination. Using a small sample size, Smith and his colleagues (2014) had young adults ride a bike vigorously for 30 minutes (Smith et al., 2014). The researchers monitored changes in the brain directly after the exercise session and again 15 minutes later. Results show that even one 30 minute session of physical activity can improve the brain's plasticity. Positive changes in the brain were sustained for 15 minutes after exercising. The more plastic the brain becomes, the better its ability to reorganize itself by modifying the number and strength of connections between nerve cells and different brain areas. This change in the brain may, in part, explain why physical activity has a positive effect on memory and higher-level functions.

Researchers from Finland found that greater levels of physical activity were associated with increased volume of the gray matter in the brain (Rottensteiner et al., 2015). The study participants were 10 pairs of identical male twins between the ages of 32 and 36 years old. In each pair of twins, one brother had exercised more over the past 3 years than the other, although they reported that they carried out similar levels of exercise earlier in their lives. On average, the more active members of twin pairs were jogging about 3 hours more per week compared to their inactive twin counterparts. The twins had MRI scans of their brains to determine the effects that physical activity had on the size of them. Results revealed that physical activity did not affect the size of the brain as a whole. However, there was a connection between more activity and more brain volume in areas related to movement (i.e., balance and coordination). The researchers concluded that these changes in the brain may have long-term health implications, such as reduced risk of falling.

Impact of Cognition on Physical Activity and Sedentary Behavior

Given that there is correlational, longitudinal, and experimental data to suggest that changes in physical activity led to enhanced cognition, we can be quite confident in saying physical activity *causes* enhancements of cognition; that the evidence of sedentary behavior and cognition is largely observational and correlational precludes the conclusion that sedentary behavior *causes* reductions in cognition. It may very well be, instead or additionally, that people with poorer cognition tend to be more sedentary and less physically active than those with better cognition.

It is reasonable to expect that a person's cognition can impact their future physical activity and sedentary behavior. It takes a lot of brain power to prioritize and plan engagement in physical activity on a regular basis, especially when things pop up that may disrupt daily life, like bad weather, feeling ill, or having assignment deadlines impending. Indeed, a building line of evidence is showing this to be the case – people with better cognitive abilities tend to be more physically active and less sedentary than those with poorer cognitive abilities. For example, Hall and colleagues (2008) found that future physical activity behavior can be explained by individual differences in executive functioning. In addition to finding a direct link between executive functioning and future behavior, this work helped us realize that executive functioning can be pivotal for following through on intentions to engage in health behaviors, such as increasing physical activity and reducing sedentary behavior. Given that the decision of how and when to use self-control is a higher-order cognitive process, it is important to consider what cognitive capacities people can contribute to changing their behavior when developing interventions to motivate increases in physical activity or reductions in sedentary behavior (Pfeffer & Strobach, 2017).

Evidence shows that those with cognitive impairments tend to be more sedentary and less active than those without cognitive impairments (Hartman et al., 2018), with one study estimating that community-dwelling dementia patients spend 66% of their time being sedentary (Alphen et al., 2016). More longitudinal and experimental research is needed to determine whether people who are more sedentary tend to have poorer cognition than those who are less sedentary or whether sedentary behavior impacts risks of poor cognition later in life.

Summary

Cognition is instrumental to our daily lives, whether it be how we organize our time, problem solve relationship quarrels, or making decisions to act in ways that keep our minds and bodies healthy. There are many things we can do that mean we aren't thinking as clearly as we could, like not getting enough sleep, consuming drugs or alcohol, or feeling stressed for a long time. Even naturally, our cognition tends to wane as we age, so it is important to understand how physical activity and sedentary behavior can play a role in keeping us sharp. The evidence seems quite clear that physical activity enhances cognition, both immediately after a single bout and chronically over time with regular physical activity engagement. The evidence is less clear for sedentary behavior, but early indications are that it depends on what we are doing while being sedentary and whether it is detrimental to cognition or not. As the body of evidence continues to evolve, we'll hopefully find ways to help people get physically active and live in ways that help them get the most out of their minds.

Vignette: Mike

Throughout grade school, I had trouble focusing. I'm not sure I was alone in this. Most kids in my class were rambunctious and struggled to sit still—more eager to make it to recess than remain inert at an uncomfortable desk. Teachers encouraged my mom to take me to a psychiatrist so that someone could verify whether or not I had ADHD and potentially, put me on medication. But my mom had a hunch there was a different approach to quelling my excess energy that didn't involve swallowing a pill.

She knew well that the days I had gym class tended to be the ones during which I was able to more easily calm down. She signed me up for an after-school sports program—one where I got to try out everything from basketball to soccer and even roller hockey. I never ended up taking any prescriptions, and mostly was able to do alright as I matured. Once I got to high school, it was pretty clear that so long as I could burn off my energy outside of classes, I could hold it together while in them.

I think my problems started cropping up in college when I didn't try out for any teams because I honestly didn't consider myself much of an athlete. Sure, I'd enjoyed sports for most of my adolescent life, but I had no delusions about being any star player. Not having a team to practice with left me with little incentive to stay fit. And I wasn't particularly practiced in walking myself through a solo workout at the school's gym.

Needless to say, my time spent exercising dwindled rapidly during my first semester. Shortly after I settled into campus life, I picked up the habit of drinking, which further dragged down my fitness. I wanted badly to fit in with my classmates. Looking back, I realize I was seeking a substitute for the camaraderie of being part of a sports team. The surest way to revive that sense of belonging seemed to be drinking beers to the point of blacking out. Exchanging war stories of how many things went wrong during the haze of alcohol-drenched evenings made me feel included and "cool."

I would joke with my college buddies that the so-called freshman 15 would have been preferable. For me, it was more like the freshman 40. By second semester of my freshman year, I'd had to buy an entirely new wardrobe—give or take the sweatpants and oversized T-shirts I could still stretch around my newly enlarged waist.

I'll never know if it was the drinking alone or the lack of healthy eating and exercise accompanying it that was to blame, but after my first winter break, I felt just like I had in elementary school, when my focus darted around the classroom, and I could barely contain my legs from bouncing underneath my desk. Too often, I'd

sit through a whole lecture fidgeting madly, biting my nails, and not remembering half of what the professor said because I was too consumed by feelings of restlessness. The only difference was that this time around I was exhausted, often hungover, and increasingly moody.

When I came home for the summer after my first year at college, I was embarrassed when I reconnected with my high school friends. Some of them joked about my weight gain. A few asked me to go for jogs with them but then stopped reaching out to me once I blew them off a couple times.

My mom was the first to swoop in and comment on my laziness. At the time, I felt that she didn't understand and was just being invasive. My dad and she staged what might be likened to an intervention one morning after I'd stumbled home following a late night out on the town. They showed me a picture from my sports playing days and asked me what changed when I left—why I'd decided to completely ignore my health (not to mention my appearance). I was definitely hurt that they were essentially telling me I'd become a really disappointing version of myself. But it was clear that they were more concerned than they were angry.

They decided we should all get a family membership at our local fitness center. The thought of working out alongside my parents was, at first blush, humiliating. But my dad arranged for me to work with a trainer and promised he and my mom wouldn't always be at the gym during the same time as me.

I hated that trainer; in part, because he was so much more fit than I ever could hope to be, even when compared to how I looked during high school, and also because he really took me to task on my drinking—enlightening me to just how many calories beer contained—while refusing to let me use being hungover as an excuse to cancel a session.

It took about 3 weeks, if I remember correctly, to actually enjoy the feeling of being physically active again. At first, it was a grueling process filled with self-loathing and anticipation of failure. But after that first week of training, I could already feel my mood improving. And by the end of the summer, I was even able to join my former high school pals for that previously turned-down jog.

My trainer and I worked to design a fitness plan for when classes started up again. I came back to school armed with some basic body weight exercises to do in my room, and I'd gotten over the intimidation factor of using all that equipment by myself at the school gym.

Being in an environment I associated with drinking made me slip back a bit during the first few weeks of my second year. But I ended up taking advantage of the student health services and seeing a psychologist to deal with the anxiety I had at the prospect of losing friends if I gave up partying. I ended up joining student senate and going to a few student support groups to make some friends who weren't as steeped in the drinking culture as those from my freshman year.

I never gave up drinking entirely. But making fitness a more regular part of my life helped reduce the appeal of alcohol—especially because alcohol interfered with my energy levels and performance. Sure, I'd miss days at the gym and feel worse about myself for it. But I never went back to not going at all. And so long as I was able to make it to the fitness center at least 3 times a week—or, if not, do some pushups in my room or take a quick jog around campus—my ability to concentrate in class vastly improved.

I ended up graduating with a double major in political science and psychology. And though the job I got out of college working at a congressional research firm is definitely a challenge to being regularly active, I continue to make time for exercise before and after work as well as on weekends. I've even joined an adult pickup basketball team started by some of my colleagues.

I know that if I cut back on physical activity, the concentration I need to get through a work week won't be there. Plus, not spending enough time moving around makes me sad, depressed, and more inclined to overdo the booze.

These days, I don't work out because it makes me look good—I've accepted that I'll likely never have the body of a sprinter or a weightlifter—but because it makes me happier and, most importantly, it enables me to get ahead in my career.

Key Terms

Alzheimer's disease A neurodegenerative disease characterized by a progressive deterioration of higher cognitive functioning in the areas of memory, problem solving, and thinking.

attention deficit/hyperactivity disorder (ADHD) One of the most common childhood disorders and can continue through adolescence and into adulthood with symptoms including difficulty staying focused and paying attention, difficulty controlling behavior, and/or hyperactivity.

brain hemispheres The two symmetrical halves of the brain.

cognition Mental processes that reflect a person's knowledge or awareness, including thinking, knowing, remembering, reasoning, decision making, learning, judging, and problem solving.

corpus callosum The connective flat neural fibers that relay information between the brain's hemispheres.

dementia A non-specific illness syndrome characterized by a serious loss of global cognitive ability in a previously unimpaired person, beyond what might be expected from normal aging.

early onset dementia Dementia that occurs before the age of 65 years.

executive functioning The cognitive process that regulates the ability to organize thoughts and activities, prioritize tasks, manage time efficiently, and make decisions.

exergaming Technology-driven physical activity.

mild cognitive impairment An intermediate stage between the expected cognitive decline of normal aging and the more pronounced decline of dementia that involves problems with memory, language, thinking, and judgment that are greater than typical age-related changes.

neurogenesis New nerve cell generation.

neurotransmitters Chemical substances that transmit nerve impulses across a synapse, the tiny communication gap between the neurons in the brain.

processing speed The speed at which the brain processes information. Faster processing speed means more efficient thinking and learning.

spatial-visual processes How we sense the interrelations of things in space around us, including navigating where we are going, and representing a concept through drawing.

Review Questions

1. What is the link between physical activity and cognition in children younger than 5 years old? How strong is the evidence?

2. How important do you think it is to consider physical activity and sedentary behavior when trying to improve academic performance in children? Why?

3. What is the state of the evidence for adults under 50 years old in terms of the impact of physical activity and sedentary behavior on cognition?

4. How would you set up a study to investigate whether exergames has benefits above and beyond physical activity? What would be important to control and how would you do that?

5. What is the difference between cognitive impairment, dementia, and Alzheimer's disease?

6. Name three potential mechanisms by which physical activity could enhance cognition.

Applying the Concepts

1. Describe how Mike's cognition was impacted by changes in physical activity. What scientific evidence can help support your claims?

2. In what ways does Mike's motivation for physical activity and sedentary behavior seem to be impacted by his cognition?

References

Aggio, D., Smith, L., Fisher, A., & Hamer, M. (2016). Context-specific associations of physical activity and sedentary behavior with cognition in children. *American Journal of Epidemiology, 183*(12), 1075–1082. https://doi .org/10.1093/aje/kww031

Alphen, H. J. M. van, Volkers, K. M., Blankevoort, C. G., Scherder, E. J. A., Hortobágyi, T., & Heuvelen, M. J. G. van. (2016). Older adults with dementia are sedentary for most of the day. *PLOS ONE, 11*(3), e0152457. https://doi .org/10.1371/journal.pone.0152457

American Psychiatric Association. (2013). *Diagnostic and statistical manual of mental disorders (DSM-5®)*. American Psychiatric Publishing.

Beckett, M. W., Ardern, C. I., & Rotondi, M. A. (2015). A meta-analysis of prospective studies on the role of physical activity and the prevention of Alzheimer's disease in older adults. *BioMed Central Geriatrics, 15*(1), 9. https://doi.org /10.1186/s12877-015-0007-2

Bloom, B. S., Engelhart, M. D., Furst, E. J., Hill, W. H., & Krathwohl, D. R. (2013). Taxonomy of educational objectives: The classification of educational goals; Handbook I: Cognitive Domain. New York: Shortmans, Green.

Brandt, V., Patalay, P., & Kerner auch Koerner, J. (2021). Predicting ADHD symptoms and diagnosis at age 14 from objective activity levels at age 7 in a large UK cohort. *European Child & Adolescent Psychiatry, 30*, 877–884.

Carson, V., Hunter, S., Kuzik, N., Wiebe, S. A., Spence, J. C., Friedman, A., Tremblay, M. S., Slater, L., & Hinkley, T. (2016). Systematic review of physical activity and cognitive development in early childhood. *Journal of Science and Medicine in Sport, 19*(7), 573–578. https://doi .org/10.1016/j.jsams.2015.07.011

Carson, V., Kuzik, N., Hunter, S., Wiebe, S. A., Spence, J. C., Friedman, A., Tremblay, M. S., Slater, L. G., & Hinkley, T. (2015). Systematic review of sedentary behavior and cognitive development in early childhood. *Preventive Medicine, 78*, 115–122. https://doi.org/10.1016/j.ypmed .2015.07.016

Carson, V., Rahman, A. A., & Wiebe, S. A. (2017). Associations of subjectively and objectively measured sedentary behavior and physical activity with cognitive development in the early years. *Mental Health and Physical Activity, 13*, 1–8. https://doi.org/10.1016/j.mhpa.2017.05.003

Centers for Disease Control and Prevention (2010). The association between school-based physical activity, including physical education, and academic performance. http://www.cdc.gov/healthyyouth/health_and_academics /pdf/pa-pe_paper.pdf

Centers for Disease Control and Prevention. (2020a). Healthy Schools. https://www.cdc.gov/healthyschools/physical activity/facts.htm

Centers for Disease Control and Prevention. (2020b). Data and Statistics About ADHD. https://www.cdc.gov/ncbddd /adhd/data.html

Chaddock, L., Pontifex, M. B., Hillman, C. H., & Kramer, A. F. (2011). A review of the relation of aerobic fitness and physical activity to brain structure and function in children. *Journal of the International Neuropsychological Society, 17*(6), 975–985. https://doi.org/10.1017/S13556 17711000567

Dawson, A. E., Wymbs, B. T., Gidycz, C. A., Pride, M., & Figueroa, W. (2017). Exploring rates of transgender individuals and mental health concerns in an online sample. *International Journal of Transgenderism, 18*(3), 295–304. https://doi.org/10.1080/15532739.2017.1314797

Dillon, K., & Prapavessis, H. (2020). Reducing Sedentary behavior among mild to moderate cognitively impaired assisted living residents: A pilot randomized controlled trial (resedent study). *Journal of Aging and Physical Activity, 29*(1), 27–35. https://doi.org/10.1123/japa.2019-0440

Donnelly, J. E., Hillman, C. H., Castelli, D., Etnier, J. L., Lee, S., Tomporowski, P., Lambourne, K., & Szabo-Reed, A. N. (2016). Physical Activity, fitness, cognitive function, and academic achievement in children: A systematic review. *Medicine and Science in Sports and Exercise, 48*(6), 1197–1222. https://doi.org/10.1249/MSS.0000000000000901

Donnelly, J. E., Hillman, C. H., Greene, J. L., Hansen, D. M., Gibson, C. A., Sullivan, D. K., Poggio, J., Mayo, M. S., Lambourne, K., Szabo-Reed, A. N., Herrmann, S. D., Honas, J. J., Scudder, M. R., Betts, J. L., Henley, K., Hunt, S. L., & Washburn, R. A. (2017). Physical activity and academic achievement across the curriculum: Results from a 3-year cluster-randomized trial. *Preventive Medicine, 99*, 140–145. https://doi.org/10.1016/j.ypmed.2017.02.006

Donnelly, J. E., & Lambourne, K. (2011). Classroom-based physical activity, cognition, and academic achievement. *Preventive Medicine, 52*, S36–S42. https://doi.org/10.1016 /j.ypmed.2011.01.021

Edwards, M. K., & Loprinzi, P. D. (2017). The association between sedentary behavior and cognitive function among older adults may be attenuated with adequate physical activity. *Journal of Physical Activity and Health, 14*(1), 52–58. https://doi.org/10.1123/jpah.2016-0313

Erickson, K. I., Hillman, C., Stillman, C. M., Ballard, R. M., Bloodgood, B., Conroy, D. E., Macko, R., Marquez, D. X., et al. (2019). Physical activity, cognition, and brain outcomes: A review of the 2018 physical activity guidelines. *Medicine and Science in Sports and Exercise, 51*(6), 1242–1251. https://doi.org/10.1249/MSS.0000000000001936

Falck, R. S., Davis, J. C., & Liu-Ambrose, T. (2017). What is the association between sedentary behaviour and cognitive function? A systematic review. *British Journal of Sports Medicine, 51*(10), 800–811. https://doi.org/10.1136 /bjsports-2015-095551

Falck, R. S., Landry, G. J., Best, J. R., Davis, J. C., Chiu, B. K., & Liu-Ambrose, T. (2017). Cross-Sectional relationships of physical activity and sedentary behavior with cognitive function in older adults with probable mild cognitive impairment. *Physical Therapy, 97*(10), 975–984. https:// doi.org/10.1093/ptj/pzx074

Fedewa, A. L., & Ahn, S. (2011). The effects of physical activity and physical fitness on children's achievement and cognitive outcomes. *Research Quarterly for Exercise and Sport, 82*(3), 521–535. https://doi.org/10.1080/02701367 .2011.10599785

Gapin, J. I., Labban, J. D., & Etnier, J. L. (2011). The effects of physical activity on attention deficit hyperactivity disorder symptoms: The evidence. *Preventive Medicine, 52*, S70–S74. https://doi.org/10.1016/j.ypmed.2011.01.022

Gijselaers, H. J. M., Kirschner, P. A., Verboon, P., & de Groot, R. H. M. (2016). Sedentary behavior and not physical activity predicts study progress in distance education. *Learning and Individual Differences, 49*, 224–229. https:// doi.org/10.1016/j.lindif.2016.06.021

Gonçalves, A.-C., Cruz, J., Marques, A., Demain, S., & Samuel, D. (2018). Evaluating physical activity in dementia: A systematic review of outcomes to inform the development of a core outcome set. *Age and Ageing, 47*(1), 34–41. https://doi.org/10.1093/ageing/afx135

Haapala, E. A., Poikkeus, A.-M., Kukkonen-Harjula, K., Tompuri, T., Lintu, N., Väistö, J., Leppänen, P. H. T., Laaksonen, D. E., Lindi, V., et al (2014). Associations of physical activity and sedentary behavior with academic skills – a follow-up study among primary school children. *PLOS ONE, 9*(9), e107031. https://doi .org/10.1371/journal.pone.0107031

Hall, P. A., Fong, G. T., Epp, L. J., & Elias, L. J. (2008). Executive function moderates the intention-behavior link for physical activity and dietary behavior. *Psychology & Health, 23*(3), 309–326. https://doi.org/10.1080/1476832070 1212099

Hamer, M., & Stamatakis, E. (2014). Prospective study of seden-tary behavior, risk of depression, and cognitive impairment. *Medicine and Science in Sports and Exercise, 46*(4), 718–723. https://doi.org/10.1249/MSS.0000000000000156

Hartman, Y. A. W., Karssemeijer, E. G. A., van Diepen, L. A. M., Olde Rikkert, M. G. M., & Thijssen, D. H. J. (2018). Dementia patients are more sedentary and less physically active than age- and sex-matched cognitively healthy older adults. *Dementia and Geriatric Cognitive Disorders, 46*(1–2), 81–89. https://doi.org/10.1159/000491995

Hillman, C. H., Erickson, K. I., & Kramer, A. F. (2008). Be smart, exercise your heart: Exercise effects on brain and cognition. *Nature Reviews Neuroscience, 9*(1), 58–65. https://doi.org/10.1038/nrn2298

Hillman, C. H., Kamijo, K., & Scudder, M. (2011). A review of chronic and acute physical activity participation on neuroelectric measures of brain health and cognition during childhood. *Preventive Medicine, 52*, S21–S28. https://doi.org/10.1016/j.ypmed.2011.01.024

Hollis, J. L., Sutherland, R., Williams, A. J., Campbell, E., Nathan, N., Wolfenden, L., Morgan, P. J., Lubans, D. R., Gillham, K., et al. (2017). A systematic review and meta-analysis of moderate-to-vigorous physical activity levels in secondary school physical education lessons. *International Journal of Behavioral Nutrition and Physical Activity, 14*(1), 52. https://doi.org/10.1186/s12966-017-0504-0

Holthoff, V. A., Marschner, K., Scharf, M., Steding, J., Meyer, S., Koch, R., & Donix, M. (2015). Effects of physical activity training in patients with alzheimer's dementia: results of a pilot RCT study. *PLOS ONE, 10*(4), e0121478. https://doi.org/10.1371/journal.pone.0121478

Lee, S. M., Burgeson, C. R., Fulton, J. E., & Spain, C. G. (2007). Physical education and physical activity: Results from the school health policies and programs study 2006. *Journal of School Health, 77*(8), 435–463. https://doi.org/10.1111/j.1746-1561.2007.00229.x

MacNeilage, P. F., Rogers, L. J., & Vallortigara, G. (2009). Origins of the left & right brain. *Scientific American, 301*(1), 60–67.

Magnon, V., Vallet, G. T., & Auxiette, C. (2018). Sedentary behavior at work and cognitive functioning: A systematic review. *Frontiers in Public Health, 6*, 239. https://doi.org/10.3389/fpubh.2018.00239

Mahar, M. T. (2011). Impact of short bouts of physical activity on attention-to-task in elementary school children. *Preventive Medicine, 52*, S60–S64. https://doi.org/10.1016/j.ypmed.2011.01.026

Northey, J. M., Cherbuin, N., Pumpa, K. L., Smee, D. J., & Rattray, B. (2018). Exercise interventions for cognitive function in adults older than 50: A systematic review with meta-analysis. *British Journal of Sports Medicine, 52*(3), 154–160. https://doi.org/10.1136/bjsports-2016-096587

Ogawa, E. F., You, T., & Leveille, S. G. (2016). Potential benefits of exergaming for cognition and dual-task function in older adults: A systematic review. *Journal of Aging and Physical Activity, 24*(2), 332–336. https://doi.org/10.1123/japa.2014-0267

O'Halloran, C. J., Kinsella, G. J., & Storey, E. (2012). The cerebellum and neuropsychological functioning: A critical review. *Journal of Clinical and Experimental Neuropsychology, 34*(1), 35–56. https://doi.org/10.1080/13803395.2011.614599

Pfeffer, I., & Strobach, T. (2017). Executive functions, trait self-control, and the intention–behavior gap in physical activity behavior. *Journal of Sport and Exercise Psychology, 39*(4), 277–292. https://doi.org/10.1123/jsep.2017-0112

Rottensteiner, M., Kujala, U. M., Leskinen, T., & Niskanen, E. (2015). Physical activity, fitness, glucose homeostasis, and brain morphology in twins. *Medicine & Science in Sports & Exercise: Official Journal of the American College of Sports Medicine, 47*(3), 509–518.

Safren, S. A., Sprich, S., Mimiaga, M. J., Surman, C., Knouse, L., Groves, M., & Otto, M. W. (2010). Cognitive behavioral therapy vs relaxation with educational support for medication-treated adults with ADHD and persistent symptoms: A randomized controlled trial. *Journal of the American Medical Association, 304*(8), 875–880. https://doi.org/10.1001/jama.2010.1192

Shaw, P., Eckstrand, K., Sharp, W., Blumenthal, J., Lerch, J. P., Greenstein, D., Clasen, L., Evans, A., et al. (2007). Attention-deficit/hyperactivity disorder is characterized by a delay in cortical maturation. *Proceedings of the National Academy of Sciences, 104*(49), 19649–19654. https://doi.org/10.1073/pnas.0707741104

Sherman, C. (2019, August 2). Right brain left brain: A misnomer. *Dana Foundation.* https://www.dana.org/article/right-brain-left-brain-really/

Singh, A., Uijtdewilligen, L., Twisk, J. W. R., van Mechelen, W., & Chinapaw, M. J. M. (2012). Physical Activity and performance at school: A Systematic review of the literature including a methodological quality assessment. *Archives of Pediatrics & Adolescent Medicine, 166*(1), 49–55. https://doi.org/10.1001/archpediatrics.2011.716

Smith, A. E., Goldsworthy, M. R., Garside, T., Wood, F. M., & Ridding, M. C. (2014). The influence of a single bout of aerobic exercise on short-interval intracortical excitability. *Experimental Brain Research, 232*(6), 1875–1882. https://doi.org/10.1007/s00221-014-3879-z

Smith, P. J., Blumenthal, J. A., Hoffman, B. M., Cooper, H., Strauman, T. A., Welsh-Bohmer, K., Browndyke, J. N., & Sherwood, A. (2010). Aerobic exercise and neurocognitive performance: A meta-analytic review of randomized controlled trials. *Psychosomatic Medicine, 72*(3), 239–252. https://doi.org/10.1097/PSY.0b013e3181d14633

Sofi, F., Valecchi, D., Bacci, D., Abbate, R., Gensini, G. F., Casini, A., & Macchi, C. (2011). Physical activity and risk of cognitive decline: A meta-analysis of prospective studies. *Journal of Internal Medicine, 269*(1), 107–117. https://doi.org/10.1111/j.1365-2796.2010.02281.x

Suarez-Manzano, S., Ruiz-Ariza, A., De La Torre-Cruz, M., & Martínez-López, E. J. (2018). Acute and chronic effect of physical activity on cognition and behaviour in young people with ADHD: A systematic review of intervention studies. *Research in Developmental Disabilities, 77*, 12–23. https://doi.org/10.1016/j.ridd.2018.03.015

Suchert, V., Pedersen, A., Hanewinkel, R., & Isensee, B. (2017). Relationship between attention-deficit/hyperactivity disorder and sedentary behavior in adolescence: A cross-sectional study. *ADHD Attention Deficit and Hyperactivity Disorders, 9*(4), 213–218. https://doi.org/10.1007/s12402-017-0229-6

Toomey, S. L., Sox, C. M., Rusinak, D., & Finkelstein, J. A. (2012). Why do children with ADHD discontinue their medication? *Clinical Pediatrics, 51*(8), 763–769.

Tremblay, M. S., LeBlanc, A. G., Kho, M. E., Saunders, T. J., Larouche, R., Colley, R. C., Goldfield, G., & Gorber, S. C. (2011). Systematic review of sedentary behaviour and health indicators in school-aged children and youth. *International Journal of Behavioral Nutrition and Physical Activity, 8*(1), 98. https://doi.org/10.1186/1479 -5868-8-98

Vaidya, C. J., Austin, G., Kirkorian, G., Ridlehuber, H. W., Desmond, J. E., Glover, G. H., & Gabrieli, J. D. E. (1998). Selective effects of methylphenidate in attention deficit hyperactivity disorder: A functional magnetic resonance study. *Proceedings of the National Academy of Sciences, 95*(24), 14494–14499. https://doi.org/10.1073 /pnas.95.24.14494

Vancampfort, D., Stubbs, B., Lara, E., Vandenbulcke, M., Swinnen, N., Smith, L., Firth, J., Herring, M. P., et al. (2018). Mild cognitive impairment and sedentary behavior: A multinational study. *Experimental Gerontology, 108*, 174–180. https://doi.org/10.1016/j.exger.2018.04.017

Vance, D. E., Wadley, V. G., Ball, K. K., Roenker, D. L., & Rizzo, M. (2005). The effects of physical activity and sedentary behavior on cognitive health in older adults. *Journal of Aging and Physical Activity, 13*(3), 294–313. https://doi.org/10.1123/japa.13.3.294

van Praag, H. (2009). Exercise and the brain: Something to chew on. *Trends in Neurosciences, 32*(5), 283–290. https:// doi.org/10.1016/j.tins.2008.12.007

Voss, M. W., Carr, L. J., Clark, R., & Weng, T. (2014). Revenge of the "sit" II: Does lifestyle impact neuronal and cognitive health through distinct mechanisms associated with sedentary behavior and physical activity? *Mental Health and Physical Activity, 7*(1), 9–24. https://doi.org/10.1016/j .mhpa.2014.01.001

Wechsler, D. (2005) Wechsler Individual Achievement Test, 2nd UK Edition. London, UK: Pearson.

Yan, S., Fu, W., Wang, C., Mao, J., Liu, B., Zou, L., & Lv, C. (2020). Association between sedentary behavior and the risk of dementia: A systematic review and meta-analysis. *Translational Psychiatry, 10*(1), 1–8. https://doi .org/10.1038/s41398-020-0799-5

Zeng, N., Ayyub, M., Sun, H., Wen, X., Xiang, P., & Gao, Z. (2017). Effects of physical activity on motor skills and cognitive development in early childhood: A systematic review. *BioMed Research International, 2017.*

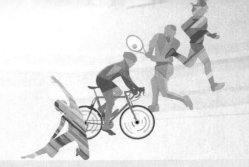

CHAPTER 9

Sleep

LEARNING OBJECTIVES

After completing this chapter, you will be able to:

- Understand why sleep is important.
- Define the stages of sleep.
- Describe how physical activity and sedentary behavior impact our sleep.
- Describe some examples of sleep disorders.
- Identify potential mechanisms for why physical activity results in improved sleep.

Introduction

Mark Twain is an American icon who has written with insight and humor. Not surprisingly then, he has been often quoted for his perspectives on a variety of topics, even exercise: "I have never taken any exercise except sleeping and resting and I never intend to take any" (Twain, 1905). As this quote indicates, Mark Twain was not a strong proponent of being physically active. Ironically, if he was alive today and consulted with healthcare professionals, he likely would be advised to exercise more frequently to improve his sleep! As Youngstedt, O'Connor, and Dishman (1997) stated, "Few behaviors are as closely linked with enhanced sleep as exercise" (p. 203). In this chapter, the suspected link between physical activity and sleep is explored. Additionally, we'll cover the evolving field of study regarding whether sedentary behavior impacts sleep. Before we examine these developing bodies of research, let's first determine what sleep is and why it is so important to our health.

What Is Sleep?

Sleep is a naturally recurring state of rest for the mind and body, in which the eyes usually close and consciousness is either completely or partially lost. When we sleep, there is a decrease in bodily movement and responsiveness to external stimuli (American Heritage Medical Dictionary, 2007). We tend to spend about one-third of our lives sleeping (National Institute of Health, 2019), but that time is far from being unproductive. Let's take a closer look at what happens to us when we sleep.

Why We Need Sleep

Until relatively recently, why we sleep has remained pretty much a mystery to scientists; however, there have been some exciting breakthroughs in our understanding of what happens to the mind and body while we sleep. Evidence now suggests purposes of sleep include saving

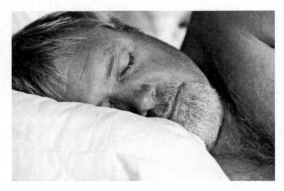

© Tish1/ShutterStock.

energy, controlling body temperature, and adaptations of our immunity system. However, the two main areas of research focus on two benefits of sleep: restoration and memory consolidation. **Restoration** allows for the body and mind to repair itself and regulate cellular functioning that can deteriorate throughout waking periods. Although this clearing out of neurotoxic waste happens gradually while we are awake, it speeds up quite rapidly while we are asleep, allowing for a more thorough restorative effect (Xie et al., 2013). **Memory consolidation** is a process in which recently encoded memory representations are reactivated and transformed into long-term memory (Rasch & Born, 2013). Without this process occurring, we would have a much harder time remembering and recalling things that are important to us. So the fact that 60% of sampled university students have pulled an all-nighter—that is, trading out a night's sleep for studying, is alarming, especially given that this behavior is associated with poorer academic performance and more depressive symptoms (Thacher, 2008). Without proper sleep, the work you put into studying may not pay off.

The Sleep Cycle

As we sleep, we follow a pattern of alternating between REM (rapid eye movement) and non-REM (non-rapid eye movement) sleep in a cycle. Factors like age, recent sleep schedules, and alcohol consumption can also lead to changes in sleep cycles (National Sleep Foundation, 2020).

Your exact sleep cycle will be different from other people's and will change throughout your life—even throughout a single night. Typically, the first sleep cycle after you fall asleep tends to be shorter (70–100 min); whereas later in the night, the cycle becomes longer (90–120 minutes). We spend about 75% of our sleep time in non-REM sleep. As we begin to fall asleep, we enter non-REM sleep, which is composed of three stages, and then enter the final stage of the sleep cycle, REM sleep:

- Stage one is the period of transition between wakefulness and the onset of sleep, and it occupies about 5% (about 10 minutes per sleep cycle) of our night's sleep. During this stage, we tend to be easily woken up and our heartbeat and breathing rates begin to relax.

- Stage two is characterized by the brain creating bursts of electricity known as **sleep spindles**, which play a pivotal role in how we process information and store memories. Stage two of non-REM sleep encompasses approximately 50% of the time (30–60 minutes per sleep cycle). Our heart and breathing rate slow even more, our body temperature drops, but we still remain in a fairly light stage of sleep.

- Stage three of non-REM sleep is the deepest, where our brain produces slow delta waves and there's no eye movement or muscle activity. This is our deepest and most restorative sleep and represents about 30% of our sleep time (20–40 minutes). It is during this stage three that our body repairs muscle and tissue. It also encourages growth, development, and improved immune functioning. It is difficult to wake someone up in this stage.

- Stage four of the sleep cycle consists of our REM sleep, which takes place about 1–2 hours after initially falling asleep. As the name suggests, this stage of sleep is characterized by rapid eye movements. It is a deeper sleep than any of the non-REM stages. During REM sleep, our eyelids flutter, and our breathing becomes irregular. Dreaming usually occurs during REM, but our brain temporarily paralyses our muscles, otherwise we may act out our dreams

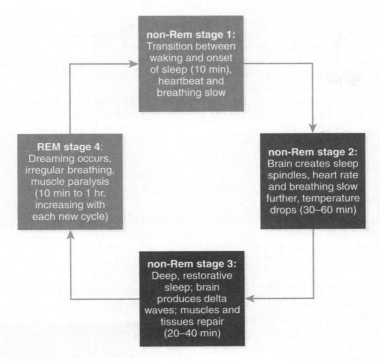

Figure 9-1 The Stages of the Sleep Cycle.

while we sleep! Time spent in REM increases with each new sleep cycle, starting at about 10 minutes and lasting up to an hour in the final cycle. REM sleep is crucial for learning, memory, daytime concentration, and mood regulation (National Sleep Foundation, 2020) (see **Figure 9-1**).

How Much Sleep Do We Need?

You can tell when you haven't gotten enough quality sleep; you have a hard time focusing and responding quickly, and you feel fatigued throughout the day. In fact, a 2020 poll reported that Americans feel sleepy 3 days per week, and many reported their sleepiness impacted their daily activities, mood, mental acuity, and productivity (National Sleep Foundation, 2021). This daytime sleepiness can have major consequences on your cognitive and academic abilities. For example, a study following more than 500 high school students for 14 days found that, regardless of how much the students studied each day, if they sacrificed sleep time to study more, they had increased trouble understanding material taught in class and were more likely to struggle on an assignment or test the following day (Gillen-O'Neel et al., 2013). So, make sure you are getting good sleep before your exercise psychology classes!

But how can you tell if you are getting sufficient sleep? There are many measures researchers and practitioners use to assess different aspects of sleep. Monitors such as actigraphs can be used to measure sleep through monitoring differences in motion and posture (Short et al., 2012). Alternatively, researchers use subjective, self-report ratings such as the Pittsburgh Sleep Quality Index (Buysse et al., 1989; Carpenter & Andrykowski, 1998). A score of five or more, indicates the need to consider some adjustments to lifestyle to ensure sufficient, quality sleep. Otherwise, the person may not function as well as they could.

The Relationship between Sleep and Academic Performance

It probably comes as no surprise to you that your sleep can impact your academic performance in university. In a study of 1,654 (55% female) full-time university undergraduate students aged 17–25 years, participants completed assessments of their sleep, academics, lifestyle, and wellbeing in the middle of a semester (Gomes et al., 2011). These variables were used to predict academic performance at the end of the semester. Here's a list of what they found significantly predicted better academic achievement:

- Better previous academic achievement
- More frequent class attendance
- More frequent nights of sufficient sleep
- Fewer night outings
- Better sleep quality

The strongest predictor was previous academic achievement, followed by class attendance. However, even after accounting for those factors, sleep had meaningful impacts on academic achievement. This is something to consider when it comes time to decide what to do tonight.

So how much sleep is enough? The first thing sleep experts will tell you is that no "magic number" exists for how much sleep we need each night This can be partly explained by the following three reasons. First, different age groups need different amounts of sleep. Although researchers cannot pinpoint the exact amount of sleep people need at different ages, **Table 9-1** shows the "rule-of-thumb" amounts of sleep different age groups need according to the Centers for Disease Control and Prevention (2019).

CRITICAL THINKING ACTIVITY 9-1

How many hours a night do you typically sleep? Are you getting enough sleep for your overall health?

Table 9-1 **Rule-of Thumb for the Amount of Sleep We Need a Day by Age from Centers for Disease Control and Prevention (2019)**

Age Group	Recommended Hours of Sleep Per Day
Newborns (0–3 months)	14–17 including naps
Infants (4–12 months)	12–16 including naps
Toddlers (1–2 years)	11–14 including naps
Preschoolers (3–5 years)	10–13 including naps
School-age children (6–12 years)	9–12
Teens (13–18 years)	8–10
Adults aged 18–60 years	7 or more
Adults aged 61–64 years	7–9
Adults aged 65 years and older	7–8

Centers for Disease Control and Prevention. (2019). How much sleep do I need? - Sleep and sleep disorders. https://www.cdc.gov/sleep/about_sleep/how_much_sleep .html. Reference to specific commercial products, manufacturers, companies, or trademarks does not constitute its endorsement or recommendation by the U.S. Government, Department of Health and Human Services, or Centers for Disease Control and Prevention.

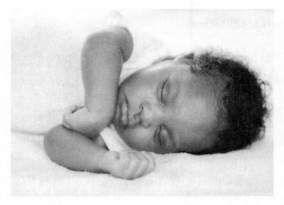

© FatCamera/E+/Getty.

Second, not only do age groups need different amounts of sleep, but sleep needs also differ by individual. Just like any other characteristics you are born with, the amount of sleep you need to perform at your best may be different for you than for someone who is of the same age. While you may be at your best sleeping 8 hours a night, someone else may only need six hours to function optimally.

The third reason is related to a person's basal sleep and sleep debt. **Basal sleep** is defined as the amount of sleep we need on a regular basis for optimal performance. **Sleep debt** is the accumulated sleep that is lost each night. Researchers have found that healthy adults have a basal sleep

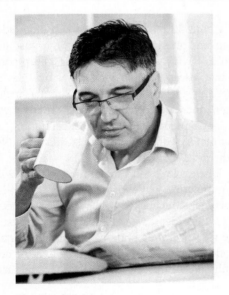

© Lucky Business/Shutterstock.

need of 7–8 hours a night. Things get complicated when you consider the interaction between basal sleep and sleep debt (Van Dongen, Rogers, & Dinges, 2003). Our basal sleep is in competition with our sleep debt; we constantly need our basal sleep to pay down our sleep debt. For example, if your basal sleep is 8 hours a night, and you only get 7 hours of sleep, you have a sleep debt of 1 hour that you need to try to make up. And this could accumulate over a week, for example, and your sleep debt would then be 7 hours. Excessive sleep debt can have many negative impacts on you, including that afternoon dip of sleepiness. Luckily, a short nap of 20 minutes can equate to 1 hour of "extra" nighttime sleep (Home, 2011), and caffeine can help reduce the feelings of sleepiness too (Horne et al., 2008).

Clinical Sleep Disorders

For most people, sleep is an inevitable, natural daily experience. However, 50–70 million Americans have a **sleep disorder** (American Sleep Association, 2021). A sleep disorder, or somnipathy, is a medical condition in which people have trouble sleeping well on a regular basis. See **Table 9-2** for a description of some common sleep disorders in accordance with the American Psychiatric Association (2021), noting that the International Classification of Sleep Disorders currently lists more than 80 distinct sleep disorders. The prevalence of sleep disorder symptoms may be higher than you would think. For example, nearly 30% of people have experienced sleepwalking at some point in their lives. Notably, though, only 1–5% of people are diagnosed with a **sleepwalking disorder**, which involves repeated episodes and distress or problems functioning as a result of regular sleepwalking. Although many people will have heard of narcolepsy (see Table 9-3), only 0.02–0.04% of people are diagnosed with it.

Other sleep disorders are far more common though. **Insomnia**, or sleeplessness, is one of the most common sleep disorders, with short-term issues reported by about 30% of adults and chronic insomnia rates of about 10% of adults (American Sleep Association, 2021). Notably, insomnia is largely comorbid, with an estimated

Table 9-2 **A Description of the Five Most Common Sleep Disorders**

Sleep Disorder	Description
Sleep apnea	Characterized by pauses in breathing or instances of shallow or infrequent breathing during sleep. To be diagnosed with sleep apnea, a clinical sleep study using polysomnography is conducted to monitor the number of episodes of absences/reductions of airflow.
Insomnia	Characterized by difficulty falling and/or staying asleep. To be diagnosed with insomnia, the sleep difficulties must occur at least three nights a week for at least three months and cause significant distress or problems in daily functioning.
Non-rapid eye movement sleep arousal disorder	Most common in children, this disorder is characterized by episodes of incomplete awakening from sleep, usually within the first third of a major sleep cycle, accompanied by sleepwalking or sleep terrors.
Restless leg syndrome	Characterized by an irresistible urge to move one's body to stop uncomfortable or odd sensations, such as feelings of creeping, crawling, tingling, burning or itching. To be diagnosed with restless leg syndrome, the symptoms must occur at least 3 times per week, continue for 3 months, and cause significant distress or problems in daily functioning.
Narcolepsy	A neurological disorder that affects the control of sleep and wakefulness. People with narcolepsy experience excessive daytime sleepiness and intermittent, uncontrollable episodes of falling asleep during the daytime. Narcolepsy is diagnosed via a spinal tap indicating loss of hypocretin producing cells.
Night terrors	Most common in children, night terrors are episodes of screaming, intense fear and flailing while still asleep. The person typically does not remember much of the dream and is unresponsive to efforts of comfort.

Data from American Psychiatric Association. (2021). What Are Sleep Disorders? American Psychiatric Association. https://www.psychiatry.org/patients-families/sleep-disorders/what-are-sleep-disorders.

40–50% of people with insomnia also diagnosed with another mental disorder. Insomnia is characterized by long-term difficulties with initiating or maintaining sleep. People with insomnia have one or more of the following symptoms: (a) difficulty falling asleep, (b) waking up often during the night and having trouble going back to sleep, (c) waking up too early in the morning, and (d) feeling tired upon waking. Thus, an individual with insomnia may have an inability to either fall asleep or stay asleep their desired length. Insomnia is often defined as a positive response to either of the following two questions:

1. "Do you experience difficulty sleeping?" or
2. "Do you have difficulty falling or staying asleep?" (Roth, 2007).

About 50% of middle-aged and older adults complain of symptoms of chronic insomnia, such as having a hard time falling asleep and/or staying asleep and having impaired daytime functioning. The results of insomnia include fatigue, increased accidents while driving a vehicle, poor mood, decreased concentration, and poor quality of life (American Academy of Sleep Medicine, 2005; Ohayon, 2012).

Restless leg syndrome impacts up to 7.2% of the population while insomnia impacts 10–15% of people. **Restless leg syndrome** is a neurological disorder characterized by an irresistible urge to move one's body to stop uncomfortable or odd sensations (Earley, 2003). It most commonly affects the legs, but can affect the arms,

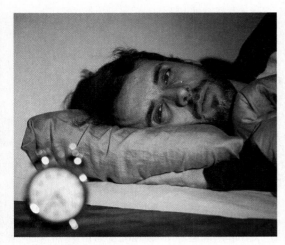

© SB Arts Media/Shutterstock.

torso, head, and even phantom limbs. The odd sensations range from pain or an aching in the muscles, to "an itch you can't scratch," an unpleasant "tickle that won't stop," or even a "crawling" feeling (Skidmore et al., 2009). The sensations typically begin or intensify during quiet wakefulness, such as when relaxing, reading, studying, or trying to sleep (Allen et al., 2003). Symptoms occur primarily at night when a person is relaxing or at rest and can increase in severity during the night. Moving the legs relieves the discomfort.

Two to 15 percent of middle-aged adults and more than one in five older adults have some form of sleep apnea (American Psychiatric Association, 2021). Obstructive sleep apnea is the most common type of sleep apnea, and it is caused by obstruction of the upper airway during sleep. This will lead to a lack of sufficient deep sleep, which is often accompanied by snoring. It is characterized by repetitive pauses in breathing during sleep, despite the effort to breathe, and it is often related to a reduction in blood oxygen saturation. These pauses in breathing, called **apneas** usually last 20 to 40 seconds. People with obstructive sleep apnea are rarely aware of having difficulty breathing, even upon awakening. Common signs of obstructive sleep apnea include unexplained daytime sleepiness, restless sleep, and loud snoring that is often followed by periods of silence followed by gasps.

Treating Clinical Sleep Disorders

Because of the prevalence and burden of sleep disorders, there is an interest—particularly on the part of people with sleep disorders—in determining how sleep can be facilitated. One common approach taken to improve the quality and quantity of sleep has been medication in the form of sleeping pills. However, sleeping pills do not seem to be the answer. In a review of the exercise and sleep literature, Buman and King (2010) noted that individuals can become dependent on pills and tolerance develops to prescribed dosages. Also, sleeping pills are often associated with profound rebound insomnia. Even more importantly, however, the regular use of sleeping pills is the mortality equivalent of smoking one to two packages of cigarettes daily. So, sleeping pills do not work well long term and their chronic use represents a health risk. Another option for the treatment of sleep disorders is cognitive behavioral therapy. A meta-analysis of 15 studies found that cognitive behavioral therapy can improve sleep initiation and maintenance when evaluated using subjective diary-based reports of sleep, but these effects were much smaller when sleep outcomes were evaluated with actigraph monitors (Mitchell et al., 2019). As we will discuss later on in this chapter, emerging evidence is revealing that changes in physical activity and sedentary behavior may help play a role in managing sleep disorder symptoms (Kline et al., 2021).

CRITICAL THINKING ACTIVITY 9-2

How would you convince someone who is taking sleep medication that exercise is a better option to treat their sleep disorder?

Sleep, Physical Activity, Sedentary Behavior, and Health Outcomes

Cappuccio et al. (2010) conducted a meta-analysis that included over 1.3 million participants to find out what the relationship is between the number of hours we sleep a night and mortality. They found that short sleepers (commonly defined as people who sleep less than 7 hours per night) have a 12% greater risk of dying than people who sleep 7–8 per night. As well, long sleepers (commonly defined as people who sleep greater than 8 or 9 hours per night) have a 30% greater risk of dying than people who sleep 7–8 per night. Researchers describe this relationship as the U-shaped curve where both sleeping too little and sleeping too much may put you at risk for increased mortality (Cappuccio et al., 2010; Grandner & Drummond, 2007; Youngstedt & Kript, 2004). Unfortunately, about 37% of U.S. adults aged 20 years or older put their health at risk by sleeping 6 hours or less a night (Frenk & Chong, 2013).

Time spent in sleep, sedentary behavior, and physical activity are co-dependent (Chastin et al., 2015); if you spend more time in one type of behavior, you are also spending less time in one of the other types of behavior. There's only 24 hours in a day after all! Despite this co-dependency, most research has separately investigated the effects of sleep, physical activity, and sedentary behavior. We are potentially missing the full picture of how changes in sleep, physical activity, and sedentary behavior are impacting us. However, there is a way to simultaneously consider how substituting one of these behaviors for another influences health outcomes – this method is called **isotemporal substitution modelling**. Isotemporal substitution modelling can be used to compare the benefits of trading time spent sleeping for either physical activity or sedentary behavior. For example, we could test if better health outcomes are associated with trading an hour of sedentary time for an hour of moderate-vigorous activity vs trading that sedentary time for an hour of extra sleep time.

A review of 56 isotemporal substitution modelling studies revealed that reallocation of sedentary time to light or moderate-vigorous physical activity was associated with a reduction in early mortality risk, but found that very few studies evaluated the impact of substituting sleep for sedentary vs physical activity behavior time (Grgic et al., 2018). In 2020, another group conducted a similar review and found again that there was little evidence regarding the values of substituting sleep for other behaviors in regards to health outcomes. This highlights the need for more research that may inform public health recommendations for combining sleep, sedentary behavior, and physical activity (Janssen et al., 2020).

There is some evidence that does indicate that sleep is important to consider in how the way we substitute our behavior impacts our health. For example, Gilchrist and colleagues (2021) found that among adolescents getting less than the recommended amount of sleep, replacing any behavior with sleep was generally associated with better health outcomes, but among those who were getting the recommended amount of sleep, few mental health benefits were gained by substituting other behaviors for sleep. Although notably, they did report that replacing screen time with any behavior, including sleep, was worthwhile for mental health amongst adolescents. Additionally, a longitudinal study of more than 200,000 Australian adults aged 45 years or older found getting sufficient sleep played an important role in how substituting time impacted risk of early mortality (Stamatakis et al., 2015). For those who slept less than 7 hours per day, lower risk of early mortality was associated with replacing sedentary time with any other option: time spent standing, walking, moderate-vigorous physical activity, or sleeping. However, for those who slept more than 7 hours per day, the same effects of reduced risk of early mortality was only found if sedentary behavior was replaced with either walking or moderate-vigorous physical activity. So, more evidence is needed to establish how substituting sleep time for other behaviors impacts us, but this evidence suggests that how much we sleep impacts how much can be gained by engaging in more physical activity and less sedentary behavior.

Sleep Hygiene

Most people are likely not getting enough sleep and that has a major public health burden, including loss of productivity, loss of quality of life, and risk of mental and physical health problems (Medicine et al., 2006). The immensity of this problem leads to the obvious question of how we can help people get more sleep. In the United States, the strongest predictor of poor sleep health and quality is stress and poor overall health (Knutson et al., 2017). Beyond these factors, there are plenty of reasons people don't get enough sleep. For example, we can lose sleep due to pets and kids, staying up too late to be on our phones, and awakening due to environmental factors (e.g., loud noises). Some of these factors are external and hard to change, but some are well within our own control. **Sleep hygiene** is a set of behavioral and environmental recommendations intended to promote healthy sleep (Hauri, 1991). Although originally developed for those with mild-moderate insomnia, sleep hygiene education interventions have been applied to many populations, including generally healthy adults without sleep disorders. Typically, sleep hygiene interventions consist of education about engaging in regular exercise, stress management, reducing bedtime noise, having regular sleep timing, and avoiding caffeine, nicotine, alcohol, and daytime naps. A review of the empirical evidence suggests there is some epidemiological and experimental research supporting a link between individual sleep hygiene recommendations and sleep, but the overall evidence of whether sleep hygiene interventions are effective in the general adult population is inconclusive (Irish et al., 2015). Amidst this overarching field of sleep hygiene research is a line of study on the impact that physical activity has on sleep. Regarding exercise, the review by Irish et al. (2015) concluded that acute and chronic

exercise can improve sleep; the extent to which different types, duration, and intensity of exercise can be specified for optimal sleep improvement; and current evidence does not support the claim that late-night exercise disrupts sleep. Next in this chapter, we'll dig into this line of research on physical activity and sleep while considering sedentary behavior as well.

Sleep, Physical Activity, and Sedentary Behavior

The National Sleep Foundation has conducted the *Sleep in America*® poll since 1991; each poll has a different focus around sleep concerns. This poll is representative of the U.S. population between the ages of 23 and 60 years. The 2013 poll that sampled 1,000 American adults focused on the relationship between sleep and physical activity (Hirschkowitz et al., 2013). They found that people who regularly were physically active reported better sleep than those who were not regularly active, but there was no difference in the self-reported amount of time they slept – their **sleep latency**. With regard to physical activity intensity, vigorous exercise appeared to produce the best sleep results. People who engaged in vigorous exercise were about twice as likely as those who didn't report *"I had a good night's sleep"* every night or almost every night during the week. As well, people who reported exercising regularly, regardless of their intensity, had better overall quality of sleep compared to those who did not regularly exercise (see **Figure 9-2**).

In 2021, Kline et al. (2021) conducted an **umbrella review**. This is a systematic review summarizing evidence from past reviews (a review of reviews) on physical activity and sleep. They reviewed evidence on the impact of physical activity on sleep outcomes across all ages and among individuals with clinical sleep disorders. Overall, this review concluded that both acute bouts of physical activity and regular engagement in physical activity improved sleep outcomes. There was moderate evidence

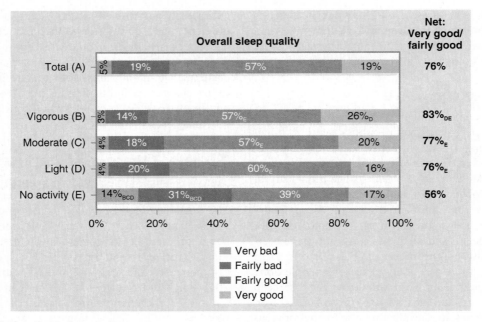

Figure 9-2 Exercise is Good for Sleep.
Data from the 2013 Sleep in America® poll overwhelmingly support the proposition that "Exercise is good for sleep." This section highlights findings showing that although those who exercise and do not exercise report very similar sleep needs and sleep patterns, those who exercise are more likely to say, "I had a good night's sleep" on both work nights and non-work nights. As shown below, the proportion of those who categorize themselves as vigorous exercisers, moderate exercisers, and light exercisers, report very good or fairly good overall sleep quality (83%, 77% and 76% respectively), which is significantly higher than those who categorize themselves as no activity or non-exercisers (56%).

Reproduced from 2013 Sleep in America® Poll: Exercise and Sleep: Summary of Findings. National Sleep Foundation. February 20, 2013. Arlington, VA. Pg. 6.

of a dose-response, meaning that longer bouts of physical activity (both acute and chronic) improved sleep, and the effect of physical activity on sleep had similar outcomes across ages and genders. Additionally, they concluded that there was moderate evidence that physical activity could enhance sleep outcomes in those with clinical sleep disorders. We will dig into all of this evidence in more detail now.

CRITICAL THINKING ACTIVITY 9-3

Do you think that if people knew that physical activity could help them sleep, they would be more inclined to engage in more physical activity? Why or why not?

Acute and Chronic Physical Activity and Sleep

The umbrella review of Kline et. al. (2021) summarized evidence of 26 reviews focused on adults, all of which reported beneficial effects of physical activity on at least one sleep outcome (see **Table 9-3**). One such review specifically focused on comparing the effects of acute and chronic physical activity on sleep (Kredlow et al., 2015). Based on their review of 66 studies, they concluded that a single bout of physical activity has small benefits on total sleep time, sleep onset latency, and sleep efficiency. Additionally, a moderately sized benefit was found for acute physical activity and wake time after sleep onset. Regular engagement in

Physical Activity and Sleep in University Students

In a review of sleep and physical activity in University students, Memon and colleagues (2021) found 29 eligible studies, representing 141,035 participants. Only four studies monitored sleep and physical activity with devices; the rest used self-reported sleep measures. Most studies did not find evidence of any association between sleep and physical activity in university students. However, more moderate-vigorous physical activity was associated with better sleep quality in accordance with the Pittsburgh Sleep Quality Index (see Table 9-1), with a small effect size ($r = -0.18$).

There is a lot to investigate about how your sleep and physical activity impact each other, especially considering that most of the evidence from studies on physical activity and sleep are cross-sectional and self-reported.

Table 9-3 **Summarized Results of Kline et al. (2021)'s Umbrella Review of Physical Activity and Sleep Research**

Review Authors	Review Findings Summary
Kredlow et al., (2015)	There were small-medium benefits found for both acute and chronic physical activity on sleep timing and quality for the general population.
Lederman et al., (2019)	Physical activity improved sleep quality in adults with mental illness.
Yang et al., (2020)	Physical activity improved sleep quality for pregnant women.
Lambert et al., (2016)	Physical activity improved sleep quality for family and caregivers.
Vanderlinden et al., (2020)	A review of 14 experimental studies of older adults revealed that all but one study showed physical activity led to favorable sleep outcomes, and there was no evidence of negative effects of physical activity on sleep.
Smagula et al., (2016)	There is mixed evidence for the benefits of physical activity for sleep outcomes amongst older adults, reflecting that many of these benefits may be dependent or interactive with demographic or other lifestyle factors including gender, ethnicity, medication, and physical and mental health comorbidities.
Antczak et al., (2020)	The evidence suggests an association between physical activity and better sleep outcomes for adolescents, although a dearth of experimental research limits how conclusive these results are.
Janssen et al., (2020)	The evidence suggests an association between physical activity and better sleep outcomes for children. Though, the scarcity of experimental research limits how conclusive these results are.
Buman et al., (2011a, 2011b)	Amongst individuals who do not have diagnosed sleep disorders but report non-clinical impaired sleep quality, 12 months of moderate-intensity exercise reduced night-to-night fluctuations in self-rated time to fall asleep, and this relationship was independent of mean-level time to fall asleep. Furthermore, the less active individuals with higher initial physical function and poorer sleep quality had the best improvements in their sleep.

Data from Kline, C. E., Hillman, C. H., Bloodgood Sheppard, B., Tennant, B., Conroy, D. E., Macko, R. F., Marquez, D. X., Petruzzello, S. J., Powell, K. E., & Erickson, K. I. (2021). Physical activity and sleep: An updated umbrella review of the 2018 Physical Activity Guidelines Advisory Committee report. *Sleep Medicine Reviews, 58*, 101489. https://doi.org/10.1016/j.smrv.2021.101489

physical activity also showed small beneficial effects on total sleep time and sleep efficiency. Additionally, regular physical activity was found to have small-to-medium benefits on sleep onset latency and medium benefits for sleep quality. The effect of physical activity on sleep may be a dose-response relationship, in that the more time is spent being physically active, the better the impacts on sleep outcomes seem to be. However, the evidence is not clear whether a specific intensity of physical activity is more or less valuable in terms of sleep outcomes (Kline et al., 2021; Kredlow et al., 2015). Overall, the result from this evidence leads to the conclusion that there are small-medium benefits of both acute and chronic physical activity on sleep timing and quality for the general population.

Some reviews have investigated similar research questions in subgroups and found similar results. For example, a review of physical activity and sleep in adults with mental illness concluded that physical activity improved sleep quality, (Lederman et al., 2019) and another review found similar benefits of physical activity on sleep for pregnant women (Yang et al., 2020) and family caregivers (Lambert et al., 2016). A review of studies of older adults has pointed to promising evidence for physical activity benefits for multiple sleep outcomes amongst 14 experimental studies (Vanderlinden et al., 2020), reporting that all but one study showed favorable results on sleep outcomes and no reports of negative effects of physical activity on sleep. Notably though, one review of studies looking at physical activity and sleep outcomes amongst older adults found mixed evidence for the benefits of physical activity on sleep, reflecting that many of these benefits may be dependent or interactive with demographic or other lifestyle factors, including gender, ethnicity, medication, and physical and mental health comorbidities (Smagula et al., 2016). Evidence of studies from children and adolescents shows strong evidence of an association between physical activity and better sleep outcomes (Antczak et al., 2020; Janssen et al., 2020); however, a dearth of experimental research of children and adolescents limits how conclusive we should be about

describing this as a causal effect, rather than as an association.

Some research has focused on people who do not have diagnosed sleep disorders but report non-clinical impaired sleep quality. For example, in a longitudinal study of adults with impaired sleep quality, Buman and his colleagues (2011a, 2011b) examined the effects of a 12-month moderate-intensity exercise program on adults' sleep quality. Under-active male and female adults aged 55 years and older with mild to moderate sleep complaints were randomized to either 12 months of a moderate-intensity endurance exercise group ($n = 36$) or a health education control group ($n = 30$). Daily sleep logs, sleep quality, and in-home polysomnographic sleep recordings were collected at baseline, 6 months, and 12 months. **Polysomnography** is a comprehensive recording of the biophysiological changes that occur during sleep. They found that 12 months of moderate-intensity exercise reduced night-to-night fluctuations in self-rated time to fall asleep, and this relationship was independent of mean-level time to fall asleep. They also found that less active individuals with higher initial physical function and poorer sleep quality had the best improvements in their sleep.

Timing of Physical Activity and Sleep

A common assumption is that engaging in vigorous bouts of exercise just prior to bedtime will disrupt a person's sleep. However, research has consistently found that engaging in either moderate or vigorous exercise in the evening does NOT impair sleep quality (Myllymaki et al., 2011). In fact, increasing either physical activity intensity or duration in the evening does not seem to disrupt sleep quality. For example, results for the 2013 *National Sleep Foundation Sleep in American Poll* revealed that evening exercise was not associated with worse sleep. In fact, most people who did vigorous evening physical activity believed that their sleep was of either equal or better quality (97%) and duration (98%) on days they engaged in physical activity (Buman et al., 2014). In other words, people who exercised close to bedtime and earlier in the day do not have a difference in their self-reported sleep quality. Some evidence shows the opposite effect, in fact.

Kredlow and colleagues (2015) reviewed study effects of acute bouts of moderate-vigorous physical activity performed more than 8 hours before bedtime, 3–8 hours before bedtime, and less than 3 hours before bedtime. They found no difference in many sleep outcomes, other than that physical activity engaged in within 3 hours of bedtime led to slightly deeper and more consolidated sleep. Another review supports this claim, finding that physical activity engaged in within 4 hours of bedtime led to deeper sleep, with the exception that vigorous physical activity ending less than an hour before bedtime might make it difficult to fall asleep initially (Stutz et al., 2019). So overall, it seems that being active in the evening will likely enhance rather than diminish sleep quality and duration in healthy adults without clinical sleep disorders. The aforementioned research clearly contradicts the long-standing sleep hygiene tip that advises not to exercise close

to bedtime. The *National Sleep Foundation* has amended its sleep recommendations for "normal" sleepers to encourage physical activity, without any caveat to time of day as long as it's not at the expense of sleep.

Sedentary Behavior and Sleep

Emerging research is revealing that sedentary behavior is negatively related to sleep quality in a variety of populations and age groups. Yang and colleagues (2017) conducted a systematic review and meta-analysis of the evidence for the association between sedentary behavior and sleep problems. 16 studies were reviewed, and it was found that sedentary behavior was associated with a 38% increase in the risk of sleep disturbances, but sedentary behavior was not found to increase the risk of daytime sleepiness or poor sleep quality. The authors concluded that, although the evidence suggests that prolonged sedentary behavior may have detrimental effects on sleep, more studies with longer follow-up periods, and experimental designs are needed to establish these effects more conclusively.

A review of screen time, sedentary behavior, physical activity, and sleep in children younger than 5 years old covered evidence from 31 studies (Janssen et al., 2020). They concluded that screen time is associated with poorer sleep outcomes in infants, toddlers, and preschoolers, recommending that parents, clinicians, and educators should promote less evening screen time for children under age five to enhance sleep outcomes. A review of screen-based sedentary behavior among adolescent girls also reported that more screen-based sedentary time was associated with more sleep problems,

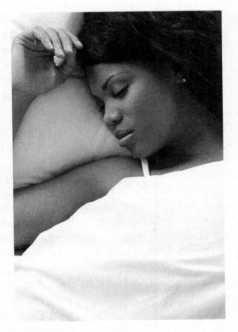

noting however that most studies do not account for physical activity, which may serve to buffer from some of these effects (Costigan et al., 2013). Although not nearly as comprehensive as the body of evidence surrounding the benefits of physical activity on sleep, these three reviews demonstrate that sedentary behavior, and screen-time in particular, may be detrimental to sleep. Given that daytime sleepiness can make sedentary behaviors more tempting, people can easily get into a bad cycle of a night of poor sleep leading to a sedentary day, leading to another night of poor sleep, and so on. Most people have personally experienced the negative effects that a night or two of poor sleep can have on all aspects of your life; however, some people have persistent negative consequences of poor sleep from clinical disorders.

Physical Activity, Sedentary Behavior, and Clinical Sleep Disorders

Historically, research investigating physical activity, sedentary behavior, and sleep has focused on people without sleep disorders. But more recently, researchers have begun to examine the effects of these behaviors on people with sleep disorders. Evidence of 2,989 American adults reveals that those who engaged in more physical activity were less likely to be diagnosed with sleep disorders and those who engaged in more sedentary behavior were more likely to be diagnosed with them (Farnsworth et al., 2015). These findings suggest these behaviors may help in the prevention of sleep disorder onset. Evidence also shows that more moderate-vigorous physical activity improves sleep for people with clinical disorders, with most evidence from studies on people with insomnia or obstructive sleep apnea (Kline et al., 2021).

Insomnia

Five reviews of 17 individual studies lead to the conclusion that physical activity enhances sleep timing and quality for people with insomnia (Kline et al., 2021). One review even found that the effects of physical activity on sleep are comparable to hypnotic medication use (Passos et al., 2012). Notably, however, is that these reviewed studies tended to be evaluations of supervised physical activity programs with 120–150 minutes of activity per week, so it is yet to be established whether these benefits of physical activity on sleep apply to people with insomnia who are active outside of a supervised, structured program.

In the review of sedentary behavior and sleep problems overall, Yang and colleagues (2017) reported on the results of five studies investigating the association between sedentary behavior and increased risk of insomnia. The meta-analysis revealed that odds of insomnia were higher for people who engaged in more sedentary behavior than people who engaged in less sedentary behavior, with a pooled odds-ratio of 1.18, meaning that prolonged sedentary behavior increases the odds of insomnia by 18%.

Obstructive Sleep Apnea

There is also moderate evidence from eight reviews of 17 unique studies that physical activity can help manage obstructive sleep apnea (Kline et al., 2021). Specifically, reviewed evidence suggests that physical activity reduces the severity of obstructive sleep apnea symptoms and daytime sleepiness, while increasing sleep efficiency among those with obstructive sleep apnea. Similar to the evidence for people with insomnia, the studies of people with obstructive sleep apnea tend to involve structured, supervised physical activity training programs. So, although the experimental design allows for strong evidence that physical activity benefits sleep, it remains untested whether these findings apply to physical activity outside of these training programs. Within these programs, however, the evidence shows there is quite a large impact on symptoms of obstructive sleep apnea. The reviews report that physical activity reduces the amount of apnea events during sleep by between 6–11 events per hour (Kline et al., 2021). That can make a substantial impact on the efficiency of people's sleep;

the estimated effect size of SMD = −0.54 shows that the impact of physical activity training programs on the burden of apnea symptoms can be reduced in an impactful way.

Although not as substantial as the evidence base for the benefits of sleep and physical activity for people with insomnia and obstructive sleep apnea, there is also building evidence to suggest physical activity can be useful in managing other sleep disorders including restless leg syndrome (Aukerman et al., 2006; Giannaki et al., 2013). Beyond the evidence establishing the value of reducing sedentary behavior for managing insomnia, little is understood about the role of sedentary behavior in managing sleep disorders.

Mechanisms of How Physical Activity and Sedentary Behavior Affect Sleep

There are several proposed mechanisms for why physical activity helps us sleep better (Buman & King, 2010; Youngstedt & Kline, 2006). Some of these commonly acceptable mechanisms are briefly reviewed below.

Anxiety Reduction

Perhaps the most plausible mechanism through which physical activity could promote sleep is anxiety reduction (Youngstedt & Kline, 2006). Disturbed sleep is a hallmark of anxiety, and chronic insomnia has been associated with increased physiological arousal. Therefore, stimuli that reduce anxiety may promote sleep. It is well-established that acute physical activity reduces anxiety and that regular physical activity results in stable reductions in anxiety.

Antidepressant Effects

Buman and King (2010) noted that depression is an important contributing factor to poor sleep, and poor sleep is a risk factor for depression. Physical activity has well-established antidepressant effects and could therefore serve as an important mediator of the depression-sleep relationship.

Thermoregulation

Our body temperature drops as we are falling asleep (Driver & Taylor, 2000). Temperature elevation (e.g., due to warm baths, saunas, or exercise prior to bedtime) can activate temperature down regulation, which is associated with deeper forms of sleep (Bauman & King, 2010). That is, increasing your body temperature before bed can improve sleep quality. Youngstedt (2005) suggested that chronic exercise could support a more efficient temperature regulation process during the sleep-wake cycle, resulting in better sleep.

Circadian Phase-shifting Effects

Circadian rhythms (commonly referred to as our body clock) are the physical, mental, and behavioral changes that follow a roughly 24-hour cycle. For example, our body temperature tends to be lowest at 4:30 a.m., we have our sharpest rise in blood pressure at 6:45 a.m., and we have greater cardiovascular and muscle strength at 5:00 p.m. Our circadian system is affected by both endogenous (e.g., body temperature, melatonin) and exogenous (e.g., bright light, exercise, meal

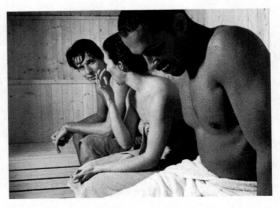

© Stockbyte/Getty Images.

timing) cues that regulate the sleep-wake cycle. Disturbed sleep may occur when endogenous and exogenous cues are not synchronized. Common circadian rhythm sleep problems that affect this sync include jet lag, shift work, and delayed sleep phase syndrome. **Jet lag** consists of symptoms that include excessive sleepiness and a lack of daytime alertness in people who travel across time zones. **Shift work** affects people who frequently rotate shifts or work at night. **Delayed sleep phase syndrome** is a disorder of sleep timing where people tend to fall asleep at very late times and have difficulty waking up in time for work, school, or social engagements.

The strongest synchronizer of our circadian rhythms is light, particularly artificial bright light, natural light, and domestic lighting conditions. Physical activity has also been implicated in such synchronization effects. While research has been hampered because of a lack of control of light and exercise characteristics, a review by Edwards et al. (2009) suggested that physical activity bouts of various intensities and durations can mediate phase shifts, independent of the effects produced by light alone.

CRITICAL THINKING ACTIVITY 9-5

How can the anxiolytic effect of physical activity help those with sleep disorders?

Summary

We are really good at filling up our days with obligations, and we typically treat sleep as a luxury instead of a priority. Research has well established that physical activity improves our sleep, both in how long we sleep and how efficient the quality of our sleep is. This mounting research supports that physical activity improves both the quality and quantity of sleep in people with and without sleep disorders. Although the evidence is less comprehensive for the impact of sedentary behavior on sleep, the preliminary evidence leans toward the conclusion that prolonged sedentary behavior can have detrimental effects on your sleep. Now that you know how essential sleep is to your functioning and well-being, it is worth prioritizing. One great way to do this is to engage in regular physical activity.

Vignette: Omar

I'm not sure when, exactly, I became such a terrible sleeper. It might have been when my family moved from a small town in Connecticut to Chicago when I was 10. My mother had been relocated for business and my father was able to start a new job. We downsized our living arrangements, so I ended up splitting a bedroom with my younger brother who was a snorer. I would frequently wake up and shake the top of the bunk bed we shared in an effort to wake him so he'd be quieter.

I started to worry I had insomnia after I began technical college in Wisconsin. I worked at a restaurant during some evenings and weekend mornings to help pay for the apartment I rented with a fellow student roommate. And on days I was on my feet a lot, running back and forth between the kitchen and tables, I'd have an easier time falling asleep. But when I spent most of my day sitting in the library, in class, or watching sports on TV during the weekend, I found myself wide awake at odd hours of the night.

My doctor at the time offered to write me a prescription for sleeping pills. He said sleeplessness could be more common among folks like myself who didn't get a lot of sunlight and kept odd hours due to work and school. I was hesitant to take them, though, having heard horror stories of friends of friends sleepwalking on Ambien. So, the bottle of pills pretty much remained tucked inside a bathroom cabinet.

One night at work, just before I was about to end my shift and head back to my apartment, I slipped on the staircase leading to the downstairs employee locker room. I landed hard on my tailbone and wrenched my spine, resulting in what I'd find out weeks later was a severely herniated disc.

The pain just kept getting worse in the days after my fall. I iced my back and took over-the-counter painkillers, but to no avail. My sleep schedule got even more interrupted, as it was barely possible to find a position to lie in that wasn't excruciating for my spine.

I was angry and frustrated at having to take time off work after I literally could no longer hold up a tray without wincing. I knew something was seriously wrong, and I was terrified that I'd have to get surgery—as a couple of different doctors I consulted with suggested. With the worker's compensation I received for the fall—turns out my employer had a series of violations that resulted in them swiftly footing my medical bills—I enrolled in physical therapy. It took almost 6 months before I was able to resume my normal life without wincing in agony with every move.

I put on a fair bit of weight during this time. And once I was okayed by the physical therapist to start an exercise program, I desperately sought her advice. She strongly suggested I take up swimming. So, in part to shed some pounds, but also to help keep my back in good shape to keep my recovery going, I started doing laps a few times a week at a local YMCA.

I felt rather ridiculous stepping into a pool in my swimming trunks considering the gut I'd grown during my time off from work. But I tried to swallow my pride and self-consciousness, dive in, and see what I could make happen.

The relief of feeling weightless in the water motivated me to come back. I was breathless within seconds of starting a forward crawl. And for the first few weeks, I could only last in the pool about 15 minutes max. Boy, was I sore from head to toe, the days after I got out of the pool. I discovered muscles in my body I didn't even know were there simply by their achiness after getting out of the pool.

But a surprisingly pleasant thing happened no later than the first night after I tried my arms and legs at swimming. I came home, had dinner, and passed out on the couch. I woke up about 5 hours later, groggy and slightly disoriented. I picked myself up and crawled back into bed for another 2 or so hours of sleep, and then woke up feeling—though incredibly sore—surprisingly refreshed.

It took me a while to get in shape. But the longer I was able to swim, the better I became at going to bed. It was almost like I didn't have a choice. My body would just be ready for bed after dinnertime, and I'd have to give in. In a few months' time, I'd nearly forgotten I ever struggled to fall and remain asleep. My roommate even asked me if I was finally taking those sleeping pills I'd told him about. I was so proud to say that I didn't even have to.

By the time I got my Associate degree in accounting, I'd been swimming regularly for almost a year. I'd mastered that crawl like you wouldn't believe! Then I got offered a job as a payroll clerk at a small accounting firm in Milwaukee after a month or so of searching, which got in the way of my workout schedule.

I had to cut back on the number of days a week I went swimming. I moved to an apartment that wasn't close to any fitness centers with pools. And as I've gotten accustomed to my new work hours, I found little time to get to and from the nearest YMCA. Not surprisingly, my sleep started getting lighter again, and I found myself desperately considering taking those pills.

I've since been searching for alternative exercise programs like treadmill walks or investing in some fitness equipment for my home. But I'm not well versed in how to go about all this. And whatever I've tried hasn't compared to the freedom I feel when propelling myself through water.

I make a point to get to the pool on weekends and I force myself to wake up early at least once during the work week to swim. I'm hoping within the next year to find a more convenient place to live—one that puts me nearer to a pool than to work. I'm not sure I realized how crucial swimming was to my health, happiness, and ability to get a good night's rest until I couldn't do it as often as I wanted.

Key Terms

apneas Pauses or reductions in breathing during sleep usually lasting between 20–40 seconds.

basal sleep The amount of sleep we need on a regular basis for optimal performance.

delayed sleep phase syndrome A disorder of sleep timing where people tend to fall asleep at very late times and have difficulty waking up in time for daily living activities.

insomnia Sleeplessness; a clinical sleep disorder characterized by long-term difficulties with initiating or maintaining sleep.

isotemporal substitution modelling A way of statistically testing how outcomes are impacted by substitution of one type of behavior for another.

jet lag Excessive sleepiness and a lack of daytime alertness in people who travel across time zones.

memory consolidation A process in which recently encoded memory representations are reactivated and transformed into long-term memory.

polysomnography Comprehensive recording of biophysiological changes that occur during sleep.

restless leg syndrome A neurological disorder characterized by an irresistible urge to move one's body to stop uncomfortable or odd sensations.

restoration Sleep that allows the body and mind to repair itself and regulate cellular functioning that can deteriorate through waking periods.

shift work A work roster that involves recurring periods in which different groups of workers do the same job at different times, including overnight.

sleep A naturally recurring state of rest for the mind and body, in which the eyes usually close and consciousness is either completely or partially lost.

sleep debt The accumulated sleep that is lost each night.

sleep disorder Medical conditions that prevent you from sleeping well on a regular basis.

sleep hygiene A set of behavioral and environmental recommendations intended to promote healthy sleep.

sleep latency Amount of time spent asleep.

sleep spindles Bursts of electricity in the brain characteristic of the second stage of sleep, which play a pivotal role in information processing and memory storage.

sleepwalking disorder Repeated episodes of sleepwalking that results in distress or problems with daily functioning.

umbrella review A systematic review summarizing evidence from other reviews (review of reviews).

Review Questions

1. Describe two benefits of sleep.
2. What is the deepest, most restorative stage of the sleep cycle?
3. How can you tell if you are getting sufficient sleep?
4. Describe the connection between sleep and academic performance.
5. What is sleep debt and how can you reduce the negative impacts of it?
6. What is insomnia and how common is it?
7. What does it mean that the relationship between sleep and the risk of dying is a U-shaped curve?
8. Describe sleep hygiene and the role that physical activity and sedentary behavior play in it.
9. What is the general consensus of the evidence on the relationship between physical activity and sleep?

Applying the Concepts

1. What advice would you give Omar about how physical activity and sedentary behavior might impact his sleep?
2. Are there aspects of Omar's story that you relate to? What is similar or different about how your sleep is impacted by physical activity or sedentary behavior?

References

Allen, R., Picchietti, D., Hening, W. A., Trenkwalder, C., Walters, A. S., & Montplaisi, J. (2003). Restless legs syndrome: diagnostic criteria, special considerations, and epidemiology: A report from the restless legs syndrome diagnosis and epidemiology workshop at the National Institutes of Health. *Sleep Medicine, 4*, 101–119.

American Academy of Sleep Medicine (2005). *International classification of sleep disorders, revised: Diagnostic and coding manual.* Westchester, IL: Diagnostic.

American Heritage Medical Dictionary (2007). *Sleep definition.* Houghton Mifflin Company.

American Psychiatric Association. (2021). *What Are Sleep Disorders?* American Psychiatric Association. https://www.psychiatry.org/patients-families/sleep-disorders/what-are-sleep-disorders

American Sleep Association. (2021). *Sleep and Sleep Disorder Statistics.* American Sleep Association. https://www.sleepassociation.org/about-sleep/sleep-statistics/

Antczak, D., Lonsdale, C., Lee, J., Hilland, T., Duncan, M. J., del Pozo Cruz, B., Hulteen, R., et al. (2020). Physical activity and sleep are inconsistently related in healthy children: A systematic review and meta-analysis. *Sleep Medicine Reviews, 51,* 101278. https://doi.org/10.1016/j.smrv.2020.101278

Aukerman, M. M., Aukerman, D., Bayard, M., Tudiver, F., Thorp, L., & Bailey, B. (2006). Exercise and restless legs syndrome: A randomized controlled trial. *Journal of the American Board of Family Medicine, 19,* 487–493.

Buman, M. P., & King, A. C. (2010). Exercise as a treatment to enhance sleep. *American Journal of Lifestyle Medicine, 6,* 500–513.

Buman, M. P., Hekler, E. B., Bliwise, D. L., & King, A. C. (2011a). Exercise effects on night-to-night fluctuations in self-rated sleep among older adults with sleep complaints. *Sleep Research, 20,* 28–37.

Buman, M. P., Hekler, E. B., Bliwise, D. L., & King, A. C. (2011b). Moderators and mediators of exercise-induced objective sleep improvements in midlife and older adults with sleep complaints. *Health Psychology, 30,* 579–587.

Buman, M. P., Phillips, B. A., Youngstedt, S. D., Kline, C. E., & Hirschkowitz, M. (2014). Does nighttime exercise really disturb sleep? Results for the 2013 National Sleep Foundation Sleep in America Pool. *Sleep Medicine, 15,* 755–761.

Buysse, D. J., Reynolds III, C. F., Monk, T. H., Berman, S. R., & Kupfer, D. J. (1989). The Pittsburgh Sleep Quality Index: A new instrument for psychiatric practice and research. *Psychiatry Research, 28*(2), 193–213.

Cappuccio, F. P., D'Elia, L., Strazzullo, P., & Miller, M. A. (2010). Sleep Duration and All-Cause Mortality: A Systematic Review and Meta-Analysis of Prospective Studies. *Sleep, 33*(5), 585–592. https://doi.org/10.1093/sleep/33.5.585

Carpenter, J. S., & Andrykowski, M. A. (1998). Psychometric evaluation of the Pittsburgh sleep quality index. *Journal of Psychosomatic Research, 45*(1), 5-13.

Centers for Disease Control and Prevention. (2019). How much sleep do I need? - Sleep and sleep disorders. https://www.cdc.gov/sleep/about_sleep/how_much_sleep.html

Chastin, S. F. M., Palarea-Albaladejo, J., Dontje, M. L., & Skelton, D. A. (2015). Combined Effects of Time Spent in Physical Activity, Sedentary Behaviors and Sleep on Obesity and Cardio-Metabolic Health Markers: A Novel Compositional Data Analysis Approach. *PLOS ONE, 10*(10), e0139984. https://doi.org/10.1371/journal.pone.0139984

Costigan, S. A., Barnett, L., Plotnikoff, R. C., & Lubans, D. R. (2013). The Health Indicators Associated With Screen-Based Sedentary Behavior Among Adolescent Girls: A Systematic Review. *Journal of Adolescent Health, 52*(4), 382–392. https://doi.org/10.1016/j.jadohealth.2012.07.018

Driver, H. S., & Taylor, S. R. (2000). Exercise and sleep. *Sleep Medicine Reviews, 4*(4), 387–402. https://doi.org/10.1053/smrv.2000.0110

Earley, C. J. (2003). Restless legs syndrome. *New England Journal of Medicine, 348,* 2103–2109.

Edwards, B. J., Reilly, T., & Waterhouse, J. (2009). Zeitgeber-effects of exercise on human circadian rhythms: What are alternative approaches to investigating the existence of a phase-response curve to exercise? *Biological Rhythm Research, 40,* 53–69.

Farnsworth, J. L., Kim, Y., & Kang, M. (2015). Sleep Disorders, Physical Activity, and Sedentary Behavior Among U.S. Adults: National Health and Nutrition Examination Survey. *Journal of Physical Activity and Health, 12*(12), 1567–1575. https://doi.org/10.1123/jpah.2014-0251

Frenk, S. M., & Chong, Y. (2013). QuickStats: sleep duration among adults aged ≥20 years, by race/ethnicity — National Health and Nutrition Examination Survey, United States, 2007–2010. *Morbidity and Mortality Weekly Report, 62,* 755.

Giannaki, C. D., Sakkas, G. K., Karatzaferi, C., Hadjigeorgiou, G. M., et al. (2013). Effect of exercise training and dopamine agonists in patients with uremic restless legs syndrome: A six-month randomized, partially double-blind, placebo-controlled comparative study. *BioMed Central Nephrology, 14,* 194.

Gilchrist, J. D., Battista, K., Patte, K. A., Faulkner, G., Carson, V., & Leatherdale, S. T. (2021). Effects of reallocating physical activity, sedentary behaviors, and sleep on mental health in adolescents. *Mental Health and Physical Activity, 20,* 100380. https://doi.org/10.1016/j.mhpa.2020.100380

Gillen-O'Neel, C., Huynh, V. W., & Fuligni, A. J. (2013). To study or to sleep? The academic costs of extra studying at the expense of sleep. *Child Development, 84*(1), 133–142.

Gomes, A. A., Tavares, J., & de Azevedo, M. H. P. (2011). Sleep and academic performance in undergraduates: A multi-measure, multi-predictor approach. *Chronobiology International, 28*(9), 786–801. https://doi.org/10.3109/07420528.2011.606518

Grandner, M. A., & Drummond, S. P. (2007). Who are the long sleepers? Towards an understanding of the mortality relationship. *Sleep Medicine Reviews, 11,* 341–360.

Grgic, J., Dumuid, D., Bengoechea, E. G., Shrestha, N., Bauman, A., Olds, T., & Pedisic, Z. (2018). Health outcomes associated with reallocations of time between sleep, sedentary behaviour, and physical activity: A systematic scoping review of isotemporal substitution studies. *International Journal of Behavioral Nutrition and Physical Activity, 15*(1), 69. https://doi.org/10.1186/s12966-018-0691-3

Hauri, P. J. (1991). Sleep hygiene, relaxation therapy, and cognitive interventions. In P. J. Hauri (Ed.), *Case Studies in Insomnia*, 65–84. Springer US. https://doi .org/10.1007/978-1-4757-9586-8_5

Hirshkowitz, M., Buman, M., Kline, C., Tulio de Mello, M., & Youngstdet, S. D. (2013). 2013 Sleep in America® poll. Exercise and Sleep. Summary of findings. National Sleep Foundation. Retrieved Dec. 5, 2013 from: https://www .thensf.org/sleep-in-america-polls/

Home, J. (2011). The end of sleep: 'sleep debt' versus biological adaptation of human sleep to waking needs. *Biological Psychology, 87*, 1–14.

Horne, J., Anderson, C., & Platten, C. (2008). Sleep extension versus nap or coffee, within the context of 'sleep debt.' *Journal of Sleep Research, 17*(4), 432–436. https://doi .org/10.1111/j.1365-2869.2008.00680.x

Institute of Medicine; Board on Health Sciences Policy; Committee on Sleep Medicine and Research (2006). Sleep Disorders and Sleep Deprivation: An Unmet Public Health Problem. National Academies Press.

Irish, L. A., Kline, C. E., Gunn, H. E., Buysse, D. J., & Hall, M. H. (2015). The role of sleep latency in promoting public health: A review of empirical evidence. *Sleep Medicine Reviews, 22*, 23–36. https://doi.org/10.1016/j .smrv.2014.10.001

Janssen, I., Clarke, A. E., Carson, V., Chaput, J.-P., Giangregorio, L. M., Kho, M. E., Poitras, V. J., Ross, R., Saunders, T. J., Ross-White, A., & Chastin, S. F. M. (2020). A systematic review of compositional data analysis studies examining associations between sleep, sedentary behaviour, and physical activity with health outcomes in adults. *Applied Physiology, Nutrition, and Metabolism, 45*(10 (Suppl. 2), S248–S257. https://doi.org/10.1139/apnm-2020-0160

Janssen, X., Martin, A., Hughes, A. R., Hill, C. M., Kotronoulas, G., & Hesketh, K. R. (2020). Associations of screen time, sedentary time and physical activity with sleep in under 5s: A systematic review and meta-analysis. *Sleep Medicine Reviews, 49*, 101226. https://doi.org/10.1016/j.smrv.2019.101226

Kline, C. E., Hillman, C. H., Bloodgood Sheppard, B., Tennant, B., Conroy, D. E., Macko, R. F., Marquez, D. X., Petruzzello, S. J., Powell, K. E., & Erickson, K. I. (2021). Physical activity and sleep: An updated umbrella review of the 2018 Physical Activity Guidelines Advisory Committee report. *Sleep Medicine Reviews, 58*, 101489. https://doi.org/10.1016/j.smrv.2021.101489

Knutson, K. L., Phelan, J., Paskow, M. J., Roach, A., Whiton, K., Langer, G., Hillygus, D. S., Mokrzycki, M., Broughton, W. A., Chokroverty, S., et al. (2017). The National Sleep Foundation's Sleep Health Index. *Sleep Health, 3*(4), 234–240. https://doi.org/10.1016/j.sleh.2017.05.011

Kredlow, M. A., Capozzoli, M. C., Hearon, B. A., Calkins, A. W., & Otto, M. W. (2015). The effects of physical activity on sleep: A meta-analytic review. *Journal of Behavioral Medicine, 38*(3), 427–449. https://doi.org/10.1007/s10865 -015-9617-6

Lambert, S. D., Duncan, L. R., Kapellas, S., Bruson, A.-M., Myrand, M., Santa Mina, D., Culos-Reed, N., & Lambrou, A. (2016). A Descriptive Systematic Review of Physical Activity Interventions for Caregivers: Effects on Caregivers' and Care Recipients' Psychosocial Outcomes, Physical Activity Levels, and Physical Health. *Annals of Behavioral Medicine, 50*(6), 907–919. https://doi.org/10.1007/s12160 -016-9819-3

Lederman, O., Ward, P. B., Firth, J., Maloney, C., Carney, R., Vancampfort, D., Stubbs, B., Kalucy, M., & Rosenbaum, S. (2019). Does exercise improve sleep quality in individuals with mental illness? A systematic review and meta-analysis. *Journal of Psychiatric Research, 109*, 96–106. https://doi.org/10.1016/j.jpsychires.2018.11.004

Memon, A. R., Gupta, C. C., Crowther, M. E., Ferguson, S. A., Tuckwell, G. A., & Vincent, G. E. (2021). Sleep and physical activity in university students: A systematic review and meta-analysis. *Sleep Medicine Reviews, 58*, 101482. https://doi.org/10.1016/j.smrv.2021.101482

Mitchell, L. J., Bisdounis, L., Ballesio, A., Omlin, X., & Kyle, S. D. (2019). The impact of cognitive behavioural therapy for insomnia on objective sleep parameters: A meta-analysis and systematic review. *Sleep Medicine Reviews, 47*, 90–102. https://doi.org/10.1016/j.smrv.2019.06.002

Myllymaki, T., Kyrolainen, H., Savolainen, K., Hokka, L., Jakonen, R., Juuti, T., et al. (2011). Effects of vigorous late-night exercise on sleep quality and cardiac autonomic activity. *Journal of Sleep Research, 20*, 146–153.

National Institute of Health. (2019). Brain Basics: Understanding Sleep (No. 17–3440c). https://www .ninds.nih.gov./health-information/public-education /brain-basics/brain-basics-understanding-sleep?search -term=understanding%20sleep

National Sleep Foundation. (2021). Sleep in America (R) Poll 2020 (No. Q1). National Sleep Foundation.

National Sleep Foundation. (2022). Stages of Sleep. https:// www.sleepfoundation.org/how-sleep-works/stages-of -sleep

Ohayon, M. M. (2002). Epidemiology of insomnia: What we know and what we still need to learn. *Sleep Medicine Reviews, 6*, 97–111.

Passos, G. S., Poyares, D. L. R., Santana, M. G., Tufik, S., & Mello, M. T. de. (2012). Is exercise an alternative treatment for chronic insomnia? *Clinics, 67*, 653–660. https://doi .org/10.6061/clinics/2012(06)17

Rasch, B., & Born, J. (2013). About Sleep's Role in Memory. *Physiological Reviews, 93*(2), 681–766. https://doi.org /10.1152/physrev.00032.2012

Roth, T. (2007). Insomnia: Definition, prevalence, etiology, and consequences. *Journal of Clinical Sleep Medicine, 3*(5 Suppl): S7–10.

Short, M. A., Gradisar, M., Lack, L. C., Wright, H., & Carskadon, M. A. (2012). The discrepancy between actigraphic and sleep diary measures of sleep in adolescents. *Sleep Medicine, 13*(4), 378–384.

Skidmore, F. M., Drago, V., Foster, P. S., & Heilman, K. M. (2009). Bilateral restless legs affecting a phantom limb, treated with dopamine agonists. *Journal of Neurology, Neurosurgery & Psychiatry, 80*(5), 569–570. https://doi.org/10.1136/jnnp.2008.152652

Smagula, S. F., Stone, K. L., Fabio, A., & Cauley, J. A. (2016). Risk factors for sleep disturbances in older adults: Evidence from prospective studies. *Sleep Medicine Reviews, 25,* 21–30. https://doi.org/10.1016/j.smrv.2015.01.003

Stamatakis, E., Rogers, K., Ding, D., Berrigan, D., Chau, J., Hamer, M., & Bauman, A. (2015). All-cause mortality effects of replacing sedentary time with physical activity and sleeping using an isotemporal substitution model: A prospective study of 201,129 mid-aged and older adults. *International Journal of Behavioral Nutrition and Physical Activity, 12*(1), 121. https://doi.org/10.1186/s12966-015-0280-7

Stutz, J., Eiholzer, R., & Spengler, C. M. (2019). Effects of Evening Exercise on Sleep in Healthy Participants: A Systematic Review and Meta-Analysis. *Sports Medicine, 49*(2), 269–287. https://doi.org/10.1007/s40279-018-1015-0

Thacher, P. V. (2008). University students and the "all nighter": correlates and patterns of students' engagement in a single night of total sleep deprivation. *Behavioral Sleep Medicine, 6*(1), 16–31. https://doi.org/10.1080/15402000701796114

Twain, M. (1905). Seventieth birthday speech. Retrieved Dec. 5, 2013 from http://www.pbs.org/marktwain/learnmore/writings_seventieth.html

Vanderlinden, J., Boen, F., & van Uffelen, J. G. Z. (2020). Effects of physical activity programs on sleep outcomes in older adults: A systematic review. *International Journal of Behavioral Nutrition and Physical Activity, 17*(1), 11. https://doi.org/10.1186/s12966-020-0913-3

Van Dongen, H. P., Rogers, N., L., & Dinges, D. (2003). Sleep debt: Theoretical and empirical issues. *Sleep and Biological Rhythms, 1,* 5–13.

Xie, L., Kang, H., Xu, Q., Chen, M. J., Liao, Y., Thiyagarajan, M., O'Donnell, J., Christensen, et al. (2013). Sleep Drives Metabolite Clearance from the Adult Brain. *Science, 342*(6156), 373–377.

Yang, S.-Y., Lan, S.-J., Yen, Y.-Y., Hsieh, Y.-P., Kung, P.-T., & Lan, S.-H. (2020). Effects of Exercise on Sleep Quality in Pregnant Women: A Systematic Review and Meta-analysis of Randomized Controlled Trials. *Asian Nursing Research, 14*(1), 1–10. https://doi.org/10.1016/j.anr.2020.01.003

Yang, Y., Shin, J. C., Li, D., & An, R. (2017). Sedentary Behavior and Sleep Problems: A Systematic Review and Meta-Analysis. *International Journal of Behavioral Medicine, 24*(4), 481–492. https://doi.org/10.1007/s12529-016-9609-0

Youngstedt, S. D. (2005). Effects of exercise on sleep. *Clinics in Sports Medicine, 24,* 355–365.

Youngstedt, S. D., & Kline, C. E. (2006). Epidemiology of exercise and sleep. *Sleep and Biological Rhythms, 4,* 215–221.

Youngstedt, S. D., & Kript, D. F. (2004). Long sleep and mortality: Rationale for sleep restriction. *Sleep Medicine Reviews, 8,* 159–174.

Youngstedt, S. D., O'Connor, R. K., & Dishman, R. K. (1997). The effects of acute exercise on sleep: A quantitative synthesis. *Sleep, 20,* 203–214.

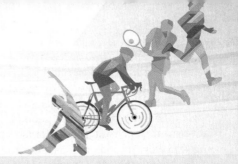

CHAPTER 10

Depression

LEARNING OBJECTIVES

After completing this chapter, you will be able to:

- Differentiate between depressed mood and major depressive disorder.
- Understand the effects of physical activity and sedentary behavior on depressive mood and major depressive disorder symptoms.
- Understand how depressive mood and major depressive disorder may impact physical activity and sedentary behavior and their motivation.

Introduction

The human mind is amazing. It can make us feel on top of the world or down in the dumps. Although feeling blue every once in a while is part of life for everyone, it can interfere with our daily functioning and the people around us if these feelings persist. Within this chapter, we will discuss the differences between feeling depressed and having a diagnosable depressive disorder. Additionally, we will consider whether changes in our physical activity and sedentary behavior may help reduce how often we feel depressed, reduce our likelihood of becoming clinically depressed, and help manage and treat depressive symptoms if we are diagnosed with **major depressive disorder**.

Depressed Mood and Major Depressive Disorder

There are important differences in feeling depressed vs being diagnosed with a major depressive disorder. A **depressed mood** is a transient mental state characterized by feeling unhappy, sad, miserable, down in the dumps, or blue. Everyone feels this way at one time or another for short periods. Depressed moods arise because of many circumstances such as the result of a death, a family break-up, a poor grade, or negative changes in job status. Notably though, depressive moods can also arise following positive events such as a birth, a graduation, a holiday period, or a major assignment. Usually, you can find a circumstance or event that elicits the depressive mood state.

Major depressive disorder is different though. Unlike depressive moods, **mood disorders** impact your general emotional well-being and your moods are usually not a reaction to something that happened (American Psychiatric Association, 2013). Whereas moods are short-lived, mood disorders are characterized by prolonged, regular occurrences of a depressed mood. Many people with these disorders will describe moods that do not align with their circumstances—feeling down even though everything is going pretty well. **Bipolar disorder** is associated with mood swings, where sometimes you feel depressed and sometimes you feel elevated (i.e., manic). Most other mood disorders are characterized by long stints of depressed mood. For example, **dysthymia** is chronic, low-grade depressed mood and/or irritability that lasts for at least 2 years. **Major depressive disorder** (also known as clinical depression disorder, unipolar depression, or unipolar disorder) is characterized by experiencing 5 or more of the symptoms listed in **Table 10-1** for at least 2 weeks, and at least one symptom is either depressed mood or loss of interest in usual activities. To be diagnosed with major depressive

disorder, these symptoms must cause significant distress and impact daily living (American Psychiatric Association, 2013).

Although there can be major life events that trigger symptoms or disorder onset, mood disorders tend to be the result of an imbalance of brain chemicals and are **heritable**—that is, susceptibility tends to run through families (Craddock & Forty, 2006). For example, estimates are that the **heritability** (i.e., the proportion of disorder risk attributable to genetics) of bipolar disorder is between 79 and 93% (Barnett & Smoller, 2009) and of major depressive disorder is 37% (Sullivan et al., 2000). Notably, this means that 63% of the risk of major depressive disorder is attributable to non-genetic, environmental influences such as exposure to stressors. So, even if someone has genetic predispositions for major depression, it may not be expressed if they never have exposure to stressful life events. Genetic predispositions should be considered as increased susceptibility to disorders, rather than a sentence for an unpreventable fate.

Major depressive disorder is a significant contributor to death, including from suicide or comorbid conditions, including cardiovascular disease and stroke (Lépine & Briley, 2011; World Health Organization, 2017). Living with major

---

Table 10-1 Major Depressive Disorder is Characterized by Experiencing Five or More of these Symptoms for at Least 2 Weeks, and at Least One Symptom Is Either Depressed Mood or Loss of Interest in Usual Activities

Depressed mood most of the day, nearly every day.

Markedly diminished interest or pleasure in all, or almost all, activities most of the day, nearly every day.

Significant weight loss when not dieting, weight gain, or decrease or increase in appetite nearly every day.

A slowing down of thought and a reduction of physical movement (observable by others, not merely subjective feelings of restlessness or being slowed down).

Fatigue or loss of energy nearly every day.

Feelings of worthlessness or excessive or inappropriate guilt nearly every day.

Diminished ability to think or concentrate, or indecisiveness, nearly every day.

Recurrent thoughts of death, recurrent suicidal ideation without a specific plan, or a suicide attempt or a specific plan for committing suicide.

depressive disorder can make it difficult to work, study, sleep, eat, and enjoy friends and activities. Not surprisingly then, major depressive disorder is a leading cause of burden around the globe, costing substantially in terms of people's quality of life, work productivity, and health care costs (Lépine & Briley, 2011; World Health Organization, 2017).

CRITICAL THINKING ACTIVITY 10-1

Describe the differences between a depressed mood and major depressive disorder. How can you tell which one you are experiencing?

Major depressive disorder is traditionally diagnosed by a psychiatric interview. In addition to psychiatric interviews, many self-report questionnaires have been used to assess symptoms. It should be noted that, although questionnaires may have established "cut-points" to identify persons who may have diagnosable major depressive disorder, such assessments are not diagnostic tools but rather measures of the presence and severity of depressive symptoms. For example, The Centre for Epidemiologic Studies Depression Scale Revised (CESD-R; Eaton et al., 2004) is a commonly used assessment of depression symptoms for use in the general public. It consists of 20 self-report items on which respondents report how often they felt that way in the past week, with response options ranging from "Not at all or less than 1 day" to "Nearly every day." See **Table 10-2** for the CESD-R. The scale is scored as a sum of all 20 responses, with higher scores indicative of more symptoms. There are also nine subscales of the CESD-R that can be calculated separately and used to assess against the major depressive disorder diagnostic criteria described earlier. They are Sadness/Dysphoria (items 2, 4, 6), Loss of Interest (items 8, 10), Appetite (items 1, 18), Sleep (items 5, 11, 19), Thinking/Concentration (items 3, 20), Guilt/Worthlessness (items 9, 17), Tired/Fatigue (items 7, 16), Movement/Agitation (items 12, 13), and Suicidal Ideation (items 14, 15).

Importantly, if you now – or at any time – feel distressed and would like to consider options for help with depression, please do reach out to your doctor, utilize call lines (e.g., National Hopeline Center: 1-800 Suicide [800 784 2433] The National Suicide Prevention Lifeline: 1-800-273-8255), or find help through relevant web resources (e.g., https://suicideprevention lifeline.org/ IMALIVE Crisis Chatline: https://www.imalive.org/). If you are in a medical emergency or suicidal crisis, call emergency services immediately (911). If you are in crisis and need referral to social and community services but are not experiencing an immediate life-threatening emergency, call 211. For details of mental health services outside of America, see: https://checkpointorg.com/global/

Some people have major depressive disorder only once in their life, while others have it several times over the course of their lifetime. Epidemiological studies suggest that about one in every 10 people will experience major depressive disorder at some point in their life, and in any 1 year, between 3–9% of people of all ages will be currently diagnosed with major depressive disorder (Centers for Disease Control and Prevention (CDC), 2010; Demyttenaere et al., 2004; World Health Organization, 2017). Women are more likely to be diagnosed with major depressive disorder than men, especially during the reproductive years (Grigoriadis & Robinson, 2007; World Health Organization, 2017). Transgender and gender-nonconforming youth tend to also have an elevated risk of being diagnosed with major depressive disorder compared to their cisgender counterparts, with one study reporting a prevalence of diagnosable major depressive disorder in 33% of the population (Chodzen et al., 2019).

Interestingly, there are also gender differences in how major depressive disorder is experienced. For example, women tend to experience more seasonal symptoms and present with **comorbid depression and anxiety** than men—that is, they experience a clinical anxiety disorder along with major depressive disorder. Across all genders, it is more likely to have comorbid depression and anxiety than to have only one—either clinical

Table 10-2 The Centre for Epidemiologic Studies Depression Scale Revised

CESD-R Items	Directions: Below is a list of the ways you might have felt or behaved. Please select the option that describes how often you have felt this way in the past week or so.				
	Not at all or Less than 1 day	1–2 days	3–4 days	5–7 days	Nearly every day for 2 weeks
1. My appetite was poor.	0	1	2	3	4
2. I could not shake off the blues.	0	1	2	3	4
3. I had trouble keeping my mind on what I was doing.	0	1	2	3	4
4. I felt depressed.	0	1	2	3	4
5. My sleep was restless.	0	1	2	3	4
6. I felt sad.	0	1	2	3	4
7. I could not get going.	0	1	2	3	4
8. Nothing made me happy.	0	1	2	3	4
9. I felt like a bad person.	0	1	2	3	4
10. I lost interest in my usual activities.	0	1	2	3	4
11. I slept much more than usual.	0	1	2	3	4
12. I felt like I was moving too slowly.	0	1	2	3	4
13. I felt fidgety.	0	1	2	3	4
14. I wished I were dead.	0	1	2	3	4
15. I wanted to hurt myself.	0	1	2	3	4
16. I was tired all the time.	0	1	2	3	4
17. I did not like myself.	0	1	2	3	4
18. I lost a lot of weight without trying to.	0	1	2	3	4
19. I had a lot of trouble getting to sleep.	0	1	2	3	4
20. I could not focus on the important things.	0	1	2	3	4

Data from Eaton, W. W., Smith, C., Ybarra, M., Muntaner, C., & Tien, A. (2004). Center for Epidemiologic Studies Depression Scale: Review and Revision (CESD and CESD-R). In *The use of psychological testing for treatment planning and outcomes assessment: Instruments for adults, Volume 3, 3rd ed* (pp. 363–377). Lawrence Erlbaum Associates Publishers.

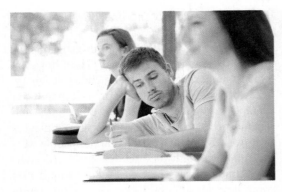

© AntonioGuillem/Getty Images.

anxiety or major depressive disorder (Brown et al., 2001).

Treatment Options for Major Depressive Disorder

The most prescribed treatments for major depressive disorder include psychotherapy and/or medications. Psychotherapy involves the person with depression talking to licensed and trained mental health care professionals in either individual or group counseling settings. The aim of psychotherapy is typically to identify factors that may be triggering depression symptoms and to aid in learning management and coping strategies. There are many types of psychotherapy that have promising evidence of success, including behavioral activation and cognitive behavioral therapy. **Behavioral activation** applies operant conditioning strategies through scheduling to encourage reconnection with environmental positive reinforcement. For example, it may be that you commit to weekly social volunteering events so that you regularly have engagement with social connectedness and a sense of purpose. Evidence suggests behavioral activation can reduce depressive symptoms by a Standardized Mean Difference (SMD) score of −0.74 (Ekers et al., 2014). That means that there is a medium-large reduction in depression symptoms as a result of the treatment. **Cognitive behavioral therapy** helps people to identity and change inaccurate perceptions that may be exacerbating symptoms. For example, you may

be asked to reflect on whether you jump to conclusions without enough information or always assume you are responsible for bad things happening. Cognitive behavioral therapy has been found to be effective in reducing depression symptoms by a small-medium effect (Cuijpers et al., 2013). Most evidence, however, shows that psychotherapy treatment is most effective for managing major depressive disorder if supplemented with anti-depressant medications (Cuijpers et al., 2014).

Evidence suggests that the effectiveness of medication for managing major depressive disorder widely varies between medications, people, and across time. For example, for people with moderate or mild symptoms, the SMD is small (< 0.20), but for people with severe symptoms, it is larger (SMD = 0.47) (Fournier et al., 2010). It can take a while to establish which medications in what dosages will work for each individual. Although a variety of medications are available for the treatment of depression, including selective serotonin reuptake inhibitors (SSRIs) and serotonin noradrenaline reuptake inhibitors (SNRIs), many patients cannot tolerate the side effects, do not respond adequately, or gradually

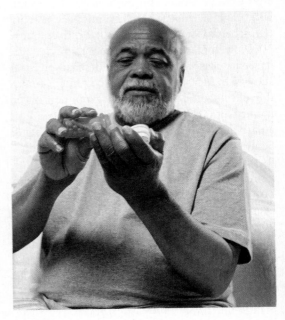

© Getty Images.

lose their response to anti-depressant medication (Fournier et al., 2010). Evidence shows that the effects of treatment are larger when medication is supplemented with other treatments, including acupuncture (Chan et al., 2015) and mindfulness training (Kuyken et al., 2016).

Depressed Mood, Physical Activity, and Sedentary Behavior

Recently, more than ever before, the role of physical activity in regulating depressive moods and in preventing and treating major depressive disorder is also being recognized. Given how many ways our feelings have been assessed in physical activity and sedentary behavior research, it is a bit difficult to tease out specific effects of physical activity and sedentary behavior on depressive mood, as opposed to effects on our general mood, feeling states, or emotions. However, there is sufficient evidence to conclude that physical activity tends to make people feel more activated and pleasant, both shortly after exercise bouts and more generally overall with regular engagement in physical activity (Evmenenko & Teixeira, 2020; Reed & Buck, 2009; Reed & Ones, 2006). From this evidence, it seems reasonable to conclude that physical activity reduces depressed mood. Interestingly, the effects of physical activity on depressive mood seem to be strongest when people are in a particularly depressed mood state (Kanning & Schlicht, 2010). Mood effects of physical activity have been shown to occur immediately after a single bout of exercise and to last at least 1 day post-exercise (Basso & Suzuki, 2017). Not all exercise is the same though. There is a convincing line of evidence to suggest that mental health benefits of physical activity are enhanced when the activity is something you enjoy doing (Abrantes et al., 2017; Berger & Motl, 2000; Pickett et al., 2017). So, rather than incidentally getting steps in through your job or while getting house chores done, it's worth taking time to find a way to regularly get some physical activity doing what you enjoy.

There is not a lot of evidence investigating the effects of sedentary behavior on mood; however, it does support the notion that more sedentary behavior is associated with depressed mood. For example, Giurgiu et al. (2019) assessed mood and sedentary behavior of 92 University employees over five days. They found the more people were sedentary, the less they felt pleasant and energized. Interestingly, these effects were found after controlling for effects of physical activity. Other studies show similar results. More time spent in sedentary behavior tends to be associated with more depressed mood (e.g., DeMello et al., 2018; Elavsky et al., 2016). It may be that mood is not only associated with overall time spent being sedentary, but also with how frequently sedentary behavior is broken up by standing and walking. Some evidence suggests that breaking up sedentary behavior frequently with walking may be beneficial for reducing depressed mood (Giurgiu, Koch, et al., 2020).

A study design that has been regularly used to assess links between physical activity, sedentary behavior, and mood is **ecological momentary assessment (EMA)**; also known as experience sampling methodology (Bolger & Laurenceau, 2013; Shiffman et al., 2008). In EMA studies, people are asked to self-report (on a smartphone app, web survey, or written diary) the targeted variables, such as their current mood, multiple times per day for several days or weeks in a row. There are four criteria of EMA studies described by Stone and Shiffman (1994):

1. Target variables are assessed as they occur (in real time).
2. Assessments are dependent upon a strategic timing schedule.
3. Assessments are intensively repeated over many observations.
4. Assessments are made in the environment that they occur in.

EMA study designs are useful for investigating what, when, and how people feel, think and act throughout their daily lives, although some evidence suggests people may act a bit different when involved in these studies than they would in normal life (Ram et al., 2017). In some EMA studies, the assessments are randomly dispersed throughout the day. By randomly sampling people's mood and experiences over time, researchers can map out typical daily profiles of the targeted variables. In other EMA studies, the assessments are **event-contingent**, meaning participants respond to assessments when a specific event occurs (such as after doing physical activity). In a review of EMA studies investigating risk factors for depressed mood states, it was found that physical activity, along with social connections, was linked to less depressed mood; whereas poor sleep, stressful events, and social conflict led to more depressed mood (Pemberton & Fuller Tyszkiewicz, 2016).

Now that it is more commonplace for people to use technology such as smartwatches that automatically records data about location, physical health, and movement, it is becoming more feasible that we could use science to predict when you will get depressed and intervene before it happens (Tuarob et al., 2017). Such interventions are called **just-in-time adaptive interventions** (Nahum-Shani et al., 2015, 2018). This type of approach may be particularly effective for people with major depressive disorder during times when help needed is crucial to avoid harm or death.

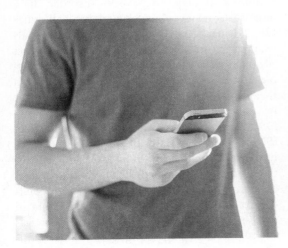

© guteksk7/Shutterstock.

CRITICAL THINKING ACTIVITY 10-2

If you were to plan a just-in-time adaptive intervention to help people avoid feeling depressed, what would you do? How would it work?

Major Depressive Disorder, Physical Activity, and Sedentary Behavior

Physical Activity and Sedentary Behavior and Prevention of Major Depressive Disorder

There has been some work on the impact of physical activity on the prevalence and incidence of major depressive disorder. **Prevalence** is the proportion of the population who have a condition at a particular time; whereas **incidence** is the proportion of the population who have experienced their first episode of the condition at a particular time. The difference is that prevalence includes all cases (new and pre-existing); whereas incidence is limited to new cases only.

The evidence of whether regular physical activity reduces the prevalence or incidence of major depressive disorder is inconclusive. Some studies suggest that physical activity participation

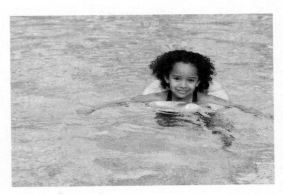

© Studio 1One/Shutterstock.

in childhood has been found to lead to reduced risks of depressive episodes in adulthood (Jacka et al., 2011; Korniloff et al., 2012). However, a systematic review of longitudinal studies found that only two of 15 studies found consistent association between regular physical activity and reduced subsequent risk of major depressive disorder (Suetani et al., 2019). Other studies have found mixed or no support for the association. Notably though, a more recent review has found that when only considering studies which measured physical activity with monitors (as opposed to self-reported activity), there was sufficient evidence that physical activity has a potential protective effect on prevalence and incidence of major depressive disorder (Gianfredi et al., 2020).

In regards to sedentary behavior, there is some evidence to suggest that less time spent in a sedentary state reduces likelihood of depression symptoms; although it remains a bit ambiguous as to whether the effects are for non-clinical depressive symptoms or the incidence and prevalence of major depressive disorder (Teychenne et al., 2010; Zhai et al., 2015). Specifically, it seems that risk of depression symptoms was most linked to time spent engaged in watching television, using a computer, or being on the internet (Zhai et al., 2015). Similar effects are seen within meta-analysis of studies of screen time and depression risk in children and adolescents. Those who spend more than 2 hours a day in front of a screen have a higher risk of depression than those who spend less time in front of a screen (Liu et al., 2016). It is important to note, though, that many of these findings do not consider the potential of bidirectional relationships. Some evidence suggests a reciprocal relationship between sedentary behavior and mood – that is, when people are sedentary, they tend to have a more depressed mood, but when people are in a depressed mood state, they are also more likely to be sedentary than physically active (DeMello et al., 2018; Giurgiu, Plotnikoff, et al., 2020). Because there are not a lot of interventions yet, we cannot rule out that the link between sedentary behavior

and risk of depression is a bidirectional association effect, rather than the result of behavior causing an increase in risk of depression. Taken together, it is difficult to make a clear call on whether increased physical activity and limited sedentary behavior will help prevent incidence and prevalence of major depressive disorder.

CRITICAL THINKING ACTIVITY 10-3

Why do you think there are so many inconsistent findings when considering if more physical activity and less sedentary behavior can reduce the prevalence and incidence of major depressive disorder? What type of study would you design to help address this unresolved scientific question?

Physical Activity and Sedentary Behavior and Treatment of Major Depressive Disorder

There has been a longstanding interest in the potential benefits of physical activity as an intervention strategy for the treatment of major depressive disorder (e.g., Franz & Hamilton, 1905). Several meta-analyses have been carried out examining the effects of physical activity on depression symptoms in people with major depressive disorder. In a large-scale review, Cooney and his colleagues (2013) meta-analytically reviewed 39 trials examining the effects of physical activity on people suffering with major depressive disorder (N = 2,326 participants). They found that when compared with the no treatment or the control interventions, physical activity had a moderate to strong treatment effect (SMD = −0.62). Many of the trials reviewed, however, had either biases or other faults. Thus, the researchers examined the effects of the exercise on depressive symptoms with only well-designed trials. When the analyses were limited to these higher quality trials, the effect was slightly weaker, suggesting only a small antidepressant effect was associated with exercise.

However, there has been criticism and rebuttal on which studies should be included in this review. The conclusion is that some of these choices led to underestimated findings of the effects of physical activity on depressive symptoms (Ekkekakis, 2015). For example, in the Cooney (2013) meta-analysis, they included studies that compared physical activity intervention groups to **active control groups**. These are groups in which a comparable standard treatment is applied. An updated estimation based on randomized controlled trials comparing physical activity to **non-active control groups** (i.e., groups in which the participants receive no comparison treatment during the study) is that the effect of physical activity on depression symptoms for people with major depressive disorder was large with a SMD = 1.14 (Schuch et al., 2016). Notably, this effect was found to be slightly larger for studies with samples of people diagnosed with major depressive disorder, as opposed to those who self-reported clinical depressive symptoms.

CRITICAL THINKING ACTIVITY 10-4

What is an example of an active control group that may be used to test whether physical activity can reduce depressive symptoms in people with major depressive disorder? What is an example of a non-active control group that may be used?

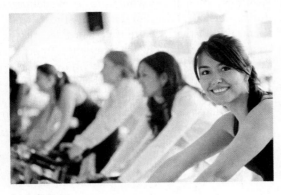

© Andresr/Shutterstock.

Beyond the mental health benefits, physical activity engagement can improve the physical health and fitness of people with major depressive disorder, a population that is particularly at risk for poor cardiovascular health and low fitness levels (Firth et al., 2019; Stanton et al., 2015, 2019). Support for physical activity in the treatment of depression is becoming more mainstream now with many clinical practice guidelines for treatment, including recommendations of physical activity.

There are evidence-based guidelines about specific frequency, intensity, duration, and physical activity type that are likely to enhance the antidepressant effects of physical activity for people with major depressive disorder. Specifically, it is recommended that treatment for major depressive disorder should include engaging in moderate-vigorous intensity physical activity at least once per week for as little as ten minutes a day, such as walking (Stanton et al., 2014).

What about patients with chronic illnesses? Both physical inactivity and comorbid depressive symptoms are prevalent among patients with a chronic illness. Herring and his colleagues (2012) meta-analytically examined whether exercise training affected depressive symptoms among patients with chronic illnesses. Their meta-analysis included 90 articles with 10,534 people with chronic illnesses such as cardiovascular disease, fibromyalgia, obesity, multiple sclerosis, and cardiometabolic disease. They found that exercise reduces depressive symptoms among people with a chronic illness. They also found that people with mild-to-moderate depressive symptoms and for whom exercise training improved function-related outcomes achieved the largest anti-depressant effects. A more recent review comparing the effects of aerobic exercise to usual care in adults living with major noncommunicable diseases, including cardiovascular disease, respiratory disease, type 2 diabetes, and cancer, found that aerobic exercise reduced depressive symptoms by an SMD of 0.50 (Béland et al., 2020). These findings provide evidence to recommend physical activity as a potential

Postpartum (or postnatal) Depression

Postpartum depression is not recognized as a separate depressive disorder, but rather women must meet the criteria for major depressive episode with an onset in either pregnancy or within 4 weeks of delivery. Postnatal depression affects about 10% of women after giving birth. Symptoms include sadness, fatigue, changes in sleeping and eating patterns, reduced libido, crying episodes, anxiety, and irritability.

A meta-analysis of 17 studies representing 93,676 women reveals that those who were physically active during pregnancy had reduced postpartum depression symptoms than those who were not active during pregnancy (Nakamura et al., 2019). Additionally, although limited in study quality, evidence of the use of physical activity in the treatment of postpartum depression symptoms reveals promising results as well (Carter et al., 2019; Daley et al., 2007). These findings suggest physical activity can prevent and help manage postpartum depression symptoms.

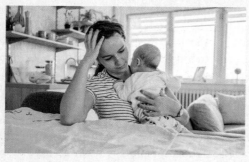

© Urbazon/E+/Getty Images.

low-risk, adjuvant treatment for depressive symptoms that may develop during chronic illness.

Although there have been plenty of correlational studies showing links between sedentary behavior and depression symptoms, there is a huge gap in the literature regarding randomized controlled trials focused on reducing depressive symptoms in people with major depressive disorder through reducing sedentary behavior. There are calls for it, and the neurophysiological evidence suggests it may feasible. But the field has not progressed far enough to make a clear-cut conclusion about whether sedentary behavior reduction can reduce depressive symptoms in people with major depressive disorder.

Depressive Symptoms in Non-Clinical Populations

Generally, evidence suggests that more physical activity and less sedentary behavior results in fewer and less severe depressive symptoms in non-clinical populations (Rebar et al., 2015; Stanton et al., 2014; Teychenne et al., 2010; Zhai et al., 2015), Interestingly, some evidence suggests these effects may differ based on the purpose of the physical activity or sedentary behavior. In a study of more than 40,000 residents of Norway, it was found that the more time people spent in physical activity during leisure time, the less depressive symptoms they presented with; however, there was no association between time spent in physical activity during work and depressive symptoms (Harvey et al., 2010). One study of more than 20,000 Swedish healthcare workers found that time spent sedentary while working was not significantly associated with frequency of depression symptoms in non-clinical populations; however, time spent sedentary while in leisure was (Hallgren et al., 2020). That is, adults who spent more than half of their leisure time in sedentary activities were more likely to experience frequent depression symptoms than those who were less sedentary during leisure time. For example, those who spent 50% of their leisure time being sedentary were 43% more likely to experience frequent depression symptoms than those who spent less than 25% of their leisure time being sedentary. So, similarly to the effects of physical activity and sedentary behavior on depressed mood, it may be that to reduce depressive symptoms in non-clinical populations, the type of activity being engaged in (e.g., leisure time vs work or chores) is more important than the movement.

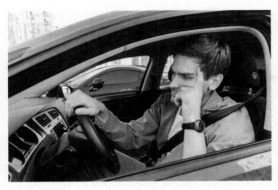

© Monstar Studio/Shutterstock.

Janssen and LeBlanc (2010) conducted a systematic review of the health benefits of physical activity in school-aged children (ages 5 to 7 years). They found that physical activity was associated with many health benefits for youth – including improvements in depression symptoms. In 2019, evidence of the mental health benefits of reducing sedentary behavior in children and adolescents was further established with a meta-analysis showing that greater amounts of sedentary behavior was associated with more depressive symptoms and higher risk of depression (Rodriguez-Ayllon et al., 2019).

Depression and Motivation for Physical Activity and Sedentary Behavior

We have just covered a very large body of scientific evidence about the antidepressant benefits for increasing physical activity and reducing sedentary behavior; however, it is important to remember that all these benefits are reliant on a person's motivation to change their behavior (Rebar & Taylor, 2017). When you feel depressed, it can be really hard to get motivated to do anything, let alone get up and go for a run (Hemmis et al., 2015; Pickett et al., 2017). There is neurophysiological research to back this up (Basso & Suzuki, 2017). Dopamine is instrumental for motivation. Depression is associated with deregulation of dopamine systems, throwing off the way we react to and anticipate rewards. So, when you feel depressed, it just may not feel "worth it" to do any physical activity and you may feel quite motivated to be sedentary.

Given the impact of depressed mood and depressive symptoms on motivation, it is not surprising that people with mental illness tend to be more sedentary and less physically active than similar people without mental illness, especially when using antidepressant medication (Vancampfort et al., 2017). One meta-analysis that looked exclusively at studies of people with major depressive disorder found that they tend to spend less time engaging in physical activity (SMD = –0.25) and more time engaging in sedentary behavior (SMD = 0.09) (Schuch et al., 2017). To ensure the antidepressant benefits are long-lasting, it is important to help motivate people to start being more physically active and to help them maintain these behaviors long-term. Some evidence suggests that intrinsic motivation, or engaging in a behavior for enjoyment, may be particularly important to motivate physical activity for people when depressive symptoms are high (Vancampfort et al., 2015, 2016). Additional evidence suggests that ensuring people with depressive symptoms maintain strong perceived control over their own behavior is instrumental for behavior change (Hemmis et al., 2015). It may be relevant to use **tailored interventions** that include features and content relevant to the people that will be using it. To help people with depression get more active and less sedentary, focusing on motivation is particularly important. See Section 4 for more reading on physical activity and sedentary behavior motivation.

CRITICAL THINKING ACTIVITY 10-5

What motivates you to be physically active? How might depressed mood or depressive symptoms interfere with your motivation? What could you do about it?

Physical Activity, Phone Use, and Depression Among University Students

A recent study found that 27.5% of University students had problematic mobile phone use (i.e., craving, dependence, tolerance, losing control, and interference with physical, mental, and social functioning). The study found that students who had problematic phone use tended to report more depressive symptoms than students who did not have problematic phone use (Tao et al., 2020). However, it was also found that engaging in physical activity helped buffer from depressive symptoms, even for students with problematic phone use. So, we're not asking you to get off your phone – but at least be active while scrolling!

Mechanisms

There have been many ways proposed in which physical activity helps to reduce depressed mood or treat and prevent major depressive disorder (Basso & Suzuki, 2017). Typically, psychological explanations are put forth in contrast to neurophysiological ones. In reality though, these are interplaying systems, so it is more likely that the neurophysiological explanations underpin or interact with the psychological mechanisms. For example, it is not that physical activity either works to reduce depression through regulation of motivation or an enhance in dopamine. Rather, it is that enhanced dopamine regulates motivation, which results in lesser depressive symptoms. To illustrate these interplaying processes further, **Table 10-3** lays out a few proposed mechanisms of the antidepressant effects of physical activity, linking neurophysiological and psychological manifestations of mechanisms. After a single bout of exercise, neurophysiological changes have been documented, including changes in neurotransmitters, metabolites, growth factors, and neuromodulators. These neurophysiological changes are associated with enhanced mood, self-beliefs, sleep, motivation, problem solving, and motivation. Likely, it is a combination of many of these effects that explains antidepressant effects of physical activity.

As is the case for any evolving scientific area, you need to be aware that there are disputes among scientists about the evidence surrounding the antidepressant effects of physical activity. For example, there is a large body of

Table 10-3 **Description of Some Potential Mechanisms of the Impact of Physical Activity on Depression**

Psychological Mechanism	Description	Neurophysiological Factors
Regulation of Coping Strategies	Regular physical activity enhances regulation of our physiological responses to stressors, which may make it less likely that depressed mood is experienced.	Plasticity of serotonergic neurons; attenuated cortisol responses to stressors.
Mood regulation and enhancement of cognitive functioning	Physical activity can enhance the neuronal plasticity that is impaired in people with major depressive disorder.	Neurotrophin factors including brain derived neurotropic factor (BDNF), insulin-like growth factor 1 (IGF-1), and vascular endothelial growth factor (VEGF) in hippocampus.
Increased positive feelings and decreased negative feelings	Physical activity can help regulate the uptake of neurotransmitters that enhance mood and regulate how we feel overall.	Change of levels of neurotransmitters such as dopamine, epinephrine, norepinephrine, acetylcholine, gamma-aminobutyric acid, and glutamate.

evidence suggesting that depression is the loss of the **brain-derived neurotrophic factor (BDNF)**. However, there is also a large body of evidence suggesting that the story is more complicated than a simple causal relationship. Rather than being the cause of major depressive disorder, it may be that BDNF plays a role in the **genesis** of the clinical disorder and how its depressive symptoms progress over time (Groves, 2007).

Summary

Scientists have had a longstanding interest in the association of physical activity with depressed moods and depressive symptoms. More recently, there is also a burgeoning line of research to understand the links between sedentary behavior and depressed moods and depressive symptoms. Thanks to advancements in science, including EMA studies, it seems quite clear that engaging in physical activity reduces depressed moods and engaging in long bouts of sedentary behavior can increase depressed moods. The evidence is a bit more unequivocal regarding whether physical activity and sedentary behavior play a role in determining whether and how severely major depressive disorder is experienced. There is no doubt, however, that physical activity is effective as an intervention strategy to reduce depression symptoms in people with major depressive disorder; whereas it remains untested if sedentary behavior reductions can be effective in the same manner. The overarching challenge within the field is that depression can undermine motivation to be physically active, making it difficult to adhere to the healthy levels of physical activity that will produce the antidepressant benefits. If enhancements in physical activity and reductions in sedentary behavior can help reduce the burden of depression for individuals and the world, then the public health impact of promoting regular physical activity amidst this target population, although a challenge, could be great.

Vignette: Laura

I have struggled with untreated depression since adolescence. I have a hunch that mental health issues run in my family, though neither my mother nor my father ever sought help for their mood swings and long stretches of sadness that sometimes kept them bedridden for days.

After I got my first job out of college as a real estate broker, I tried therapy. But it just seemed to make me sadder. And I found it too hard to commit to the twice weekly sessions the professional I was seeing recommended. Searching for deals and showing clients apartments took up too much time and I wanted to be good at my job.

Though my job often required me to be on my feet a lot, I never was one to pursue fitness. Many of my colleagues often referred to the gyms they went to throughout the city I worked in, and there was constant talk in my office of trending yoga classes, CrossFit, and spin.

So that I wouldn't burst into tears during normal business hours, I decided to go on antidepressants. I took them for about 4 years. But after tiring of their accompanying loss of sex drive and weight gain, I gradually decreased the milligrams of Sertraline I was taking until I was completely drug free at 31 years old.

Throughout the course of my coming off the pills, I didn't feel my mood crash drastically—at least, not right away. But I did feel increasingly anxious, perhaps due to the chemical let down as well as the hesitation that I wouldn't be able to function in the absence of a prescription.

Then my living situation changed. To have some extra income, I decided to rent out the spare bedroom in my apartment. A young woman moved in who taught fitness classes at an upscale gym in our neighborhood. For months, she kept beseeching me to drop into one of her yoga or cycling sessions. But I kept telling her, "No, I'll make an idiot of myself."

What made me finally bite the bullet and attend an extremely overcrowded Saturday afternoon spin class wasn't the desire to be healthy, per se. It was a realization that the weight I thought would miraculously fall off after I stopped the antidepressants wasn't budging at all. Wanting to look a bit better, fit into my "skinny" clothes again, and possibly boost my self-esteem in the process, I bought a pair of exercise pants, a sports bra, and found the most secluded bike in the classroom.

I can honestly say that my first spin class was the most brutal, unenjoyable 45 minutes of my life. I would even go so far as to place it on par with the depressive episodes I fell into that left me listless, hopeless, and, in my worst hours, suicidal. But after I got off that bike, every inch of my flesh dripping with sweat, I felt that I'd accomplished something as rewarding as closing a real estate deal. I guess you could call it my first exercise high.

I came back the following weekend. I needed about 7 days to get over the insane amount of soreness in my leg muscles, lower back, and even my arms. Though it was just as hard as the first time, once I got to the end, I still felt that same rush.

I must say, it was addicting—but in a good way. My depressive episodes tend to come in waves, often during the colder seasons or when my sleep schedule gets off track. Getting a membership at a cycling studio—which I finally did last March as a little birthday present to myself—made me feel that in order to get my money's worth, I should really commit to at least three classes a week. Often—due to the constraints of my work schedule—this required me to be on a bike around 6:30 in the morning. Having this obligation helped me get to bed at an earlier hour and keep to a more regular routine.

It would be too far reaching to say that my new exercise habits have cured my depression for good. I still experience really low moods when I encounter setbacks at work, or when my new attempts to date don't go well. But I will say that despite my desire to, on some days, stay in bed until the afternoon or itemize all the things I hate about the world, I know if I just make it to an exercise class—even if I sit in the back and pedal slowly—I'll feel a little bit better.

Key Terms

active control groups Study groups in which a comparable standard treatment is applied. Active control groups are usually used to test whether the intervention treatment is better than other forms of known effective treatments.

behavioral activation A form of psychotherapy in which operant conditioning strategies are used through scheduling in order to encourage reconnection with environmental positive reinforcement.

bipolar disorder A psychological condition in which a person has periods of depression and periods of being extremely happy or being cross or irritable.

brain-derived neurotrophic factor (BDNF) A protein found in the brain that is related to nerve survival and growth.

cognitive behavioral therapy A form of psychotherapy that helps people to identify and change inaccurate perceptions that may exacerbate symptoms.

comorbid depression and anxiety The shared experience of a clinical anxiety disorder with major depressive disorder. It is more common to have comorbid depression and anxiety than either disorder in isolation.

depressed mood A transient mental state characterized by feeling unhappy, sad, miserable, down in the dumps, or blue.

dysthymia A depressed mood that occurs for most of the day, for more days than not, for at least 2 years (at least one year for children and adolescents).

ecological momentary assessment (EMA) A study design in which the target variables are assessed as they occur (in real time) and assessments are dependent upon a strategic timing schedule, intensively repeated over many observations, and made in the environment they occur in. It is also known as experience sampling methodology.

event-contingent A type of ecological momentary assessment study in which participants respond to assessments when a specific event occurs.

genesis The progression of the onset and development of symptoms throughout a disorder.

heritable Something that tends to run in families, shared through common genes.

heritability The proportion of disorder risk attributable to genetics.

incidence The proportion of the population who have experienced their first episode of a condition at a particular time.

just-in-time adaptive interventions Intervention programs aiming to provide the right type and amount of support at the time when the support is most needed.

major depressive disorder A psychological disorder characterized by persistent feelings of sadness and/or loss of interest that can interfere with your daily functioning.

mood disorders Psychiatric disorders characterized by a distorted mood that is inconsistent with your circumstances and interferes with daily functioning.

non-active control groups Study groups in which the participants receive no comparison treatment during the study. These are usually used to test whether the intervention treatment is effective at all.

postpartum depression Moderate to severe depression in a woman after she has given birth.

prevalence The proportion of the population who have experienced their first episode of the condition at a particular time.

tailored interventions Intervention programs that include features and content made specifically to be relevant to the people who will be using it.

Review Questions

1. What is the difference between a depressed mood and a depressive disorder?
2. How can a person determine if they have a mood disorder or not?
3. What resource might you provide to someone who may need help with depression (including yourself)?
4. Describe three treatment options for depression.
5. How does physical activity and sedentary behavior impact immediate and long-term depressive mood states?
6. What is a just-in-time adaptive intervention and how might it be applied to help people with mood disorders?
7. What is the difference between prevalence and incidence?
8. How can physical activity play a role in the treatment of Major Depressive Disorder?
9. What impact does depression have on motivation for physical activity and sedentary behavior?

Applying the Concepts

1. What scientific evidence that you read about in this chapter supports some of the things described by Laura?
2. Describe the impact that Laura's enjoyment of physical activity had on her motivation and her mental health.

References

Abrantes, A. M., Farris, S. G., Garnaat, S. L., Minto, A., Brown, R. A., Price, L. H., & Uebelacker, L. A. (2017). The role of physical activity enjoyment on the acute mood experience of exercise among smokers with elevated depressive symptoms. *Mental Health and Physical Activity, 12*, 37–43. https://doi.org/10.1016/j.mhpa.2017.02.001

American Psychiatric Association. (2013). *Diagnostic and statistical manual of mental disorders (DSM-5®)*. American Psychiatric Publishing.

Barnett, J. H., & Smoller, J. W. (2009). The genetics of bipolar disorder. *Neuroscience, 164*(1), 331–343. https://doi.org/10.1016/j.neuroscience.2009.03.080

Basso, J. C., & Suzuki, W. A. (2017). The Effects of acute exercise on mood, cognition, neurophysiology, and neurochemical pathways: A review. *Brain Plasticity, 2*(2), 127–152. https://doi.org/10.3233/BPL-160040

Béland, M., Lavoie, K. L., Briand, S., White, U. J., Gemme, C., & Bacon, S. L. (2020). Aerobic exercise alleviates depressive symptoms in patients with a major non-communicable chronic disease: A systematic review and meta-analysis. *British Journal of Sports Medicine, 54*, 272–278. https://doi.org/10.1136/bjsports-2018-099360

Berger, B. G., & Motl, R. W. (2000). Exercise and mood: A selective review and synthesis of research employing the profile of mood states. *Journal of Applied Sport Psychology, 12*(1), 69–92.

Bolger, N., & Laurenceau, J. P. (2013). *Intensive longitudinal methods: An introduction to diary and experience sampling research*. Guilford Press.

Brown, T. A., Campbell, L. A., Lehman, C. L., Grisham, J. R., & Mancill, R. B. (2001). Current and lifetime comorbidity of the DSM-IV anxiety and mood disorders in a large clinical sample. *Journal of Abnormal Psychology, 110*(4), 585–599.

Carter, T., Bastounis, A., Guo, B., & Jane Morrell, C. (2019). The effectiveness of exercise-based interventions for preventing or treating postpartum depression: A systematic review and meta-analysis. *Archives of Women's Mental Health, 22*(1), 37–53. https://doi.org/10.1007/s00737-018-0869-3

Centers for Disease Control and Prevention (CDC). (2010). Current depression among adults—United States, 2006 and 2008. *MMWR. Morbidity and Mortality Weekly Report, 59*(38), 1229–1235.

Chan, Y. Y., Lo, W. Y., Yang, S. N., Chen, Y. H., & Lin, J. G. (2015). The benefit of combined acupuncture and antidepressant medication for depression: A systematic review and meta-analysis. *Journal of Affective Disorders, 176*, 106–117. https://doi.org/10.1016/j.jad.2015.01.048

Chodzen, G., Hidalgo, M. A., Chen, D., & Garofalo, R. (2019). Minority stress factors associated with depression and anxiety among transgender and gender-nonconforming youth. *Journal of Adolescent Health, 64*(4), 467–471. https://doi.org/10.1016/j.jadohealth.2018.07.006

Cooney, G. M., Dwan, K., Greig, C. A., Lawlor, D. A., Rimer, J., Waugh, F. R., McMurdo, M., & Mead, G. E. (2013). Exercise for depression. *Cochrane Database of Systematic Reviews, 9*(CD004366). https://doi.org/10.1002/14651858.CD004366.pub6

Craddock, N., & Forty, L. (2006). Genetics of affective (mood) disorders. *European Journal of Human Genetics, 14*(6), 660–668. https://doi.org/10.1038/sj.ejhg.5201549

Cuijpers, P., Berking, M., Andersson, G., Quigley, L., Kleiboer, A., & Dobson, K. S. (2013). A meta-analysis of cognitive-behavioural therapy for adult depression, alone and in comparison with other treatments. *The Canadian Journal of Psychiatry, 58*(7), 376–385. https://doi.org/10.1177/070674371305800702

Cuijpers, P., Sijbrandij, M., Koole, S. L., Andersson, G., Beekman, A. T., & Reynolds III, C. F. (2014). Adding psychotherapy to antidepressant medication in depression and anxiety disorders: A meta-analysis. *Focus, 12*(3), 347–358.

Daley, A. J., MacArthur, C., & Winter, H. (2007). The role of exercise in treating postpartum depression: A review of the literature. *Journal of Midwifery & Women's Health, 52*(1), 56–62. https://doi.org/10.1016/j.jmwh.2006.08.017

DeMello, M. M., Pinto, B. M., Dunsiger, S. I., Shook, R. P., Burgess, S., Hand, G. A., & Blair, S. N. (2018). Reciprocal relationship between sedentary behavior and mood in young adults over one-year duration. *Mental Health and Physical Activity, 14*, 157–162. https://doi.org/10.1016/j.mhpa.2017.12.001

Eaton, W. W., Smith, C., Ybarra, M., Muntaner, C., & Tien, A. (2004). Center for Epidemiologic Studies Depression Scale: Review and Revision (CESD and CESD-R). In *The use of psychological testing for treatment planning and outcomes assessment: Instruments for adults, Volume 3, 3rd ed* (pp. 363–377). Lawrence Erlbaum Associates Publishers.

Ekers, D., Webster, L., Straten, A. V., Cuijpers, P., Richards, D., & Gilbody, S. (2014). Behavioural activation for depression; an update of meta-analysis of effectiveness and sub group analysis. *PLOS ONE, 9*(6), e100100. https://doi.org/10.1371/journal.pone.0100100

Ekkekakis, P. (2015). Honey, I shrunk the pooled SMD! Guide to critical appraisal of systematic reviews and meta-analyses using the Cochrane review on exercise for depression as example. *Mental Health and Physical Activity, 8*, 21–36. https://doi.org/10.1016/j.mhpa.2014.12.001

Elavsky, S., Kishida, M., & Mogle, J. A. (2016). Concurrent and lagged relations between momentary affect and sedentary behavior in middle-aged women. *Menopause (New York, N.Y.), 23*(8), 919–923. https://doi.org/10.1097/GME.0000000000000645

Evmenenko, A., & Teixeira, D. S. (2020). The circumplex model of affect in physical activity contexts: A systematic review. *International Journal of Sport and Exercise Psychology, 0*(0), 1–34. https://doi.org/10.1080/1612197X.2020.1854818

Firth, J., Siddiqi, N., Koyanagi, A., Siskind, D., Rosenbaum, S., Galletly, C., Allan, S., Caneo, C., Carney, R., Carvalho, A. F.,

Chatterton, M. L., Correll, C. U., Curtis, J., Gaughran, F., Heald, A., Hoare, E., Jackson, S. E., Kisely, S., Lovell, K., … Stubbs, B. (2019). The Lancet Psychiatry Commission: A blueprint for protecting physical health in people with mental illness. *The Lancet Psychiatry, 6*(8), 675–712. https://doi.org/10.1016/S2215-0366(19)30132-4

Fournier, J. C., DeRubeis, R. J., Hollon, S. D., Dimidjian, S., Amsterdam, J. D., Shelton, R. C., & Fawcett, J. (2010). Antidepressant drug effects and depression severity: A patient-level meta-analysis. *JAMA, 303*(1), 47–53. https://doi.org/10.1001/jama.2009.1943

Franz, S. I., & Hamilton, G. V. (1905). The effects of exercise upon the retardation in conditions of depression. *American Journal of Psychiatry, 62*(2), 239–256. https://doi.org/10.1176/ajp.62.2.239

Gianfredi, V., Blandi, L., Cacitti, S., Minelli, M., Signorelli, C., Amerio, A., & Odone, A. (2020). Depression and objectively measured physical activity: A systematic review and meta-analysis. *International Journal of Environmental Research and Public Health, 17*(10), 3738. https://doi.org/10.3390/ijerph17103738

Giurgiu, M., Koch, E. D., Ottenbacher, J., Plotnikoff, R. C., Ebner-Priemer, U. W., & Reichert, M. (2019). Sedentary behavior in everyday life relates negatively to mood: An ambulatory assessment study. *Scandinavian Journal of Medicine & Science in Sports, 29*(9), 1340–1351. https://doi.org/10.1111/sms.13448

Giurgiu, M., Koch, E. D., Plotnikoff, R. C., Ebner-Priemer, U. W., & Reichert, M. (2020). Breaking up sedentary behavior optimally to enhance mood. *Medicine and Science in Sports and Exercise, 52*(2), 457–465.

Giurgiu, M., Plotnikoff, R. C., Nigg, C. R., Koch, E. D., Ebner-Priemer, U. W., & Reichert, M. (2020). Momentary mood predicts upcoming real-life sedentary behavior. *Scandinavian Journal of Medicine & Science in Sports, 30*(7), 1276–1286. https://doi.org/10.1111/sms.13652

Grigoriadis, S., & Robinson, G. E. (2007). Gender issues in depression. *Annals of Clinical Psychiatry, 19*(4), 247–255. https://doi.org/10.1080/10401230701653294

Groves, J. O. (2007). Is it time to reassess the BDNF hypothesis of depression? *Molecular Psychiatry, 12*(12), 1079–1088. https://doi.org/10.1038/sj.mp.4002075

Hallgren, M., Nguyen, T. -T. -D., Owen, N., Vancampfort, D., Dunstan, D. W., Wallin, P., Andersson, G., & Ekblom-Bak, E. (2020). Associations of sedentary behavior in leisure and occupational contexts with symptoms of depression and anxiety. *Preventive Medicine, 133*, 106021. https://doi.org/10.1016/j.ypmed.2020.106021

Harvey, S. B., Hotopf, M., Øverland, S., & Mykletun, A. (2010). Physical activity and common mental disorders. *The British Journal of Psychiatry, 197*(5), 357–364.

Hemmis, L., de Vries, H., Vandelanotte, C., Short, C. E., Duncan, M. J., Burton, N. W., & Rebar, A. L. (2015). Depressive symptoms associated with psychological correlates of physical activity and perceived helpfulness of intervention features. *Mental Health and Physical Activity, 9*, 16–23. https://doi.org/10.1016/j.mhpa.2015.08.001

Herring, M. P., Puetz, T. W., O'Connor, P. J., & Dishman, R. K. (2012). Effect of exercise training on depressive symptoms among patients with a chronic illness: A systematic review and meta-analysis of randomized controlled trials. *Archives of Internal Medicine, 172*(2), 101–111. https://doi.org/10.1001/archinternmed.2011.696

Jacka, F. N., Pasco, J. A., Williams, L. J., Leslie, E. R., Dodd, S., Nicholson, G. C., Kotowicz, M. A., & Berk, M. (2011). Lower levels of physical activity in childhood associated with adult depression. *Journal of Science and Medicine in Sport, 14*(3), 222–226.

Janssen, I., & LeBlanc, A. G. (2010). Systematic review of the health benefits of physical activity and fitness in school-aged children and youth. *International Journal of Behavioral Nutrition and Physical Activity, 7*(1), 40. https://doi.org/10.1186/1479-5868-7-40

Kanning, M., & Schlicht, W. (2010). Be active and become happy: An ecological momentary assessment of physical activity and mood. *Journal of Sport and Exercise Psychology, 32*(2), 253–261. https://doi.org/10.1123/jsep.32.2.253

Korniloff, K., Vanhala, M., Kautiainen, H., Koponen, H., Peltonen, M., Mäntyselkä, P., Oksa, H., Kampman, O., & Häkkinen, A. (2012). Lifetime leisure-time physical activity and the risk of depressive symptoms at the ages of 65–74 years: The FIN-D2D survey. *Preventive Medicine, 54*(5), 313–315. https://doi.org/10.1016/j.ypmed.2012.02.008

Kuyken, W., Warren, F. C., Taylor, R. S., Whalley, B., Crane, C., Bondolfi, G., Hayes, R., Huijbers, M., Ma, H., Schweizer, S., Segal, Z., Speckens, A., Teasdale, J. D., Van Heeringen, K., Williams, M., Byford, S., Byng, R., & Dalgleish, T. (2016). Efficacy of mindfulness-based cognitive therapy in prevention of depressive relapse: An individual patient data meta-analysis from randomized trials. *JAMA Psychiatry, 73*(6), 565–574. https://doi.org/10.1001/jamapsychiatry.2016.0076

Lépine, J. P., & Briley, M. (2011). The increasing burden of depression. *Neuropsychiatric Disease and Treatment, 7*(Suppl 1), 3–7. https://doi.org/10.2147/NDT.S19617

Liu, M., Wu, L., & Yao, S. (2016). Dose–response association of screen time-based sedentary behaviour in children and adolescents and depression: A meta-analysis of observational studies. *British Journal of Sports Medicine, 50*(20), 1252–1258. https://doi.org/10.1136/bjsports-2015-095084

Nahum-Shani, I., Hekler, E. B., & Spruijt-Metz, D. (2015). Building health behavior models to guide the development of just-in-time adaptive interventions: A pragmatic framework. *Health Psychology, 34*(S), 1209.

Nahum-Shani, I., Smith, S. N., Spring, B. J., Collins, L. M., Witkiewitz, K., Tewari, A., & Murphy, S. A. (2018). Just-in-time adaptive interventions (JITAIs) in mobile health: Key components and design principles for ongoing health behavior support. *Annals of Behavioral Medicine, 52*(6), 446–462.

Nakamura, A., van der Waerden, J., Melchior, M., Bolze, C., El-Khoury, F., & Pryor, L. (2019). Physical activity during pregnancy and postpartum depression: Systematic review and meta-analysis. *Journal of Affective Disorders, 246*, 29–41. https://doi.org/10.1016/j.jad.2018.12.009

Pemberton, R., & Fuller Tyszkiewicz, M. D. (2016). Factors contributing to depressive mood states in everyday life: A systematic review. *Journal of Affective Disorders, 200*, 103–110. https://doi.org/10.1016/j.jad.2016.04.023

Pickett, K., Kendrick, T., & Yardley, L. (2017). "A forward movement into life": A qualitative study of how, why and when physical activity may benefit depression. *Mental Health and Physical Activity, 12*, 100–109. https://doi.org/10.1016/j.mhpa.2017.03.004

Ram, N., Brinberg, M., Pincus, A. L., & Conroy, D. E. (2017). The questionable ecological validity of ecological momentary assessment: Considerations for design and analysis. *Research in Human Development, 14*(3), 253–270. https://doi.org/10.1080/15427609.2017.1340052

Rebar, A. L., Stanton, R., Geard, D., Short, C., Duncan, M. J., & Vandelanotte, C. (2015). A meta-meta-analysis of the effect of physical activity on depression and anxiety in non-clinical adult populations. *Health Psychology Review, 9*(3), 366–378.

Rebar, A. L., & Taylor, A. (2017). Physical activity and mental health; it is more than just a prescription. *Mental Health and Physical Activity, 13*, 77–82. https://doi.org/10.1016/j.mhpa.2017.10.004

Reed, J., & Buck, S. (2009). The effect of regular aerobic exercise on positive-activated affect: A meta-analysis. *Psychology of Sport and Exercise, 10*(6), 581–594.

Reed, J., & Ones, D. S. (2006). The effect of acute aerobic exercise on positive activated affect: A meta-analysis. *Psychology of Sport and Exercise, 7*(5), 477–514. https://doi.org/10.1016/j.psychsport.2005.11.003

Rodriguez-Ayllon, M., Cadenas-Sánchez, C., Estévez-López, F., Muñoz, N. E., Mora-Gonzalez, J., Migueles, J. H., Molina-García, P., Henriksson, H., Mena-Molina, A., Martínez-Vizcaíno, V., Catena, A., Löf, M., Erickson, K. I., Lubans, D. R., Ortega, F. B., & Esteban-Cornejo, I. (2019). Role of physical activity and sedentary behavior in the mental health of preschoolers, children and adolescents: A systematic review and meta-analysis. *Sports Medicine, 49*(9), 1383–1410. https://doi.org/10.1007/s40279-019-01099-5

Schuch, F. B., Vancampfort, D., Richards, J., Rosenbaum, S., Ward, P. B., & Stubbs, B. (2016). Exercise as a treatment for depression: A meta-analysis adjusting for publication bias. *Journal of Psychiatric Research, 77*, 42–51.

Schuch, F., Vancampfort, D., Firth, J., Rosenbaum, S., Ward, P., Reichert, T., Bagatini, N. C., Bgeginski, R., & Stubbs, B. (2017). Physical activity and sedentary behavior in people with major depressive disorder: A systematic review and meta-analysis. *Journal of Affective Disorders, 210*, 139–150. https://doi.org/10.1016/j.jad.2016.10.050

Shiffman, S., Stone, A. A., & Hufford, M. R. (2008). Ecological momentary assessment. *Annual Review of Clinical Psychology, 4*, 1–32.

Stanton, R., Happell, B., & Reaburn, P. (2014). The mental health benefits of regular physical activity, and its role in preventing future depressive illness. *Nursing: Research and Reviews, 4*, 45–53. https://doi.org/10.2147/NRR.S41956

Stanton, R., Rosenbaum, S., Kalucy, M., Reaburn, P., & Happell, B. (2015). A call to action: Exercise as treatment for patients with mental illness. *Australian Journal of Primary Health, 21*(2), 120–125. https://doi.org/10.1071/PY14054

Stanton, R., Rosenbaum, S., Rebar, A., & Happell, B. (2019). Prevalence of chronic health conditions in Australian adults with depression and/or anxiety. *Issues in Mental Health Nursing, 40*(10), 902–907. https://doi.org/10.1080/01612840.2019.1613701

Stone, A. A., & Shiffman, S. (1994). Ecological momentary assessment (EMA) in behavorial medicine. *Annals of Behavioral Medicine, 16*(3), 199–202. https://doi.org/10.1093/abm/16.3.199

Suetani, S., Stubbs, B., McGrath, J. J., & Scott, J. G. (2019). Physical activity of people with mental disorders compared to the general population: A systematic review of longitudinal cohort studies. *Social Psychiatry and Psychiatric Epidemiology*, 1–15.

Sullivan, P. F., Neale, M. C., & Kendler, K. S. (2000). Genetic epidemiology of major depression: review and meta-analysis. *American Journal of Psychiatry, 157*(10), 1552–1562. https://doi.org/10.1176/appi.ajp.157.10.1552

Tao, S., Wu, X., Yang, Y., & Tao, F. (2020). The moderating effect of physical activity in the relation between problematic mobile phone use and depression among university students. *Journal of Affective Disorders, 273*, 167–172. https://doi.org/10.1016/j.jad.2020.04.012

Teychenne, M., Ball, K., & Salmon, J. (2010). Sedentary behavior and depression among adults: A review. *International Journal of Behavioral Medicine, 17*(4), 246–254. https://doi.org/10.1007/s12529-010-9075-z

The WHO World Mental Health Survey Consortium. (2004). Prevalence, severity, and unmet need for treatment of mental disorders in the World Health Organization World Mental Health Surveys. *JAMA, 291*(21), 2581–2590. https://doi.org/10.1001/jama.291.21.2581

Tuarob, S., Tucker, C. S., Kumara, S., Giles, C. L., Pincus, A. L., Conroy, D. E., & Ram, N. (2017). How are you feeling? A personalized methodology for predicting mental states from temporally observable physical and behavioral information. *Journal of Biomedical Informatics, 68*, 1–19. https://doi.org/10.1016/j.jbi.2017.02.010

Vancampfort, D., Firth, J., Schuch, F. B., Rosenbaum, S., Mugisha, J., Hallgren, M., Probst, M., Ward, P. B., Gaughran, F., Hert, M. D., Carvalho, A. F., & Stubbs, B. (2017). Sedentary behavior and physical activity levels in people with schizophrenia, bipolar disorder and major depressive disorder: A global systematic review and meta-analysis. *World Psychiatry, 16*(3), 308–315. https://doi.org/10.1002/wps.20458

Vancampfort, D., Moens, H., Madou, T., De Backer, T., Vallons, V., Bruyninx, P., Vanheuverzwijn, S., Mota, C. T., Soundy, A., & Probst, M. (2016). Autonomous motivation is associated with the maintenance stage of behaviour change in people with affective disorders. *Psychiatry Research, 240*, 267–271. https://doi.org/10.1016/j.psychres.2016.04.005

Vancampfort, D., Stubbs, B., Venigalla, S. K., & Probst, M. (2015). Adopting and maintaining physical activity behaviours in people with severe mental illness: The importance of autonomous motivation. *Preventive Medicine, 81*, 216–220. https://doi.org/10.1016/j.ypmed.2015.09.006

World Health Organization. (2017). *Depression and other common mental disorders: Global health estimates*. World Health Organization. https://apps.who.int/iris/bitstream/handle/10665/254610/WHO-MSD-MER-2017.2-eng.pdf

Zhai, L., Zhang, Y., & Zhang, D. (2015). Sedentary behaviour and the risk of depression: A meta-analysis. *British Journal of Sports Medicine, 49*(11), 705–709. https://doi.org/10.1136/bjsports-2014-093613

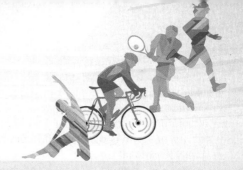

CHAPTER 11

Anxiety and Stress

LEARNING OBJECTIVES

After completing this chapter you will be able to:

- Differentiate between stress, anxiety, and stressors.
- Understand the differences between anxiety symptoms and clinical anxiety disorders.
- Describe the state of evidence on physical activity and sedentary behavior and stress, both in laboratory settings and in real life.
- Understand whether physical activity and sedentary behavior play roles in the prevention and treatment of anxiety disorders.

Introduction

Everyone can feel anxious and experiences stress. Some people feel stressed or anxious occasionally, while others feel anxious seemingly all of the time, and others have diagnosable clinical anxiety disorders. Stress is a normal part of everyday life's challenges, but how we manage and react to stressful situations differs among people and can change over time. In this chapter, we will examine anxiety, stress, and clinical anxiety disorders and consider evidence of how physical activity and sedentary behavior may impact them. Conversely, we will also consider how stress and anxiety may impact our physical activity and sedentary behavior. We will consider research into laboratory and real-life **stressors** as well as research using physical activity as a prevention and treatment for clinical anxiety disorders.

Stress and Anxiety

What is the Difference Between Stress and Anxiety?

Just think about how many times you have said *I am stressed* or *I feel anxious*. Stress or anxiety can result from daily annoyances (like forgetting your phone or wallet at your house); the consequences of overstretched, time-pressured lifestyles; and to events such as illness, loss, and natural disasters. Although most people can recognize when they are feeling stressed or anxious, it can be difficult to describe what distinguishes one from the other. Both stress and anxiety are responses to when we feel challenged or threatened but **stress** is the response to threats or challenges, whereas **anxiety** is the anticipation of a future threat (American Psychiatric Association, 2013).

Anxiety tends to arise when we are uncertain about how something will play out and is just one type of stress response. So, we may be stressed by an upcoming exam, which may include feelings of anxiety or feelings of focus and commitment (and maybe even all three).

Stress is a normal response to events that make you feel either threatened or upset your balance in some way. Importantly, stress won't arise unless you feel like you aren't capable of coping with actual or imagined challenges (Selye, 1950). These challenges can be demands that are physical, such as running a marathon; mental, such as memorizing text; or emotional, such as a relationship problem. When you sense danger—whether it is real or imagined—your body's defenses kick into high gear in a rapid, automatic process known as the **fight-or-flight response** or the stress response. When you perceive a threat, your sympathetic nervous system responds to the challenge by releasing a flood of stress hormones, including adrenaline and cortisol. These hormones rouse the body for emergency action and are characterized by increased heart rate, increased blood flow to the brain and muscles, raised sugar levels, sweaty palms and soles, dilated pupils, and erect hairs. In other words, when you are under stress, your heart pounds faster, your muscles tighten, your blood pressure rises, your breath quickens, and your senses become sharper. These physical changes increase your strength and stamina, speed your reaction time, and enhance your focus—preparing you to either fight or flee from the stressor at hand.

Selye (1950) describes our responses to stress as general adaptation of our body and mind trying to recover to its "natural" state of calmness or balance, referred to as **homeostasis**. He argues that when we are exposed to a stressor, it causes an imbalance out of homeostasis, and our body and mind respond to stress with physiologic and psychological reactions with the aim of returning back to a homeostatic state. There are three stages of Selye's (1950) general adaptation responses to stress:

1. **Alarm:** Occurs immediately upon perception of stress, and the body's fight-or-flight response is activated; very draining physically and mentally

2. **Resistance:** Occurs with continued perceived stress, and the body stays in an activated state; mental and physical resources will be depleted if this state is long

3. **Exhaustion:** Mental and physical depletion occurs as a result of prolonged exposure to stress; can lead to suppressed immune system and poor functioning and increased likelihoods of depression, heart disease, digestive problems, and diabetes

The stress response is the body's way of protecting you. When working properly, it helps you stay focused, energetic, and alert. In emergency situations, stress can save your life—giving you extra strength to defend yourself or spurring you to slam on the brakes to avoid an accident. The stress response also helps you rise to meet challenges. Stress is what keeps you on your toes during a presentation at work, sharpens your concentration when you are attempting a free throw, or drives you to complete an assignment or exam when you would rather be watching television or socializing. But stress can also elicit negative feelings or unhelpful responses like anxiety.

Anxiety is a negative psychological and physiologic state characterized by feelings of nervousness, worry, fatigue, concentration problems, apprehension, and arousal. The physical effects of anxiety may include heart palpitations, sweating, trembling, muscle weakness and tension, fatigue, nausea, chest pain, shortness of breath, stomach aches, or headaches. Anxiety stress responses are typically short-lived and are referred to as **state anxiety** (Endler & Kocovski, 2001; Speilberger, 1983). State anxiety is what we experience, for example, when we are doing a presentation, writing an exam, and watching a closely matched sporting event. After the "threat" has subsided, the anxiety state lessens until we feel "normal" again.

All people feel high levels of state anxiety at some point in their lives. However, some people regularly experience high states of anxiety to the point that it could be considered a part of their personality; this is referred to as having high **trait anxiety** (Endler & Kocovski, 2001; Speilberger, 1983). Trait anxiety varies according to how people have conditioned themselves to respond to and manage their stress. People with high trait anxiety often feel anxious in many different types of situations; whereas someone with low trait anxiety may be able to keep their calm regardless of what's going on around them. A person's trait anxiety can be important to be aware of because having high trait anxiety may make you more susceptible to other consequences. For example, evidence suggests that athletes with high trait anxiety may be at increased risk for musculoskeletal injuries (Cagle et al., 2017).

CRITICAL THINKING ACTIVITY 11-1

What is the difference between anxiety and stress? Provide examples of each from your everyday life.

The *State-Trait Anxiety Inventory* (Speilberger et al., 1983) is a self-report psychological questionnaire that is commonly used to assess state and trait anxiety. The State-Trait Anxiety Inventory has 20 items for assessing trait anxiety (*how you generally feel*) and 20 items for assessing state anxiety (*how you feel right now, that is, at this moment*). See **Table 11-1** for sample items for the State-Trait Anxiety Inventory. Each item is answered on a Likert-type, and higher scores indicate greater anxiety. If you have high trait anxiety, you have a predisposition to regularly experience high levels of state anxiety, but you will not feel anxious unless there is the perception of a threat or challenge with an unsure outcome—a stressor.

Stressors refer to outside forces that we must deal with. It is both the stressors in our lives and our responses to these stressors that determine the severity of stress and persistence of anxiety in our lives. We can experience both active and

Table 11-1 Sample Items from the State-Trait Anxiety Inventory

State Anxiety Items	**Directions:** Select the appropriate number to indicate how you feel *right now*, that is, *at this moment*.			
	Not at all	Somewhat	Moderately So	Very Much So
I am tense	1	2	3	4
I am worried	1	2	3	4
I feel anxious	1	2	3	4
I feel jittery	1	2	3	4
Trait Anxiety Items	**Directions:** Select the appropriate number to indicate how you *generally* feel.			
	Not at all	Somewhat	Moderately So	Very Much So
I worry too much over something that really doesn't matter	1	2	3	4
I feel nervous and restless	1	2	3	4
I lack confidence	1	2	3	4
Some unimportant thoughts run through my mind and bother me	1	2	3	4

Data from Speilberger, C. D., Gorsuch, R., Lushene, R., Vagg, P. R., & Jacobs, G. A. (1983). *Manual for the state trait anxiety inventory (Form Y) Consulting Psychologists Press:* Palo Alto, CA.

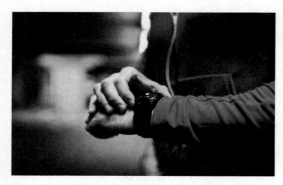

© Bbernard/Shutterstock.

The Stroop Task

PINK	YELLOW	BROWN
BLACK	GRAY	GREEN
BROWN	ORANGE	RED
ORANGE	GREEN	BLUE
YELLOW	RED	PURPLE
PURPLE	PINK	ORANGE
BLUE	BROWN	GRAY

Figure 11-1 Stroop color word task.

CRITICAL THINKING ACTIVITY 11-2

Complete the Stroop Color Word text. There are several that you can find on the Internet. How long did it take you to complete the task? Did you find this task stressful? What type of stressor is this?

passive stressors that can be further divided into laboratory and real-life stressors. See **Table 11-2** for examples of these types of stressors. Active stressors are tasks or situations in which the person's response leads to a particular outcome. In other words, the response is under the individual's control. An example of a common laboratory active stressor is the Stroop color word task in which colored words are presented with a conflict (see **Figure 11-1**). That is, the name of the color (e.g., blue, red, green) is printed in a color not denoted by the name (e.g., the word "red" printed in blue ink instead of red ink). In this reaction time stress test, the person is supposed to ignore the word and state the color of the letters of the word. In contrast, passive stressors are tasks or situations in which the individual's response has no bearing on the outcome. For example, they have no control over a situation involving pain or noise.

Stress, Physical Activity and Sedentary Behavior

Stress is a subjective experience. Much of the stress we experience is based on our own perception of a situation; therefore, sources of stress can vary greatly from one person to another. The following two factors largely determine how we respond to stressful situations: (a) the way we perceive the situation, and (b) our general state of physical health. Evidence suggests that physical activity can impact stress by regulating both how we react to stressful situations (i.e., our reactivity to stress) and our physical capacity for coping with stressors.

Crews and Landers (1987) suggested that two general processes through which physical activity could serve to reduce stress are coping and inoculation. Insofar as coping is concerned, physical activity could provide a more efficient system by reducing recovery time in the autonomic nervous system. Similarly, inoculation might occur if chronic physical activity enhances the individual's physical and psychological abilities to deal with stress. So, for example, when an individual is faced with a stressor, the autonomic

Table 11-2 Types of Stressors

Stressor	Laboratory	Real-life
Passive	Films that elicit emotional reactions Exposure to unpleasant sounds	Dental procedure In-flight emergency
Active	Stroop color word task Reaction time Mental arithmetic	Public speaking Exam Parachuting Defending dissertation

nervous system responds with its "flight or fight response." For those individuals who are physically active, the stress response might be of less magnitude (i.e., at a lower level) and/or less time might be spent in a state of stress because of a faster recovery from the stress response.

Laboratory Stress Research

Considerable laboratory research has been undertaken to examine the association between physical activity and reactivity to stressors. Typically, participants are exposed to a stressor such as electric shock, a loud noise, or cognitive tasks to be performed under time pressure. The question of interest is whether involvement in physical activity or increased fitness helps protect the individual from the effects of a stressor (i.e., by reducing their reactivity) and/or help the person recover more quickly than inactive or less fit persons (Landers & Petruzzello, 1994).

One commonly used lab-based stress test is the Trier Social Stress Test (Kirschbaum et al., 1993; Kudielka et al., 2007). The test consists of a brief preparation period, during which a panel of judges asks you (the participant) to prepare a presentation, usually set up as a job interview scenario. You are allowed a pen and paper during this time. Then, unexpectedly, the pen and paper are taken from you and the judges quietly observe your effort at a 5-minute presentation in front of the panel of judges, in a room with an imposing microphone and visible video recording device. If your presentation is shorter than 5 minutes, the judges will urge you to keep going until the 5 minutes are up. Following the presentation, right when you are ready to feel at ease, you are asked to conduct a mental arithmetic challenge such as counting backwards from 2,023 by sets of 17 for another 5 minutes. When you make a mistake, you'll hear, "Stop—mistake—start over at 2,023, please." You can just imagine how this task could evoke a stress response, especially if you're hooked up to various monitors to assess your cortisol, blood pressure, and/or heart rate!

Using the Trier Social Stress Test, Rimmele and colleagues (2007, 2009) exposed groups of male elite athletes and groups of healthy, untrained men to the lab-based stressor and measured their physiologic (e.g., cortisol, heart rate) and psychological (e.g., mood, anxiety) responses. They found that responses to the stress test were experienced to a lesser extent by the elite athletes compared with the untrained men. These findings indicate that sport, fitness, or high levels of physical activity, might buffer people from some of the potential negative psychological and physiological responses to stressors. Although notably, in a review of the impact of physical activity and fitness on stress reactivity to the Trier Social Stress, Mücke and colleagues (2018) found that higher physical activity or fitness was associated with buffered physiologic or psychological stress responses in only half of the studies they reviewed. These mixed findings may be an indication that the effects of physical activity levels or fitness on stress are not reliable. Before ruling on the state of the evidence either way though, we need to consider evidence from studies that manipulate physical activity and measures within-person change in responses, instead of comparing groups of active vs. less-active people.

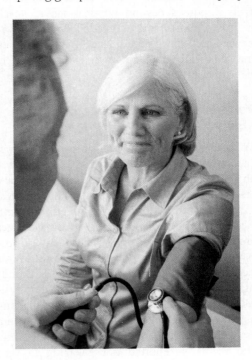

© Brand X Pictures/Thinkstock.

Hamer and his colleagues (2006) conducted a review of randomized controlled trials that examined the effects of acute aerobic exercise on blood pressure responses to psychosocial laboratory tasks. The stressor tasks used in the studies reviewed included the Stroop color task, mental arithmetic, public speech, and cold pressor. Of the 15 studies reviewed, 10 had significant reductions in postexercise stress-related blood pressure responses compared with the control. The mean effect sizes for systolic and diastolic blood pressure of 0.38 and 0.40, respectively. Of importance, Hamer et al., (2006) found that exercise dose moderated the size of the effect, with greater exercise doses showing larger effects. In other words, more physical activity resulted in better responses to the stressor. The researchers concluded that an acute episode of aerobic exercise has a beneficial impact on the blood pressure response to a psychosocial stressor.

Quite notably, there is an absence of evidence testing whether sedentary behavior impacts laboratory-based stress responses. Before we can say whether sedentary behavior has effects on stress responses beyond physical activity levels or fitness, more work is needed. Who knows? Maybe someday you'll lead this important line of research and be in the next edition of the textbook!

Real-life Stress, Anxiety, and Physical Activity Research

To investigate whether the impact of physical activity on stress responses seen in the lab generalize to real-life, researchers have observed people's stress, anxiety, and physical activity over time. In a study by Puterman and colleagues (2017), more than 2,000 United States adults reported their daily physical activity, how they felt, and their responses to stressful events each night for 8 consecutive nights. The findings revealed that those who were more physically active tended to have less negative feeling responses to daily stress than those who were less active. There were some people in the study who regularly reported not engaging in very

Research with Undergraduate Students Highlight Tracking Stress Reactions

Flueckiger et al. (2016) found that when students were more physically active than was typical for them, stress had less of an impact on how pleasant or unpleasant they felt. To rule out that these effects are present as a result of alternative variables about people who tend to be more active than others (e.g., personality, self-control, fitness), Von Haaren and colleagues (2015) conducted an intervention and randomly allocated people to either have immediate access to a 20-week aerobic exercise training program or to wait until the study was done to have access to the program (i.e., a waitlist control). Their findings showed that the physical activity training program reduced University students' emotional stress responses to the real-life stressful situation of an academic examination.

much physical activity and an interesting finding emerged for those people—the buffering effect of physical activity on negative feeling responses to daily stressors was stronger if the stressful event happened soon after they were engaged in the physical activity. This study points to both acute and long-term benefits of physical activity as a buffer from negative reactions to real-life stressors. Feeding into this line of evidence are two studies that tracked how university students reacted to stress across an academic year shown in the box above.

Several meta-analyses have statistically summarized the research on physical activity and stress or anxiety (Conn, 2010; Kugler et al., 1994; Landers & Petruzzello, 1994; Long & Stavel, 1995; Petruzzello et al., 1991; Sarris et al., 2012; Wipfli et al., 2008). The number and types of studies included in those meta-analyses have varied widely. In fact, so many meta-analyses have been conducted that there are now meta-analyses of these meta-analyses. Rebar et al., (2015) conducted a meta-meta-analysis of 306 study effects with 10,755 participants for the effect of physical activity on anxiety. They found that physical activity reduced anxiety symptoms by a small effect of –0.38.

Researchers have also found that physical activity and exercise interventions are effective in reducing anxiety or stress in several special populations such as cancer patients undergoing treatment, cancer survivors (Lim et al., 2012), patients with systemic lupus erythematosus (Zhang et al., 2012), children, and young people (Carter et al., 2021).

Up to this point, we've focused on how physical activity and sedentary behavior impact stress responses, but it is also worth considering the reciprocal relationship—how stress can impact movement behavior. Researchers from Finland examined which stressful life-events are related to physical activity (Engberg et al., 2012). They conducted a systematic review of the literature examining the effects of life-events on changes in physical activity behavior. More specifically, they examined how the following positive and negative major life-change events affect physical activity: transition to university; change in employment status; marital transitions and changes in relationships; pregnancy/having a child; experiencing harassment at work, violence or disaster; and moving into an institution. The researchers found that for men and women, transition to university, having a child, remarriage, and mass urban disaster results in decreased physical activity levels. In comparison, retirement resulted in increased physical activity levels.

They also found that in young women, beginning work, changing work conditions, changing from being single to cohabiting, getting married, pregnancy, divorce/separation, and reduced income resulted in decreased physical activity behavior. In contrast, starting a new personal relationship, returning to study, and harassment at work increased physical activity behavior for young women.

In middle-aged women, changing work conditions, reduced income, personal achievement and death of a spouse/partner increased physical activity, while experiencing violence and a family member being arrested or jailed decreased physical activity. In older women, moving into

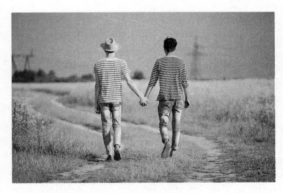

© Olesia Bilkei/Shutterstock.

an institution and interpersonal loss decreased exercise, while longer-term widowhood increased exercise. In addition, experiencing multiple simultaneous life events decreased physical activity in men and women. The researchers concluded that people experiencing life events could be an important target group for physical activity promotion (Engberg et al., 2012).

CRITICAL THINKING ACTIVITY 11-3

How does stress and anxiety affect your physical activity behavior? How does your physical activity behavior impact your stress and anxiety?

Real-life Stress, Anxiety, and Sedentary Behavior Research

Compared with that of physical activity and fitness, far less has been investigated on the role of sedentary behavior in real-life stress responses. However, the evidence tends to suggest more sedentary behavior may lead to elevated mood and physiologic stress responses. For example, Endrighi, Steptoe, and Hamer (2016) found that when people increased their sedentary behavior (M increase of 32 min/day), their negative mood elevated and stress induced inflammatory responses. A study tracking university students over 6 months showed that daily academic and general stress were associated positively with daily sedentary behavior and negatively with daily physical activity, findings that were partially explained through physiologic stress responses measured via hair cortisol concentration (Lines et al., 2021).

The evidence base of the links between daily-life sedentary behavior and stress or anxiety are a bit more advanced. Teychenne and colleagues (2019) conducted a systematic review of the association between sedentary behavior and stress. Of the 26 studies, reporting on 72,795 people, only 37% reported more sedentary behavior was associated with higher stress; 10% reported the inverse association—that more sedentary behavior was associated with lower anxiety, and 53% reported no significant association between sedentary behavior and stress. It was concluded that there was insufficient evidence that overall time spent in sedentary behavior was associated with stress. This means that there is no strong evidence either way as to whether sedentary behavior is linked to stress or not. However, when considering only studies that used monitors to assess sedentary behavior instead of self-report, it was found that there was strong evidence of no significant association between sedentary behavior and anxiety. Interestingly, there was also strong evidence of no association between TV viewing or computer use and stress. So—good news—maybe all the time you're spending vegging on the couch isn't to blame for your stress!

However, when reflecting on how much you sit during the day, it's worth considering findings from Diaz and colleagues (2018). They monitored sedentary behavior of New York City metro residents over an entire year and asked people daily how stressful their day was. They found that people who were more stressed were not more or less sedentary than those who were less stressed; however, when they focused on the cause of the stress, things got interesting. They found that stress from arguments was associated with more time spent being sedentary; whereas (not surprisingly) stress from running late or work-related stress was associated with less time spent sedentary. Overall, the evidence

of sedentary behavior and stress suggests that these effects differ, depending on where the stress came from, who the person is who is managing the stress, and what type of activity the person is engaging in while sedentary. Whereas most of this evidence is correlational, there is also some experimental work showing that a 1-week sedentary behavior-inducing intervention leads to increases in anxiety among young adults (Edwards & Loprinzi, 2016).

Most studies in this area have focused on high-income countries, but some evidence suggests similar patterns from lower income countries around the world. In a study of more than 40,000 people in low- and middle-income countries, it was found that people who reported problems with anxiety regularly in the past 30 days were two times as likely to be sedentary for more than 8 hours/day than those who reported having fewer problems with anxiety (Vancampfort et al., 2018). Overall, the evidence suggests that more physical activity leads to less anxiety and stress, whereas sedentary behavior leads to more anxiety and stress. Importantly, these studies are in general population samples or what we call **nonclinical populations**, consisting of people who have not been diagnosed with a clinical anxiety disorder. There is an entire other body of evidence considering the role of physical activity and sedentary behavior among people with clinical anxiety disorders.

Clinical Anxiety Disorders

Anxiety disorders are diagnosable health conditions, distinct from the feelings of anxiety or stress that everyone experiences in that they involve excessive fear or anxiety. People experience anxiety disorders as a range of psychological and physiologic symptoms varied from mild to severe in intensity. Generally, anxiety disorders manifest as excessive rumination, worrying, uneasiness, and fear about future uncertainties that are either based on real or imagined events. For a person to be diagnosed with an anxiety disorder, fear or anxiety must be out of proportion to the situation or age inappropriate and hinder day-to-day living for at least 6 months (American Psychiatric Association, 2013).

Anxiety disorders are becoming more common around the globe at any age, with the global prevalence of anxiety disorders at 3.6%—that's more than 260 million people! (World Health Organization, 2017). Anxiety disorders include generalized anxiety disorder, specific phobias, panic disorder, social anxiety disorder, separation anxiety disorder, and agorophobia. See **Table 11-3** for a description of these clinical anxiety disorders.

Some segments of the population are particularly vulnerable to anxiety disorders, including transgender people (Millet et al., 2017), pregnant women (Fawcett et al., 2019), those with physical health conditions such as irritable bowel syndrome (Zamani et al., 2019), or other mental illnesses, including depression (Rebar et al., 2017). In fact, it is more common to have additional physical or mental health comorbidities with an anxiety disorder than not (Firth et al., 2019; World Health Organization, 2003). In the United States, the prevalence of anxiety disorders in women is twice as common as in men. It is important to note that anxiety disorders are diagnosable (i.e., able to be diagnosed) but estimates are that most anxiety disorders go undiagnosed and unreported (Bandelow et al., 2017; Kroenke et al., 2007). It may be that gender differences in willingness to report anxiety disorders and stigmas around mental illness may explain why there is such disparity in the prevalence rates of anxiety disorders in men and women in the United States.

Treatment and Prevention of Anxiety Disorders

Anxiety disorders are mostly treated on an outpatient basis without requiring hospitalization, except in extreme circumstances. Treatment recommendations include psychoeducation (information about their diagnosis), psychotherapy (e.g., cognitive behavioral therapy), pharmacotherapy (e.g., selective serotonin reuptake inhibiting or selective serotonin norepinephrine reuptake inhibiting drugs), and changes in lifestyle behaviors such as meditation and exercise (Bandelow et al., 2017). Importantly, the best treatment depends largely on the preferences, needs, and comorbidities of the specific person. Evidence suggests that physical activity may be a good approach for management and treatment of anxiety disorders, with the added benefit that it will help regulate the physical and mental health

Table 11-3 Description of Clinical Anxiety Disorders

Anxiety Disorder	Description
Generalized anxiety disorder	Long-lasting anxiety that is not focused on any one object or situation. Nonspecific persistent fear and worry and becoming overly concerned with everyday matters
Specific phobias	Fear and anxiety are triggered by a specific stimulus or situation
Panic disorder	Brief attacks of intense terror and apprehension, often marked by trembling, shaking, confusion, dizziness, nausea, and difficulty breathing
Social anxiety disorder	Intense fear and avoidance of negative public scrutiny, public embarrassment, humiliation, or social interaction
Separation anxiety disorder	Excessive anxiety regarding separation from home or from people to whom the person has a strong emotional attachment such as a parent, guardian, grandparents, or siblings
Agoraphobia	Anxiety in situations where the person perceives certain environments as dangerous or uncomfortable (e.g., bridges, shopping malls, airports)

comorbidities that are common for people with anxiety disorders (e.g., cardiovascular disease, obesity, depression) (Firth et al., 2019; Kandola et al., 2018). Additionally, unlike some of the other anxiety disorder treatment options, physical activity can be a freely accessible, universally available option. Physical activity may be a means for helping the many people who miss out on the treatment they need for anxiety disorders because of the country in which they live, their financial insecurity, or avoidance of the stigma of seeking mental health support.

Epidemiological surveys have found that regular physical activity is associated with reduced anxiety symptoms in people with a clinical anxiety disorder (Kandola et al., 2018). For example, using cross-sectional data from the World Health Survey of 237,964 individuals across 47 countries, Stubbs et al. (2017) found that people who engaged in less physical activity were 1.32 times more likely to have an anxiety disorder than those who engaged in high amounts of physical activity. A limitation, however, with cross-sectional studies is their inability to be used to explain the direction of the physical activity and anxiety disorder relationship. That is, do people who engage in more physical activity have fewer anxiety disorders or does regular physical activity result in the reduction of anxiety disorders? Probably, the answer is that the relationship is "bi-directional"—physical activity behavior probably prevents anxiety disorder symptoms but anxiety disorder symptoms also likely impact future physical activity behavior. Anxiety disorders are associated with many symptoms that are related to low physical activity adherence (e.g., fatigue, poor motivation, and social isolation; Assis et al., 2008). Not surprisingly then, it is also found that people with anxiety disorders tend to spend more time being sedentary than those without anxiety disorders, although this research field is still in its infancy (Teychenne et al., 2015).

Exercise training or increases in physical activity are effective for enhancing treatment for anxiety disorders. A meta-analysis of the anxiolytic effects of exercise for people with anxiety disorders reviewed six randomized controlled trials investigating exercise conditions vs. control conditions such as treatment as usual or waitlist controls (Stubbs, Vancampfort, et al., 2017). The findings revealed that exercise significantly reduced anxiety symptoms to a medium-sized effect (SMD = –0.58). The authors use this evidence to recommend that exercise should be considered an evidence-based option for anxiety symptoms among people with anxiety disorders. Similar findings are present when focusing on specific anxiety disorders. For example, physical activity shows initial promise as a treatment for patients with social anxiety disorder (Jazaieri et al., 2012), generalized anxiety disorder (Herring et al., 2012), and panic disorder (Broocks et al., 1998; Hovland et al., 2013).

Potential Mechanisms

The exact mechanisms by which physical activity and sedentary behavior influence stress, anxiety, and anxiety disorder symptoms are unknown. However, there are some lines of research suggesting it is likely a blending of neurobiologic and psychosocial effects.

Neurobiological Effects

From a neurobiologic perspective, there is reason to suspect that these behaviors might impact the regulation of the stress and reward responses of the body and brain. For example, the vagus nerve is the longest nerve of the body that feeds into the brain; it coordinates the body's reactivity to and recovery from stress. Physical activity improves vagal nerve functioning and sedentary behavior leads to reduced vagal nerve functioning (Dedoncker et al., 2021). Another potential neurobiological reason for why the positive effects of exercise on stress reactivity may be related to stress hormones. Heaney et al. (2014) examined the relationship between regular physical activity, life events stress, and the cortisol and dehydroepiandrosterone (DHEA) ratios in older adults. Cortisol and DHEA are **stress hormones**. The constant release of these stress hormones, in response to continuous stressors people experience, can result in hormonal imbalances and adrenal dysfunction. The ultimate result of the release of these stress hormones over time has negative effects on people's overall health such as sleep, mood disturbances, and suppressed immune system.

Psychosocial Effects

Potential psychosocial mechanisms include improved self-regulation or self-control (Oaten & Cheng, 2005), improved sleep, aggregated positive effects of acute exercise on mood (Reed & Buck, 2009), reduced tension, and increased feelings of control (Salmon, 2001). Several explanations have been advanced, but most likely, the effects of physical activity and sedentary

behavior on stress, anxiety, and anxiety disorder symptoms are the result of complex interactions between neurobiologic and psychosocial processes. (Asmundson et al., 2013; Landers & Arent, 2007).

Summary

Feelings of stress arise when we perceive an imbalance between the demands of the situation and our ability to meet those demands. The body responds with a "flight-or-fight" response and changes in the autonomic nervous system: increased heart rate, increased blood pressure, and so on. Sometimes, these stress responses can include feelings of anxiety—the worry and anticipation of a threat. Some people are more prone than others to feeling anxiety more often and some have stress and anxiety interfere so much with daily life that it is a diagnosable anxiety disorder. The good news, however, is that increases in physical activity and reductions in sedentary behavior are likely to not only enhance our ability to deal with stress but also prevent and manage anxiety disorder symptoms.

CRITICAL THINKING ACTIVITY 11-4

Can you describe some reasons why physical activity and sedentary behavior may impact stress or anxiety? Make sure you think about some psychosocial and neurobiologic explanations.

Vignette: Wáng

Everyone keeps telling me how good my life is and how lucky I am to have this life. And sometimes I feel the same way—I am lucky. I got into a great University, I'm doing well in school, and I work really hard to be competitive for graduate programs through volunteering and part-time gig at the café. But every once in a while, I feel like giving it all up. Sometimes I wake up in the night and just feel so overwhelmed with my never-ending to do list that I just feel like I don't even know where to begin. But then I get so worried about what my dad will think if I don't get into grad school and how disappointed my professors will be if I don't live up to their expectations—so I keep going. Even though my heart races and I feel like I can't take a deep breathe, I keep going. Eventually, I'll catch up with

things enough to take a break, but it sure can't be for the next 4 years!

Last night, I had such a horrible sense of things piling up high and a lack of control that I had to get help. I called the University's student support services and I've got an appointment to meet with them next week. Just calling for help makes me feel better even though they haven't even done anything yet. Well, that's not right. They did tell me to get outside and go for a run. I haven't run in so long and it felt so good. My heart was beating fast while I was doing it and my breathe was quick, but once I was done, I had these realizations that the things I was worrying about don't seem so bad anymore. I feel like I can cope. Although it doesn't solve any of my problems necessarily, at least I know I can always go for a run just to get my stress under control.

I used to run a lot in high school, but I just couldn't find the time with University studying and work. It just wasn't a priority for me anymore. Maybe my stress and anxiety were my body's reminder that it's time to do things for myself again. Maybe it's time to make running a priority. Even though it takes an hour every day to get ready for the run, run, then shower and dress afterward, it surprisingly hasn't put me behind on anything. It seems like I'm more productive after a run than if I had just sat and powered through my work and skipped a run. It's definitely not a cure-all, but it's a cure-some for my worries and some days, that's huge!

Key Terms

anxiety A cognitive and emotional stress response that includes anticipation of a future threat.

anxiety disorders Diagnosable health conditions, distinct from feelings of anxiety or stress, characterized by a range of psychological and physiologic symptoms, including excessive rumination, worrying, uneasiness, and fear about future uncertainties.

fight-or-flight response The response of the sympathetic nervous system to a stressful event, preparing the body to fight or flee, and associated with the release of stress hormones.

homeostasis The natural state of our body and mind, characterized by calmness and balance that is disrupted by stress responses.

nonclinical populations Consisting of people who have not been diagnosed with a clinical disorder.

state anxiety Temporary state of high anxiety.

stress The process by which we perceive and respond to events, called stressors, that we appraise as threatening or challenging.

stress hormones Hormones such as cortisol and epinephrine released by the body in situations that are interpreted as being potentially dangerous.

stressor Any event or situation that triggers coping adjustments.

trait anxiety Individual differences in tendencies to experience frequent high levels of state anxiety.

Review Questions

1. What is the difference between stress and anxiety?
2. What is the distinction between anxiety and clinical anxiety disorders?
3. Describe the proposed mechanisms of how physical activity is associated with stress and anxiety. Does physical activity impact stress and anxiety? Does stress and anxiety impact physical activity?
4. What type of study could you set up to investigate whether time spent being sedentary influences daily anxiety? How would that study be different if you wanted to investigate whether time spent being sedentary influenced your risk of being diagnosed with a clinical anxiety disorder?
5. Describe three clinical anxiety disorders and how they are distinct.
6. How would you describe the evidence about whether physical activity is a good treatment option for clinical anxiety disorders? What about the literature concerning sedentary behavior and clinical anxiety disorders?

Applying the Concepts

1. What do you think Wáng is experiencing when he runs? How is that helping how he feels and what is the scientific explanation behind it?
2. Will Wáng's stress get better if he runs regularly compared with just when he feels overwhelmed? Why or why not?

References

American Psychiatric Association. (2013). *Diagnostic and statistical manual of mental disorders (DSM-5®)*. American Psychiatric Publishing.

Asmundson, G. J., Fetzner, M. G., DeBoer, L. B., Powers, M. B., Otto, M. W., & Smits, J. A. (2013). Let's get physical: A contemporary review of the anxiolytic effects of exercise for anxiety and its disorders. *Depression & Anxiety, 30*(4), 362–373. https://doi.org/10.1002/da.22043

de Assis, M. A., de Mello, M. F., Scorza, F. A., Cadrobbi, M. P., Schooedl, A. F., da Silva, S. G., de Albuquerque, M., da Silva, A. C., & Arida, R. M. (2008). Evaluation of physical activity habits in patients with posttraumatic stress disorder. *Clinics, 63*(4), 473–478. https://doi.org/10.1590/S1807-59322008000400010

Bandelow, B., Michaelis, S., & Wedekind, D. (2017). Treatment of anxiety disorders. *Dialogues in Clinical Neuroscience, 19*(2), 93–107.

Broocks, A., Bandelow, B., Pekrun, G., George, A., Meyer, T., Bartmann, U., Hillmer-Vogel, U., & Rüther, E. (1998). Comparison of aerobic exercise, clomipramine, and placebo in the treatment of panic disorder. *The American Journal of Psychiatry, 155*(5), 603–609. https://doi.org/10.1176/ajp.155.5.603

Cagle, J. A., Overcash, K. B., Rowe, D. P., & Needle, A. R. (2017). Trait anxiety as a risk factor for musculoskeletal injury in athletes: A critically appraised topic. *International Journal of Athletic Therapy & Training, 22*(3), 26–31.

Carter, T., Pascoe, M., Bastounis, A., Morres, I. D., Callaghan, P., & Parker, A. G. (2021). The effect of physical activity on anxiety in children and young people: A systematic review and meta-analysis. *Journal of Affective Disorders, 285*, 10–21. https://doi.org/10.1016/j.jad.2021.02.026

Conn, V. S. (2010). Anxiety outcomes after physical activity interventions: Meta-analysis findings. *Nursing Research, 59*(3), 224–231. https://doi.org/10.1097/NNR.0b013e3181dbb2f8

Crews, D. J., & Landers, D. M. (1987). A meta-analytic review of aerobic fitness and reactivity to psychosocial stressors. *Medicine & Science in Sports & Exercise, 19*(5, Suppl), 114–120. https://doi.org/10.1249/00005768-198710001-00004

Dedoncker, J., Vanderhasselt, M-A., Ottaviani, C., & Slavich, G. M. (2021). Mental health during the COVID-19 pandemic and beyond: The importance of the vagus nerve for biopsychosocial resilience. *Neuroscience & Biobehavioral Reviews, 125*, 1–10. https://doi.org/10.1016/j.neubiorev.2021.02.010

Diaz, K. M., Thanataveerat, A., Parsons, F. E., Yoon, S., Cheung, Y. K., Alcantara, C., Duran, A. T., Ensari, I., Krupka, D. J., Schwartz, J. E., Burg, M. M., & Davidson, K. W. (2018). The influence of daily stress on sedentary behavior: Group and person (N of 1) level results of a 1-year observational study. *Psychosomatic Medicine, 80*(7), 620–627. https://doi.org/10.1097/PSY.0000000000000610

Edwards, M. K., & Loprinzi, P. D. (2016). Experimentally increasing sedentary behavior results in increased anxiety in an active young adult population. *Journal of Affective Disorders, 204*, 166–173. https://doi.org/10.1016/j.jad.2016.06.045

Endler, N. S., & Kocovski, N. L. (2001). State and trait anxiety revisited. *Journal of Anxiety Disorders, 15*(3), 231–245. https://doi.org/10.1016/S0887-6185(01)00060-3

Endrighi, R., Steptoe, A., & Hamer, M. (2016). The effect of experimentally induced sedentariness on mood and psychobiological responses to mental stress. *The British Journal of Psychiatry, 208*(3), 245–251. https://doi.org/10.1192/bjp.bp.114.150755

Fawcett, E. J., Fairbrother, N., Cox, M. L., White, I. R., & Fawcett, J. M. (2019). The prevalence of anxiety disorders during pregnancy and the postpartum period: A multivariate Bayesian meta-analysis. *The Journal of Clinical Psychiatry, (80*(4): 18r12527.) https://doi.org/10.4088/JCP.18r12527

Firth, J., Siddiqi, N., Koyanagi, A., Siskind, D., Rosenbaum, S., Galletly, C., Allan, S., Caneo, C., Carney, R., Carvalho, A. F., Chatterton, M. L., Correll, C. U., Curtis, J., Gaughran, F., Heald, A., Hoare, E., Jackson, S. E., Kisely, S., Lovell, K., . . . Stubbs, B. (2019). The *Lancet Psychiatry* Commission: A blueprint for protecting physical health in people with mental illness. *The Lancet Psychiatry, 6*(8), 675–712. https://doi.org/10.1016/S2215-0366(19)30132-4

Flueckiger, L., Lieb, R., Meyer, A. H., Witthauer, C., & Mata, J. (2016). The importance of physical activity and sleep for affect on stressful days: Two intensive longitudinal studies. *Emotion, 16*(4), 488–497. https://doi.org/10.1037/emo0000143

Herring, M. P., Puetz, T. W., O'Connor, P. J., & Dishman, R. K. (2012). Effect of exercise training on depressive symptoms among patients with a chronic illness: A systematic review and meta-analysis of randomized controlled trials. *Archives of Internal Medicine, 172*(2), 101–111. https://doi.org/10.1001/archinternmed.2011.696

Hovland, A., Nordhus, I. H., Sjøbø, T., Gjestad, B. A., Birknes, B., Martinsen, E. W., Torsheim, T., & Pallesen, S. (2013). Comparing physical exercise in groups to group cognitive behaviour therapy for the treatment of panic disorder in a randomized controlled trial. *Behavioural and Cognitive Psychotherapy, 41*(4), 408–432. https://doi.org/10.1017/S1352465812000446

Jazaieri, H., Goldin, P. R., Werner, K., Ziv, M., & Gross, J. J. (2012). A randomized trial of MBSR versus aerobic exercise for Social Anxiety Disorder. *Journal of Clinical Psychology, 68*(7), 715–731. https://doi.org/10.1002/jclp.21863

Kandola, A., Vancampfort, D., Herring, M., Rebar, A., Hallgren, M., Firth, J., & Stubbs, B. (2018). Moving to beat anxiety: Epidemiology and therapeutic issues with physical activity for anxiety. *Current Psychiatry Reports, 20*(63). https://doi.org/10.1007/s11920-018-0923-x

Kirschbaum, C., Pirke, K-M., & Hellhammer, D. H. (1993). The 'Trier Social Stress Test'–A tool for investigating psychobiological stress responses in a laboratory setting. *Neuropsychobiology, 28*(1–2), 76–81.

Kroenke, K., Spitzer, R. L., Williams, J. B., Monahan, P. O., & Löwe, B. (2007). Anxiety disorders in primary care: Prevalence, impairment, comorbidity, and detection. *Annals of Internal Medicine, 146*(5), 317–325. https://doi.org/10.7326/0003-4819-146-5-200703060-00004

Kudielka, B. M., Hellhammer, D. H., & Kirschbaum, C. (2007). *Ten Years of Research with the Trier Social Stress Test–Revisited.*

Kugler, J., Seelbach, H., & Krüskemper, G. M. (1994). Effects of rehabilitation exercise programmes on anxiety and depression in coronary patients: A meta-analysis. *British Journal of Clinical Psychology, 33*(3), 401–410. https://doi.org/10.1111/j.2044-8260.1994.tb01136.x

Landers, D. M., & Arent, S. M. (2007). Physical activity and mental health. In *Handbook of Sport Psychology, 3rd ed* (pp. 469–491). John Wiley & Sons, Inc.

Landers, D. M., & Petruzzello, S. J. (1994). Physical activity, fitness, and anxiety. In *Physical activity, fitness, and health: International proceedings and consensus statement* (pp. 868–882). Human Kinetics Publishers.

Lim, S. S., Vos, T., Flaxman, A. D., Danaei, G., Shibuya, K., Adair-Rohani, H., AlMazroa, M. A., Amann, M., Anderson, H. R., Andrews, K. G., Aryee, M., Atkinson, C., Bacchus, L. J., Bahalim, A. N., Balakrishnan, K., Balmes, J., Barker-Collo, S., Baxter, A., Bell, M. L., . . . Ezzati, M. (2012). A comparative risk assessment of burden of disease and injury attributable to 67 risk factors and risk factor clusters in 21 regions, 1990–2010: A systematic analysis for the Global Burden of Disease Study 2010. *The Lancet, 380*(9859), 2224–2260. https://doi.org/10.1016/S0140-6736(12)61766-8

Lines, R. L., Ducker, K. J., Ntoumanis, N., Thøgersen-Ntoumani, C., Fletcher, D., & Gucciardi, D. F. (2021). Stress, physical activity, sedentary behavior, and resilience—The effects of naturalistic periods of elevated stress: A measurement-burst study. *Psychophysiology, 58*(8), e13846. https://doi.org/10.1111/psyp.13846

Long, B. C., & van Stavel, R. (1995). Effects of exercise training on anxiety: A meta-analysis. *Journal of Applied Sport Psychology, 7*(2), 167–189. https://doi.org/10.1080/10413209508406963

Millet, N., Longworth, J., & Arcelus, J. (2017). Prevalence of anxiety symptoms and disorders in the transgender population: A systematic review of the literature. *International Journal of Transgenderism, 18*(1), 27–38.

Mücke, M., Ludyga, S., Colledge, F., & Gerber, M. (2018). Influence of regular physical activity and fitness on stress reactivity as measured with the trier social stress test protocol: A systematic review. *Sports Medicine, 48*(11), 2607–2622. https://doi.org/10.1007/s40279-018-0979-0

Oaten, M., & Cheng, K. (2005). Academic examination stress impairs self–control. *Journal of Social and Clinical Psychology, 24*(2), 254–279.

Petruzzello, S. J., Landers, D. M., Hatfield, B. D., Kubitz, K. A., & Salazar, W. (1991). A meta-analysis on the anxiety-reducing effects of acute and chronic exercise. *Sports Medicine, 11*(3), 143–182. https://doi.org/10.2165/00007256-199111030-00002

Puterman, E., Weiss, J., Beauchamp, M. R., Mogle, J. A., & Almeida, D. M. (2017). Physical activity and negative affective reactivity in daily life. *Health Psychology, 36*(12), 1186–1194. https://doi.org/10.1037/hea0000532

Rebar, A. L., Stanton, R., Geard, D., Short, C., Duncan, M. J., & Vandelanotte, C. (2015). A meta-meta-analysis of the effect of physical activity on depression and anxiety in non-clinical adult populations. *Health Psychology Review, 9*(3), 366–378.

Rebar, A. L., Stanton, R., & Rosenbaum, S. (2017). Comorbidity of depression and anxiety in exercise research. *The Lancet Psychiatry, 4*(7), 519. https://doi.org/10.1016/S2215-0366(17)30164-5

Reed, J., & Buck, S. (2009). The effect of regular aerobic exercise on positive-activated affect: A meta-analysis. *Psychology of Sport and Exercise, 10*(6), 581–594.

Rimmele, U., Seiler, R., Marti, B., Wirtz, P. H., Ehlert, U., & Heinrichs, M. (2009). The level of physical activity affects adrenal and cardiovascular reactivity to psychosocial stress. *Psychoneuroendocrinology, 34*(2), 190–198. https://doi.org/10.1016/j.psyneuen.2008.08.023

Rimmele, U., Zellweger, B. C., Marti, B., Seiler, R., Mohiyeddini, C., Ehlert, U., & Heinrichs, M. (2007). Trained men show lower cortisol, heart rate and psychological responses to psychosocial stress compared with untrained men. *Psychoneuroendocrinology, 32*(6), 627–635. https://doi.org/10.1016/j.psyneuen.2007.04.005

Salmon, P. (2001). Effects of physical exercise on anxiety, depression, and sensitivity to stress: A unifying theory. *Clinical Psychology Review, 21*(1), 33–61.

Sarris, J., Moylan, S., Camfield, D. A., Pase, M. P., Mischoulon, D., Berk, M., Jacka, F. N., & Schweitzer, I. (2012). Complementary medicine, exercise, meditation, diet, and lifestyle modification for anxiety disorders: A review of current evidence. *Evidence-Based Complementary and Alternative Medicine, 2012*, e809653. https://doi.org/10.1155/2012/809653

Selye, H. (1950). Stress and the general adaptation syndrome. *British Medicine Journal, 1*(4667), 1383–1392. https://doi.org/10.1136/bmj.1.4667.1383

Speilberger, C. D. (1983). *Manual for the State Trait Anxiety Inventory (Form Y) Consulting Psychologists Press: Palo Alto. CA.*

Stubbs, B., Koyanagi, A., Hallgren, M., Firth, J., Richards, J., Schuch, F., Rosenbaum, S., Mugisha, J., Veronese, N., Lahti, J., & Vancampfort, D. (2017). Physical activity and anxiety: A perspective from the World Health Survey. *Journal of Affective Disorders, 208*, 545–552. https://doi.org/10.1016/j.jad.2016.10.028

Stubbs, B., Vancampfort, D., Rosenbaum, S., Firth, J., Cosco, T., Veronese, N., Salum, G. A., & Schuch, F. B. (2017). An examination of the anxiolytic effects of exercise for people with anxiety and stress-related disorders: A meta-analysis. *Psychiatry Research, 249*, 102–108. https://doi.org/10.1016/j.psychres.2016.12.020

Teychenne, M., Costigan, S. A., & Parker, K. (2015). The association between sedentary behaviour and risk of anxiety: A systematic review. *BMC Public Health, 15*(513), 2–8. https://doi.org/10.1186/s12889-015-1843-x

Teychenne, M., Stephens, L. D., Costigan, S. A., Olstad, D. L., Stubbs, B., & Turner, A. I. (2019). The association between sedentary behaviour and indicators of stress: A systematic review. *BioMed Central Public Health, 19*(1357), 2–15. https://doi.org/10.1186/s12889-019-7717-x

Vancampfort, D., Stubbs, B., Herring, M. P., Hallgren, M., & Koyanagi, A. (2018). Sedentary behavior and anxiety: Association and influential factors among 42,469 community-dwelling adults in six low- and middle-income countries. *General Hospital Psychiatry, 50*, 26–32. https://doi.org/10.1016/j.genhosppsych.2017.09.006

von Haaren, B., Haertel, S., Stumpp, J., Hey, S., & Ebner-Priemer, U. (2015). Reduced emotional stress reactivity to a real-life academic examination stressor in students participating in a 20-week aerobic exercise training: A randomised controlled trial using Ambulatory Assessment.

Psychology of Sport and Exercise, 20, 67–75. https://doi.org/10.1016/j.psychsport.2015.04.004

Wipfli, B. M., Rethorst, C. D., & Landers, D. M. (2008). The anxiolytic effects of exercise: A meta-analysis of randomized trials and dose–response analysis. *Journal of Sport and Exercise Psychology, 30*(4), 392–410.

World Health Organization. (2003). *Investing in mental health.* World Health Organization.

World Health Organization. (2017). *Depression and other common mental disorders: Global health estimates.* World Health Organization. https://apps.who.int/iris/bitstream/handle/10665/254610/WHO-MSD-MER-2017.2-eng.pdf

Zamani, M., Alizadeh-Tabari, S., & Zamani, V. (2019). Systematic review with meta-analysis: The prevalence of anxiety and depression in patients with irritable bowel syndrome. *Alimentary Pharmacology and Therapeutics, 50*(2), 132–143. https://doi.org/10.1111/apt.15325

Zhang, J., Wei, W., & Wang, C. (2012). Effects of psychological interventions for patients with systemic lupus erythematosus: A systematic review and meta-analysis. *Lupus, 21*(10), 1077–1087. https://doi.org/10.1177/0961203312447667

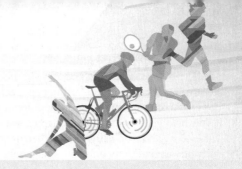

CHAPTER 12

Self-Esteem and Body Image

LEARNING OBJECTIVES

After completing this chapter, you will be able to:

- Better understand the meaning of the term body image.
- Examine the role that exercise and sedentary behavior plays in changing body image.
- Differentiate among terms used to describe the self, such as self-esteem and self-concept.
- Discuss the role of physical activity and sedentary behavior in modifying self-esteem.
- Understand the relationship between physical activity and individual attitudes and beliefs about the body.
- Describe the relationship between social physique anxiety and physical activity.

Introduction

Few psychological constructs have received as much research attention as **self-esteem**, and for good reason. High self-esteem is associated with emotional stability, happiness, and resilience to stress. In contrast, low self-esteem is related to mental illnesses such as depression, anxiety, and eating disorders. Thus, self-esteem is a critical component of human functioning and performance. Not surprisingly, researchers have examined various components of self-esteem and how it affects overall health, including physical activity and sedentary behavior.

Body image is one such component of self-esteem. Body image represents the mental picture you have of your body. That is, what your body looks like, what you believe about your

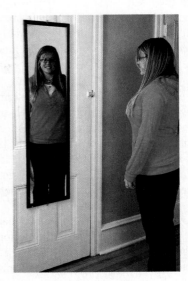

© Cjmckendry/iStock/Getty Images Plus/Getty Images.

body, and how you feel about your body. Self-esteem and body image influence each other. For example, it is hard to feel good about yourself if you hate your body. In this chapter, we examine self-esteem and body image and their relationship with physical activity and sedentary behavior.

Self-Esteem

Self-esteem represents a stable global positive or negative evaluative of a person's own self-worth. That is, the degree to which a person possesses positive and negative self-perceptions. Positive self-perceptions include the ability to make statements like "I am competent" or "I am a good person." In comparison, negative self-perceptions are reflected in statements such as "I am incompetent" or "I am worthless."

The terms self-esteem and **self-concept** are often used interchangeably, but they have distinct meanings. The statement "I am a good person" is evaluative in nature, and thus, it is a manifestation of the person's self-esteem. In comparison, self-concept refers to the many attributes and the roles that people use to evaluate themselves to establish their self-esteem. In other words, one's self-concept is a collection of beliefs about oneself that includes such things as academic performance, athletic performance, age, and racial identity. Generally, self-concept embodies the answer to "Who am I?" The statement "I am a regular exerciser," because it is self-descriptive in nature, would reflect the individual's self-concept.

Self-esteem has received a great deal of research attention, largely because it is positively related to psychological health, physical health, and overall quality of life. Self-esteem is associated with many positive achievements and socially related behaviors, including leadership ability, satisfaction, decreased anxiety, and improved academic and physical performance (Liu, Tian, Yang, Want, & Luo, 2022).

Historically, the conception and measurement of self-esteem were unidimensional. Self-esteem was considered, and thus was measured, as one overall global index. The implicit assumption made with a unidimensional self-esteem

approach was that a single measure would provide insight into a person's evaluative self-worth in a wide range of settings. This measurement approach was imprecise because it assessed a general sense of self-worth without considering the role of other contributors to self-esteem.

More recently, researchers have acknowledged that self-esteem should be viewed in both a multidimensional and hierarchical manner. Common domains that contribute to a person's global self-esteem are social acceptance, physical appearance, academic competence, athletic competence, romantic appeal, close friendships, job competence, and behavioral conduct. Thus, your perceptions of your physical self may be dramatically different from your perceptions of your academic self. Consistent with a multidimensional approach, theoreticians now suggest that self-perceptions be organized into a hierarchical structure (Białecka-Pikul, Stępień-Nycz, Sikorska, Topolewska-Siedzik, & Cieciuch, 2019).

One such hierarchical structure is the exercise and self-esteem model (Sonstroem & Morgan, 1989). In this model, changes in physical activity and associated physical parameters (e.g., fitness, weight) that are brought about by physical activity (e.g., walking, running) are proposed to have indirect effects on global self-esteem. In this model, changes in self-efficacy related to changes in activity are proposed to affect the subdomains of physical esteem, such as perceptions of physical conditioning, attractive body, and strength. Then these more-specific

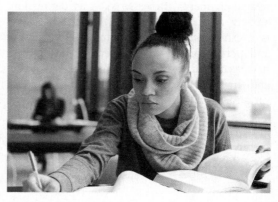

© Jacoblund/iStock/Getty Images Plus/Getty Images.

perceptions are theorized to be related to physical self-worth, which is the immediate precursor of global esteem (McAuley et al., 2005).

The top of the hierarchy is global self-esteem. In turn, global self-esteem develops as a result of evaluative perceptions arising from a number of life areas such as the physical self, the social self, the spiritual self, and the academic self. Therefore, changes in global self-esteem are the result of prior changes that have occurred in the facets of self-esteem, because these are at the bottom of the multidimensional hierarchical model, whereas global self-esteem is at the top of this model. As a result, when changes in the facets of self-esteem are not significant, no significant changes will occur in global self-esteem (Sonstroem & Morgan, 1989).

Furthermore, the aspects of self-esteem that are considered important by the person will have a significant impact on their global self-esteem. For example, an adolescent girl may perform well in school (i.e., her academic self), but at the same time, she may feel socially isolated from her peers (i.e., her social self). Because she wants to be popular among her peers, her low social self-esteem will have a greater influence on her global self-esteem. See **Figure 12-1** for a hierarchical model of self-esteem.

CRITICAL THINKING ACTIVITY 12-1

What domains of self-esteem have the greatest influence on your global self-esteem? Describe these in detail.

Physical Self-Esteem

Based on this hierarchical model of self-esteem, the physical self has the most implications for physical activity and sedentary behavior. Fox and Corbin (1989) developed the **physical self-perception profile**, which enabled the physical component of self-esteem to be examined in more detail. See **Figures 12-2** and **12-3** for descriptions of physical self-esteem.

The physical self-perception profile (Fox & Corbin, 1989; Ruiz-Montero, Chiva-Bartoll, Baena-Extremera, & Hortigüela-Alcalá, 2020) is based on a hierarchical, multidimensional theoretical model of self-esteem, in which self-perceptions are categorized as superordinate (i.e., global self-esteem), domain (e.g., physical self-worth), subdomain (e.g., body attractiveness), facet (e.g., figure/physique), subfacet (e.g., slim waistline), and state (e.g., "I feel lean today"). Self-perceptions are general and enduring at the top of the hierarchy. At lower levels, self-perceptions become increasingly specific and unstable. The model holds that the extent to which we feel good about ourselves physically will contribute to how we feel about ourselves in general.

More specifically, the physical self-perception profile model states that physical self-worth (i.e., general feelings of pride, satisfaction, happiness, and confidence in the physical self) is formed through the contribution of the following four subdomains of physical self-perceptions: (1) physical conditioning, (2) body attractiveness, (3) physical strength, and (4) sport competence. A detailed description of these subdomains can be found in **Table 12-1**. These four subdomains

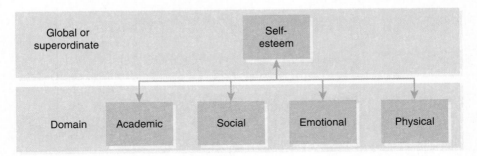

Figure 12-1 Multidimensional and Hierarchical Self-Esteem.

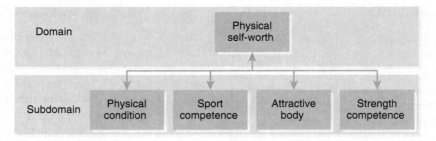

Figure 12-2 Physical Self-Esteem.

are subordinate to global physical self-esteem and global general self-esteem. Self-perceptions can vary from one level to another, for example, from the superordinate (global self-esteem), domain (physical), subdomain (sport competence), facet (soccer ability), subfacet (shooting ability), and state ("I can score this goal").

For example, total weight may contribute to feelings of being fat, which, in turn, may contribute to social physique anxiety and, subsequently, to poor body image. That poor body image, in turn, would influence the individual's physical self-esteem, which, in turn, would influence the individual's overall self-esteem. Although all dimensions (e.g., social self-esteem, academic self-esteem) contribute to global self-esteem, physical self-esteem plays a preeminent role.

Fox and Corbin (1989) developed the physical self-perception profile to measure the four subdomains of the physical self, along with a subscale to measure general overall physical self-worth. With this tool, a person is asked to read a pair of contrasting statements and decide which of the two statements is most characteristic of themselves. The person then checks a box, denoting the extent to which the statement is characteristic of themselves by indicating whether the item is "Sort of true for me" or "Really true for me." The physical self-perception profile has been successfully applied to a variety of populations and cultures. Sample items of each of the subscales can be found in **Table 12-2**. Let's take a closer look at the research examining the effects of physical activity and sedentary behavior on self-esteem.

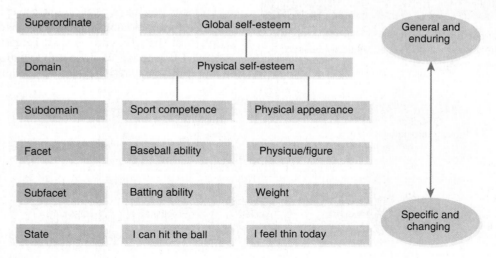

Figure 12-3 Levels of Physical Self-Perception.

Table 12-1 **Physical Self-Perception Profile Subdomains**

Subdomain	Description
Physical condition	Perceptions of level of physical condition, stamina and fitness, ability to maintain exercise, confidence in exercise setting
Body attractiveness	Perceived attractiveness of figure or physique, ability to maintain an attractive body, confidence in appearance
Physical strength	Perceived strength, muscle development, confidence in situations requiring strength
Sport competence	Perceptions of sport and athletic ability, ability to learn sport skills, confidence in sport environment

Effects of Physical Activity and Sedentary Behavior on Self-Esteem

Self-esteem is a predictor of many psychosocial well-being constructs. For example, self-esteem is positively related to self-efficacy, body satisfaction, and leadership; and it is negatively related to levels of anxiety and depression (Fernandes et al., 2022). Not surprisingly, a large body of research has examined the relationship between self-esteem and physical activity. In particular, researchers have focused on the effects of physical activity on children and adolescents' self-esteem. Typically, these studies involve a comparison of the self-esteem of young people before and after a physical activity intervention program. Meta-analyses and systematic reviews of this research support that physical activity is positively associated, and sedentary behavior is negatively associated, with self-esteem in children and adolescents (Rodriguez-Ayllon et al., 2019; Visier-Alfonso et al., 2022). This consistent finding has led researchers to conclude that physical activity improves self-esteem (Collins, Booth, Duncan, Fawkner, & Niven, 2019). This

Table 12-2 **Sample Items from the Physical Self-Perception Profile**

Subdomain	Sample Item
Physical condition	Some people make certain they take part in some form of regular vigorous physical exercise BUT others don't often manage to keep up regular vigorous physical exercise.
Body attractiveness	Some people feel that compared with most, they have attractive bodies BUT others feel that compared with most, their bodies are not quite so attractive.
Physical strength	Some people feel that their muscles are much stronger than most others of their sex BUT others feel that on the whole, their muscles are not quite as strong as most others of their sex.
Sport competence	Some people feel that they are among the best when it comes to athletic ability BUT others feel that they are not among the most able when it comes to athletics.
Physical self-worth	Some people feel extremely satisfied with the kind of person they are physically BUT others sometimes feel a little dissatisfied with their physical selves.

Data from Fox, K. R., & Corbin, C. B. (1989). The physical self-perception profile: development and preliminary validation. *Journal of Sport and Exercise Psychology, 11,* 408–430.

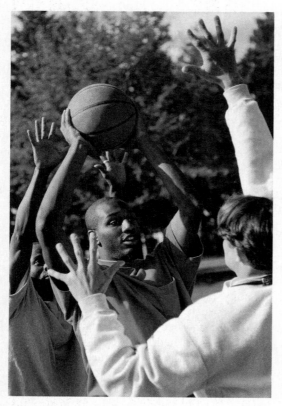

© Doug Menuez/Photodisc/Getty Images.

positive association is also evident with over-weight or obese children and adolescents. In their review of the literature, Andrade, Correaia, and Coimbra (2019) found that exergaming had a small positive effect on self-esteem with this special population.

It is important to note that the aforementioned studies tend to focus on global self-esteem. As Figures 12-1 and 12-2 illustrate, physical self-esteem develops as a result of evaluative perceptions arising from a number of dimensions, including sport competence, physical strength, physical condition, and body image. Indeed, within the context of physical activity, researchers have revealed that self-esteem should be considered multidimensional and hierarchical (Sonstroem et al., 1994); that is, exercise can promote positive changes in physical self-perceptions that can manifest as an increase in global self-esteem.

Moore and his colleagues (2011) assessed self-esteem using the hierarchical framework of the exercise and self-esteem model (Sonstroem & Morgan, 1989). The aim of their study was to determine whether resistance training could cause changes in global (i.e., physical self-worth) and subdomain levels (e.g., aerobic condition, attractive body, sport competence, strength) of self-esteem. They had 120 college students complete measures of the physical subdomains (i.e., strength, endurance, physical attractiveness, and sport competence) and global self-esteem before and after a 12-week resistance exercise training program.

They found that the students had significant improvements in their self-perception constructs at all levels of the exercise and self-esteem model. The hierarchical structure of self-esteem was partially supported because successively smaller improvements at each level of the model were found. For example, global self-esteem showed lesser improvements than physical self-worth.

Based on the research we have discussed thus far, it is not clear whether increasing self-esteem leads to more physical activity or whether increasing physical activity leads to higher self-esteem. To address the direction of the self-esteem and physical activity relationship, Schmalz and her colleagues (2007) used data from a longitudinal study to explore the relationship between physical activity and global self-esteem among 197 girls from childhood into early adolescence. The girls' physical activity and self-esteem were assessed when they were 9, 11, and 13 years old.

The researchers found that more physical activity at ages 9 and 11 years predicted higher self-esteem at ages 11 and 13 years. Of importance, the effects of physical activity on self-esteem were most apparent at age 11 and for girls with higher body mass index (BMI). The authors concluded that participating in physical activity can lead to positive self-esteem among adolescent girls, particularly for younger girls and those at greatest risk of being overweight. Their findings support other longitudinal research conducted in older populations that physical activity has positive effects on both global and subdomain self-esteem levels of physical condition and body attractiveness.

As well, a review of over 15,000 participants found that low levels of physical activity and sleep and high levels of sedentary behavior were unfavorably associated with adiposity outcomes, behavioral problems, depression, and self-esteem (Alanazi et al., 2021).

Is physical activity related to self-esteem for both genders? Yes, increased levels of physical activity are beneficial for global self-esteem by enhancing both girls' and boys' perceptions of physical self-esteem. However, the influence of physical appearance on global self-worth is stronger for female than for male populations (Haugen, Safvenborn, & Ommundsen, 2011).

What about other types of physical activity? Collins and his colleagues (2019) conducted a systematic and meta-analytic review of the research examining the effects of resistance training on various aspects of self-esteem with school children between the ages of 5 to 18 years. They found that resistance training resulted in improvements in the self-esteem components of physical strength and physical self-worth. No significant improvements, however, were found for body attractiveness, physical condition, and sport competence. The findings indicate that resistance training has a positive impact on some components of self-esteem in youth.

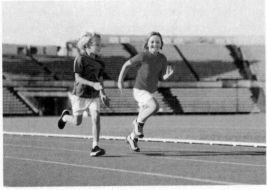

© FamVeld/Shutterstock.

Body Image

As shown in Figure 12-2, one integral component contributing to a person's physical self-esteem (which, in turn, has a major impact on global self-esteem) is body image. As the term suggests, body image refers to the self-perceptions, attitudes, feelings, and behaviors an individual holds with respect to their body and physical appearance. Body image is defined as the subjective picture or mental image of one's own body. Increasingly, the lean and fit body for women and the lean and muscular body for men have been endorsed as ideal body types in the media. Males and females who deviate from the sometimes impossible "ideal" and internalize this ideal may experience body image problems.

Body image is a multidimensional subjective experience composed of five dimensions: perceptual, cognitive, affective, subjective, and behavioral (see **Table 12-3**). These dimensions interact with and influence each other. Our body image perception is based on the mental images we have of our appearance, as well as the sensations of being in our bodies. Sometimes our perception is accurate—our mental image matches up with the reality of our appearance and how others perceive our appearance—but sometimes it is distorted, and we see something

Table 12-3 **Dimensions of Body Image**

Dimension	Description
Perceptual	Mental images we have of our appearance and the sensations of being in our body.
Cognitive	Beliefs about our appearance.
Affective	Feelings associated with body image.
Subjective	General evaluated form of body image. Often assessed via body satisfaction/dissatisfaction.
Behavioral	Behaviors in which people engage with regard to their body image, such as excessive checking and body avoidance.

very different from what others see. When our perception is distorted, we may overestimate our overall body size, size of specific body parts, or evaluate our bodies differently from others— usually more harshly or with a magnified focus.

The affective dimension represents feelings associated with body image and can cover the emotional spectrum. In body image disturbance, these feelings tend to take the form of shame, disgust, fear, or sadness. Such feelings may be a constant backdrop, causing significant distress and preoccupation.

The cognitive dimension represents beliefs about our appearance (e.g., "being too big or round"), as well as the meaning of our appearance (e.g., "therefore, I am unacceptable or worthless"). In body image disturbance, people tend to equate appearance with overall self-worth. Thus, if these individuals are dissatisfied with their appearance, they are dissatisfied with themselves as a whole. Research shows that when young women think about their appearance while taking a math test, their performance is markedly worse than young women who do not think about their appearance. For individuals with body image disturbance, thoughts about appearance persist throughout the day and detract from concentration and enjoyment of everyday activities.

The subjective evaluation dimension is more general in nature and tends to encompass body satisfaction (dissatisfaction), for example, in a person being satisfied (or dissatisfied) with their body as a whole or with specific body parts (e.g., arms, legs, buttocks).

Finally, the behavioral aspect of body image involves behaviors people engage in with regard to their body image, such as excessive checking and body avoidance. Body checking can take many forms, such as weighing, measuring, pinching, or looking in the mirror. Body checking is driven by the desire to get information or reassurance about one's appearance or body size in an attempt to alleviate anxiety. On the opposite end of the spectrum is body avoidance, which involves avoiding exposure (of the self or others) to one's appearance. Examples of body avoidance behaviors include wearing baggy clothes, avoiding mirrors, and preferring not to be touched. The purpose is to avoid upsetting information about one's appearance or body size, and it is fueled by dissatisfaction and the sense that one's body is unacceptable. Someone who is highly body dissatisfied may avoid going to the beach because they do not want to be seen in public in a bathing suit. As well, people who are body dissatisfied may not work out at the gym for fear that others are looking at their bodies negatively.

CRITICAL THINKING ACTIVITY 12-2

How are body image and self-esteem related? Is one of these constructs more important than the other?

Scope and Significance of Body Image

Although body dissatisfaction is common in male and female populations, women and girls tend to be more body dissatisfied than men and boys. And body dissatisfaction is related to low self-esteem. Consistent with the ideal physique portrayed in the media of a thin and toned physique for women and a lean and muscular body for men, girls typically wanted to be thinner and boys frequently wanted to be more muscular (Karazsia et al., 2017).

There is nothing wrong with people caring about the body image and level of muscularity. However, for some people, the investment in their appearance may become all-consuming, and it may have negative health outcomes. Negative body image can have detrimental physical, social, psychological, and economic consequences. More specifically, negative body image is related to emotional distress, higher body mass index, smoking, dramatic measures to alter appearance (e.g., steroid use), social anxiety, impaired sexual functioning, depression, and eating disorders. In short, body dissatisfaction is common, and it can adversely affect a person's psychosocial functioning and quality of life.

The differences in the prevalence of body dissatisfaction shown by women and men in the studies presented is not atypical. Generally, across a wide variety of studies with participants who varied in age, women were found to have greater dissatisfaction with their physical appearance than men. Also, additional research has shown that women, compared with men, are more likely to diet, see themselves as overweight despite objective evidence to the contrary, overestimate their body size, and exercise for weight-related reasons (Bouzas et al., 2019).

CRITICAL THINKING ACTIVITY 12-3

Why do women have more body image disturbance than men? Describe the possible psychological, social, and physical reasons for this gender difference.

In contrast to women who tend to experience pressure to be slender, men often experience pressure to maintain an athletic and muscular body type. For example, men represented as prestigious in popular magazines are often lean and muscular. Although women report more body dissatisfaction than men, it is still common in men. For example, a large-scale survey of 52,677 visitors to a popular U.S. news website found that 48% of men reported that they felt dissatisfied with their weight, 11% felt physically unattractive, and 16% were so uncomfortable with their bodies that they avoided wearing a bathing suit in public (Frederick et al., 2007).

Failure to achieve a lean and muscular build, a prominent characteristic of masculinity for many, may lead to body dissatisfaction. Frederick and his colleagues (2007) used a figure-rating scale—a tool used to measure body dissatisfaction—to determine men's satisfaction with their muscularity and body fat in a series of international studies conducted in the United States, Ukraine, and Ghana. The researchers found widespread desire for increased muscularity among men, with over half of the U.S. men surveyed (range = 51 to 71%) reporting that they were not satisfied with their body fat level. They also found that over 90% of U.S. undergraduate men wanted to be more muscular, as did many Ukrainian (69%) and Ghanaian (49%) men. In the United States, men's ratings of their current and ideal muscularity were associated with endorsement of the male role, and many men desired increased muscularity for reasons related to increased dominance and attractiveness to women.

Widespread body image disturbance for men and women is associated with consumers spending billions of dollars annually for products aimed at changing their body size and shape, such as diet pills, unnecessary cosmetic surgery, beauty products, and fitness products. Because of the detrimental outcomes associated with negative body image and its malleable and subjective nature, society could benefit from a better understanding of the efficacy of interventions aimed at improving body image.

Body image interventions typically consist of psychoeducational, cognitive behavioral, or drug therapies (e.g., weight loss pills/programs; Mahon & Seekis, 2022). Because many of these interventions are expensive, in short supply, and often not suitable for young populations, other, more practical strategies should be examined and promoted. One promising alternative mode of intervention for negative body image is exercise. Let's take a look at the research examining the effects of physical activity on body image.

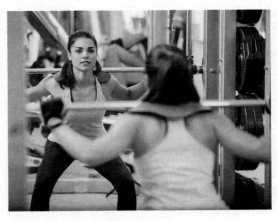

© Antonio_Diaz/iStock/Getty Images Plus/Getty Images.

Body Image and Physical Activity

A meta-analysis by Campbell and Hausenblas (2009) provides support for the suggestion that physical activity improves body image. In their meta-analysis, they examined the impact that exercise interventions had on people's body image. They reviewed 57 interventions and found a small effect size (.29) that indicated that exercise resulted in improved body image from pre- to postintervention for the exercise group compared with the nonexercise control group.

Campbell and Hausenblas (2009) concluded that exercise represents a practical and widely accessible intervention for negative body image. Although the effect size was small, exercise has advantages over other types of therapy, such as cognitive behavioral therapy. For example, exercise has the ability to reach and benefit many people. Other practical advantages of exercise are that, compared with other interventions, it is low cost, has minimal side-effects, and is a socially acceptable behavior. These benefits may result in exercise receiving greater acceptance as a treatment. Finally, exercise is self-sustaining because it can be maintained once the basic skills are learned.

The positive effect of exercise on body image has been evident in a variety of populations, both male and female, individuals with overweight and obesity, and pregnant women (Bassett-Gunter, McEwan, & Kamarhie, 2017; Carraça et al., 2021; Sun, Chen, Wang, Liu, & Zhang, 2018; Tebar et al., 2021).

However, an important research question is to examine what specific types of physical activities are related to improved body image. Regarding activity mode, researchers have found that both aerobic and resistance types of exercise resulted in improved body image (SantaBarbara, Whitworth, & Ciccolo, 2017). Regarding the distance and intensity of physical activity, researchers have found that walking longer distances and engaging in moderate to vigorous physical activity have stronger effects on body image than lifestyle physical activity (Rote, Swartz, & Klos, 2013). Even brief, four-session

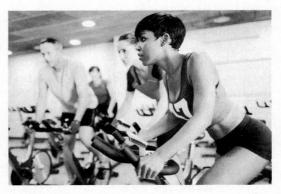

© Tempura/E+/Getty Images.

yoga interventions resulted in improved body image in young women (Halliwell, Dawson, & Burkey, 2019). Compared with the control group, participants in the yoga condition reported significant increases in body appreciation, body connectedness, body satisfaction, and positive mood at the end of the intervention as well as at the 4-week follow-up. There were no significant changes in negative mood or body surveillance.

Another question is whether a person's body image acts as either a motivator or barrier to physical activity participation. A study by Brudzynski and Ebben (2013) sheds light on the relationship between motivation and barriers to engage in physical activity and body image. They examined the relationship between body image and physical activity motivation, barriers, and frequency and location of physical activity behavior of 1,044 university students. They found that 78.6% of the students in their study could be classified as regularly active. They also found that body image was related to increased physical activity amounts for the regularly active, with 58% reporting that body image influenced the amount of physical activity in which they engaged.

Negative body image was a primary motive for physical activity participation with students when they felt overweight, when they wanted to improve appearance, and when they wanted to change a specific body area. Body image was also identified as a barrier to physical activity location, with most exercisers reporting a preference for private locations. Those not regularly active (34.2%) were satisfied with their overall appearance and did not identify body image as a significant barrier to physical activity. The researchers concluded that body image is a motivator for physical activity amount and a barrier to physical activity location for those regularly active, but that it is not a barrier to physical activity for those not regularly active. Body dissatisfaction may also result in exercise addiction characteristics. A review of 33 studies (n = 8747) found a moderate effect size, indicating that body dissatisfaction is related to exercise addiction.

CRITICAL THINKING ACTIVITY 12-4

How can physical activity be both a motivator and demotivator for physical activity behavior?

An interesting question is what happens to regular exercisers' body dissatisfaction during brief periods of nonexercise. Regular exercisers who take even 3 days off of exercise report increases in body dissatisfaction (Niven, Rendell, & Chisholm, 2008). This finding reveals the transient nature of body image, and indicates that body image may be an important motivator for regular exercise.

Appearance-based exercise motivation (i.e., the extent that exercise is pursued to influence weight or shape) affects both body image and exercise frequency in women. Exercise frequency has been shown to be related to higher positive body image, but high levels of appearance-based exercise motivation weakened these relationships (Homan & Tylka, 2014). Thus, messages promoting exercise need to deemphasize weight loss and appearance and promote positive body image. For example, **fitspiration** is any message (usually in the form of an image with a quote included) designed to inspire people to attain a fitness goal (Limniou et al., 2021). The results of the aforementioned study suggest that fitspiration messages should not focus on appearance-related images, such as six-pack abs. Of importance, body dissatisfaction may be a causal factor in excessive exercise and

exercise addiction (Alcaraz-Ibáñez, Paterna, Sicilia, & Griffiths, 2021).

Body image can also vary by college major. Norwegian researchers (2021) examined the relationship of two types of body image (i.e., body appreciation and body appearance pressure) in university students with various majors. Body appreciation is accepting and holding favorable opinions toward, and respecting one's body, as well as resisting the sociocultural pressures to internalize the stereotyped beauty standards and appreciating the functionality and health of the body. In comparison, body appearance pressure is the pressure one experiences to obtain an idealized body.

The researchers found that female exercise science students had better body appreciation compared with teaching, engineering, or business students. No group difference was found with male students. A high percentage of students reported experiencing body appearance pressure, with 69 and 85% among male and female exercise science students, and 57 and 83% among male and female teaching, engineering, or business students.

A visit to university fitness centers explains this seemingly contradictory observation. Fitness centers were the settings where most students experienced body appearance pressure. Even though female exercise science students are exposed to highly body-oriented environments, they also report characteristics that might protect their body image. The researchers concluded that the female exercise science students findings could be explained by their higher levels of physical activity, which had had a positive influence on their body composition, resulting in more body satisfaction. Despite the high levels of body appreciation reported, exercise science students experienced just as much body appearance pressure, and for males slightly more pressure, compared to other students. As such, body appearance pressure represents a challenge on college campuses. Actions to promote body appreciation and prevent body appearance pressure such as media literacy, body functionality, and exercise within educational programs are in need.

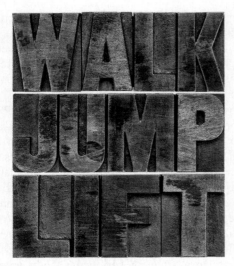

© Marekuliasz/iStock/Getty Images Plus/Getty Images.

Self-Presentational Anxiety

Self-presentation is the process by which people attempt to control and monitor how they are perceived and evaluated by others (Leary, 1992). People generally want others to view them in desirable ways. Thus, they attempt to control the inferences made by others by only presenting information about themselves that will bring about the desired impression, while hiding things that would be inconsistent with this desired image. The impressions that we make on other individuals affect how they treat us; therefore, self-presentation underlies most of our social interactions. Some people, however, are more apprehensive about incurring negative evaluation and are more prone to self-presentational concerns than their less-apprehensive counterparts.

When the individual doubts that they will be able to generate a positive impression or forestall an undesirable impression, social anxiety results (Leary, 1992). Because physical appearance is such an important component of both physical self-esteem and global self-esteem, social anxiety can arise as a result of concerns about the self-presentation of one's body. Self-presentation is also an important determinant of physical activity because it affects people's physical activity cognitions, attitudes,

Table 12-4 Social Physique Anxiety Scale

1 = Not at all characteristic
2 = Slightly characteristic
3 = Moderately characteristic
4 = Very characteristic
5 = Extremely characteristic

1. I wish I wasn't so uptight about my physique/figure. _____
2. I am bothered by thoughts that other people are evaluating my weight or muscular development negatively. _____
3. Unattractive features of my physique/figure make me nervous in certain social setting. _____
4. In the presence of others, I feel apprehensive about my physique/figure. _____
5. I am comfortable with how fit my body appears to others. _____
6. It would make me uncomfortable to know others are evaluating my physique/figure. _____
7. When it comes to displaying my physique/figure to others, I am a shy person. _____
8. I usually feel relaxed when it is obvious that others are looking at my physique/figure. _____
9. When in exercise clothes, I often feel nervous about the shape of my body. _____

Scoring

1. Reverse score: Items 5 and 8.
2. Add up the 9 items. Score range = 9 to 45.
3. High score = high social physique anxiety.

Data from Martin, K. A., Rejeski, W. J., Leary, M. R., McAuley, E., & Bain, S. (1997). Is the Social Physique Anxiety Scale really multidimensional? Conceptual and statistical arguments for a unidimensional model. *Journal of Sport and Exercise Psychology, 19,* 359–367.

and behaviors. Self-presentational anxiety about your own body or physique is called social physique anxiety. **Table 12-4** provides the items from the Social Physique Anxiety Scale (Martin et al., 1997), which can be used to assess this trait.

High social physique anxiety is associated with less physical activity in individuals with obesity (Baillot, Black, Brunet, & Romain, 2020). Also, Crawford and Eklund (1994) noted that women who are higher in the trait of social physique anxiety also reported a greater tendency to exercise for self-presentation reasons, such as weight control, body tone, and physical attractiveness. Conversely, women lower in the trait of social physique anxiety were more likely to exercise for motives generally unrelated to self-presentation, such as fitness, mood enhancement, health, and enjoyment.

A similar result was found when Hausenblas and Martin (2000) measured levels of social physique anxiety and exercise behavior in 286 female aerobics instructors. Instructors who were involved in leading classes primarily for self-presentation reasons (e.g., weight loss, improved body tone) had higher levels of social physique anxiety. In comparison, instructors who were involved in leading classes for leadership opportunities (i.e., to educate or to lead) or to affect enhancement (i.e., to have fun or to reduce stress) possessed a lower degree of social physique anxiety.

Focht and Hausenblas (2003, 2004) found that social physique anxiety can also affect how women feel during and after exercise. They examined the influence of different exercise environments upon state anxiety and positive feeling states in women with high social physique anxiety. The participants completed the following three conditions: (1) exercise in a self-presentational environment that involved working out in a coed gym in front of mirrors, (2) exercise in a laboratory alone, and (3) quiet rest in a laboratory alone. Participants completed assessments of their state anxiety and feeling states before, during, and after each condition.

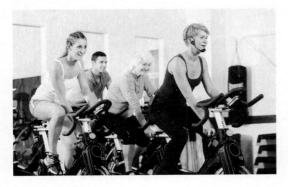

© Kzenon/Alamy Stock Photo.

These researchers found that only the exercise environment perceived to be high in evaluative threat (i.e., self-presentational environment) was associated with elevated in-task state anxiety (see **Figure 12-4**). Also, significant reductions in state anxiety were observed from pre-exercise to 5 minutes post-exercise in both the self-representational and laboratory exercise environments. The reduction in state anxiety, however, was significantly larger in the self-presentational environment. Whereas the anxiolytic response persisted through the 120-minute post-exercise assessment following the laboratory environment, state anxiety did not differ significantly from baseline at any of the remaining assessments following exercise in the self-presentational exercise environment. No significant changes in state anxiety were detected following quiet rest. In summary, state anxiety increased during exercise in the self-presentational environment, and the anxiolytic effect observed 5 minutes after both exercise conditions only persisted following exercise in the laboratory environment.

Focht and Hausenblas (2003, 2004) also found that increases in positive feeling states emerged following exercise but not following quiet rest. Finally, they reported that whereas feeling states returned to baseline within 1 hour following the self-presentational exercise condition, improvements in feeling states persisted for 2 hours following exercise in the lab condition. They concluded that the psychological benefits of acute exercise may not generalize to women with high social physique anxiety. In other words, the negative feeling states that emerged during exercise in the self-presentational environment support the idea that psychological distress experienced with public exercise settings may deter women with social physique anxiety from exercising. Thus, given that negative in-task feeling states only emerged during the self-presentational environment, exercising in settings where evaluative threatening aspects of the environment can be modified (e.g., locations of mirrors, privacy) would be advantageous for women with social physique anxiety, particularly

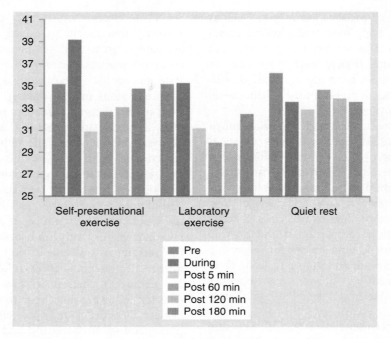

Figure 12-4 State Anxiety Levels Before, During, and Following the Three Conditions.

Data from Focht, B. C., & Hausenblas, H. A. (2004). Perceived evaluative threat and state anxiety during exercise in women with high social physique anxiety. *Journal of Applied Sport Psychology, 16,* 361–368; Focht B. C., & Hausenblas, H. A. (2006). Exercising in public and private environments: Effects on feeling states in women with social physique anxiety. *Journal of Applied Behavioral Research, 11,* 147–165.

during the adoption phase of a physical activity program (Focht & Hausenblas, 2006). Initiating physical activity in settings that minimize evaluative threat may allow women with social physique anxiety to avoid self-presentational anxiety while at the same time providing them with the opportunity to enhance their perceptions of their exercise abilities and body image.

CRITICAL THINKING ACTIVITY 12-5

You need to design an exercise intervention for a female adult who has high social physique anxiety. What type of intervention would you design and why? Justify your answer based on current research on this topic.

What are the effects of regular exercise on social physique anxiety? Pearson, Hall, and Gammage (2013) found that an exercise intervention results in improved social physique

anxiety in sedentary women with overweight and obesity. As well, Martin Ginis and colleagues (2014) found that an 8-week exercise program for women with body-image concerns resulted in significant reductions in social physique anxiety and other related body image measures. Of importance, women who were assigned

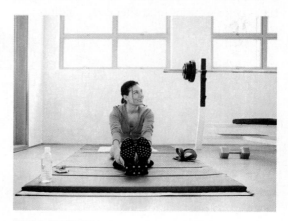

© Siri Stafford/DigitalVision/Getty Images.

to the aerobic training condition had greater improvements in social physique anxiety and appearance evaluation compared with women in the strength-training condition.

Summary

Self-esteem and body image are important constructs for physical activity. Researchers have continually demonstrated that physical activity is associated with improved self-esteem and body image. In other words, people who are physically active have higher self-esteem, are less preoccupied with body measurements, and have better body image than nonactive people (Korn et al., 2013). The emerging research is revealing that sedentary behavior is negatively related with self-esteem and body image. In summary, physical activity can be used to enhance self-esteem and body image. It has a positive impact on males and females of all ages, but the greatest effects of physical activity are shown in people with low levels of self-esteem, body image, and physical activity.

Vignette: Divya

During adolescence, I stopped fitting in with the other girls in my grade. I was a late bloomer whose body remained boxy and flat while the rest of my former friends' physiques grew shapely. Their newly feminine forms garnered more attention from the boys in our school. I don't recall getting that type of attention at all. I was repeatedly teased for not having a womanly figure. During recess, one of the popular girls at the time even accused me of being a boy because I wouldn't show the rest of the girls my bra. It wasn't unusual for my female classmates to showcase their new purchases from lingerie stores, as if flaunting their need for underwire support in my face. (I didn't wear one at the time because I had no need, so I refused to lift up my shirt out of shame.)

Whereas the rest of the girls in my class wore tight-fitting tank tops to school, I opted for baggier shirts to hide my lack of shapeliness. By the time we all entered high school, I was convinced I was physically unattractive and destined to be forever excluded because I didn't look ladylike, like everyone else.

Once I did begin to fill out—rapidly during the summer after eighth grade—I put on more weight than the other girls. And to top it all off, I had acne.

I was too afraid to be seen in shorts or even to change in front of my peers in any locker room. So I'd hug the walls in gym class, avoid trying out for sports teams, and rarely do anything physical after school. I read and watched television—sometimes zoning out in front of the screen for hours just to take my mind off the agony involved in being such an outsider at school.

I felt increasingly worse throughout high school, and I eventually found refuge in dark rock and metal music, vibrantly unnatural hair colors, and a group of friends who held a very dismal view of humanity. All of us dressed to express this. Our clothing was all black, all the time—and grungy.

I'd say that the most exercise I got before college was the rock concerts I'd go to with my new friends. Lost in a crowd of equally angry, disaffected teens and young adults, I could jump around, thrash my arms, and dance without the anxiety-provoking apprehension that everyone was watching and judging my body.

When it came time to prepare for college, I specifically pinpointed my top choices based on location. I didn't want to be in a warm area, where the weather would call for shorts rather than long pants and jackets. I was accepted early decision to a school in the Northeast. And for the next 4 years, I hid my body under layers and layers of sweatshirts, sweatpants, and a parka.

Unexpectedly, I lost a great deal of weight once I began classes, in part, because I had been given a prescription to help me focus for long stretches of time. Also, the food at the college I ended up attending wasn't very palatable. And as far as drinking went, I never developed a taste for alcohol—especially not beer or hard liquor, which were popular among my college peers. So the dreaded freshman 15 didn't end up applying to me.

I became heavily involved in theater during my sophomore year—but mostly from the tech and production end, not the stage. By junior year I was trying my hand at directing and writing scripts. And in between meeting the rest of my requirements, I was trying to hide a burgeoning crush on the supporting actor I casted in the play I wrote for my senior thesis.

He had no idea I was falling in love with him, even if I did gush about his allure to my fellow theater friends. It had been suggested to me—as kindly as possible—that I try to catch his eye by pulling myself together a bit by buying some nicer, tighter-fitting clothes and possibly toning up my arms, thighs, and abdomen at the campus gym. But I had no idea where to start. I was horrified at the idea of wearing anything smaller than a large, even though I'd come to realize that some medium-sized tops were still loose on my frame.

A friend of mine attempted to drag me to the campus gym and teach me how to use the elliptical several times over the years but to no avail. I hated being seen in exercise clothes. I was convinced the entire gym was judging me. (I could barely stand how I looked in them, and so I just assumed everyone else would agree, if not think even lower of me than I did of myself.) Even worse, I feared I'd run into my crush and risk being seen by him at my worst. Often, I'd put makeup on and then get worried about sweating it off. It always ended up being futile.

There was an alternative, however. And that was a women's-only fitness studio that I could walk to from campus in under a half hour. Sure, the trudge was trying during the colder days of the winter. But I thought at least the walking would shape me up in some way and contribute to the body I wanted to have in order to be more attractive.

The woman's gym was different from my campus fitness center. It didn't have too many mirrors. And during yoga classes—as well as the other class I'd later take involving huge straps hanging from the ceiling, called TRX—the lights in the workout room were dim. Plus, the bodies I was surrounded by weren't obnoxiously slim or insanely muscular, as I'd feared going in. They were average. In fact, I'd say I was on the skinner side of the class gamut.

But a strange thing happened as my muscles grew accustomed to the motions in the classroom. The more able I was to do the yoga postures—and, later, to move my limbs through various rotations on that TRX—the less concerned I became with how I looked while in motion. Gradually, my focus was increasingly absorbed by how it felt to master those movements. And the more of them I could figure out and repeat without flailing, the better I started to feel about myself.

In terms of weight loss, I didn't notice any drastic changes. But I did start to see the muscles in my arms and legs become a bit more prominent. Most of all, I felt my spine elongate during the days, and the way I walked became more confident. After a couple months of classes, I decided to take a risk and buy a slim-fitting pair of jeans alongside a form-fitting V-neck.

"Divya!" My theater friends exclaimed when I tried to keep my chin up as I strode into rehearsal dressed like this for the first time. I was worried they might finish that sentence with a line like, "What did you do to yourself?" or "What on earth are you wearing!?" But instead, holding my breath, I heard "My god, you look amazing!"

That social validation helped motivate me so much to persist in my efforts at the fitness center. And before I graduated, I was able to get over my fears of exercising in the campus gym. Sure, it was extremely intimidating to see girls in there who were completely comfortable inhabiting skin-tight yoga pants and stretchy workout tees. But I tried my best to just stick to what I knew I could do, inhabit my own strength, and keep my head up.

In fact, it was after one of those campus gym sessions that the lead actor in my play ended up asking me out for the first time. (I banked on the fact that he'd attribute the flush in my cheeks and the thump in my chest while we were talking to the jump squats I had just done on the set, rather than as a reaction to him acknowledging my presence with so much enthusiasm!)

We ended up dating until the end of school, after which we parted ways to return to our respective home towns and lead separate lives. But until this day, years since I've gone on to work at a small theater company in upstate New York and remain active at my local community fitness center, I've never forgotten something he said to me during our third or fourth date. "Divya, I always noticed you; even before you started changing your wardrobe. I just don't think you were aware of my interest until you learned how to notice yourself."

Key Terms

body image The self-perceptions and attitudes an individual holds with respect to their body and physical appearance.

fitspiration A message, usually in the form of an image with a quote included, designed to inspire people to attain a fitness goal.

Physical Self-Perception Profile An assessment tool based on a hierarchical, multi-dimensional theoretical model of self-esteem in which self-perceptions can be categorized as superordinate, domain, subdomain, facet, sub-facet, and state.

self-concept The multitude of attributes and roles through which a person evaluates themselves to establish self-esteem judgments.

self-esteem A stable global positive or negative evaluative of one's own worth.

self-presentation The process by which people attempt to control and monitor how they are perceived and evaluated by others.

Review Questions

1. What is the difference between self-esteem and self-concept?
2. Describe the Physical Self-Perception Profile.
3. Describe the study conducted by Justin Moore and colleagues (2011). What was the main conclusion from this study?
4. Define body image. How does body image differ from self-esteem?
5. Describe the "ideal" physique for men vs. women.
6. What is the relationship between body image and physical activity?
7. What is social physique anxiety? What is the relationship between social physique anxiety and physical activity behavior?
8. How does body image affect physical activity motivation?
9. Define the term fitspiration. Do you think that fitspirations are effective in increasing people's motivation to engage in physical activity?

Applying the Concepts

1. What concepts help explain how and why Divya's preoccupation with the way others perceived her impacted her exercise habits?
2. Why was Divya able to exercise in the woman's fitness facility more readily than at her school's gym?
3. Describe the shift in Divya's attitude toward exercise and her self-awareness while engaging in it. How might this help explain the benefits she derived from her active lifestyle?
4. How did Divya's self-concept change once she became active? How did these changes impact her self-esteem and body image?

References

Alanazi, Y. A., Sousa-Sá, E., Chong, K. H., Parrish, A., & Okely, A. D. (2021). Systematic review of the relationships between 24-hour movement behaviours and health indicators in school-aged children from Arab-speaking countries. *International Journal of Environmental Research and Public Health, 18*(16):8640. https://www.mdpi.com/1660-4601/18/16/8640

Alcaraz-Ibáñez, M., Paterna, A., Sicilia, A., & Griffiths, M. D. (2021). A systematic review and meta-analysis on the relationship between body dissatisfaction and morbid exercise behaviour. *International Journal of Environmental Research and Public Health, 18*(2), 585.

Andrade, A., Correia, C. K., & Coimbra, D. R. (2019). The psychological effects of exergames for children and adolescents with obesity: A systematic review and meta-analysis. *Cyberpsychology Behavior and Social Networking, 22*(11), 724–735. https://doi.org/10.1089/cyber.2019.0341

Baillot, A., Black, M., Brunet, J., & Romain, A. J. (2020). Biopsychosocial correlates of physical activity and sedentary time in adults with severe obesity. *Clinical Obesity, 10*(3), e12355. https://doi.org/10.1111/cob.12355

Bassett-Gunter, R., McEwan, D., & Kamarhie, A. (2017). Physical activity and body image among men and boys: A meta-analysis. *Body Image, 22*, 114–128. https://doi.org/10.1016/j.bodyim.2017.06.007

Białecka-Pikul, M., Stępień-Nycz, N., Sikorska, I., Topolewska-Siedzik, E., & Cieciuch, J. (2019). Change and consistency of self-esteem in early and middle adolescence in the context of school transition. *Journal of Youth and Adolescence, 48*, 1605–1618.

Bouzas, C., Bibiloni, M., & Tur, J. A. (2019). Relationship between body image and body weight control in overweight ≥55-year-old adults: A systematic review. *International Journal of Environmental Research and Public Health, 16*(9), 1622. https://doi.org/10.3390/ijerph16091622

Brudzynski, L. R., & Ebben, W. (2010). Body image as a motivator and barrier to exercise participation. *International Journal of Exercise Science, 3*(1), 14–24.

Campbell, A., & Hausenblas, H. A. (2009). Effects of exercise interventions on body image: A meta-analysis. *Journal of Health Psychology, 14*(6), 780–793.

Carraça, E. V., Encantado, J., Battista, F., Beaulieu, K., Blundell, J. E., Busetto, L., van Baak, M., Dicker, D., Ermolao, A., Farpour-Lambert N., Pramono, A., Woodward, E., Bellicha, A., & Oppert, J-M. (2021). Effect of exercise training on psychological outcomes in adults with overweight or obesity: A systematic review and meta-analysis. *Obesity Reviews, 22*(S4), e13261. https://doi.org/10.1111/obr.13261

Collins, H., Booth, J. N., Duncan, A., Fawkner, S., & Niven, A. (2019). The effect of resistance training interventions on 'The Self' in youth: A systematic review and meta-analysis.

Sports Medicine Open, 5(29). https://doi.org/10.1186/s40798-019-0205-0

Crawford, S., & Eklund, R. C. (1994). Social physique anxiety, reasons for exercise, and attitudes toward exercise settings. *Journal of Sport and Exercise Psychology, 16*(1), 70–82.

Ekeland, E., Heian, F., & Hagen, K. B. (2005). Can exercise improve self-esteem in children and young people? A systematic review of randomized controlled trials. *British Journal of Sports Medicine, 39*, 792–798.

Fernandes, B., Newton, J., & Essau, C. A. (2022). The mediating effects of self-esteem on anxiety and emotion regulation. *Psychological Reports, 125*(2), 787–803. https://doi.org/10.1177/0033294121996991. Epub 2021 Feb 24.

Focht, B. C., & Hausenblas, H. A. (2003). State anxiety responses to acute exercise in women with high social physique anxiety. *Journal of Sport & Exercise Psychology, 25*(2), 123–144.

Focht, B. C., & Hausenblas, H. A. (2004). Perceived evaluative threat and state anxiety during exercise in women with high social physique anxiety. *Journal of Applied Sport Psychology, 16*(4), 361–368.

Focht B. C., & Hausenblas, H. A. (2006). Exercising in public and private environments: Effects on feeling states in women with social physique anxiety. *Journal of Applied Behavioral Research, 11*(3–4), 147–165.

Fox, K. R., & Corbin, C. B. (1989). The physical self-perception profile: Development and preliminary validation. *Journal of Sport and Exercise Psychology, 11*(4), 408–430.

Frederick, D., A. Buchanan, G. M., Sadehgi-Azar, L., Peplau, L. A., Haselton, M. G., Berezovskaya, A., & Lipinski, R. E. (2007). Desiring the muscular ideal: Men's body satisfaction in the United States, Ukraine, and Ghana. *Psychology of Men & Masculinity, 8*(2), 103–117.

Halliwell, E., Dawson, K., & Burkey, S. (2019). A randomized experimental evaluation of a yoga-based body image intervention. *Body Image, 28*, 119–127.

Haugen, T., Säfvenborn, R., & Ommundsen, Y. (2011). Physical activity and global self-worth: The role of physical self-esteem indices and gender. *Mental Health and Physical Activity, 4*(2), 49–56.

Hausenblas, H. A., & Martin, K. A. (2000). Bodies on display. Predictors of social physique anxiety in female aerobic instructors. *Women in Sport and Physical Activity Journal, 9*, 1–14.

Homan, K. J., & Tylka, T. L. (2014). Appearance-based exercise motivation moderates the relationship between exercise frequency and positive body image. *Body Image, 11*(2), 101–108.

Karazsia, B. T., Murnen, S. K., & Tylka, T. L. (2017). Is body dissatisfaction changing across time? A cross-temporal meta-analysis. *Psychological Bulletin, 143*(3), 293–320.

Korn, L., Gonen, E., Shaked, Y., & Golan, M. (2013). Health perceptions, self and body image, physical activity, and nutrition among undergraduate students in Israel. *PLos One*, 8:e58543. https://doi.org/10.1371/journal.pone.0058543

Leary, M. J. (1992). Self-presentation in exercise and sport. *Journal of Sport and Exercise Psychology, 14*, 339–351.

Limniou, M., Mahoney, C., & Knox, M. (2021). Is Fitspiration the healthy Internet trend it claims to be? A British students' case study. *International Journal of Environmental Research and Public Health*, 2021 *18*(4), 1837. https://doi.org/10.3390/ijerph18041837

Liu, B., Tian, L., Yang, S., Wang, X., & Luo, J. (2022). Effects of multidimensional self-esteems on health promotion behaviors in adolescents. *Frontiers in Public Health, 26*;10:847740. https://doi.org/10.3389/fpubh.2022.847740

Mahon, C., & Seekis, V. (2022). Systematic review of digital interventions for adolescent and young adult women's body image. *Frontiers in Global Women's Health*, 3:832805. https://doi.org/10.3389/fgwh.2022.832805. eCollection 2022.

Martin, K. A., Rejeski, W. J., Leary, M. R., McAuley, E., & Bain, S. (1997). Is the Social Physique Anxiety Scale really multidimensional? Conceptual and statistical arguments for a unidimensional model. *Journal of Sport and Exercise Psychology, 19*(4), 359–367.

Martin Ginis, K. A., Strong, H. A., Arent, S. M., Bray, S. R., & Bassett-Gunter, R. L. (2014). The effects of aerobic- versus strength-training on body image among young women with pre-existing body image concerns. *Body Image, 11*(3), 219–227.

McAuley, E., Elavsky, S., Motl, R. W., Konopack, J. F., Hu, L., & Marquez D. X. (2005). Physical activity, self-efficacy, and self-esteem: Longitudinal relationships in older adults. *The Journals of Gerontology, 60B*(5), P268–P275.

Moore, J. B., Mitchell, N. G., Bibeau, W. S., & Bartholomew, J. B. (2011). Effects of a 12-week resistance exercise program on physical self-perceptions in college students. *Research Quarterly for Exercise and Sport, 82*(2), 291–301.

Niven, A., Rendell, E., & Chisholm, L. (2008). Effects of 72-h of exercise abstinence on affect and body dissatisfaction in healthy female regular exercisers. *Journal of Sports Science, 26*(11), 1235–1242.

Pearson, E. S., Hall, C. R., & Gammage, K. L. (2013). Self-presentation in exercise: Changes over a 12-week cardiovascular programme for overweight and obese sedentary females. *European Journal of Sport Sciences, 13*(4), 407–413.

Rodriguez-Ayllon, M., Cadenas-Sánchez, C., Estévez-López, F., Muñoz, N. E., Mora-Gonzalez, J. Migueles, J. H., Molina-García, P., Henriksson, H., Mena-Molina, A., Martínez-Vizcaíno, V., Catena, A., Löf, M., Erickson, K. I., Lubans, D. R., Ortega, F. B., & Esteban-Cornejo, I. (2019). Role of physical activity and sedentary behavior in the mental health of preschoolers, children and adolescents: A systematic review and meta-analysis. *Sports Medicine,*

49(9), 1383–1410. https://doi.org/10.1007/s40279-019-01099-5

Rote, A. E., Swartz, A. M., & Klos, L. A. (2013). Associations between lifestyle activity and body image attitudes among women. *Women & Health, 53*(3), 282–297.

Ruiz-Montero, P. J., Chiva-Bartoll, O., Baena-Extremera, A., Hortigüela-Alcalá, D. (2020). Gender, physical self-perception and overall physical fitness in secondary school students: A multiple mediation model. *International Journal of Environmental Research and Public Health, 17*(18), 6871. https://doi.org/10.3390/ijerph17186871

SantaBarbara, N. J., Whitworth, J. W., & Ciccolo, J. T. (2017). A systematic review of the effects of resistance training on body image. *Journal of Strength and Conditioning Research, 31*(10), 2880–2888. https://doi.org/10.1519/JSC.0000000000002135

Schmalz, D. L., Deane, G. D., Birch, L. L., & Krahnstoever Davison, K. (2007). A longitudinal assessment of the links between physical and self-esteem in early adolescent non-Hispanic females. *Journal of Adolescent Health, 41*(6), 559–565.

Shavelson, R. J., Hubner, J. J., & Stanton, G. C. (1976). Self-concept: Validation of construct interpretations. *Review of Educational Research, 46*(3), 407–441.

Sonstroem, R. J., & Morgan, W. P. (1989). Exercise and self-esteem: Rationale and model. *Medicine and Science in Sports and Exercise, 21*(3), 329–337.

Sun, W., Chen, D., Wang, J., Liu, N., & Zhang, W. (2018). Physical activity and body image dissatisfaction among pregnant women: A systematic review and meta-analysis of cohort studies. *European Journal of Obstetrics, Gynecology, and Reproductive Biology, 229*, 38–44. https://doi.org/10.1016/j.ejogrb.2018.07.021. Epub 2018 Jul 20.

Sundgot-Borgen, C., Sundgot-Borgen, J., Bratland-Sanda, S., Kolle, E., Torstveit, M. K., Svantorp-Tveiten, K. M., & Fostervold Mathisen, T. (2021). Body appreciation and body appearance pressure in Norwegian university students comparing exercise science students and other students. *BioMed Central Public Health, 21*(532), 2–11. https://link.springer.com/content/pdf/10.1186/s12889-021-10550-0.pdf

Tebar, W., Gil, F. C. S., Scarabottolo, C. C., Codogno, J. S., Fernandes, R. A. & Christofaro, D. G. (2020). Body size dissatisfaction associated with dietary pattern, overweight, and physical activity in adolescents: A cross-sectional study. *Nursing and Health Sciences, 22*(3), 749–757.

Visier-Alfonso, M. E., Sánchez-López, M., Álvarez-Bueno, C., Ruiz-Hermosa, A., Nieto-López, M., & Martínez-Vizcaíno, V. (2022). Mediators between physical activity and academic achievement: A systematic review. *Scandinavian Journal of Medicine & Science in Sports, 32*(3), 452–464. https://doi.org/10.1111/sms.14107. Epub 2021 Dec 5.

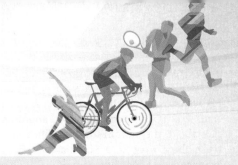

CHAPTER 13

Excessive and Addictive Exercise

LEARNING OBJECTIVES

After completing this chapter, you will be able to:

- Describe the criteria for exercise addiction, anorexia nervosa, bulimia nervosa, and muscle dysmorphia.
- Describe the relationship between physical activity and eating disorders.
- Outline the psychological effects of muscle dysmorphia.
- Understand the difference between primary and secondary exercise addiction.

Introduction

Since the "fitness boom" of the 1970s, much has been written about the benefits of exercise. Everywhere we turn, we hear that we should be more physically active, and with good reason given all the physiological, psychological, and social benefits of exercising. Does an activity with so many health benefits have the potential to be harmful? The answer is yes. For a small number of people, their exercise behavior is excessive and may possibly be an addiction. The following quote by Carl Gustav Jung, the founder of **analytical psychology**, held the belief that any type of addiction is negative. According to Jung (1957), "Every form of addiction is bad, no matter whether the narcotic be alcohol, morphine, or idealism." Although he did not specifically address exercise addiction, presumably, he would view it as negative.

It's important to emphasize that while exercise may represent an addictive behavior for a small number of people who engage in it to an extreme and unhealthy level, frequent exercise is not inherently abusive. This chapter focuses on the following three issues that are associated with excessive physical activity: (1) exercise addiction, (2) eating disorders, and (3) muscle dysmorphia. In this chapter, we will define these three excessive exercise issues, describe their significance, and examine the role that physical activity plays in each.

Exercise Addiction

Does Exercise Have Negative Health Effects?

Current exercise guidelines identify the minimum amount of exercise needed to experience health benefits. For the general adult population, most guidelines call for 150 to 300 minutes per week of moderate physical activity or 75 to 150 minutes per week of vigorous physical activity, or some equivalent combination of both intensities (Bull et al., 2020). Although increased amounts of exercise above the minimum guidelines are encouraged, there may be a point at which too much exercise may have detrimental health effects.

The idea that there's an ideal amount of exercise for health has been around for thousands of years. Hippocrates taught that "if we could give every individual the right amount of nourishment and exercise—not too little and not too much—we would have found the safest way to health." In support of Hippocrates statement, large observational studies reveal that there's likely an upper threshold for the benefits of exercise whereby higher doses of physical activity are associated with increased risk of disease and premature death (Buckley, Lip, & Thijssen, 2020; Kim et al., 2021; O'Keefe et al., 2020).

Research has also shed some preliminary insight into the question of "how much is too much" from a mental health perspective. Studies conducted with adolescents and adults revealed that very high levels of exercise results in decreased well-being (Kim et al., 2012). And a systematic review found that individuals at risk for excessive exercise show a broad range of mental disorders such as eating disorders, depression, anxiety, other substance-related and addictive disorders, and borderline personality disorder (Colledge, Sattler, Schillin, Gerber, Pühse, & Walte, 2020). Further research is needed to determine, however,

at which point physical activity may become detrimental to one's physical and mental health in varying populations.

CRITICAL THINKING ACTIVITY 13-1

Do you think there is a point at which one can engage in too much exercise? In other words, is there a point at which increased exercise duration, frequency, or intensity may have negative health outcomes?

We do know that for a very small number of people, physical activity is excessive. Rather than exercise enhancing people's lives, it ends up assuming a life of its own (Hausenblas, Schrieber, & Smoliga, 2017). These people continue to exercise despite injuries, mental health issues, and physical exhaustion. They may even watch their careers crumble and their family and friends drift away. This perspective is illustrated in the following two quotes:

> I have learned there is no need for haste, no need to worry, no need to agonize over the future . . . The world will wait. Job, family, friends will wait; in fact, they must wait on the outcome. And that outcome depends upon the lifetime that is in every day of running . . . Can anything have a higher priority than running? It defines me, adds to me, makes me whole. I have a job and a family and friends that can attest to that.
>
> (Quote from avid runner, Dr. George Sheehan, in Waters, 1981, p. 51)

As the years went on, I inevitably developed those aches and pains brought about by refusing to rest and pushing through discomfort . . . Against my doctor's orders, I stuck to my rigorous, daily workouts of 2 (or more) hours a day. The vast majority of that time was spent hunched over an elliptical machine, pursing my lips and wincing

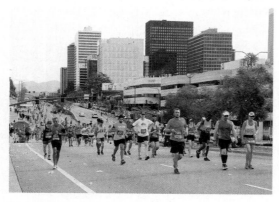

© Stella Levi/iSock/Getty Images.

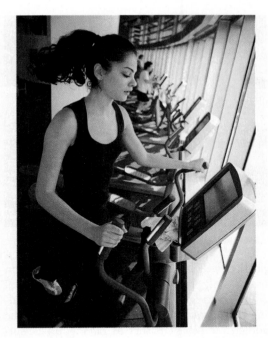

© Webphotographeer/E+/Getty Images.

Table 13-1 Adult Guidelines by Physical Activity Level and Health Benefit

Physical Activity Level	Moderate-Intensity Minutes per Week	Health Benefit
Inactive	None	None
Low	<150	Some
Medium	150–300	Substantial
High	>300	Additional

through pain. I refused to have surgery, as was clinically recommended, because it would mean too much time off from the gym.

(Schreiber & Hausenblas, 2015, p. 81)

The term often used to describe this compulsive behavior is exercise addiction. In this section, we discuss exercise addiction with regard to how it is defined, what researchers have to say about it, and how it might be treated.

Exercise Addiction Defined

Current exercise guidelines identify the minimum amount of physical activity needed to experience health benefits (see **Table 13-1**). The guidelines also recommend that an increased amount of physical activity is associated with additional benefits. For example, exercising for more than 300 minutes a week at a moderate intensity is associated with additional health benefits. Although increases above the minimum guidelines are encouraged, no cutoff exists for "how much is too much." Is there an upper limit of activity above which there are no additional health benefits?

Determining when regular exercise becomes excessive, and thus detrimental to an individual's physical and psychological health, is referred to as **exercise addiction**. Simply stated, exercise addiction is a craving for leisure-time physical activity that results in uncontrollably excessive exercise behavior that manifests itself in physiological (e.g., tolerance) and/or psychological (e.g., withdrawal) symptoms (Hausenblas & Symons Downs, 2002a). Characteristics of exercise addiction include exercising despite either injury or illness; increasing exercise volume to avoid feeling lazy; an inability to reduce exercise volume; experiencing withdrawal effects when unable to exercise (e.g., increase anxiety, tension, anger, and depression); lying to family and friends about time spent exercising; and giving up social, occupational, and family obligations to exercise (Colledge et al., 2020; Hausenblas & Symons Downs, 2002a).

It is important to emphasize that just because, for example, someone runs 6 days a week for 45 minutes a session or has been regularly weight-lifting for several years doesn't mean that they are addicted to exercise. In fact, there are thousands of people who are physically active 5, 6, or even 7 days a week who are not addicted to exercise. Addiction is not only indicated by the behavior but also by the psychological reasons underlying the behavior. One of the most difficult issues is to distinguish healthy, frequent exercise from excessive and addictive exercise.

Exercise addiction is often classified as a multidimensional maladaptive pattern of physical activity, leading to significant impairment or distress, as manifested by three or more criteria from a list of seven (APA, 2013; Hausenblas & Symons Downs (2002a). The seven criteria for exercise addiction are listed in **Table 13-2**. For example, if a person reports feelings of anxiety and depression when unable to exercise, spends little to no time with family or friends because of physical activity involvement, and continues to run despite a doctor's advice to allow an overused injury to heal, they could potentially be exercise addicted.

We often think of addiction within the context of physical addiction to drugs and alcohol. However, addiction can occur without a substance entering the body. We're talking about behavioral addiction, which simulates the same phenomenon in which a person compulsively engages in activities or behaviors despite their detrimental impact on their mental and/or

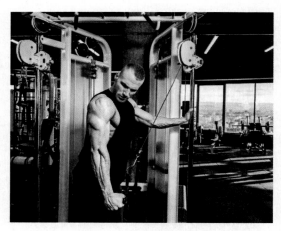

© Srdjan Randjelovic/Shutterstock.

physical well-being. Although gambling addiction is the only recognized diagnosable behavioral addiction, a growing body of research is finding that a small number of people may become addicted to behaviors such as gaming, plastic surgery, sex, social media, shopping, and exercise.

Table 13-2 Exercise Addiction Criteria

Criteria	Description	Example
Tolerance	Need for increased exercise levels to achieve the desired effect, or diminished effects experienced from the same exercise level.	Running 5 miles no longer results in improved mood.
Withdrawal	Negative symptoms are evidenced with cessation of exercise, or exercise is used to relieve or forestall the onset of these symptoms.	Anxiety, depression, and/or fatigue experienced when unable to exercise.
Intention	Exercise is undertaken with greater intensity, frequency, or duration than was intended.	Intended to run for 5 miles, but ran for 7 miles instead.
Lack of control	Exercise is maintained despite a persistent desire to cut down or control it.	Ran during lunch break despite trying to not exercise during work hours.
Time	Considerable time is spent in activities essential to exercise maintenance.	Vacations are exercise related, such as skiing or hiking.
Reduction in other activities	Social, occupational, or recreational pursuits are reduced or dropped because of exercise.	Running rather than going out with friends for dinner.
Continuance	Exercise is maintained despite the awareness of a persistent physical or psychological problem.	Running despite shin splints.

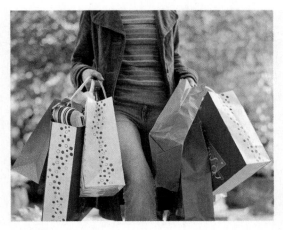

© Dylan Ellis/DigitalVision/Getty Images.

CRITICAL THINKING ACTIVITY 13-2

Do you think that exercise addiction should be a behavioral mental health addiction?

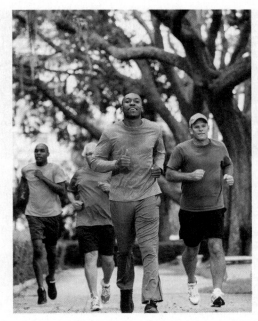

© Kali9/E+/Getty Images.

Origins of Research on Exercise Addiction

Exercise addiction was first identified by accident by Baekeland about 50 years ago. He wanted to study the common belief that exercise promotes deep sleep. To test this hypothesis, he designed a 1-month longitudinal study to examine the effects of exercise deprivation (i.e., no physical activity) on adults' sleep. Two key study findings led him to the conclusion that some people may become addicted to physical activity.

First, he encountered great difficulty recruiting high-volume male exercisers who were willing to stop exercising for 1 month. He defined high-volume as people who exercised 5 or 6 days a week. In fact, offering an increase in participant payment wasn't enticing enough to persuade these runners to stop exercising for a month. He finally was able to recruit men who regularly exercised 3 to 4 days a week. Second, during the 1-month deprivation period, the participants reported decreased psychological well-being.

Baekeland (1970) realized the importance of these complaints and designed a self-report questionnaire to assess the participants' negative moods. He found that the participants retrospectively reported that their 1 month of exercise deprivation caused increased anxiety, nighttime sleep awakening and arousal, and decreased sexual drive. In short, Baekeland found that these high volume runners refused to abstain from physical activity for a 1-month period, and regular runners reported withdrawal symptoms during physical activity deprivation.

A variety of terms have been used to describe exercise addiction such as exercise dependence, obligatory exercise, compulsive exercise, committed exercisers, morbid exercise, exercise abuse, and chronic exercise. (Hausenblas & Symons Downs, 2002a). Despite a slow and controversial beginning, in recent years, increased interest in exercise addiction has occurred because of standardized definitions and psychometrically sound measures. The exercise addiction research is characterized by four general approaches: (1) comparing exercisers to eating disorder patients, (2) determining the prevalence of exercise addiction in various populations, (3) examining correlates of exercise addiction,

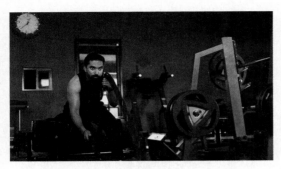

© WESTOCK PRODUCTIONS/Shutterstock.

and (4) examining the effects of exercise deprivation on mood. Each of these research areas will be discussed in more detail below.

Prevalence of Exercise Addiction

Prevalence represents the proportion of a population found to have a condition. Many researchers have been interested in trying to determine how many people are addicted to exercise. Hausenblas and Symons Downs (2002b) examined the prevalence of exercise dependence symptoms in over 2,300 exercisers. The Exercise Dependence Scale (see **Table 13-3** for sample items from this measure) was used

to assess the prevalence of exercise addiction in this physically active population. This scale operationalizes exercise addiction based on the DSM-IV criteria for substance dependence. When completing the scale, participants were asked to refer to their current exercise beliefs and behaviors that had occurred in the past 3 months. The researchers found that approximately 7% of the exercisers were classified as at-risk for exercise addiction, 61% as nonaddicted-symptomatic (i.e., displayed some exercise addiction symptoms), and 32% as non-addicted-asymptomatic (i.e., displayed no exercise addiction symptoms).

Hausenblas and Symons Downs (2002b) also found a hierarchy of responses for vigorous exercise level, self-efficacy, and **perfectionism**. Participants classified as at-risk for exercise addiction scored higher on self-efficacy and perfectionism and engaged in more vigorous exercise than those classified as nonaddicted-symptomatic and individuals classified as non-addicted-symptomatic scored higher than those classified as nonaddicted-asymptomatic. This correlational study used self-report measures, thus, cause–effect conclusions aren't possible. We can't say, for example, that being perfectionistic causes an individual to be exercise addicted.

Table 13-3 Sample Items from the Exercise Dependence Scale

Subscale	Item
Tolerance	I continually increase my exercise duration to achieve the desired effects/benefits.
Withdrawal effects	I exercise to avoid feeling tense.
Continuance	I exercise despite persistent physical problems.
Lack of control	I am unable to reduce how intensely I exercise.
Reduction in other activities	I choose to exercise so that I can get out of spending time with family/friends.
Time	A great deal of my time is spent exercising.
Intention effects	I exercise longer than I plan.

Data from Hausenblas, H. A., & Symons Downs, D. (2002b). How much is too much? The development and validation of the Exercise Dependence Scale. *Psychology and Health: An International Journal, 17*, 387–404.

Reviews of prevalence research have found that exercise addiction varies by population and activity (Trott et al., 2020, 2021). For example, the prevalence of exercise addiction was about 8% among general exercisers, 5% for amateur competitive athletes, and 5.5% for university students. For sport type, endurance athletes were found to be most at risk (14.2%) followed by ball game athletes (10.4%), fitness center attendees (8.2%), and power athletes (6.4%; Di Lodovico, Poulnais, & Gorwood, 2019). Also, the prevalence of exercise addiction may vary among university majors with students in nutrition, exercise, and health-related fields potentially being at higher risk (Rocks et al., 2017).

Researchers have also determined the prevalence of exercise addiction with other types of addictions. In other words, do people who are addicted to exercise also have a higher chance of being addicted to other behaviors (e.g., shopping, Internet use, gambling, smartphone use) or substances (e.g., nicotine, alcohol)? A high co-occurrence of exercise addiction with other types of addictions exists (Ertl et al., 2022). For example, in a sample of 2,853 Italian high school students, Villella and colleagues (2011) found that exercise addiction, compulsive buying, internet addiction, and work addiction were positively related. The strong relationship among these different addictions is in line with the hypothesis of a common psychopathological dimension underlying them.

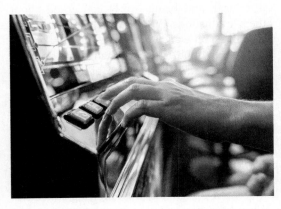

© Tomasz Zajda/EyeEm/Getty Images.

Correlates of Exercise Addiction

Researchers have been interested in examining correlates or variables that will help identify if someone may be at risk for exercise addiction. Several demographic, social, behavioral, and psychological correlates of exercise addiction have been identified (Alcaraz-Ibáñez, Paterna, Sicilia, & Griffiths, 2021; Bueno-Antequera, et al., 2020; Colledge et al., 2020; Grima, Estrada-Marcén, & Montero-Marín, 2019; Lukács, Sasvári, Varga, & Maye, 2019). These exercise addiction correlates are described in more detail in the following section and summarized in **Table 13-4**.

Psychological Correlates

Exercise addiction symptoms are associated with certain personality characteristics such as anxiety, hostility, and harm-avoidance behaviors. Researchers have also found a positive relationship of exercise addiction with extraversion and neuroticism, and a negative relationship with agreeableness. In other words, people reporting high exercise addiction symptoms may be more extraverted, more neurotic, and less agreeable than individuals low in exercise addiction symptoms (Andereassen et al., 2013).

What are some potential explanations for why agreeableness, extraversion, and neuroticism are related to exercise addiction? Highly neurotic people have limited impulse control, cope poorly with stress, and are often irrational. It is plausible that people reporting high exercise addiction symptoms may be using exercise as a maladaptive coping strategy for their stress. People who display high neuroticism scores may be prone to excessive worry or concern over their appearance or their health. In an effort

Table 13-4 Correlates of Exercise Addiction Symptoms

Category	Correlate	Relationship
Demographic	Age	Younger adults at increased risk over older adults
	Attention Deficient Hyperactivity Disorder (ADHD)	Positive relationship between childhood ADHD
Psychological	Extraversion	Positive
	Neuroticism	Positive
	Agreeableness	Negative
	Perfectionism	Positive
	Self-esteem	Negative Positive
	Anxiety	Positive
	Depression	Positive
	Social Physique Anxiety	Positive
	Body dissatisfaction	Positive
	Exercise identity	Positive
Behavioral	Exercise volume	Positive
	Participating in childhood sports	Positive
	Pain and overuse injuries	Positive
Social	Loneliness	Positive

to reduce these concerns, neurotic individuals may use excessive exercise as a maladaptive coping strategy to either avoid or relieve their withdrawal symptoms.

People with high extraversion are characterized as assertive, energetic, active, upbeat, and as liking excitement. Because a behavioral component of exercise addiction is excessive exercise, it may not be surprising that these individuals report being energetic, active, and upbeat. Finally, people low in agreeableness tend to be egocentric, skeptical of others' intentions, and competitive. These people may also view flattery or deception as a necessary social skill. Thus, less sympathetic, altruistic, and cooperative people tend to have more exercise addiction symptoms.

Perfectionism is a personality trait characterized by a person's striving for flawlessness, setting high performance standards, being extremely self-critical, and being overly concerned about others' evaluations. A positive relationship exists between exercise addiction symptoms and perfectionism (Hausenblas & Symons Downs, 2002b). Individuals classified as at-risk for exercise addiction scored higher on perfectionism than those classified as nonaddicted-symptomatic, whereas the latter scored higher than those classified as nonaddicted-asymptomatic.

Exercise identity is the extent that exercise is descriptive of one's self-concept. Someone who has high exercise identity would most likely strongly agree to the following statement: "When I describe myself to other people, I usually include my involvement in physical exercise" (Anderson & Cychosz, 1994). Not surprisingly, exercise identity is an important determinant of regular exercise behavior and exercise addiction symptoms. Researchers have found that a stronger exercise identity is associated with greater odds of experiencing exercise addiction symptoms (Lu et al., 2012).

Self-esteem may be a protective factor against exercise addiction (Gori et al., 2021). Low self-esteem is a characteristic of an addictive personality, and **social physique anxiety** (i.e., anxiety related to the public presentation of one's image) is positively related to exercise addiction (Cook et al., 2015).

Demographic Correlates

Regarding the relationship between age and exercise addiction, most studies have examined college students. Depending on the sample size and the degree of sophistication of the research design, this can produce valuable information and insights regarding exercise addiction in general. However, the focus on college students and the absence of cross-sectional analyses from different age groups of exercisers makes it difficult to explore risk factors for exercise addiction prevalence by age. The prevalence for exercise addiction tends to decline with age as older exercisers develop a more balanced lifestyle. This is not surprising considering the negative relationship between exercise behavior and age, with older adults being less likely to exercise than younger populations. This may be due to the fact that physical activity levels decrease with age and that older adults may be able to regulate their emotions better than younger adults, thus reducing their risk of exercise addiction.

Attention-deficit hyperactivity disorder (ADHD) is one of the most common childhood disorders and can continue through adolescence and into adulthood. Symptoms include difficulty staying focused and paying attention, difficulty controlling behavior, and hyperactivity. The symptoms of ADHD usually cause functional impairment in social, occupational, and academic activities.

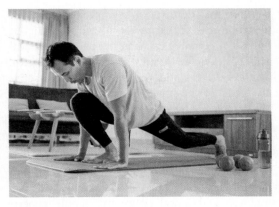

© Odua Images/Shutterstock.

Using a retrospective design, Berger and his colleagues (2014) examined the associations of ADHD with exercise addiction symptoms in 1,615 German adults. The adults completed a retrospective assessment of both their childhood and adult ADHD. Their exercise addiction symptoms were assessed via the Exercise Dependence Scale. Adults with childhood-only ADHD had a higher frequency of exercise addiction symptoms than adults without ADHD. More specifically, 9% of the adults with childhood-only ADHD displayed exercise addiction symptoms, compared with only 2.7% of adults without childhood ADHD. These results reveal that excessive exercising is overrepresented in people in which ADHD symptoms in childhood have not persisted into adulthood. It is plausible that some adults may suppress ADHD symptoms by excessive exercise.

Exercise Deprivation

Exercise deprivation sensations (also referred to as exercise withdrawal symptoms) are cardinal identifying components of exercise addiction. These sensations represent the psychological and physiological effects that occur when regular exercisers either reduce or stop exercising. The individual may either experience withdrawal symptoms, such as anxiety and fatigue, because of a lack of exercise, or engage in exercise to either relieve or avoid the onset of the withdrawal symptoms.

Exercise deprivation symptoms arise for the same reason that regular exercise results in positive psychological states. That is, physical activity leads to positive psychological states, whereas the cessation of regular physical activity leads to negative psychological states or reductions in the positive psychological states. The most frequently reported feelings resulting from exercise deprivation are guilt, depression, irritability, restlessness, tension, stress, anxiety, confusion, anger, and sluggishness (Weinstein, Koehmstedt, & Kop, 2017). **Table 13-5** lists common withdrawal symptoms people experience during exercise deprivation. It's important to emphasize that exercise deprivation sensations are experienced by both nonaddicted and addicted exercisers, with larger withdrawal effects experienced by addicted exercisers (Antunes et al., 2016).

One noteworthy study of exercise deprivation was undertaken by Gregory Mondin and his colleagues (1996) at the University of Madison-Wisconsin. They examined the effects of 3 days of exercise deprivation on mood states and anxiety in 10 male and female regular runners. Participants had to run at least 6 to 7 days a week for a minimum duration of 45 minutes per session to be classified as a regular runner.

In this study, the runners completed their regular workout on the Monday, refrained from physical activity on the Tuesday, Wednesday, and Thursday, and then resumed their regular physical activity on the Friday. Also, on the no-exercising days, the participants limited their lifestyle physical activity. For example, they were asked to take the bus instead of biking to work, park close to buildings to minimize walking, and take the elevator instead of the stairs. Mood and state anxiety were assessed each day. The researchers found that the participants displayed increased mood disturbance and anxiety during the no-exercise days. When physical activity was resumed on the Friday, participants' positive mood improved and their anxiety decreased. See **Figure 13-1** for a graphic display of the anxiety results. The researchers concluded that a brief period of physical activity deprivation in regular exercisers results in mood disturbance within 24 hours.

Eating Disorders

Excessive physical activity is a potential eating disorder symptom. Unfortunately, there is no consensus on how to define and conceptualize excessive amounts of exercise with regard to eating disorders. In this section, we describe two eating disorders, anorexia nervosa and bulimia nervosa, and the role that excessive exercise plays in their development and maintenance.

Table 13-5 Exercise Deprivation Symptoms

Affective	Cognitive	Physiological	Social
Anxiety	Confusion	Muscle soreness	Increased need for social interaction
Depression	Impaired concentration	Disturbed sleep	
Irritability		Lethargy	
Hostility		Fatigue	
Anger		Increased galvanic skin response	
Tension		Gastrointestinal problems	
Guilt		Decreased vigor	
Frustration		Increased pain	
Sexual tension			
Decreased self-esteem			

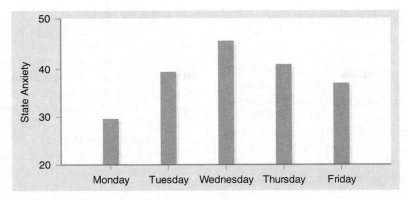

Figure 13-1 Exercise Deprivation Study: State Anxiety Scores Across the Week.

Data from Mondin, G. W., Morgan, W. P., Piering, P. N., Stegner, A. J., Stotesbery, C. L., Trine, M. R., & Wu, M. (1996). Psychological consequences of exercise deprivation in habitual exercisers. *Medicine and Science in Sports and Exercise, 28*, 1199–1203.

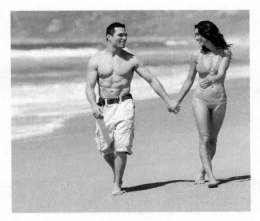

© Jacob Wackerhausen/iStock/Getty Images Plus/Getty Images.

Anorexia Nervosa

The criteria for **anorexia nervosa** includes an intense and unrealistic fear of becoming fat and engaging in behaviors intended to produce distinct weight loss (see **Table 13-6**). The disturbance of self-evaluation and consequential denial of the severity of one's low weight are defined as maintaining a weight that is less than 85% of what is considered an ideal body weight for that person (APA, 2015). Although anorexia nervosa can affect men and women of any age, race, and socioeconomic and cultural background, anorexia nervosa is 10 times more common in female than male populations.

Table 13-6 Diagnostic Criteria for Anorexia Nervosa and Bulimia Nervosa

Anorexia Nervosa	Bulimia Nervosa
Persistent restriction of energy intake leading to significantly low body weight (in context of what is minimally expected for age, sex, developmental trajectory, and physical health).	Recurrent episodes of binge eating.
Either an intense fear of gaining weight or of becoming fat, persistent behavior that interferes with weight gain (even though significantly low weight).	Recurrent inappropriate compensatory behavior in order to prevent weight gain (e.g., self-induced vomiting, excessive exercise).
Disturbance in the way one's body weight or shape is experienced, undue influence of body shape and weight on self-evaluation, or persistent lack of recognition of the seriousness of the current low body weight.	Binge eating and inappropriate compensatory behaviors occuring, on average, at least once a week for 3 months.
	Body image disturbance.

Bulimia Nervosa

The criteria for **bulimia nervosa** are an intense fear of becoming fat, powerful urges to overeat, and subsequent binges that are followed by engaging in some sort of purging or compensatory behavior in an attempt to avoid the fattening effects of excessive caloric intake (see Table 13-6). Similar to anorexia nervosa, the fear that people experience with bulimia nervosa is in regard to self-evaluation resulting in compensatory behaviors in an attempt to avoid weight gain. The paradox is the presence of **binge eating**, which is defined as uncontrollable urges to overeat. These binges must occur within 2 hours and include an amount of food that is larger than most people would consume in a similar setting with a sense of lack of control during the binge. Compensatory behaviors are separated into purging type (i.e., self-induced vomiting; use of laxatives, diuretics, or enemas; or medication abuse) and nonpurging type (i.e., other compensatory behaviors, such as fasting or exercising excessively). Unlike anorexia nervosa, there is no criterion defining maintenance of body weight or presence of amenorrhea.

Bulimia nervosa is considered to be less life threatening than anorexia nervosa; however, the occurrence of bulimia nervosa is higher. Bulimia nervosa is nine times more likely to occur in women than men. Most people with bulimia nervosa are normal weight. Antidepressants are widely used in treating bulimia nervosa. Patients who have bulimia nervosa often also have impulsive behaviors involving overspending and sexual behaviors, as well as family histories of alcohol and substance abuse and mood and eating disorders.

Eating Disorders and Exercise Addiction

People with eating disorders have a 3.5× increased risk of developing exercise addiction than people without an eating disorders (Trott et al., 2020, 2021). A distinction is often made between primary exercise addiction and secondary exercise addiction with regard to eating disorders.

Primary exercise addiction is defined as meeting the criteria for exercise addiction and exercising solely for the psychological gratification resulting from the exercise behavior itself. **Secondary exercise addiction** is defined as meeting the criteria for exercise addiction but using excessive exercise to accomplish some other end (e.g., weight loss or body composition changes) that is related to an eating disorder. Thus, for secondary exercise addiction, the excessive exercise is secondary to an eating disorder and the main motivation for physical activity is to control and/or change body composition.

Male populations tend to display more primary exercise addiction symptoms than female populations. Although the prevalence of primary exercise dependence tends to be lower among women, the severity of their symptoms is comparable to that in men.

CRITICAL THINKING ACTIVITY 13-4

What are some plausible explanations for why male populations are more at risk for primary exercise addiction than female populations?

CRITICAL THINKING ACTIVITY 13-5

What is the difference between primary and secondary exercise addiction? Why is it important From a treatment standpoint to differentiate between the two types of exercise addiction?

Despite a lack of compelling empirical evidence, a misconception exists that excessive exercise leads to developing an eating disorder. In fact, despite that earlier models of treatment recommended complete abstinence from exercise in eating-disorder populations, recent guidelines advocate for the gradual inclusion of healthier forms of exercise into an overall treatment plan (Hausenblas, Cook, & Chittester, 2008; Martenstyn, Touyz, & Maguire, 2021).

In an attempt to understand the relationship between exercise and eating disorders,

Hausenblas and colleagues (2008) developed the exercise and eating disorders model (see **Figure 13-2**). The exercise and eating disorders model states that regular exercise is associated with improvements in several physiological measures (i.e., cardiovascular health, metabolism, adiposity, and bone density), psychological measures (i.e., body image, depression, anxiety, stress reactivity, and self-esteem), and social benefits that are risk and maintenance factors for eating disorders. The exercise and eating disorders model has consolidated and supported several narrative and meta-analytic reviews that highlight that exercise makes positive improvements on eating disorder risk, development, and maintenance factors.

The model also extends our current understanding of the relationship between exercise and health status by including exercise addiction, which may explain why developing an eating disorder may supersede the benefits of exercise. Simply stated, this model posits that, in the absence of pathological psychological factors such as exercise addiction, the benefits conveyed by regular exercise (e.g., improvements in depression, anxiety, stress reactivity, self-esteem, body composition) may counteract the risk factors for eating disorders (e.g., body dissatisfaction, depression, anxiety, increased body mass).

Researchers have found initial support for the exercise and eating disorder model. For example, Cook and colleagues (2011) had 539 university students complete self-report measures of physical and psychological quality of life, exercise behavior, eating disorder risk, and exercise dependence symptoms. Structural

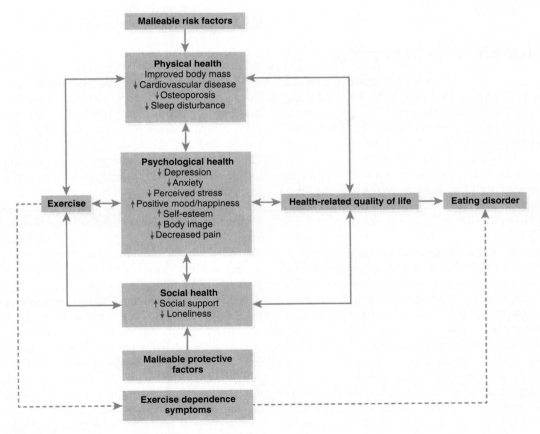

Figure 13-2 Exercise and Eating Disorders Model.

equation modeling analysis found support for the mediation effect of exercise dependence on eating disorders, as well as the effect of psychological well-being on eating disorders. Together, exercise behavior, psychological well-being, and exercise dependence symptoms predicted 23% of the variation in eating disorders. These results indicated that the psychological health benefits conveyed by exercise reduced eating disorder risk.

Initial tests of the exercise and eating disorders model suggest that the model may combine two divergent lines of research (Cook, Hausenblas, Crosby, Cao, & Wonderlich, 2015); that is, exercise may play a role in developing an eating disorder when exercise addiction is simultaneously present. Similarly, the psychological health benefits of exercise may also reduce eating disorder risk for individuals without exercise addiction.

Muscle Dysmorphia

Muscle dysmorphia is an illness characterized by an intense preoccupation that one is not big enough or sufficiently muscular, despite often being larger and more muscular than the average person. Although this phenomenon is recognized in bodybuilding communities under the term bigorexia since the 1980s, it did not receive scientific attention until Harvard researchers identified that approximately 10% of the bodybuilders they were studying had irrational beliefs that they were too small (Pope et al., 1997). They labeled this disorder as reverse anorexia. It was later renamed as muscle dysmorphia, and a set of diagnostic criteria was proposed that placed the compulsive need to exercise at the crux of muscle dysmorphia symptomology. Although the literature on muscle dysmorphia is still in its infancy, it's considered a subtype of the obsessive mental disorder called body dysmorphic disorder.

In muscle dysmorphia, the delusional or exaggerated belief is that one's own body is too small, too skinny, insufficiently muscular, or insufficiently lean, although in most cases, the individual's build is normal or even large

and muscular. In other words, a person suffering with muscle dysmorphia will most likely perceive themselves to lack muscles despite being very muscular. These delusions lead to the pathological pursuit of muscularity through excessive exercise (often resistance training) and dietary practices that take precedence over other important areas of life (Cooper et al., 2020).

Pope and colleagues (1997), in their discussion of muscle dysmorphia, provided the following example:

> All of his waking hours are consumed with preoccupations of getting bigger. He tries to resist these thoughts but reports success only half of the time. He weighs himself 2–3 times daily and checks mirrors 10–12 times a day to monitor his physique. He wears baggy sweatshirts and long pants even in the heat of summer to disguise his perceived smallness. (p. 554)

Many terms have been used to describe muscle dysmorphia, including bodybuilding anorexia, inverse anorexia, reverse anorexia, megorexia nervosa, bigameraria, and vigorexia. People with muscle dysmorphia are: (1) pathologically preoccupied with the appearance of the whole body; (2) concerned that they are not sufficiently large or muscular; and (3) are consumed by weightlifting, dieting, and steroid abuse. As a consequence, these people experience profound distress about having their bodies seen in public, exhibit impaired social and occupational functioning, and may abuse anabolic steroids and other drugs.

Other behavioral signs of muscle dysmorphia, include excessively working out and lifting weights; repeatedly counting calories; avoiding eating out at restaurants due to perceived lack of control over food content; balancing carbohydrates, fats, proteins, and vitamins to achieve a "perfect" formula; eating multiple meals throughout the day at rigidly adhered to schedules; excessively checking mirrors or other reflective surfaces; avoiding mirrors or other reflective surfaces; and avoiding social situations where bodies may be on display, such as at the beach or pool.

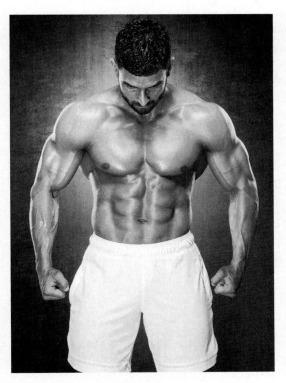

© MR.BIG-PHOTOGRAPHY/iStock/Getty Images Plus/Getty Images.

Correlates of Muscle Dsymorphia

A positive relationship exists between Muscle dysmorphia and **drive for muscularity**, general anxiety, social physique anxiety, body dissatisfaction, disordered eating, anabolic steroid abuse, mood disorders, depression, neuroticism, perfectionism, exercise addiction, and mood intolerance all have a positive relationship. In comparison, a negative relationship exists between muscle dysmorphia and perceived body attractiveness and self-esteem. Also, the severity of muscle dsymorphia is greatest in competing bodybuilders compared with noncompeting bodybuilders. Finally, men are more at-risk for muscle dysmorphia than women (Bégin, Turcotte, & Rodrigue, 2019; Cooper et al., 2020).

A study by Italian researchers found that 5% of university students had traits of muscle dysmorphia (Gorrasi et al., 2020). They also found

that students in the sport sciences had higher levels of muscle dysmorphia than students in the health sciences, business, and humanities. Additionally, students with muscle dysmorphia traits were more likely to be on a diet and were at increased risk for an eating disorder. Exercise is a main focus for individuals with muscle dysmorphia. In particular, resistance exercise (i.e., weightlifting and bodybuilding) is often undertaken to attain increased muscle mass and decreased fat mass. Ironically, exercise amounts and intensities are often increased despite the fact that people with muscle dysmorphia often possess a large muscular physique that actually meets or exceeds the cultural ideal. Because the preoccupation with one's body is pathological, reaching a level of satisfaction with one's body is not attained despite a muscular appearance. The resulting increases in musculature from increased amounts of exercise often plateau, thus further contributing to body dissatisfaction. Consequently, physically active individuals with muscle dysmorphia often follow a diet of high-protein and low-fat foods along with dietary and ergogenic supplements to reduce body fat.

Muscle Dysmorphia Measures

As with other psychological issues, muscle dysmorphia is often measured with self-report measures. **Table 13-7** provides sample items from commonly used measures of muscle dysmorphia and drive for muscularity.

Summary

This chapter examined some potential negative effects of exercise: exercise addiction, eating disorders, and muscle dysmorphia. For some people, exercise may represent a negative behavior when it becomes excessive, and it can be associated with pathological behaviors such as binging, purging, extreme body dissatisfaction, and steroid use. It is important to emphasize, however, that exercise is largely a positive behavior—a behavior that few adults engage in on a regular basis.

Table 13-7 Examples of Muscle Dysmorphia Measure Items

Scale	Sample Items
Drive for Muscularity Attitudes Questionnaire (Morrison & Morrison, 2004) Measured on a Likert-type scale (1 "strongly disagree" to 5 "strongly agree").	Being muscular gives me confidence. I would like to be more muscular in the future. I feel less of a man when I have small muscles than when I have large muscles. I think I need to gain a few pounds of "bulk" (muscle mass).
Drive for Muscularity Scale (McCreary & Sasse, 2000) Measured on a Likert-type scale (1 "always" to 6 "never").	I wish that I were more muscular. I lift weights to build up muscle. I use protein or energy supplements. I think about taking anabolic steroids. I think that my legs are not muscular enough.

Vignette: Katie

It began when I was living with 14 other girls at a residential facility in Connecticut designed to provide support to emotionally troubled teens. In the 45 minutes a day that I was permitted privacy in my own room, I spun through 100 repetitions of lunges, squats, jumping jacks, crunches, and as many pushups as I could manage. This was all in the hopes of proving to myself and to my body, that I had control over something: that I could make myself smaller.

I'd arrived at the residential facility following a 9-week stay at a boot camp program in Naples, Idaho, that my parents believed might put an end to my pot smoking, my self-harm, and my promiscuity. I was barely 13. Their confusion and concern and their own painful divorce added up to me being too much for either of them to handle. So they sent me away.

Since middle school, I saw my body as defective. I was the last girl in my grade to develop breasts, and the first to be excluded from popular lunch tables and after-school gatherings buzzing with queen bees. I intuited something was inherently wrong with me. And that belief took root in my nascent identity, growing over time into a lifelong self-loathing, fueled by a hypervigilance

toward how big or how loud or how unattractive I might, at any moment, suddenly become. I did not believe I could let my guard down. Ever. I felt I always had to be doing something to make myself better. Relaxation and pleasure quickly became enemies.

The first culprit was my face. In sixth grade, I'd hide in the bathroom with a turtleneck sweater pulled up over my lips and my nose, refusing to return to class for fear I was too ugly to be seen. The second culprit was my legs—too chicken-like, I thought. I wanted a round backside. Thicker thighs, like my female classmates who got to bask in male attention. I thought if I looked more like them, I wouldn't be as inferior—so unlovable.

Ironically, I strove toward putting on weight at first, hoping to be softer around my edges like the girls at the top of the social totem pole. Then, as time went on and I learned what society deemed attractive—heard the praise heaped on those who could keep their figures in check—my drive to grow larger reversed course. Minimization—reaching my smallest possible size—took precedence above all other goals.

I grew up in Manhattan, a city stuffed to the brim with conspicuous thinness. Women were lauded for svelte physiques and shamed for even the slightest suggestions of corpulence. My father chastised my mother for how high the numbers got on our bathroom scale after she gave birth to me.

"I just stopped finding her attractive," he would say to me over phone calls after he'd moved out.

And when I reached for a box of cookies in his new apartment, he looked at me coldly and said, "You don't want to look like your mother, do you?"

After I left the residential facility and returned to high school—sober now and hell-bent on getting perfect grades so as to disprove my teachers' assumptions that I would be some kind of failure—I discovered the gym. Here was another tool to aid me in manipulating my body—in pummeling myself into something tighter, smaller, more productively controlled. Even better, I could use "having to work out" as an excuse to escape the social anxiety I felt whenever friends asked me to "hang out."

The gym organized me. It gave me a schedule. It justified and dictated whatever I ate. Carbs were permissible if used as fuel. Protein and fat for recovery. Several months into a regular routine, I began to find satisfaction in what I saw in the mirror. To like my own reflection was intoxicating enough to keep me coming back. I was not used to taking pride in my body. And I clung to this new transient confidence, terrified to return to its absence. This meant hitting the gym constantly. Daily. Avoiding stillness at all costs.

Working out wove itself into the fabric of who I was. "Gym rat." "Yoga freak." "Exercise addict," people would call me. All compliments to my stubborn prioritization of burning calories over developing meaningful relationships or spending any modicum of extended time with my family.

By the time I entered college, my world revolved around the gym. No sooner would I finish a class than I'd dash off to the campus fitness center. I'd dabbled in treatment at an outpatient eating disorder clinic prior to my freshman year, but I was unsatisfied by their focus on food. Sure, I had issues surrounding what I ate. But my main problem was my compulsive zeal for physical activity. I had to get to the gym or else anxiety, depression, self-hatred, and a crumbling sense of helplessness would consume me. No matter how tired or sick or stressed or busy I was, I would go. Getting on that elliptical machine, going for that run, lifting those weights, or cycling through that yoga routine was nonnegotiable. Few treatment professionals I met with seemed to understand this and approach it as its own unique disorder.

By the time I graduated college, 99 pounds gripping my 5-foot, 6-inch frame, I could count on two hands the number of friendships and career opportunities I'd lost due to being barely available outside of my exercise schedule.

Injuries ensued. By 26, I'd weathered two herniated discs in my spine, a stress fracture in my left foot, and a persistent exhaustion that, no matter how much sleep I got in between gym sessions, never abated. Although I would seek treatment for exercise addiction time and again, my obsession with burning calories and lifting weights would creep back into my life, leaking around the edges of whatever job or hobby or interest outside physical activity I managed to take hold of.

Although I have been able to find love and connection, my ability to participate in relationships is severely limited by my obsession with working out. I feel lucky to have a life partner who tries his best not to take my compulsions personally, and squeezes himself into the narrow time slots left around my hours spent exercising.

Traveling is incredibly difficult for me. My obsessiveness surrounding my routines has grown so thick that even most hotel gym equipment won't suffice. I crave the specificities of my home gym's setup. So enmeshed have I become in my routine that I am terrified to face change, to be uprooted from that which I know offers me a respite from anxiety—over my appearance, at the prospect of losing control, or the overwhelming nature of any given day's tasks. I am equally addicted to the familiarity of my rituals surrounding physical activity as I am to its physiological effects. I know that the behavior has more control over me than I have over it. Yet, it is so much of who I am that I can't unravel myself from the transient solace that comes after each daily exercise session.

I want to believe there will be a day when I can sit still in my skin. When I won't wake up dreading the 2-hour workouts I can't seem to say no to, despite the havoc they wreak on my schedule, my mental stability, and my connections to other people. But I know from over 25 years of being in this body, being trapped in this cycle,

that it's going to take years to undo the habitual self-abuse that is my daily routine. And to me, the saddest part of all of this is that no matter how haggard I look at the gym, or how sick I feel myself to be, there is always someone—a fellow gym-goer, a trainer—who waits for me to come out of a handstand or demount an elliptical machine to tell me, "whatever you're doing, keep it up—it's great."

Key Terms

analytical psychology The psychoanalytic system of psychology developed and practiced by Carl Jung.

anorexia nervosa Eating disorder characterized by an intense and unrealistic fear of becoming fat and engaging in behaviors intended to produce distinct weight loss.

binge eating Eating a large amount of food in a discrete period of time.

bulimia nervosa Eating disorder characterized by recurrent overeating and use of inappropriate measures to prevent weight gain afterward, such as purging, fasting, or exercising excessively.

drive for muscularity Individual's perception that they are not muscular enough and that bulk should be added to their body frame in the form of muscle mass (irrespective of a person's percentage of actual muscle mass or body fat).

exercise addiction Craving for leisure-time physical activity that results in uncontrollably excessive exercise behavior that manifests itself in

physiological (e.g., tolerance) and/or psychological (e.g., withdrawal) symptoms.

exercise identity The extent that exercise is descriptive of one's self-concept.

muscle dysmorphia Psychological disorder characterized by the preoccupation with the idea that one's body is not lean and muscular.

perfectionism Striving for flawlessness and perfection and accompanied by critical self-evaluations.

primary exercise addiction Meeting the criteria for exercise addiction and exercising solely for the psychological gratification resulting from the exercise behavior itself.

secondary exercise addiction Meeting the criteria for exercise addiction, but using excessive exercise to accomplish some other end (e.g., weight loss or body composition changes) that is related to an eating disorder.

social physique anxiety Anxiety related to the public presentation of one's image.

Review Questions

1. Define exercise addiction. What are the seven criteria for a diagnosis of exercise addiction?

2. What is the relationship between personality and exercise addiction?

3. Describe exercise deprivation and the symptoms that exercise-addicted individuals may experience when deprived of exercise.

4. Describe the diagnostic criteria for anorexia nervosa and bulimia nervosa.

5. What is the difference between primary and secondary exercise addiction?

6. Describe the exercise and eating disorder model developed by Hausenblas and colleagues. What does the research tell us about this model?

7. Define muscle dysmorphia. What other terms are used to describe muscle dysmorphia?

Applying the Concepts

1. Do you think that Katie exhibits primary or secondary exercise addiction? What aspects of her behavior indicate one over the other?

2. What criteria of exercise addiction does Katie exhibit?

References

Alcaraz-Ibáñez, M., Paterna, A., Sicilia, A., & Griffiths, M. D. (2021). A systematic review and meta-analysis on the relationship between body dissatisfaction and morbid exercise behaviour. *International Journal of Environmental Research and Public Health, 18*(2), 585.

American Psychiatric Association. (2013). Diagnostic and statistical manual of mental disorders (5th ed.).

Anderson, D. F., & Cychosz, C. M. (1994). Development of an exercise identity scale. *Perceptual and Motor Skills, 78*(3), 747–751.

Antunes, H. K., Leite, G. S., Lee, K. S., Barreto, A. T., dos Santos, R. V., de Souza, H., Tufik S., & de Mello, M. T. (2016). Exercise deprivation increases negative mood in exercise-addicted subjects and modifies their biochemical markers. *Physiology & Behavior, 156*, 182–190. https://doi .org/10.1016/j.physbeh.2016.01.028. Epub 2016 Jan 23.

Baekeland, F. (1970). Exercise deprivation: Sleep and psychological reactions. *Archives of General Psychiatry, 22*(4), 365–369.

Bégin, C., Turcotte, O., & Rodrigue, C. (2019). Psychosocial factors underlying symptoms of muscle dysmorphia in a non-clinical sample of men. *Psychiatry Research, 272*, 319–325. https://doi.org/10.1016/j.psychres.2018.12.120

Berger, N. A., Müller, A., Brähler, E., Philipsen, A., & de Zwaan, M. (2014). Association of symptoms of attention-deficit/hyperactivity disorder with symptoms of excessive exercising in an adult general population sample. *BioMed Central Psychiatry, 14*(250). https://doi.org/10.1186 /s12888-014-0250-7

Buckley, B. J., Lip, G. Y., & Thijssen, D. H. (2020). The counterintuitive role of exercise in the prevention and cause of atrial fibrillation. *American Journal of Physiology. Heart and Circulation Physiology, 319*(5), H1051–H1058. https://doi.org/10.1152/ajpheart.00509.2020

Bueno-Antequera, J., Mayolas-Pi, C., Reverter-Masià, J., López-Laval, I., Oviedo-Caro, M. A., Munguia-Izquierdo D., Ruidiaz-Peña M., & Legaz-Arrese, A. (2020). Exercise addiction and its relationship with health outcomes in indoor cycling practitioners in fitness centers. *International Journal of Environmental Research and Public Health, 17*(11), 4159. https://doi.org/10.3390/ijerph17114159

Bull, F. C., Al-Ansari, S. S., Biddle, S., Borodulin, K., Buman, M. P., . . . Willumsen, J. F. (2020). World Health Organization 2020 guidelines on physical activity and sedentary behaviour. *British Journal of Sports Medicine, 54*(24), 1451–1462.

Colledge, R., Cody, R., Buchner, U. G., Schmidt, A., Pühse, U., Gerber, M., Wiesbeck, G., Lang, U. E., & Walter, M. (2020). Excessive exercise—A meta-review. *Frontiers in Psychiatry, 11*, (521572), https://doi.org/10.3389/fpsyt .2020.521572

Colledge, F., Sattler, I., Schilling, H., Gerber, M., Pühse, U., Walter, M. (2020). Mental disorders in individuals at risk for exercise addiction—A systematic review. *Addictive Behavioral Reports, 12*, 100314. https://doi.org/10.1016/j .abrep.2020.100314. eCollection 2020 Dec.

Cook, B. J., Hausenblas, H., Crosby, R. D., Cao, L., & Wonderlich, S. A. (2015). Exercise dependence as a mediator of the exercise and eating disorders relationship: A pilot study. *Eating Behaviors, 16*, 9–12.

Cook, B., Karr, T. M., Zunker, C., Mitchell, J. E., Thompson, R., Sherman, R., Erickson, A., Cao, L., & Crosby, R. D. (2015). The influence of exercise identity and social physique anxiety on exercise dependence. *Journal of Behavioral Addictions, 4*(3), 195–199.

Cook, B., Hausenblas, H., Tuccitto, D., & Giacobbi, P. Jr. (2011). Eating disorders and exercise: A structural equation modelling analysis of a conceptual model. *European Eating Disorders Review, 19*(3), 216–225.

Cooper, M., Eddy, K. T., Thomas, J. J., Franko, D. L., Carron-Arthur, B. et al. (2020). Muscle dysmorphia: A systematic and meta-analytic review of the literature to assess diagnostic validity. *International Journal of Eating Disorders, 53*(10), 1583–1604. https://doi.org/10.1002 /eat.23349

Di Lodovico, L., Poulnais, S., & Gorwood, P. (2019). Which sports are more at risk of physical exercise addiction: A systematic review. *Addictive Behaviors, 93*, 257–262. https://doi.org/10.1016/j.addbeh.2018.12.030. Epub 2018 Dec 23.

Ertl, M., Pazienza, R., Cannon, M., Cabrera Tineo, Y. A., Fresquez, C. L., McDonough, A. K., Bozek, D. M., Ozmat, E. E., Ladouceur, G. M., Planz, E. K., & Martin, J. L. (2022). Associations between impulsivity and exercise addiction, disordered eating, and alcohol use behaviors: A latent profile analysis. *Substance Use & Misuse, 57*(6), 886–896.

Gori, A., Topino, E., & Griffiths, M. (2021). Protective and risk factors in exercise addiction: A series of moderated mediation analyses. *International Journal of Environmental Research and Public Health, 18*(18):9706. https://doi.org /10.3390/ijerph18189706

Gorrasi, I. S., Bonetta, S., Roppolo, M., Daga, G. A., Bo, S., Tagliabue, A., ... Carraro E. (2020). Traits of orthorexia nervosa and muscle dysmorphia in Italian university students: A multicentre study. *Eating and Weight Disorders – Studies on Anorexia, Bulimia and Obesity, 25*, 1413–1423. https://doi.org/10.1007/s40519-019-00779-5

Hausenblas, H. A., Cook, B. J., & Chittester, N. I. (2008). Can exercise treat eating disorders? *Exercise and Sport Sciences Reviews, 36*(1), 43–47. https://doi.org/10.1097/jes.0b013e31815e4040

Hausenblas, H. A., Schreiber, K., & Smoliga, J. M. (2017). Addiction to exercise. *British Medical Journal, 357*, j1745. https://doi.org/10.1136/bmj.j1745

Hausenblas, H. A., & Symons Downs, D. (2002a). Exercise dependence: A systematic review. *Psychology of Sport and Exercise,* (2), 89–123.

Hausenblas, H. A., & Symons Downs, D. (2002b). How much is too much? The development and validation of the Exercise Dependence Scale. *Psychology & Health, 17*(4), 387–404.

Jung, C. G. (1957). Memories, dreams, reflections. New York, NY: Vintage.

Kim, Y. S., Park, Y. S., Allegrante, J. P., Marks, R., Ok, H., Ok Cho, K., & Garber, C. E. (2012). Relationship between physical activity and general mental health. *Preventive Medicine, 55*(5), 458–463.

Kim, K. H., Choi, S., Kim, K., Chang, J., Kim, S. M., Kim, S. R., Cho, Y., Oh, Y. H., Lee, G., Son, J. S., & Park, S. M. (2021). Association between physical activity and subsequent cardiovascular disease among 5-year breast cancer survivors. *Breast Cancer Research and Treatment, 188*, 203–214. https://doi.org/10.1007/s10549-021-06140-8

Lukács, A., Sasvári, P., Varga, B., & Mayer, K. (2019). Exercise addiction and its related factors in amateur runners. *Journal of Behavioral Addictions, 8*(2), 343–349. https://doi.org/10.1556/2006.8.2019.28

Martenstyn, J. A., Touyz, S., & Maguire, S. (2021). Treatment of compulsive exercise in eating disorders and muscle dysmorphia: Protocol for a systematic review. *Journal of Eating Disorders, 9*(19). https://doi.org/10.1186/s40337-021-00375-y

McCreary, D. R., & Sasse, D. K. (2000). An exploration of the drive for muscularity in adolescent boys and girls. *Journal of American College Health, 48*(6), 297–304.

Mondin, G. W., Morgan, W. P., Piering, P. N., Stegner, A. J., Stotesbery, C. L., Trine, M. R., & Wu, M. (1996). Psychological consequences of exercise deprivation in habitual exercisers. *Medicine and Science in Sports & Exercise, 28*(9), 1199–1203.

Morrison, T. G., & Morrison, M. A. (2004). Scale examining drive for muscularity in males. *Psychology of Men and Muscularity, 5*(1), 30–39.

O'Keefe, E. L., Torres-Acosta, N., O'Keefe, J. H., & Lavie, C. L. (2020). Training for longevity: The reverse J-Curve for exercise. *Missouri Medicine, 117*(4), 355–361.

Pope, H. G., Gruber, A. J., Choi, P., Olivardia, R., & Phillips, K. A. (1997). Muscle dysmorphia: An underrecognized form of body dysmorphic disorder. *Psychosomatics, 38*(6), 548–557.

Rocks, T., Pelly, F., Slater, G., & Martin, L. A. (2017). Prevalence of exercise addiction symptomology and disordered eating in Australian students studying nutrition and dietetics. *Journal of the Academy of Nutrition and Dietetics, 117*(10), 1628–1636.

Santarnecchi, E., & Dèttore, D. (2012). Muscle dysmorphia in different degrees of bodybuilding activities: Validation of the Italian version of Muscle Dysmorphia Disorder Inventory and Bodybuilder Image Grid. *Body Image, 9*(3), 396–403.

Simón-Grima, J., Estrada-Marcén, N., & Montero-Marín, J. (2018). Exercise addiction measure through the *Exercise Addiction Inventory* (EAI) and health in habitual exercisers. A systematic review and meta-analysis. *Adicciones,* 31(3):233–249. https://doi.org/10.20882/adicciones.990

Trott, M., Jackson, S. E., Firth, J., Jacob, L., Grabovac, I., Stubbs, B., & Smith, L. (2020). A comparative meta-analysis of the prevalence of exercise addiction in adults with and without indicated eating disorders. *Eating and Weight Disorders, 26*, 37–46. https://doi.org/10.1007/s40519-019-00842-1

Trott, M., Yang, L., Jackson, S. E., Firth, J., Gillvray, C., Stubbs, B., & Smith, L. (2020). Prevalence and correlates of exercise addiction in the presence vs. absence of indicated eating disorders. *Frontiers in Sports and Active Living, 2*(84), 1–13. https://doi.org/10.3389/fspor.2020.00084

Villella, C., Martinotti, G., Di NiCola, M., Cassano, M., La Torre, G., Gliubuzzi, M. D., Messeri, I., Petruccelli, F., Luigi Janiri, B., & Conte, G. (2011). Behavioural addictions in adolescents and young adults: Results from a prevalence study. *Journal of Gambling Studies, 27*, 203–214.

Waters, B. (1981). Defining the runner's personality. *Runner's World, 16*, 48–51.

Weinstein, A. A., Koehmstedt, C., & Kop, W. J. (2017). Mental health consequences of exercise withdrawal: A systematic review. *General Hospital Psychiatry, 49*, 11–18. https://doi.org/10.1016/j.genhosppsych.2017.06.001 Epub 2017 Jun 6.

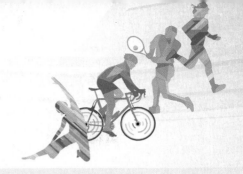

SECTION 4

Theoretical Models for Physical Activity and Sedentary Behavior

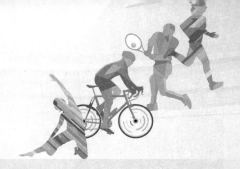

CHAPTER 14

Social Cognitive Theory and Theory of Planned Behavior

LEARNING OBJECTIVES

After completing this chapter, you will be able to:

- Describe the main factors that have been proposed to influence self-efficacy.
- Explain how self-efficacy can be measured.
- Outline the relationship between social cognitive theory and physical activity/sedentary behavior.
- Describe the current evidence for using social cognitive theory to change physical activity.
- Define the theory of planned behavior variables that explain physical activity and sedentary behavior intention.
- Define the theory of planned behavior variables that explain behavior.
- Outline the methods used in an elicitation study.
- Describe the theory of planned behavior beliefs.

Introduction

A shift in thinking from a behaviorist (i.e., stimulus causes response) to a cognitive (i.e., stimulus causes thinking, which then causes a response) focus in the second half of the 20th century sparked the development of social cognitive approaches to understanding behavior and behavior change. In this chapter, we overview two of the most popular and well-researched social cognitive approaches that have been applied to understand physical activity and sedentary behavior: social cognitive theory and theory of planned behavior.

Social cognitive theory, as currently conceptualized (Bandura, 2004), is a model that includes goals, sociostructural factors, and outcome expectations, but the central mediator of the model is the construct of self-efficacy. **Self-efficacy** is the belief that an individual has the ability to do what is needed to achieve a certain outcome (Bandura, 1997). However, in social cognitive theory, self-efficacy is the foundation for human behavior. Albert Bandura (1997) highlighted the importance of self-efficacy, because there is little motivation to enact a behavior if a person does not believe they can act to produce desired results.

Self-efficacy is thought to influence the course of action an individual chooses. Will you jog or cycle with friends or attend a box aerobics

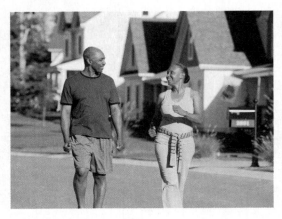

© Siri Stafford/Lifesize/Thinkstock.

class? Or avoid all of these activities? A belief that you have the capability to successfully carry out any or all of these activities will influence your decision. Also, the amount of effort you expend in these activities will be influenced by your efficacy belief. With a weak belief in your personal capability to keep up or perform successfully, it is likely that you will be more tentative. Self-efficacy also will influence the degree of perseverance you demonstrate when obstacles and adversities arise. It will impact whether your thought patterns hinder or facilitate your performance. Expectations of failure generally serve as a self-fulfilling prophecy. Similarly, individuals with low self-efficacy are more likely to feel anxious, stressed, or depressed if environmental demands become high. Finally, as a result of all of the above, if your self-efficacy is low, social cognitive theory

suggests that your level of accomplishment will be detrimentally affected.

Given the important role that self-efficacy is thought to play in human behavior generally, it is hardly surprising that numerous researchers have studied its specific role in physical activity. Indeed, it is likely the most frequently applied construct in physical activity psychology research (Beauchamp et al., 2019). Issues that have been examined include whether self-efficacy is related to the intention to become active, the initiation and continuation of a more physically active lifestyle, resisting a sedentary lifestyle, effort expended on physical activity, and thought patterns about physical activity. The results from that research are discussed below.

Self-Efficacy in Social Cognitive Theory

Self-efficacy is an integral component of social cognitive theory, a conceptual approach useful for understanding human behavior. Social cognitive theory combines aspects of operant conditioning, social learning theory, and cognitive psychology. **Figure 14-1** provides a schematic illustration of the main tenets of the theory, as proposed by Bandura (1998).

In social cognitive theory, self-efficacy affects behavior directly through its impact on outcome expectations, sociostructural factors, and goals.

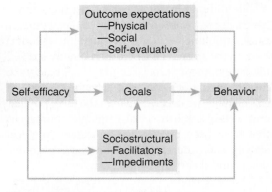

Figure 14-1 Social Cognitive Theory.

Data from Bandura, A. (1998). Health promotion from the perspective of social cognitive theory. *Psychology & Health, 13*(4), 623–649.

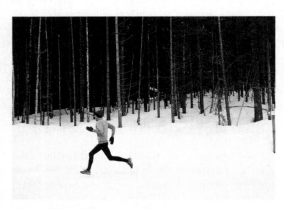

© Michael Blann/DigitalVision/Getty Images.

Outcome expectations are the expectations an individual has about the outcomes of a behavior. These can be physical (e.g., performing exercise would be painful), social (e.g., my friends will be pleased if I go to aerobics class with them), or self-evaluative (e.g., I will feel proud of myself for sticking to my running schedule). The outcome expectation construct has had mixed evidence as a correlate of physical activity, with reviews and meta-analyses showing small (Bohlen et al., 2021) to negligible (Young et al., 2014) effects. Self-efficacy is also thought to impact sociostructural factors (i.e., facilitators and barriers) that play a role in behavior change. A person must hold a strong enough level of self-efficacy to overcome these barriers. However, the evidence for the relationship between sociostructural factors and physical activity in applications of social cognitive theory has not been reported often and may be negligible (Young et al., 2014). It has also been contended that sociostructural factors may be a cause of self-efficacy (i.e., one will likely believe they are less capable when environments have many barriers to action), even though this is not included in the current social cognitive theory model (Beauchamp et al., 2019). Finally, personal goals related to behavior can be formed through the combination of self-efficacy, outcome expectations, and sociostructural factors. This proposition in social cognitive theory has had strong support in physical activity research (Young et al., 2014; McEwan et al., 2016; see the section below on theory of planned behavior and intention).

The basis of the social cognitive theory is the concept of triadic **reciprocal determinism** (Bandura, 1977). Specifically, three classes of determinants—behavior, internal personal factors, and external environment—are assumed to coexist. Behavior (i.e., its type, frequency, duration, and context) is influenced by and influences internal personal factors (i.e., individual cognitions such as self-efficacy, outcome expectations, and goals). An individual's outcome expectation and self-efficacy beliefs, for example, would influence dieting behavior. In turn, the effectiveness (or ineffectiveness) of dieting behavior would serve to shape the person's outcome expectations. As another example, an athlete's teammates (i.e., environment) might influence their self-efficacy about dieting behavior. Again, in turn, the athlete's own outcome expectations would have a reciprocal influence on their teammates (see **Figure 14-2**).

What are some of the implications of accepting a triadic reciprocal causation perspective? One implication is relatively straightforward: cognitions such as self-efficacy are assumed to

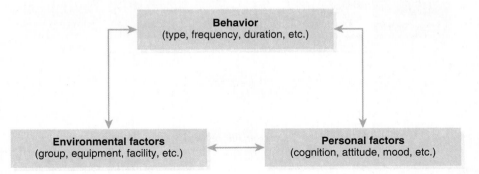

Figure 14-2 Reciprocal Determinism.

play a role in behavior. A cardiac rehabilitation patient may be physically capable of moderate physical activity. However, if they do not possess the belief that this is the case, physical activity behavior is unlikely. A patient also could learn through the consequences of their own actions. A cardiac rehabilitation patient who engages safely in physical activity would gain self-efficacy from the experience.

A third implication is that an individual's beliefs can be influenced by external environmental factors. A person does not have to engage directly in a behavior to develop the belief about personal capabilities. In short, self-efficacy can be influenced through social persuasion as well as the success of (similar) others. That same cardiac rehabilitation patient may gain efficacy by coming to a class and observing other patients with similar health problems engaging in physical activities.

CRITICAL THINKING ACTIVITY 14-2

Triadic reciprocal determinism makes sense, but it definitely makes it difficult to understand what comes first in a "chicken-or-egg" type scenario because the environment, the individual, and behavior are all thought to cause each other. What do you think comes first in terms of physical activity? If you were asked to develop a physical activity intervention, what factor would you start with in your program?

Sources of Self-Efficacy Beliefs

As **Figure 14-3** shows, self-efficacy can arise from a number of sources (Bandura, 1997). According to social cognitive theory, the most important, potent source of self-efficacy is personal **mastery experiences**. Carrying out a task successfully helps to cement the belief in the person that they have the capabilities necessary. In this regard, success is obviously important for self-efficacy to develop. However, Bandura has pointed out that an efficacy belief is more resilient if the individual has also had to overcome obstacles and adversity—and has done so successfully. Similarly, of course, self-efficacy can be fragile; initial failure experiences can serve to undermine efficacy beliefs. The power of personal experiences can, therefore, shape self-efficacy for better or worse.

Another source of efficacy is **vicarious experiences**, or observational learning. The behavior (and successes or failures) of others can be used as a comparative standard for the individual. Observing others who are similar achieve success increases self-efficacy, while observing them fail is thought to diminish it. Essentially, the individual is thought to be persuaded if a similar other has the capability and does well.

Bandura also has pointed out that while vicarious experiences are generally a less-powerful source of self-efficacy beliefs than mastery experiences, there are conditions under which this

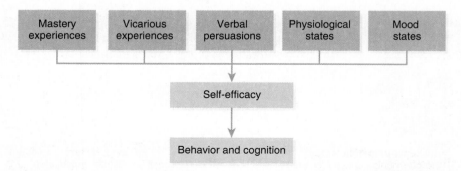

Figure 14-3 Proposed Sources of Self-Efficacy.

Data from Bandura, A. (1997). Self-efficacy, the exercise of control. New York, NY: Freeman.

is not the case. For example, a woman may experience failure in her initial attempts to use a stair-climber and, as a result, lose self-efficacy. However, observing a friend who is perceived to be similar (or less fit), exercise successfully could serve as a catalyst to enhance self-efficacy.

A specialized form of vicarious experiences is cognitive self-modeling; that is, imagery experiences. Here, the individual uses visualization to repeatedly and successfully confront and master challenging situations.

A third source of information that has an impact on self-efficacy is **verbal persuasion**. Its influence is generally thought to be weaker than observational vicarious experiences or personal experiences. However, Bandura (1997) pointed out that verbal persuasion may not lead to lasting improvement in self-efficacy, but can play an important role in self-change if a person perceives the verbal persuasion as realistic. Generally, verbal persuasion has its greatest impact on self-efficacy on those individuals who have some reason to believe that they could be successful if they persist.

The fourth source of information for self-efficacy beliefs is the individual's **physiological state**. Bodily sensations such as increased heart rate, increased sweating, and increased respiratory rate can serve to provide a signal to the individual about their current level of efficacy. Bandura emphasized that the individual's physiologic state—like performance experiences, vicarious experiences, and verbal persuasion—is not, by itself, an indicator of self-efficacy. The individual's appraisal of the information is crucial. If, for

example, an elevated heart rate is interpreted as confirmation of a suspected poor physical condition, it could serve to reduce self-efficacy. In contrast, if an elevated heart rate is interpreted as evidence of being adequately warmed-up, it could serve to enhance self-efficacy.

The final factor, **mood states**, can influence self-efficacy through either affective priming or cognitive priming. Affective priming occurs because previous successes and failures are stored in memory (and recalled) with associated mood states. Thus, when we are successful, we store that experience in memory along with the feelings of joy, elation, vigor, and so on that initially accompanied it. Similarly, when we fail, we store that experience in memory with the feelings of frustration, sorrow, depression, and so on that initially accompanied it. Therefore, the presence of a negative mood state prior to an effect serves to prime memories of failures, thereby serving to reduce self-efficacy.

The cognitive priming perspective is similar but with a subtle distinction. Memory of a failure might be stored with the negative mood state, but it is also stored with an accompanying cognition—an attribution for example. Consider the athlete who has just had a poor performance in a 10K race. The memory of that performance, the emotion associated with it (e.g., feeling depressed), and any accompanying attribution (e.g., "my failure to arrive 1 hour prior to the start was one reason for my poor performance") would be stored in memory together. Given similar or related experiences in a subsequent race, the cognition of the earlier causal event (arriving too close to the start time) would prime both the emotion (feeling depressed) and memory of the failure. The result would be diminished self-efficacy.

Nature and Measurement of Self-Efficacy

Theoreticians have stated that self-efficacy is a complex construct that can vary along three dimensions. One dimension, the level of self-efficacy,

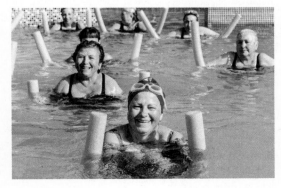

© Karelnoppe/Shutterstock.

reflects a belief in personal ability to accomplish a particular task or component of a task. Generally, when people consider self-efficacy, this is the dimension that comes to mind. However, an individual's self-efficacy can also vary in strength; that is, the degree of conviction that a particular task or component of a task can be carried out successfully. Thus, for example, an individual might hold the belief that they can complete a 30-minute aerobics class (i.e., the level of self-efficacy). However, they also might only be 75% (not 100%) confident about this belief (i.e., the strength of self-efficacy). The third dimension, generality, reflects the degree to which efficacy beliefs transfer to related tasks. An individual who has high self-efficacy for an aerobics class may also have similarly high efficacy in all activities requiring aerobic fitness.

One of the measurement challenges in self-efficacy research is separating one's capability from one's motivation. Self-efficacy is an assessment of capability, but confidence can easily be misinterpreted or misconstrued as motivation independent of ability (Cahill, Gallo, Lisman, & Weinstein, 2006; Kirsch, 1982; Rhodes & Blanchard, 2007). For example, people could report that they are not confident that they can exercise regularly because they do not like to exercise, even if they feel they actually would have the ability to do so. This appraisal assesses an outcome expectation (I would enjoy/not enjoy exercise), rather than a judgment of efficacy (Bandura, 1977; Cahill et al., 2006). Williams and Rhodes (2014, 2016) suggest this often happens due to how people colloquialize the wording of "I can" in popular speech. For example, if someone asks you whether you can go to the movies tonight, you may answer that you can't. This likely has to do with other priorities or commitments and not a literal interpretation that you are physically or mentally unable to go to the movies. Indeed, when Rhodes and Blanchard (2007) asked college students why they were confident that they could or could not exercise, almost half of the reasons were motivational in nature (enjoyment, health, motivation), while the other half were about capability (time, skill). To help reduce the chances of this mistaken meaning, Rhodes and colleagues

have argued and demonstrated that "confidence" items with a motivational qualifier (e.g., "if I wanted to") help measure ability instead of outcome expectations (Rhodes & Blanchard, 2007; Rhodes & Courneya, 2003, 2004). More recently, Rhodes and colleagues have also shown that questionnaires, including a vignette that illustrates how we use colloquial language around the word "I can," followed by instructions to answer self-efficacy questions with the literal meaning of "I can" may assist in self-efficacy measurement (Lithopoulos et al., 2019; Rhodes et al., 2016). Still, the challenge for physical activity scientists remains an attempt to separate motivation and outcome expectancies from self-efficacy expectations (Beauchamp et al., 2019; Williams & Rhodes, 2016).

Self-Efficacy in Physical Activity Contexts

Because self-efficacy is a situation-specific construct, different manifestations (operational definitions of self-efficacy) have been assessed, depending on the context and interest of the researcher. The best way to operationalize self-efficacy for physical activity has received research attention because it helps us understand where our promotion efforts should be focused. Several researchers have contributed to this area, and the two forms of efficacy highlighted in the following discussion do not represent a comprehensive list, but rather are among the most common in physical activity research.

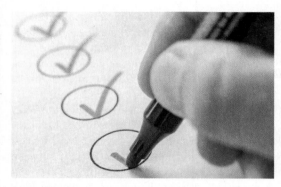

One of the most common forms of self-efficacy is sometimes referred to as **barrier efficacy** (McAuley & Mihalko, 1998). It represents an individual's beliefs about possessing the capability to overcome obstacles to physical activity. These obstacles/barriers could be social, such as spousal lack of encouragement; or personal, such as time limitations; or environmental, such as bad weather that might interfere with physical activity. Respondents indicate, for example, their confidence that they can attend exercise classes three times a week in spite of inclement weather. A special form of barrier efficacy is **scheduling efficacy**. It reflects the individual's confidence that physical activity can be scheduled into a daily or weekly routine.

Another form of self-efficacy used commonly in the physical activity literature is **task efficacy**. An early debate among self-efficacy theorists centered around self-efficacy and its role in repeated/complex behaviors such as regular exercise (Bandura, 1995; Kirsch, 1995; Maddux, 1995). The main debate focused on whether self-efficacy is about confidence to perform the act itself (walking involves putting one foot in front of the other) or the confidence to regulate the action. In physical activity, this has given rise to specific measurements of task efficacy (Blanchard et al., 2007). Task efficacy is the confidence to perform the specific physical activity itself. As you could imagine, many people may feel that they have high task efficacy with simple activities (e.g., walking), but this would change as the difficulty of the activity increases (e.g., mountain climbing). In addition, task efficacy may be very

important for clinical or physically compromised populations (Blanchard et al., 2007; Blanchard, Rodgers, Courneya, Daub, & Knapik, 2002). Finally, task self-efficacy may be more important for the initial adoption of physical activity, but barrier efficacy may become more important as one attempts to maintain a physically active lifestyle (Higgins, Middleton, Winner, & Janelle, 2014).

Self-Efficacy and Physical Activity Behavior

Figure 14-3 shows that various factors contribute to self-efficacy. In turn, when self-efficacy is present, it is positively associated with behavior. A meta-analysis of 67 studies showed that 60% of the tests supported a significant direct relationship between self-efficacy and physical activity (Young et al., 2014). To contextualize the size of this effect, Spence and colleagues (2006) showed the effect size as r = 0.35, which makes it one of the largest and most reliable correlates of physical activity. However, the indirect effects of self-efficacy on physical activity through other social cognitive constructs in the model (e.g., sociostructural factors, outcome expectations) have considerably less evidence, with only 36% of studies showing this effect. Thus, self-efficacy has the most evidence as a direct predictor of physical activity.

Initiation and Maintenance of Physical Activity

Changes in behavior often unfold slowly. One reason is that people perceive the presence of a number of (real or perceived) barriers, and they are not confident about their ability to overcome those barriers. Not surprisingly, barrier efficacy plays a role insofar as initiating a lifestyle that involves being physically active. Early research showed that people who intend to become more active in the immediate future (but have not actually done so) have greater barrier efficacy than people who have no intention of adopting a physically active lifestyle (Armstrong, Sallis, Hovell, & Hofstetter, 1993). Oman and King (1998) conducted a 2-year randomized trial where 63 participants were randomly assigned to a condition for participation in an aerobic exercise program (higher-intensity, home-based exercise; higher-intensity, class-based exercise; or lower-intensity, home-based exercise). Results from the study indicated that independent of treatment group, baseline self-efficacy was a significant predictor of exercise behavior during adoption but not during the maintenance phase.

Still, exercise efficacy also plays a role insofar as maintaining a physically active lifestyle is concerned. In a review paper on self-efficacy and exercise, this positive, significant relationship has been illustrated among a variety of populations (clinical and nonclinical) and ages (ranging between adolescents and older adults) (McAuley & Blissmer, 2000). For example, a study of 174 older adults participating in an exercise program (randomized to an aerobic group or stretching and toning group) measured both exercise self-efficacy and physical efficacy levels across a 12-month trial (McAuley et al., 1999). Results showed that a curvilinear growth of self-efficacy occurred across the trial, with declines at the follow-up stage (postexercise program). Participants, therefore, had increases in self-efficacy throughout the program, but then declines occurred at the follow-up. As a result of the interplay between physical activity participation and self-efficacy, it becomes essential for practitioners to develop physical activity opportunities that help to build personal self-efficacy levels.

Effort Expended in Physical Activity

It was pointed out earlier in the chapter that one expected consequence of self-efficacy pertains to the amount of effort expended; that is, efficacious individuals could be expected to try harder. Research has supported this expected relationship with regard to physical activity. A variety of indices of physical effort or exertion, such as perceived exertion, self-reports of activity intensity, peak heart rate, vital capacity, expiratory volume, and time to reach 70% of maximal heart rate, have been found to be related to exercise efficacy, as well as disease- and health-related efficacy (see McAuley and Mihalko, 1998, for an overview of this research).

It was pointed out earlier (see also Figure 14-2) that the strongest, most viable source of efficacy beliefs are expected to be mastery experiences. Thus, not surprisingly, the relationship between self-efficacy and involvement in physical activity is reciprocal. Efficacy beliefs are associated with the initiation and maintenance of physical activity. In turn, both acute and long-term involvement in a program of physical activity lead to significant gains in self-efficacy (McAuley & Blissmer, 2000).

The positive effects of physical activity on self-efficacy are not restricted to general populations only. Individuals involved in cardiac rehabilitation programs (Blanchard, Rodgers, Courneya, Daub, & Knapik, 2002) and other clinical populations have reported increased efficacy beliefs following a program of physical activity (McAuley & Blissmer, 2000).

Self-Efficacy and Mental States

Figure 14-3 is intended to illustrate schematically that when self-efficacy beliefs are stronger, cognitions about physical activity are greater, more active, and more positive. Research on the role that efficacy beliefs play in physical activity has demonstrated this relationship.

It has been shown by Albert Bandura (1986) that individuals who possess greater self-efficacy also have lower depression and anxiety than those reporting lower self-efficacy. Similarly, efficacy beliefs are interrelated with emotional responses following acute sessions of physical activity. For example, individuals possessing greater exercise efficacy report more positive and less negative affect (McAuley, Shaffer, & Rudolph, 1995) following an acute bout of activity. Similarly, they also report enjoying the experience more (McAuley, Wraith, & Duncan, 1991).

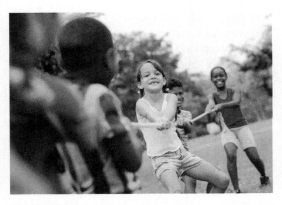

© Stefanolunardi/Shutterstock.

Efficacy beliefs are also associated with a number of positive intrapersonal characteristics. For example, Kavussanu and McAuley (1995) noted that individuals with greater self-efficacy tend to be more optimistic. As another example, exercise efficacy has been positively associated with self-esteem (Sonstroem, Harlow, & Josephs, 1994).

Enhancing Self-Efficacy: Experimental Evidence

The previous sections served to highlight the important role that efficacy beliefs play in involvement in physical activity. An important question is, how can efficacy be enhanced in individuals uncertain about their capability to organize and execute the actions associated with a physically active lifestyle?

Despite Bandura's clear, logical, and prescriptive grounds for how to change self-efficacy, the literature surrounding physical activity interventions has mixed support (Baranowski, Anderson, & Carmack, 1998; Lubans, Foster, & Biddle, 2008; Rhodes & Pfaeffli, 2010; Rhodes et al., 2021). For example, in Rhodes and Pfaeffli's (2010) examination of whether self-efficacy interventions could account for changes in physical activity, only 1 of 19 studies supported a complete link between changes in self-efficacy and changes in physical activity. An updated meta-analysis of

this literature showed that interventions changing self-efficacy, and the resulting effect on physical activity was very small ($ab = 0.04$) but significant (Rhodes et al., 2021). Thus, self-efficacy has some support for its role as a mediator of physical activity changes due to interventions. The same findings were noted for interventions that employed the full social cognitive theory model to change physical activity (Rhodes et al., 2021).

The experimental evidence for the importance of various sources of self-efficacy to impart change also has relatively mixed evidence (Conn, Hafdahl, & Mehr, 2011; McEwan et al., 2019; Prestwich et al., 2014). A series of meta-analyses by French and colleagues that mapped behavior change techniques to self-efficacy interventions and physical activity have best illustrated these mixed results (Ashford et al., 2010; French et al., 2014; Williams and French, 2011). Ashford, Edmunds, and French (2010), and Williams and French (2011) reviewed 27 physical activity interventions that used sources of self-efficacy in order to change exercise self-efficacy ($d = 0.16$) and behavior ($d = 0.21$), but they only showed modest effects. This was also replicated in a meta-analysis separating barrier ($d = 0.13$) and task ($d = 0.21$) efficacy interventions (Higgins et al., 2014). Interestingly, mastery experiences were also not found to be the most effective way to change self-efficacy; positive feedback and vicarious experience were shown as more effective (Ashford et al., 2010). The results of this review had relatively low numbers of studies with specific techniques (i.e., most studies employed a variety of sources, which could confound these results). Analysis of whether self-efficacy change techniques can change self-efficacy has also been performed with samples of older adults (French, Olander, Chisholm, & Mc Sharry, 2014). Overall, interventions were able to change self-efficacy ($d = 0.37$), but similar to past results, these changes did not link well to changes in behavior ($d = 0.16$). The results also showed no clear mechanism that was effective in changing self-efficacy, and positive feedback and vicarious experience were associated with less change. What is so interesting in these studies is that many of the changes in self-efficacy were associated with techniques that did not align with the four sources of self-efficacy. Rhodes and Williams (2017) suggest these results may be from self-efficacy measures assessing motivation and self-efficacy (thus more behavior change techniques could be effective), yet the key findings suggest that changing self-efficacy may represent only a small component of what is needed to promote and sustain changes in physical activity.

Social Cognitive Theory Applied to Sedentary Behavior

Unlike physical activity, the study of sedentary behavior from the perspective of social cognitive theory is in its relatively early stages. Still, one cannot assume that the same principles and findings for social cognitive theory and physical activity can be used to understand sedentary behavior. The most obvious difference would be self-efficacy and its relationship with sedentary behavior. While physical activity is a complex behavior that often requires skill and control over various other temptations (i.e., high self-efficacy), sedentary behaviors are often known for their ease and tempting outcomes. Thus, low confidence to sit in a comfy chair and watch a screen hardly seems like a driving factor that would explain the variations in sedentary behavior! Indeed, research has generally demonstrated no relationship between control factors like self-efficacy and sedentary behavior (Rhodes, Temmel, & Mark, 2012; O'Donoghue et al., 2016; Prince et al., 2017), with the one caveat being video games, where skill is associated with play hours (Terlecki et al., 2011). Instead, social cognitive theory, when applied to sedentary behaviors, is often phrased in terms of limiting the behavior. For example, self-efficacy might be phrased as confidence to limit TV time or time spent online (Van Dyck et al., 2011).

Applications of social cognitive theory to sedentary behavior are too few at present to render any definitive judgment on how it applies to sedentary behavior, but early work does demonstrate that it may have a use. For example,

Van Dyck and colleagues (2011) showed that outcome expectations about both the benefits of TV and Internet use and the cons of not limiting TV and Internet use correlate with self-reported TV and Internet use in a sample of adults from Belgium. They also showed that self-efficacy to limit these sedentary behaviors was a large correlate (negative relationship) with behavior. Motl and colleagues (2019) explored the application of social cognitive theory to limit sedentary behavior to 275 people with multiple sclerosis using accelerometry measurement of sitting time. Only self-efficacy ($b = 0.32$) explained variance in sedentary behavior, as there was no independent association with outcome expectations, barriers, or goal setting. Perhaps most interesting is the potential link between screen viewing and families. A study by Jago, Sebire, Edwards, and Thompson (2013) showed that children were five times more likely to engage in excessive screen time behavior if their parents also reported high screen time themselves. Furthermore, the researchers found that parental self-efficacy to limit screen time had a large link to child-reported screen time. The findings illustrate how social cognitive theory may interact with reciprocal determination (parental behavior to child behavior) in a family setting.

There have also been promising results in intervention trials to reduce sedentary behavior using approaches that target social cognitive theory constructs, such as outcome expectations and self-efficacy. Studies including adults (Nigg et al., 2021), older adults (Gardiner, Eakin, Healy, & Owen, 2011), cancer survivors (Mama et al., 2017), adolescents (Bergh et al., 2012; Dewar et al., 2014), and preschool children (Zimmerman, Ortiz, Christakis, & Elkun, 2012) have all shown that social cognitive theory–based interventions can reduce sedentary behavior. The exact mechanism, however, for the behavior change is less understood. For example, while Zimmerman and colleagues work with preschool children and their parents showed that screen time was limited via a change in the negative outcome expectation from letting children watch TV, the studies with adolescents were unable to show why sedentary behavior decreased. None of these studies have yet linked these changes to self-efficacy, which is considered the most important variable in social cognitive theory.

Theory of Planned Behavior

The **theory of planned behavior** (Ajzen, 1991) is an extension of the **theory of reasoned action** developed by Martin Fishbein and Icek Ajzen (Ajzen & Fishbein, 1980; Fishbein & Ajzen, 1975). Since its introduction approximately 30 years ago, the theory of planned behavior, like social cognitive theory, has become one of the most frequently cited and influential models for predicting human behavior.

The theory of planned behavior is concerned with the link between our attitudes and our behaviors. The following quote by William James (1842–1910), a pioneering American psychologist, highlights the effects that our attitudes have on our behaviors: "It is our attitude at the beginning of a difficult task, which, more than anything else, will affect its successful outcome (n.d.)." The theory of planned behavior also assumes that individuals are capable of forethought and making rational decisions about their behavior and its consequences.

The theory of planned behavior specifies that the following four psychological variables may influence our behavior: **intention**, **attitude**,

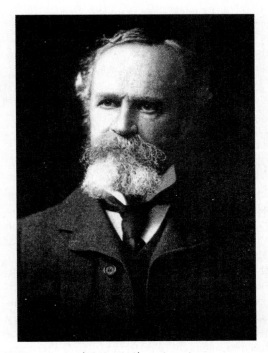

William James (1842–1910), an American philosopher and psychologist, is often called the Father of American Psychology.

Courtesy of US National Library of Medicine.

subjective norm, and **perceived behavioral control**. The combination of an individual's expectations about performing a particular behavior and the value attached to that behavior form the conceptual basis of this theory. This expectation-by-value approach provides a framework for understanding the relationship between people's attitudes and their underlying beliefs.

Theory of Planned Behavior Variables

Figure 14-4 presents the main variables of the theory of planned behavior. Let's take a look at each of these main variables in more detail.

Intention

In the theory of planned behavior, a person's intention to perform a behavior is the central determinant of whether they engage in that behavior.

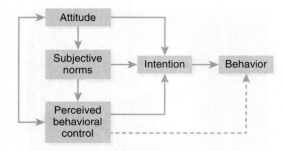

Figure 14-4 Theory of Planned Behavior.

Intention comprises two components: a decisional aspect that provides direction (i.e., *decisional intention*) and the intensity of determination to act in that direction (i.e., *intention strength*) (Rhodes & Rebar, 2017). Ajzen (1991) defines intention using the latter component as a person's willingness and how much effort they are planning to exert to perform the behavior. The stronger a person's intention to perform a behavior, the more likely they will be to engage in that behavior. Thus, if someone has a strong intent to go for a walk this afternoon, they are likely to go for that walk. In comparison, if a person has a strong intent to watch television after work today, they will most likely be sitting on the couch and enjoying a television show.

Attitude

Attitude represents an individual's positive or negative evaluation of performing a behavior. Do you find regular exercise useless or useful, harmful or beneficial, boring or interesting? An older adult may have a negative attitude toward engaging in a vigorous physical activity, such as running, but have a positive attitude toward walking in the neighborhood. Our attitude toward a specific behavior is a function of our **behavioral beliefs**, which are the perceived consequences of carrying out a specific action and our evaluation of each of these consequences. A college student's beliefs about playing doubles tennis could be represented by both positive expectations (e.g., it will improve my social life because I will meet lots of people) and negative expectations (e.g., it will reduce my time to study). In shaping a physical activity behavior, the person evaluates the consequences attached to each of these beliefs. Common behavioral beliefs

for physical activity include that it improves fitness/health, enhances physical appearance, provides enjoyment, increases social interactions, and improves psychological health (Symons Downs & Hausenblas, 2005a).

Subjective Norm

Subjective norm reflects the perceived social pressure that individuals feel to perform or not perform a particular behavior. Subjective norm is believed to be a function of **normative beliefs**, which are determined by the perceived expectations of important significant others (e.g., family, friends, physician, priest) or groups (e.g., classmates, teammates, church members) and by the individual's motivation to comply with the expectations of these important significant others. For example, an individual may feel that his doctor thinks he should exercise three times a week. That individual, however, may not be inclined to act according to these perceived beliefs if the doctor's comments are not highly valued. Common normative beliefs for physical activity include family members, friends, and healthcare professionals (Symons Downs & Hausenblas, 2005a).

Perceived Behavioral Control

Perceived behavioral control represents the perceived ease or difficulty of performing a behavior. Perceived behavioral control influences behavior either directly or indirectly through intention. People may hold positive attitudes toward a behavior and believe that important others would approve of their behavior. However, they are not likely to form a strong intention to perform that behavior if they believe they do not have the resources or opportunities to do so (Ajzen, 1991). You may have a positive attitude and enjoy swimming; however, if you do not have access to a pool, you will not be able to perform this behavior.

Perceived behavioral control is a function of **control beliefs**. Control beliefs represent the perceived presence or absence of required resources and opportunities (e.g., there is a road race this weekend), the anticipated obstacles or

Table 14-1 Theory of Planned Behavior Sample Items for Exercise

Construct	Item	Scaling
Attitude	For me to exercise regularly during the winter will be:	Useless Useful 1 2 3 4 5 6 7
Intention	I intend to exercise regularly during the winter.	Strongly disagree Strongly agree 1 2 3 4 5 6 7
Subjective norm	Most people who are important to me would like me to exercise regularly during the winter.	Strongly disagree Strongly agree 1 2 3 4 5 6 7
Perceived behavioral control	How much control do I have over exercising during the winter?	Very little control Complete control 1 2 3 4 5 6 7

impediments to behavior (e.g., the probability of rain on the weekend is 90%), and the perceived power of a particular control factor to facilitate or inhibit performance of the behavior (e.g., even if it rains this weekend, I can still participate in the road race; Ajzen & Driver, 1991). The most common control beliefs for physical activity include lack of time, lack of energy, and lack of motivation (Symons Downs & Hausenblas, 2005a). **Table 14-1** contains sample items for measuring the theory of planned behavior constructs in relation to regularly exercising during

the winter. **Figure 14-5** highlights the relationships among the beliefs and the other theory of planned behavior constructs.

CRITICAL THINKING ACTIVITY 14-5

Read the vignette about Rachel at the end of this chapter. Describe in detail her attitude, perceived behavioral control, subjective norm, and intention. How did these constructs change over time to influence her exercise behavior?

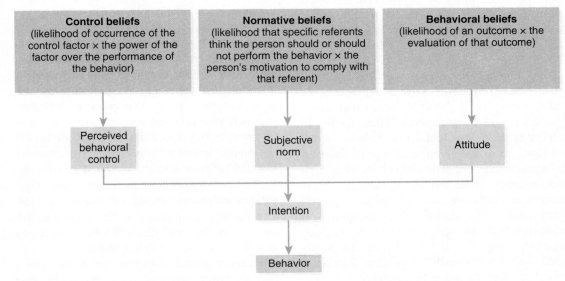

Figure 14-5 Relationship of the Theory of Planned Behavior Constructs (including beliefs) with Behavior.

Reproduced from Ajzen, I. (1985). From intentions to actions: A theory of planned behavior. In J. Kuhl & J. Beckman (Eds.), *Action-control: From cognition to behavior* (pp. 11–39). With permission of Springer Science+Business Media.

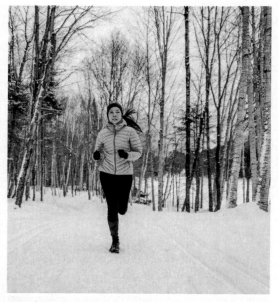

© Maridav/Shutterstock.

Theory of Planned Behavior and Physical Activity

Several meta-analytic and narrative reviews have supported the theory of planned behavior for explaining and predicting a variety of physical activities in a variety of populations, including ethnic minorities, youth, pregnant women, cancer patients, diabetic adults, university students, and older adults, just to name a few (Blanchard et al., 2008; Conner, 2020; Hagger & Chatzisarantis, 2009; Hausenblas, Carron, & Mack, 1997; Hausenblas & Symons Downs, 2004; Jones et al., 2007; Karvinen et al., 2007; McEachan et al., 2011; Symons Downs & Hausenblas, 2005a, 2005b). In general, research has found that intention is the strongest predictor of physical activity, followed by a smaller effect of perceived behavioral control. For example, McEachan and colleagues (2011) performed a meta-analysis of 103 studies (>23,000 participants) and showed that intention was associated with physical activity in the medium effect size range (b = 0.42) and perceived behavioral control had a small independent association (b = 0.11) after controlling for intention.

In addition, our intention to perform physical activity is associated with our attitude and perceived behavioral control, followed by subjective norm. In the same meta-analysis by McEachan and colleagues noted above, attitude (b = 0.40) and perceived behavioral control (b = 0.33) had medium sized associations with intention, while subjective norm (b = 0.12) had a smaller association. This information may be important for designing physical activity interventions because it illustrates how people evaluate physical activity (i.e., their attitude) and how their sense of control over their performance (perceived behavioral control) have the greatest association with whether they will intend to do the behavior. It is important to note, however, that the influence of each of the theory of planned behavior constructs can vary based on the population and context.

Sedentary Behavior Research

Fewer researchers have attempted to study the theory of planned behavior with regard to sedentary behavior, yet there are some indications that the theory has utility. In one of the first studies to apply the theory of planned behavior to sedentary behaviors, Rhodes and Dean (2019) used the model to predict computer use, reading, television viewing, and sedentary socializing among undergraduate students and a community sample of the Canadian population. The researchers found that all four behaviors were predicted by intention, and intention was predicted by attitude. Subjective norm also predicted intention to watch television and socialize in the community sample, but perceived behavioral control did not predict intention or behavior. The theory of planned behavior was also explored as a predictor of sedentary behavior in 31 advanced cancer patients with brain metastases (Lowe et al., 2015). The patients completed a survey interview that assessed the theory of planned behavior variables as well as medical and demographic information. The cancer patients also wore an accelerometer that objectively recorded their time spent lying down (i.e., supine), sitting, standing, and stepping during 7 days of active treatment.

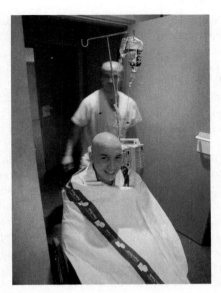

© National Geographic Image Collection/Alamy Stock Photo.

The researchers found that the time spent lying down or sitting was correlated with attitude toward physical activity. More specifically, patients who sat or were supine for greater than 20.7 hours per day reported significantly lower attitudes than patients who sat less. As well, patients who were older than 60 years of age spent more time sitting or being supine.

In another study, Prapavessis and his colleagues (2015) examined the utility of the theory of planned behavior for predicting sedentary intention and sedentary time with 372 adults. Using a Web-based survey design, the participants completed a modified version of the Sedentary Behavior Questionnaire. In addition, the participants self-reported their attitude, subjective norm, intention, and perceived behavioral control toward sedentary behavior (see **Table 14-2** for sample questionnaire items).

Table 14-2 **Sample Theory of Planned Behavior Items for Sedentary Behavior**

Construct	Sample Item
Intention	How much time do you intend to spend sitting for work, school, or leisure or recreational pursuits (e.g., watching TV; using the computer; doing office or school work; reading; talking on the phone; sitting in lectures or meetings; sitting in a car, train, or bus; eating; socializing; sitting for religious or spiritual pursuits) per day in the coming week?
Attitude	For you to sit for work, school, or leisure or recreational pursuits (e.g., watching TV; using the computer; doing office or school work; reading; talking on the phone; sitting in lectures or meetings; sitting in a car, train, or bus; eating; socializing; sitting for religious or spiritual pursuits) for 0–4 hours per day (none to one-quarter of your waking hours) would be. . . Pleasant Unpleasant 1 2 3 4 5 6 7
Subjective norm	The people in my life whose opinions I value would approve of my sitting for work, school, or leisure or recreational pursuits (e.g., watching TV; using the computer; doing office or school work; reading; talking on the phone; sitting in lectures or meetings; sitting in a car, train, or bus; eating; socializing; sitting for religious or spiritual pursuits) for _____ per day.
Perceived behavioral control	How much control do you have over the amount of time you spend sitting for work, school, or leisure or recreational pursuits (e.g., watching TV; using the computer; doing office or school work; reading; talking on the phone; sitting in lectures or meetings; sitting in a car, train, or bus; eating; socializing; sitting for religious or spiritual pursuits) per day? No control Complete control 1 2 3 4 5 6 7

Data from Prapavessis, H., Gaston, A., & DeJesus, S. (2015). The theory of planned behavior as a model for understanding sedentary behavior. *Psychology of Sport and Exercise, 19,* 23–32.

The researchers found more positive cognitions and greater intentions to engage in leisure and recreation sedentary pursuits on weekends vs. weekdays. The authors suggested that this may stem from the fact that Western society values academic and career success, and weekdays are typically reserved for work, school, or family responsibilities. The researchers also found that the strongest and most consistent predictor of sedentary intention and behavior were subjective norm and intentions.

CRITICAL THINKING ACTIVITY 14-6

Which of the theory of planned behavior constructs are most effective in predicting exercise behavior?

Elicitation Studies

A main strength of the theory of planned behavior is that an elicitation study forms the basis for developing questions to assess the theory's variables in a specific population. The elicitation study enables a practitioner to determine the specific beliefs for a specific population. This is important because we know that beliefs vary by population and even by activity. For example, the main behavioral beliefs for breast cancer survivors are that exercise gets their mind off cancer and treatment, makes them feel better, improves their well-being, and helps them maintain a normal lifestyle (Courneya, Jones, Mackey, & Fairey, 2006). In comparison, the main behavioral beliefs for pregnant women are related to pregnancy-specific issues, such as having a healthier pregnancy and an easier labor and delivery (Hausenblas, Giacobbi, Cook, Rhodes, & Cruz, 2011).

Because beliefs vary by population, researchers and practitioners are encouraged to refer to research that has already determined the physical activity beliefs of their specific intervention population (e.g., postpartum women, cancer survivors, high school students). If physical activity beliefs for a specific population of interest have not been determined, it is recommended that the practitioner or researcher conduct an elicitation study to determine the main beliefs for the population of interest. **Table 14-3** provides an example of open-ended items used to assess the beliefs of pregnant women during their first trimester. Women during their first trimester would be asked to list about three to five questions for each of the items. Then a content analysis (i.e., a simple frequency count) is undertaken to determine which beliefs are most salient. Finally, a structured belief questionnaire is developed based on the salient beliefs that were identified.

Structured items that arise from the elicitation study should be specific to the target at

Table 14-3 **Assessing the Theory of Planned Behavior Beliefs in Pregnant Women During Their First Trimester**

Belief	Item
Behavioral beliefs	List the main advantages of exercising during your first trimester.
	List the main disadvantages of exercising during your first trimester.
Control beliefs	List the main factors that prevented you from exercising during your first trimester.
	List the main factors that helped you to exercise during your first trimester.
Normative beliefs	List the individuals or groups who were/are most important to you when you thought/think about exercising during your first trimester.

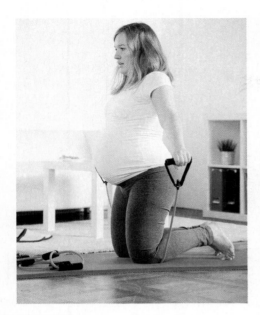

© AzmanL/E+/Getty Images.

which the behavior is directed, the action or specificity of the behavior under study, and the context and time in which the behavior is being performed (Ajzen & Fishbein, 1980). This means, for example, that when trying to develop a walking intervention for older adults, you should ask a sample of older adults to "List the advantages of walking briskly three times a week for 30 minutes outside during the summer." This information will help researchers to develop an intervention based on the salient behavioral beliefs of these older adults that is specific to the behavior. According to the theory of planned behavior, once beliefs are modified, intention will be altered, and the desired behavior change will occur (Symons Downs & Hausenblas, 2005a, 2005b). The relative contribution of the theory of planned behavior constructs may fluctuate from context to context. Thus, before interventions using this framework are implemented, the predictive ability of these constructs with the specific population and specific context should first be tested. **Table 14-4** contains belief items that assess the main variables of the theory of planned behavior for pregnant women (Hausenblas et al., 2011).

CRITICAL THINKING ACTIVITY 14-7

Describe how the theory of planned behavior beliefs may vary from pregnant women to older adults. What implications does this have for developing exercise interventions with these two populations?

Using Theory for Practice

The theory of planned behavior (Ajzen, 1991) is one of the most validated theories for explaining and predicting physical activity behavior, as evidenced by meta-analyses that reveal the strong descriptive and predictive ability (Hagger, Chatzisarantis, & Biddle, 2002; Hausenblas, Carron, & Mack, 1997; McEachan et al., 2011 Symons Downs & Hausenblas, 2005a, 2005b). However, promoting physical activity and reducing sedentary behavior involves changing behavior through intervention. Overall, the application of the theory of planned behavior to change physical activity through intervention has been far more limited than observational studies where behavior was merely predicted. This paucity of evidence has been a critique of the theory (Sniehotta et al., 2014), because behavior change is such an important part of why health behavior research is even conducted in the first place.

There is some emerging evidence, however, that the theory of planned behavior is as effective in changing behavior as other theories, such as social cognitive theory noted above, self-determination theory (see Chapter 15), or the transtheoretical model (see Chapter 16). Gourlan and colleagues (2016), for example, conducted a meta-analysis of these different theories and found eight studies that have used the theory of planned behavior for physical activity intervention. They showed that theory of planned behavior interventions had a small ($d = 0.26$) yet significant effect on physical activity changes and this was not significantly different from other theoretical approaches. In a more recent meta-analysis, Rhodes and colleagues

Table 14-4 Example of Theory of Planned Behavior Belief Items for Pregnant Women

Instructions. The following questions pertain to your **first trimester** exercise behavior. Using the scales below, please indicate your answer by placing it in the space provided after each statement.

1	2	3	4	5	6	7
Extremely Unlikely						Extremely Likely

Behavioral beliefs: Exercising regularly in my first trimester will:

Help control my weight _____

Improve my physical health _____

Make me feel better _____

Increase my energy _____

Improve my appearance/body image _____

Improve my fitness _____

Make my labor and delivery easier _____

Get me outside (fresh air) _____

Relieve my stress _____

Reduce my nausea _____

Improve my baby's health _____

Improve my circulation/blood flow _____

Take too much time _____

Increase my risk of injury _____

1	2	3	4	5	6	7
Strongly Disagree						Strongly Agree

Normative beliefs: Would the following people approve of me exercising regularly in my first trimester:

Spouse/Significant Other _____

Friends _____

Children _____

Co-workers _____

Parents _____

Doctors _____

Siblings _____

1	2	3	4	5	6	7
Strongly Disagree						Strongly Agree

Control beliefs: I will be able to exercise regularly during my first trimester despite:

Health issues (injury/pain) _____

No time to exercise _____

Being tired (having no energy) _____

Bad weather _____

Limited knowledge about exercising during my pregnancy _____

Other children to care for _____

Limited social support _____

Pregnancy-specific discomforts (e.g., breast soreness) _____

Fear of miscarriage/harming baby _____

Headaches _____

Morning sickness/nausea _____

(2021) showed that four studies had data available to show that the intervention on theory of planned behavior variables could be tracked significantly to physical activity changes ($ab = 0.05$) with a small effect size. Similar to Gourlan and colleagues, this effect was comparable to interventions based on other theories. At this time, the evidence is too limited to assess whether the theory of planned behavior is a useful theory for changing sedentary behavior.

CRITICAL THINKING ACTIVITY 14-8

Using the theory of planned behavior as a guide, how would you assess the constructs for sedentary behavior and then apply the findings to conduct a sedentary behavior intervention?

Extending the Theory of Planned Behavior: The Reasoned Action Approach

Although the theory of planned behavior has been successful in explaining and predicting physical activity behavior, limitations of research examining the theory exist (Sniehotta, Presseau, & Araujo-Sores, 2014). As Icek Ajzen (2011) stated: "Yet, for all its popularity, or perhaps because of it, the theory of planned behavior [TPB] has also been the target of much criticism and debate" (p. 1113). Two of the most common criticisms of the approach (and these can also be applied to social cognitive theory) include the gap between intentions (or goals) and behavior and the failure to consider less rational/premeditative determinants of behavior, which will be covered in Chapters 16 and 17, respectively. However, some of the most interesting research conducted with the theory of planned behavior over the last 20 years has been to discern more information and focus from its attitude, subjective norm, and perceived control constructs.

Attitude researchers, including Ajzen and Fishbein, have long considered an attitude to include both instrumental (evaluation of the long-term utility of a behavior) and affective/experiential (evaluation of the pleasure, enjoyment of the behavior) properties (e.g., Fishbein, 1967; Fishbein & Ajzen, 1974; Zanna & Rempel, 1988). These components have been typically aggregated together to form a generalized attitude construct, such as the one conceived in the theory of planned behavior. However, for the last 20 years, there has been convincing evidence that the affective component of a physical activity attitude is a much larger predictor of physical activity intention and subsequent behavior than the instrumental component (Lowe et al., 2002; French et al., 2005). Put in a straightforward way, how we feel about the experience of engaging in physical activity is more important to our intentions and subsequent behavior than what we expect to get from the long-term benefits derived from physical activity. This effect has now been well established through reviews and meta-analyses (e.g., Rhodes, Fiala & Conner, 2009; Rhodes, 2017; McEachan et al., 2016).

CRITICAL THINKING ACTIVITY 14-9

What do you think are the main reasons for your intentions to be active or sedentary? Is how you feel about the activity more important than what you think you will get from it in the long-run? What are the implications of this when trying to promote physical activity and limit sedentary behavior?

Similar reconsideration pertains to the construct of subjective norm. Consistent throughout physical activity literature, the theory of planned behavior variables of attitude and perceived behavioral control have been significant predictors of intention. Subjective norm, however, is generally a weaker predictor of intention (McEachan et al., 2011). One reason may be that significant others may not be important in encouraging participation of physically active individuals (Culos-Reed, Gyurcsik, & Brawley, 2001; Rhodes & Nigg, 2011). A second reason for the weak contribution of subjective norm to the prediction of physical activity might lie in its operationalization (Manning, 2009). In this area, researchers have pointed to two distinct factors in the subjective norm construct that include the perception of what a person thinks important others want them to do (known as injunctive norm) and observing what important others do themselves (known as descriptive norm) (Cialdini et al., 1991). Early evidence applying these two constructs within the context of physical activity showed that descriptive norms may be the more important predictors of intention and even behavior (Okun et al., 2002).

Finally, there is also ambiguity regarding how to define perceived behavioral control, and this creates measurement problems (see Ajzen, 2002a). In fact, Estabrooks and Carron (1998) noted that Ajzen (1985, 1991) has been inconsistent in the manner in which he has defined perceived behavioral control, representing it as both self-efficacy and as the perceived ease or difficulty of performing the specific behavior. Ajzen (2002a) has since noted that perceived behavioral control is composed of the following two components: (1) self-efficacy (i.e., ease or difficulty of performing the behavior)

and (2) controllability (i.e., beliefs about the extent to which performing the behavior is up to the person). Early research applying these multiple components to physical activity has tended to support the self-efficacy component as a critical predictor more than the controllability component (e.g., Terry and O'Leary, 1995).

Based on this ongoing research with the theory of planned behavior constructs, Fishbein and Ajzen (2010) have amended the model to include the two component structures of attitude, subjective norm, and perceived behavioral control. This amended model is called the Reasoned Action Approach (see **Figure 14-6**). Attitude toward the behavior is assumed to consist of experiential (a relabel from affective attitude) and instrumental attitudes; perceived norm (a relabel from subjective norm) is assumed to consist of injunctive and descriptive norms; and perceived behavioral control is assumed to consist of capacity and autonomy (a relabel of self-efficacy and controllability, respectively).

The earliest test of this model in the physical activity domain—long before it was coined the reasoned action approach—was conducted

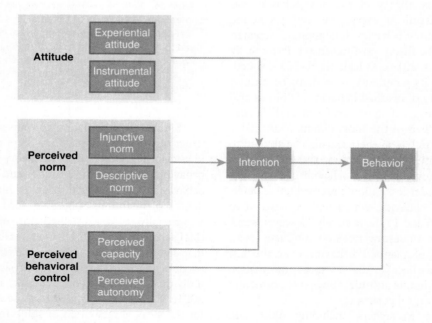

Figure 14-6 Reasoned Action Approach.

by Rhodes and Courneya (2003) with samples of undergraduate students and cancer survivors. These researchers found that affective attitude and capacity were the main predictors of intention, while injunctive and descriptive norm contributed equally to predicting intention but with much smaller effects. Since that time, McEachan and colleagues (2016) have conducted a meta-analysis of 14 health behaviors that could be coded using the reasoned action approach model. The results showed that affective (or experiential) attitude (b = 0.40) and perceived capacity (b = 0.27) had roughly medium-sized effects on intention, while instrumental attitude (b = 0.19), injunctive norm (b = 0.10), and descriptive norm (b = 0.07) had small effects, and autonomy did not have a significant effect. As expected, intention was the largest predictor of behavior (b = 0.44), but there were also significant small effects from affective attitude (b = 0.05), perceived capacity (b = 0.09), and descriptive norm (b = 0.11). The research is too limited at present to assess prediction of sedentary behavior.

Summary

A shift in thinking from a behaviorist to a cognitive focus sparked the development of social cognitive approaches to understanding behavior and behavior change. This chapter included two prominent theories applying this social cognitive approach. Bandura (1997) has defined self-efficacy as the belief that one is capable of organizing and executing the courses of action required to produce an outcome. It is thought to be influenced by a variety of factors, including mastery experiences, vicarious experiences (i.e., observational learning), imagery experiences, verbal persuasion, physiologic states, and mood. Efficacy plays an important role in exercise and physical activity and may play a role in limiting sedentary behavior. For example, it has been shown to be positively associated with physical activity generally, as well as with the initiation of a program of physical activity, maintenance of involvement, and expenditure of effort during participation. Despite these findings, there are still some areas of self-efficacy research with mixed findings. Some researchers have demonstrated that self-efficacy may measure motivation and willingness more than capability. The experimental evidence on self-efficacy and physical activity is also mixed, showing that correlations are not necessarily causation. Changing self-efficacy has proven difficult in our current interventions, and changes in self-efficacy do not always link to subsequent changes in behavior. Furthermore, contemporary evidence suggests that vicarious experience and positive feedback may be even stronger sources of self-efficacy than graded mastery experiences.

Researchers have applied the theory of planned behavior and found support for the utility of attitudes, perceived behavioral control, and, to a lesser extent, subjective norms in explaining people's intention to become physically active. Emerging research is revealing that the theory of planned behavior may be effective in explaining and predicting sedentary behavior. In general, there is strong evidence that the theory of planned behavior can explain and predict people's physical activity intentions and behaviors. Because of the success of the theory of planned behavior to explain and predict exercise behavior, it may also serve as a useful framework to guide physical activity interventions.

Vignette: Rachel

One of the first things my mother said to me after I told her I'd finally gotten pregnant was, "Well, then you should probably stop running."

About 6 months before my husband and I verified our forthcoming baby's heartbeat,

I completed my first marathon. I was thrilled when I finally crossed the finish line! Learning how to stay properly fueled and come into race day fully prepared was an incredible learning process—terrifying at times (not to mention arduous), but ultimately one of the most reward-ing periods of my life.

My mother did not approve of my marathon training. She was concerned it would reignite the eating disorder I briefly grappled with during college—even though this episode of my life had taken place over a decade ago.

I'd always been the chubby girl in middle and high school. So once I moved across country for undergrad, I was hell bent on proving to my new friends that I, too, could squeeze into a pair of size 2 jeans. I went overboard on restricting what I ate, in part, because I wasn't exactly sure what a healthy diet should entail. And I was unaware there were severe health consequences associated with massively reducing your caloric intake like I did.

I had tried out for the track team shortly after beginning my first semester of classes because I thought this would help keep my weight down. But once my weight fell so low that I stopped getting my period, I had to quit. I didn't have the stamina, and my body simply couldn't take the daily meets.

After working with a nutritionist and psy-chologist at my college's health center, I was able to figure out a more moderate daily meal plan. I never had to leave school or take any drastic measures to get better, like enrolling in an inpa-tient clinic. I got my weight back up to a normal level and resumed running. This time with the cross-country team.

I've managed to keep a steady training reg-imen ever since graduating, paying particular attention to my nutritional needs so as not to mess up my system again. If nothing else, I feel that my running schedule has helped improve my body image concerns, because the mileage I cover each week makes me feel more empow-ered in my skin.

But doubt began wending its way into my devotion to running when my husband and I ini-tially tried to conceive. Because it didn't happen immediately, I started to worry that my daily runs might be interfering with the process of getting pregnant. It was hard not to think that my exercise habits were to blame, even though I was regularly menstruating and maintaining a healthy BMI.

But my OB/GYN, an exercise physiologist I worked with, and a nutritionist all told me it was okay to keep exercising as I had been while attempting to get pregnant. I wanted to trust them, but weekly insinuations from mom that running was rendering me unable to foster new life inside of me really messed with my head.

I guess habit won out, though. No, I didn't jump into gearing up for marathon number two once I switched into baby mode, but until my pregnancy tests turned up positive, I was log-ging between 5 and 8 miles on most days of the week. I dialed down my mileage after getting the good news. I'll admit, I was nervous that hitting the trail near my home might induce a miscar-riage, even though my OB/GYN reiterated that the chances of this were so low as to be negligible. But throughout my first trimester, I was still able to complete a 5K.

What truly changed my behavior wasn't the social stigma of being told I was insane for not staunching my runs (and not just by my mother but also by other family members and some col-leagues at work), it was the morning sickness and fatigue that got in the way. And once the second trimester rolled around, the discomfort in my lower back—coupled with an elevated need for trips to the ladies' room during my workouts—eventually took me back to walking and taking advantage of the elliptical machine at my gym.

Despite the fear and the negative attitudes from my family and some coworkers, I really did believe in my ability to make it through my pregnancy without giving up physical activity altogether. Though during the final few weeks of it, I was really only able to do prenatal Pilates and yoga in between a few light spurts on the elliptical. I started each morning with the inten-tion to do whatever I could.

I gave birth to a healthy baby girl on sched-ule and with no complications. (I had worried that, like my mother had to do when I was born, I would have to deliver via a C-section. But this wasn't necessary.)

That baby girl is now turning 5 and I've got-ten back to running 10Ks ever since she was a year old. And the only reason I'm not training for another marathon is that her brother is now on his way into the world.

The best part? Over the holidays the discussion of running came up over a family dinner with my mother. I watched her open her mouth as she looked from her new granddaughter to my husband, then to me. "You know how I feel about you still doing those races," she said to me. Then added, "but I guess you proved me wrong."

Key Terms

attitude An individual's positive or negative evaluation of performing a behavior.

barrier efficacy An individual's beliefs about possessing the capability to overcome obstacles to physical activity.

behavioral beliefs Perceived consequences of carrying out a specific action and a person's evaluation of each of these consequences.

control beliefs Perceived presence or absence of required resources and opportunities, the anticipated obstacles or impediments to behavior, and the perceived power of a particular control factor to facilitate or inhibit performance of the behavior.

first trimester Begins on the first day of a woman's last period and lasts until the end of week 12.

intention Person's willingness and how much effort they are planning to exert to perform a behavior.

mastery experiences Personal experiences with carrying out a task successfully; thought to be the most important cause of self-efficacy beliefs.

mood states A source of self-efficacy beliefs whereby previous successes and failures are stored in memory (and recalled) with associated feelings.

normative beliefs Perceived expectations of important significant others or groups and the individual's motivation to comply with the expectations of these important significant others.

outcome expectations Expectations an individual has about the outcomes of a particular behavior.

perceived behavioral control Perceived ease or difficulty of performing a behavior.

physiological state Bodily sensations, such as increased heart rate, increased sweating, and increased respiratory rate.

reciprocal determinism The interdependency and codetermination of behavior, internal personal factors, and external environmental factors.

scheduling efficacy An individual's beliefs about possessing the capability to schedule physical activity into a daily or weekly routine.

self-efficacy Belief in one's capabilities to organize and execute the course of action required to produce a certain outcome.

social support The perception and actuality that one is cared for by others, has assistance available from other people, and that one is part of a supportive social network.

subjective norm Perceived social pressure that individuals feel to perform or not perform a particular behavior.

task efficacy An individual's beliefs about possessing the capability to perform a behavioral act.

theory of planned behavior A theory about the link between beliefs and behavior.

theory of reasoned action A theory about the link between volitional behavior and intention.

verbal persuasion A source of self-efficacy beliefs whereby positive verbal statements ("you can do it") increase self-efficacy. Greatest impact on self-efficacy is found in those individuals who have some reason to believe that they could be successful with a task if they persist.

vicarious experiences Observational learning from the successful or unsuccessful behavior of others used as a comparative standard; thought to be a powerful cause of self-efficacy beliefs.

Review Questions

1. According to Bandura's social cognitive theory, what are the most important reasons for performing or not performing physical activity?

2. What are the main causes of self-efficacy beliefs? Which causes are most important?

3. Explain the three dimensions of self-efficacy measurement.

4. What types of self-efficacy are important to physical activity?

Applying the Concepts

1. Which variable(s) of the theory of planned behavior best explains Rachel's ability to stick to her running regimen throughout her pregnancy?

2. Apart from the variables in the theory of planned behavior, what else might account for Rachel's ability to maintain her commitment to running?

References

Ajzen, I. (1985). From intentions to actions: A theory of planned behavior. In J. Kuhl, & J. Beckman (Eds.), *Action-control: From cognition to behavior* (pp. 11–39). Heidelberg: Springer.

Ajzen, I. (1991). The theory of planned behavior. *Organizational Behavior and Human Decision Processes, 50*(2), 179–211.

Ajzen, I. (2002a). Perceived behavioral control, self-efficacy, locus of control, and the theory of planned behavior. *Journal of Applied Social Psychology, 32*(4), 665–683.

Ajzen, I. (2002b). Construction of a standard questionnaire for the theory of planned behavior. Retrieved August 2002 from http://www.unix.oit.umass.edu/~aizen

Ajzen, I., & Driver, B. L. (1991). Prediction of leisure participation from behavioral, normative, and control beliefs: An application of the theory of planned behavior. *Leisure Sciences, 13*(3), 185–204.

Armstrong, C. A., Sallis, J. F., Hovell, M. F., & Hofstetter, C. R. (1993). Stages of change, self-efficacy, and the adoption of vigorous exercise: A prospective analysis. *Journal of Sport and Exercise Psychology, 15*(4), 390–402.

Ashford, S., Edmunds, J., & French, D. P. (2010). What is the best way to change self-efficacy to promote lifestyle and recreational physical activity? A systematic review with meta-analysis. *British Journal of Health Psychology, 15*(2), 265–288.

Bandura, A. (1977). Self-efficacy: Toward a unifying theory of behavioral change. *Psychological Review, 84*(2), 191–215.

Bandura, A. (1986). Social foundations of thought and action: A social-cognitive theory. Englewood Cliffs, NJ: Prentice-Hall.

Bandura, A. (1995). On rectifying conceptual ecumenism. In J. E. Maddux (Ed.), *Self-efficacy, adaptation, and adjustment: Theory, research, and application.* New York, NY: Plenum.

Bandura, A. (1997). *Self-efficacy, the exercise of control.* New York, NY: Freeman.

Bandura, A. (1998). Health promotion from the perspective of social cognitive theory. *Psychology & Health, 134,* 623–649.

Baranowski, T., Anderson, C., & Carmack, C. (1998). Mediating variable framework in physical activity interventions: How are we doing? How might we do better? *American Journal of Preventive Medicine, 15*(4), 266–297.

Beauchamp, M. R., Crawford, K. L., & Jackson, B. (2019). Social cognitive theory and physical activity: Mechanisms of behavior change, critique, and legacy. *Psychology of Sport and Exercise, 42,* 110–117.

Bergh, I. H., Bjelland, M., Grydeland, M., Lien, N., Andersen, L. F., Klepp, K. I., Anderssen, S. A., & Ommundsen, Y. (2012). Mid-way and post-intervention effects on potential determinants of physical activity and sedentary behavior, results of the HEIA study—a multi-component school-based randomized trial. *International Journal of Behavioral Nutrition and Physical Activity, 9*(63).

Blanchard, C. M., Fortier, M. S., Sweet, S., O'Sullivan, T., Hogg, W., Reid, R. D., & Sigal, R. J. (2007). Explaining physical activity levels from a self-efficacy perspective: The physical activity counseling trial. *Annals of Behavioral Medicine, 34*(3), 323–328.

Blanchard, C. M., Rodgers, W., Courneya, K. S., Daub, B., & Knapik, G. (2002). Does barrier efficacy mediate the gender/exercise adherence relationship during phase II cardiac rehabilitation? *Rehabilitation Psychology, 47*(1), 106–120.

Cahill, S. P., Gallo, L. A., Lisman, S. A., & Weinstein, A. (2006). Willing or able? The meanings of self-efficacy. *Journal of Social and Clinical Psychology, 25*(2), 196–209.

Cialdini, R. B., Kallgren, C. A., & Reno, R. R. (1991). A focus theory of normative conduct: A theoretical refinement and reevaluation of the role of norms in human behavior. *Advances in Experimental Social Psychology, 24,* 201–234.

Conn, V. S., Hafdahl, A. R., & Mehr, D. R. (2011). Interventions to increase physical activity among healthy adults: Meta-analysis of outcomes. *American Journal of Public Health, 101*, 751–758.

Conner, M. (2020). Theory of planned behavior. In G. Tenenbaum, & R. C. Eklund (Eds.), *Handbook of Sports Psychology (4th Edition)* (pp. 3–18). Wiley.

Courneya, K. S., Jones, L. W., Mackey, J. R., & Fairey, A. S. (2006). Exercise beliefs of breast cancer survivors before and after participation in a randomized controlled trial. *International Journal of Behavioral Medicine, 13*, 259–264.

Dewar, D. L., Morgan, P. J., Plotnikoff, R. C., Okely, A. D., Batterham, M., & Lubans, D. R. (2014). Exploring changes in physical activity, sedentary behaviors and hypothesized mediators in the NEAT girls group randomized controlled trial. *Journal of Science and Medicine in Sport, 17*(1), 39–46.

Fishbein, M. (1967). Attitude and the prediction of behavior. In M. Fishbein (Ed.), *Readings in attitude theory and measurement* (pp. 477–492). Wiley.

Fishbein, M., & Ajzen, I. (1975). *Belief, attitude, intention, and behavior.* Don Mills, NY: Addison-Wesley.

Fishbein, M., & Ajzen, I. (2010). Predicting and changing behavior: The reasoned action approach. Psychology Press.

French, D. P., Sutton, S., Hennings, S. J., Mitchell, J., Wareham, N. J., Griffin, S., Hardeman, W., & Kinmonth, A. L. (2005). The importance of affective beliefs and attitudes in the theory of planned behavior: Predicting intention to increase physical activity. *Journal of Applied Social Psychology, 35*(9), 1824–1848.

French, D. P., Olander, E. K., Chisholm, A., & Mc Sharry, J. (2014). Which behaviour change techniques are most effective at increasing older adults' self-efficacy and physical activity behaviour? A systematic review. *Annals of Behavioral Medicine, 48*(2), 225–234.

Gardiner, P. A., Eakin, E. G., Healy, G. N., & Owen, N. (2011). Feasibility of reducing older adults' sedentary time. *American Journal of Preventive Medicine, 41*(2), 174–177.

Gebel, K., Bauman, A. E., Reger-Nash, B., & Leydon, K. M. (2011). Does the environment moderate the impact of a mass media campaign to promote walking? *American Journal of Health Promotion, 26*(1), 45–48.

Gourlan, M., Bernard, P., Bortolon, C., Romain, A. J., Lareyre, O., Carayol, M., Ninot, G., & Boiché, J. (2016). Efficacy of theory-based interventions to promote physical activity. A meta-analysis of randomised controlled trials. *Health Psychology Review, 10*(1), 50–66.

Hagger, M. S., Chatzisarantis, N. L., & Biddle, S. J. (2002). The influence of autonomous and controlling motives on physical activity intentions with the theory of planned behavior. *British Journal of Health Psychology, 7*(3), 283–297.

Hagger, M. S., & Chatzisarantis, N. L. (2009). Integrating the theory of planned behaviour and self-determination theory in health behaviour: A meta-analysis. *British Journal of Health Psychology, 14*(2), 275–302.

Hausenblas, H. A., Carron, A. V., & Mack, D. E. (1997). Application of theories of reasoned action and planned behavior to exercise behavior: A meta-analysis. *Journal of Sport and Exercise Psychology, 19*(1), 36–51.

Hausenblas, H., Giacobbi, P., Cook, B., Rhodes, R., & Cruz, A. (2011). Prospective examination of pregnant and nonpregnant women's physical activity beliefs and behaviours. *Journal of Infant and Reproductive Psychology, 29*(4), 308–319.

Hausenblas, H. A., & Symons Downs, D. (2004). Prospective examination of the theory of planned behavior applied to exercise behavior during women's first trimester of pregnancy. *Journal of Reproductive and Infant Psychology, 22*(3), 199–210.

Higgins, T. J., Middleton, K. R., Winner, L., & Janelle, C. M. (2014). Physical activity interventions differentially affect exercise task and barrier self-efficacy: A meta-analysis. *Health Psychology, 33*(8), 891–903.

Jago, R., Sebire, S. J., Edwards, M. J., & Thompson, J. L. (2013). Parental TV viewing, parental self- efficacy, media equipment, and TV viewing among preschool children. *European Journal of Pediatrics, 172*, 1543–1545.

James, W. (n. d.). *BrainyQuote.com*. Retrieved August 19, 2015, from BrainyQuote.com website: http://www.brainyquote .com/quotes/quotes/w/williamjam157168.html. Read more at http://www.brainyquote.com/citation/quotes/quotes/w /williamjam157168.html#x8DpS5ooSp37bJjR.99

Jones, L. W., Guill, B., Keir, S. T., Carter, K., Friedman, H. S., Bigner, D. D., & Reardon, D. A. (2007).Using the theory of planned behavior to understand the determinants of exercise intention in patients diagnosed with primary brain cancer. *Psycho-Oncology, 16*(3), 232–240.

Karvinen, K. H., Courneya, K. S., Campbell, K. L., Pearcey, R. G., Dundas, G., Capstick, V., & Tonkin, K. (2007). Correlates of exercise motivation and behavior in a population-based sample of endometrial cancer survivors: An application of the theory of planned behavior. *International Journal of Behavioral Nutrition and Physical Activity, 4*(21), 20–30.

Kavussanu, M., & McAuley, E. (1995). Exercise and optimism: Are highly active individuals more optimistic? *Journal of Sport and Exercise Psychology, 17*(3), 246–258.

Kirsch, I. (1982). Efficacy expectations or response predictions: The meaning of efficacy ratings as a function of task characteristics. *Journal of Personality and Social Psychology, 42*(1), 132–136. https://doi.org/10.1037/0022-3514.42 .1.132

Kirsch, I. (1995). Self-efficacy and outcome expectancy: A concluding commentary. In J. E. Maddux (Ed.), *Self-efficacy, adaptation, and adjustment: Theory, research, and application* (pp. 341–345). New York, NY: Plenum.

Lithopoulos, A., Grant, S. J., Williams, D. M., & Rhodes, R. E. (2020). Experimental comparison of physical activity self-efficacy measurement: Do vignettes reduce motivational confounding? *Psychology of Sport and Exercise, 47*, 101642.

Lowe, R., Eves, F., & Carroll, D. (2002). The influence of affective and instrumental beliefs on exercise intentions and behavior: A longitudinal analysis. *Journal of Applied Social Psychology, 32*(6), 1241–1252.

Lowe, S. S., Danielson, B. B., Beaumont, C., Watanabe, S. M., Baracos, V. E., & Courneya, K. S. (2015). Correlates of objectively measured sedentary behavior in cancer patients with brain metastases: An application of the theory of planned behavior. *Psycho-Oncology, 24*(7), 757–762. https://doi.org/10.1002/pon.3641

Lubans, D. R., Foster, C., & Biddle, S. J. (2008). A review of mediators of behavior in interventions to promote physical activity among children and adolescents. *Preventive Medicine, 47*(5), 463–470.

Maddux, J. E. (1995). Looking for common ground: A comment on Kirsch and Bandura. In J. E. Maddux (Ed.), *Self-efficacy, adaptation, and adjustment: Theory, research, and application* (pp. 377–386). New York, NY: Plenum.

Mama, S. K., Song, J., Ortiz, A., Tirado-Gomez, M., Palacios, C., Hughes, D. C., & Basen-Engquist, K. (2017). Longitudinal social cognitive influences on physical activity and sedentary time in Hispanic breast cancer survivors. *Psycho-Oncology, 26*(2), 214–221.

McAuley, E., & Blissmer, B. (2000). Self-efficacy determinants and consequences of physical activity. *Exercise and Sport Sciences Reviews, 28*(2), 85–88.

McAuley, E., Katula, J. A., Mihalko, S. L., Blissmer, B., Duncan, T. E., Pena, M., & Dunn, E. (1999). Mode of physical activity and self-efficacy in older adults: A latent growth curve analysis. *Journal of Gerontology, 54B*(5), 283–292.

McAuley, E., & Mihalko, S. (1998). Measuring exercise-related self-efficacy. In J. Duda (Ed.), *Advances in sport and exercise psychology* (pp. 371–390). Morgantown, WV: Fitness Information Technology.

McAuley, E., Shaffer, S. M., & Rudolph, D. (1995). Affective responses to acute exercise in elderly impaired males: The moderating effects of self-efficacy and age. *International Journal of Aging and Human Development, 41*(1), 13–27.

McAuley, E., Wraith, S., & Duncan, T. E. (1991). Self-efficacy, perceptions of success, and intrinsic motivation for exercise. *Journal of Applied Social Psychology, 21*(2), 139–155.

McEachan, R. R., Conner, M., Taylor, N. J., & Lawton, R. J. (2011). Prospective prediction of health-related behaviors with the theory of planned behaviour: A meta-analysis. *Health Psychology Review, 5*(2), 97–144.

McEachan, R., Taylor, N., Harrison, R., Lawton, R., Gardner, P., & Conner, M. (2016). Meta-analysis of the reasoned action approach (RAA) to understanding health behaviors. *Annals of Behavioral Medicine, 50*(4), 592–612.

McEwan, D., Beauchamp, M. R., Kouvousis, C., Ray, C., Wyrough, A., & Rhodes, R. E. (2019). Examining the active ingredients of physical activity interventions underpinned by theory versus no stated theory: A meta-analysis. *Health Psychology Review, 13*(1), 1–17.

Motl, R. W., Sasaki, J. E., Cederberg, K. L., & Jeng, B. (2019). Social-cognitive theory variables as correlates of sedentary behavior in multiple sclerosis: Preliminary evidence. *Disability and Health Journal, 12*(4), 622–627.

Nigg, C. R., Aneas Zurkinden, N. L., Beck, D. A., Bisang, X. J. B., Charbonnet, B., Dütschler, B., . . ., & Zutter, M. T. (2021). Promoting more physical activity and less sedentary behaviour during the COVID19 situation–SportStudisMoveYou (SSMY): A randomized controlled trial. *Health Psychology Bulletin, 5*, 1–11.

O'Donoghue, G., Perchoux, C., Mensah, K., Lakerveld, J., van der Ploeg, H., Bernaards, C., Chastin, S. F. M., Simon, C., O'Gorman, D., & Nazare, J. A. (2016). A systematic review of the correlates of sedentary behaviour in adults aged 18–65 years: a socio-ecological approach. *BioMed Central Public Health, 16*, 163.

Oman, R. F., & King, A. C. (1998). Predicting the adoption and maintenance of exercise participation using self-efficacy and previous exercise participation rates. *American Journal of Health Promotion, 12*, 154–161.

Prapavessis, H., Gaston, A., & DeJesus, S. (2015). The theory of planned behavior as a model for understanding sedentary behavior. *Psychology of Sport and Exercise, 19*, 23–32.

Prestwich, A., Sniehotta, F. F., Whittington, C., Dombrowski, S. U., Rogers, L., & Michie, S. (2014). Does theory influence the effectiveness of health behavior interventions? Meta-analysis. *Health Psychology, 33*(5), 465–474.

Prince, S. A., Reed, J. L., McFetridge, C., Tremblay, M. S., & Reid, R. D. (2017). Correlates of sedentary behaviour in adults: a systematic review. *Obesity Reviews, 18*(8), 915–935.

Rhodes, R. E., & Blanchard, C. M. (2007). What do confidence items measure in the physical activity domain? *Journal of Applied Social Psychology, 37*(4), 759–774.

Rhodes, R. E., & Courneya, K. S. (2003). Self-efficacy, controllability, and intention in the theory of planned behavior: Measurement redundancy or causal independence? *Psychology and Health, 18*(1), 79–91.

Rhodes, R. E., & Courneya, K. S. (2003). Investigating multiple components of attitude, subjective norm, and perceived behavioral control: An examination of the theory of planned behavior in the exercise domain. *British Journal of Social Psychology, 42*(1), 129–146.

Rhodes, R. E., & Courneya, K. S. (2004). Differentiating motivation and control in the theory of planned behavior. *Psychology, Health, & Medicine, 9*(2), 205–215.

Rhodes, R. E., & Pfaeffli, L. A. (2010). Mediators of physical activity behaviour change among adult non-clinical populations: A review update. *International Journal of Behavioral Nutrition and Physical Activity, 7*(37).

Rhodes, R. E. (2017). The evolving understanding of physical activity behavior: A multi-process action control approach. In A. J. Elliot (Ed.), *Advances in Motivation Science* (Vol. 4, pp. 171–205). Elsevier Academic Press.

Rhodes, R. E., Boudreau, P., Weman Josefsson, K., & Ivarsson, A. (2021). Mediators of physical activity behavior change interventions among adults: A systematic review and meta-analysis. *Health Psychology Review, 15*(2), 272–286.

Rhodes, R. E., Fiala, B., & Conner, M. (2009). Affective judgments and physical activity: A review and meta-analysis. *Annals of Behavioral Medicine, 38*(3), 180–204.

Rhodes, R. E., & Nigg, C. R. (2011). Advancing physical activity theory: A review and future directions. *Exercise and Sports Sciences Reviews, 39*(3), 113–119.

Rhodes, R. E., & Rebar, A. L. (2017). Conceptualizing and defining the intention construct for future physical activity research. *Exercise and Sports Sciences Reviews, 45*(4), 209–216.

Rhodes, R. E., Williams, D. M., & Mistry, C. D. (2016). Using short vignettes to disentangle perceived capability from motivation: A test using walking and resistance training behaviors. *Psychology, Health & Medicine, 21*(5), 639–651.

Rhodes, R. E., Mark, R., & Temmel, C. (2012). Correlates of adult sedentary behaviour: A systematic review. *American Journal of Preventive Medicine, 43*, e3–e28.

Sonstroem, R. J., Harlow, L. L., & Josephs, L. (1994). Exercise and self-esteem: Validity of model expansion and exercise associations. *Journal of Sport and Exercise Psychology, 16*(1), 29–42.

Spence, J. C., Burgess, J. A., Cutumisu, N., Lee, J. G., Moylan, B., Taylor, L., & Witcher, C. S. (2006). Self-efficacy and physical activity: A quantitative review. *Journal of Sport and Exercise Psychology, 28*, S172.

Symons Downs, D., & Hausenblas, H. A. (2005a). Elicitation studies and the theory of planned behavior: A systematic review of exercise beliefs. *Psychology of Sport and Exercise, 6*(1), 1–31.

Symons Downs, D., & Hausenblas, H. A. (2005b). Exercise behavior and the theories of reasoned action and planned behavior: A meta-analytic update. *Journal of Physical Activity and Health, 2*, 76–97.

Sniehotta, F. F., Presseau, J., & Araujo-Soares, V. (2014). Time to retire the theory of planned behaviour. *Health Psychology Review, 8*, 1–7.

Sweet, S. N., Martin Ginis, K. A., & Latimer-Cheung, A. E. (2012). Examining physical activity trajectories for people with spinal cord injury. *Health Psychology, 31*(6), 728–732. https://doi.org/10.1037/a0027795

Terlecki, M., Brown, J., Harner-Steciw, L., Irvin-Hannum, J., Marchetto-Ryan, N., Ruhl, L., & Wiggins, J. (2011). Sex differences and similarities in video game experience, preferences, and self-efficacy: Implications for the gaming industry. *Current Psychology, 30*, 22–33.

Vallance, J. K., Courneya, K. S., Plotnikoff, R. C., & Mackey, J. R. (2008). Analyzing theoretical mechanisms of physical activity behavior change in breast cancer survivors: Results from the activity promotion (ACTION) trial. *Annals of Behavioral Medicine, 35*(2), 150–158.

Van Dyck, D., Cardon, G., Deforche, B., Owen, N., De Cocker, K., Wijndaele, K., & De Bourdeaudhuij. I(2011). Socio-demographic, psychosocial, and home environmental attributes associated with adults' domestic screen time. *BioMed Central Public Health, 11*(668).

Wegner, D. M. (2002). *The illusion of conscious will.* Cambridge, MA: MIT Press.

Williams, S., & French, D. P. (2011). What are the most effective intervention techniques for changing physical activity self-efficacy and physical activity behaviour—and are they the same? *Health Education Research, 26*(2), 308–322.

Williams, D. M., & Rhodes, R. E. (2016). The confounded self-efficacy construct: Review, conceptual analysis, and recommendations for future research. *Health Psychology Review, 10*(2), 113–128.

Young, M. D., Plotnikoff, R. C., Collins, C., Callister, R., & Morgan, P. J. (2014). Social cognitive theory and physical activity: A systematic review and meta-analysis. *Obesity Reviews, 12*, 983–995.

Zimmerman, F. J., Ortiz, S. E., Christakis, D. A., & Elkun, D. (2012). The value of social-cognitive theory to reducing preschool TV viewing: A pilot randomized trial. *Preventive Medicine, 54*, 212–218.

Zanna, M. P., & Rempel, J. K. (1988). Attitudes: A new look at an old concept. In D. Bar-Tal, & A. W. Kruglanski (Eds.), *The social psychology of knowledge* Cambridge University Press.

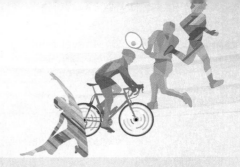

CHAPTER 15

Motivational Theories

LEARNING OBJECTIVES

After completing this chapter, you will be able to:

- Describe the constructs of the health belief model, protection motivation theory, and self-determination theory.
- Describe research that has applied these theories to physical activity.
- Discuss the advantages and limitations of the health belief model, protection motivation theory, and self-determination theory.

Introduction

Fred Kerlinger (1973), in a discussion on the scientific process, noted that "the basic aim of science is theory . . . perhaps less cryptic, the basic aim of science is to explain natural phenomena" (p. 8). A similar observation was made by Leonardo da Vinci hundreds of years ago. "Science generally, and the theories of science specifically, provide the rudder or compass to guide practice." In this chapter, we highlight one of the first theories applied to understand physical activity and finish the chapter with a theory that has begun to receive much contemporary research.

A natural phenomenon that scientists and public health practitioners are trying to explain is why more people are not physically active. Physically inactive people are at risk for several chronic disorders, such as heart disease, stroke, obesity, and diabetes (Warburton & Bredin, 2017). Even though these individuals are at risk, they may not experience any symptoms associated with these diseases. Thus, they may not consider it necessary to discuss their inactive lifestyle with a physician or increase their physical activity levels. Three scientific theories—the health belief model (Rosenstock, 1974), protection motivation theory (Rogers, 1983), and self-determination theory (Deci & Ryan, 2000)—have been used to explain physical (in)activity from a health perspective (see Chapters 14, 16, and 17 for other perspectives).

Health Belief Model

The health belief model is generally acknowledged as the first model that adapted theory from the behavioral sciences to health problems, and it remains one of the most widely recognized conceptual frameworks for health behavior. It was introduced in the 1950s by social psychologists Godfrey Hochbaum, Stephen Kegels, and Irwin Rosenstock, who all worked for the United States Public Health Service. During the early 1950s,

© Norbert9/Shutterstock; © sergeymansurov/Shutterstock.

317

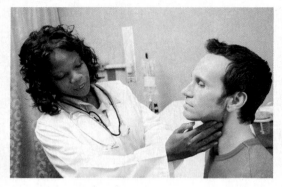

© Jupiterimages/Thinkstock.

the Public Health Service was oriented toward prevention of disease rather than treatment of disease. Thus, the originators of the health belief model were concerned with the widespread failure of individuals to engage in preventive health measures, such as getting a flu vaccine. They postulated that individuals will comply with preventive regimens if they possess minimal levels of relevant health motivation and knowledge, perceive themselves as potentially vulnerable, view the disease as severe, are convinced that the preventive regimen is effective, and see few difficulties or barriers in undertaking the regimen. In addition, internal or external cues that individuals associate with taking health-related actions are considered to be an essential catalyst.

The first research based on the health belief model was initiated by Godfrey Hochbaum (1952). He attempted to identify factors underlying the decision to obtain the then-available preventive service of a chest x-ray for the early detection of tuberculosis. Subsequently, the model has been applied to screening utilization rates for high blood pressure, cervical cancer, dental disease, polio, influenza, and most recently, COVID-19 (e.g., Sheppard & Thomas, 2021; Walrave et al., 2020). It has been applied to predict patient responses to symptoms (Kirscht, 1974) and to comply with prescribed medical and health regimens (Becker, 1974), such as hypertension medication, diet, and physical activity (Aho, 1979; Frewen, Schomer, & Dunne, 1994; Hayslick, Weigand, Weinberg, Richardson, & Jackson, 1996; Tirrell & Hart, 1980). In short, the

health belief model became a major framework for explaining and predicting the reasons people engage in a variety of preventive health behaviors.

Health Belief Model Constructs

The basic components of the health belief model suggest that behavior depends mainly on two variables: (1) the value placed by an individual on a particular behavioral goal, and (2) the individual's estimate of the likelihood that a given action will achieve that goal (Janz & Becker, 1984). When these two variables were conceptualized in the context of health-related behavior, the focus was on either (1) the desire to avoid illness, or if ill, to get well, or (2) the belief that a specific health action will prevent illness or hasten recovery.

The model was originally composed of the following four constructs: perceived susceptibility, perceived severity, **perceived benefits**, and perceived barriers. These concepts were proposed as accounting for people's "readiness to act." An added concept, **cues to action**, would activate that readiness and stimulate the actual behavior. A more recent addition to the model is self-efficacy, or one's confidence in the ability to successfully perform a behavior (see Chapter 14). Self-efficacy was included in the model by Irwin Rosenstock and his colleagues (Rosenstock, Stretcher, & Becker, 1988) to accommodate the challenges of changing unhealthy behaviors, such as being sedentary, smoking, or overeating, to healthy behaviors. In addition to these constructs, the following three other groups of variables are considered important for predicting health behavior: (1) demographic factors, such as age, sex, and race; (2) psychosocial factors, such as personality and peer pressure; and (3) structural factors, such as knowledge (Rosenstock et al., 1988). **Figure 15-1** provides a schematic of the health belief model. Each of the model's constructs is described in detail in the following discussion. (Also see **Table 15-1** for definitions and applications of the health belief model constructs.)

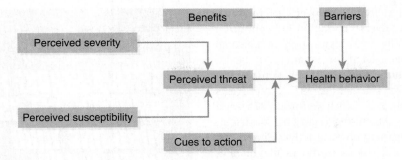

Figure 15-1 Health Belief Model.

Data from Janz, N., & Becker, M. (1984). The health belief model: A decade later. *Health Education Quarterly, 11*, 1–47.

Perceived Susceptibility

To engage in a behavior and thereby avoid an illness, an individual must first believe that they are personally susceptible to that illness. Individuals vary in their **perceived susceptibility** to a disease or condition (e.g., Venema & Pfattheicher,

2021; Scarinci et al., 2021). Those people at the low-end of perceived susceptibility deny the possibility of contracting an adverse condition. Individuals in a moderate category admit to a possibility of disease susceptibility. Finally, those individuals at the high-end of perceived

Table 15-1 Definitions, Applications, and Examples of the Health Belief Model Constructs

Construct	Definition	Application	Example
Perceived susceptibility	Person's opinion of the chances of getting a disease.	Define populations at risk. Personalize risk based on a person's features or behavior. Heighten perceived susceptibility if too low.	My chances of getting cardiovascular disease are high because I am sedentary and overweight.
Perceived severity	Person's opinion of the seriousness of a condition and its consequences.	Specify consequences of the risk and condition.	Cardiovascular disease is a serious illness that may cost me my life.
Perceived benefits	Person's opinion of the efficacy of the advised action to reduce risk or seriousness of impact.	Define when, where, and how to take action. Clarify the positive effects to be expected.	I will walk for a half-hour 6 days a week. Becoming physically active will make me healthier and reduce my chances of a heart attack.
Perceived barriers	Person's opinion of the physical and psychological costs of the advised action.	Identify and reduce barriers through reassurance, incentives, and assistance.	Becoming physically active will take time away from others things I enjoy doing.
Cues to action	Strategies to activate "readiness."	Provide how-to information, promote awareness, give reminders.	I will buy physical activity videos and magazines and post reminder notes on the fridge.
Self-efficacy	Confidence in one's ability to take action.	Provide training and guidance in performing action.	I will start slow and gradually increase my frequency, intensity, and duration of walking.

susceptibility feel there is danger that they will experience an adverse condition or contract a disease. An individual's perception of personal susceptibility is related to a variety of health behaviors, including immunization (Cummings, Jette, Brock, & Haefner, 1979), dental visits (Becker, Kaback, Rosenstock, & Ruth, 1975), and screening for tuberculosis (Haefner & Kirscht, 1970). With regard to physical activity, if a person believes they are at-risk for cardiovascular disease, they may begin an exercise regimen to reduce their perceived susceptibility to the disease.

Perceived Seriousness or Severity

Perceived severity refers to an individual's feelings concerning the seriousness of a health condition if it is contracted or treatment is not obtained, or both. Feelings concerning the seriousness of contracting an illness (or leaving it untreated) also vary from person to person. These feelings can be considered from the point of view of the difficulties that an illness (or potential illness) would create. For example, an individual may evaluate the severity of cancer in terms of the following: (1) medical consequences, such as pain, discomfort, disability, and death; (2) social consequences, such as difficulties with family, friends, and significant others; and (3) occupational consequences, such as loss of work time and financial burdens (Rosenstock, 1990).

Perceived Benefits of Taking Action

Perceived benefit is the efficacy of the advised action to reduce risk or seriousness of impact. The direction of action that a person chooses will be influenced by their beliefs regarding the action. For example, an inactive individual at high risk for cardiovascular disease would not be expected to increase their physical activity level unless it was perceived as feasible and efficacious. Perceived benefits are conceptually identical to the outcome expectation construct of Bandura's social cognitive theory (Bandura, 2004; see Chapter 14).

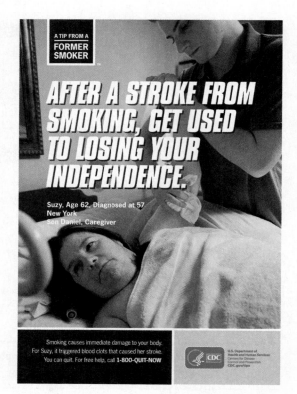

Courtesy of the Centers for Disease Control and Prevention 2014 Tips From Former Smokers campaign. Reference to specific commercial products, manufacturers, companies, or trademarks does not constitute its endorsement or recommendation by the U.S. Government, Department of Health and Human Services, or Centers for Disease Control and Prevention.

Self-Efficacy

Self-efficacy is a judgment regarding one's ability to perform a behavior required to achieve a certain outcome, and it is an important component of behavior change (Bandura, 1997). Researchers who have examined self-efficacy within the health belief model have found overwhelming support for it. For example, Chen, Neufeld, Feely, and Skinner (1998) found that self-efficacy was the only health belief model construct to predict exercise compliance among patients with upper-extremity impairment.

Perceived Barriers to Take Action

It is important to note that action may not take place even though the individual believes that the benefits to taking action are effective, and they possess self-efficacy about performing that behavior. This inactivity may be due to **perceived barriers**. Common barriers to undertaking physical activity include low motivation, inconvenience of facilities, expense, lack of time, and discomfort (e.g., muscle soreness). These barriers may cause a person to not engage in the health behavior. For example, individuals may acknowledge the severity of type 2 diabetes and know that they are at risk for the disease. They may also believe that physical activity will reduce their chance of developing diabetes. However, they may not become active due to the perceived barrier of lack of time to engage in physical activity.

Cues to Action

An individual's perception of the degree of both susceptibility and severity determines their desire to take action, and the perceptions of benefits determine the preferred path of action. However, an event or cue is necessary to trigger the decision-making process and motivate an individual's readiness to take action. These cues to action might be internal, external, or both. Internal cues could include perceptions of bodily states such as dizziness, elevated heart rate, and shortness of breath. External cues could include mass media communications (e.g., watching a physical activity video or television commercial) or receiving a postcard from a physician that outlines the health benefits of exercise (Rosenstock, 1974). Such factors as use of mass media, postcard reminders, and the presence of symptoms have been found to influence people to take a recommended health action (Rosenstock, 1974).

The following example illustrates how the components of the health belief model are hypothesized to predict behavior. An inactive person believes that they could have a heart attack (is susceptible), that inactivity can lead to heart attack (the severity is great), and that becoming physically active will reduce the risk (benefits) without negative side effects or excessive difficulty (barriers). Print materials and letters of reminder sent to the person might promote physical activity adherence (cues to action). And, if the individual has had a hard time being active in the past, a strategy involving the use of behavioral contracts could be used to establish achievable short-term goals so that the person's confidence (self-efficacy) to engage in physical activity increases.

CRITICAL THINKING ACTIVITY 15-1

The cues to action construct is relatively unique to the health belief model. It suggests that there are defining events in our lives that push us into action to change our behavior. Consider your own life and any big changes you have made over the last 2 years. Were there any cues to action?

Application of the Health Belief Model to Physical Activity

Harrison, Mullen, and Green (1992) conducted a meta-analysis of studies using the health belief model with adults. The conclusions of this review were that there is a lack of standardized definitions/measurement of the six constructs of the health belief model and as a result, the rigor of the theory as a psychological framework is decreased. The review found small and varied effect sizes for the link between physical activity behavior and the constructs of the health belief model. It was also found that retrospective studies had significantly larger effect sizes than prospective studies.

Researchers have also found that health beliefs differ across health behaviors. This was illustrated in a study by Janelle O'Connell and his colleagues (1985). They tested 69 adolescents with obesity and 100 adolescents without obesity to determine if both dieting and physical activity behavior could be predicted using the health belief model constructs. The health beliefs examined included knowledge of the (1) etiology, pathology, and demographic variables associated with obesity; (2) proper means of losing weight by dieting and exercising; (3) perceived severity of obesity; (4) perceived susceptibility to the causes of obesity; (5) cues to losing weight by dieting and exercising; (6) benefits of losing weight by dieting and exercising; (7) barriers

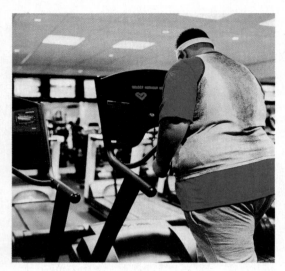

© Digital Vision/Photodisc/Thinkstock.

to losing weight by dieting and exercising; and (8) social support for dieting and exercise. To determine salient beliefs within the health belief model, an elicitation study was undertaken with 58 obese and nonobese adolescents. The most prevalent responses elicited were then used to construct a health belief model questionnaire.

It was found that knowledge of the benefits of dieting was the most powerful predictor of dieting for the adolescents with obesity, whereas knowledge of the susceptibility to the causes of obesity best explained the current dieting practices of the nonobese adolescents. Physical activity behavior of teenagers with obesity was best explained by cues to exercising. The salient cues for exercising included the external cue of peer pressure and the internal cues of poor health and poor muscle tone. None of the health belief model constructs were significant predictors of physical activity behavior of nonobese adolescents. The authors concluded that weight-control programs for children with obesity should attempt to emphasize cues to exercising to encourage participation in aerobic exercise. The cues should be provided in the form of both internal and external stimuli for maximal results. The authors also concluded; however, that the utility of the health belief model was limited for explaining exercise behavior.

In another prospective study, Neil Oldridge and David Streiner (1990) examined the ability of the health belief model to predict exercise compliance and dropout in a cardiac rehabilitation population. They also examined whether the model added predictive utility to routinely assessed patient demographics and health behaviors such as age, weight, occupation type, and smoking status. The health beliefs of 120 male patients with coronary artery disease assessed were the severity of the disease, perceptions of susceptibility to the disease, perceptions of effectiveness of exercise, barriers to exercise, and cues to action. A 6-month exercise program was introduced consisting of twice-weekly supervised exercise sessions lasting approximately 90 minutes. Home-based exercise also was recommended for at least 3 days a week. At the end of the program, the patients were divided into either compliers or dropouts. Dropouts were defined as those participants who either missed more than 50% of all the sessions or more than eight consecutive sessions. Dropouts were then further classified as either unavoidable or avoidable. Reasons for unavoidable dropout included cardiac complications, death, and moving away. Reasons for avoidable dropouts included loss of motivation/interest, inconvenience, and fatigue.

They found that 62 patients (52%) dropped out of the program. Of those who dropped out, 34 were categorized as avoidable and 28 were classified as unavoidable. Compliers were more likely to be nonsmokers, have a white-collar occupation, have active leisure habits, and be younger than the dropouts. With regard to the health belief model constructs, the only significant difference between the compliers and dropouts was in perceptions of the severity of the disease, but this was in the opposite direction of what was hypothesized; that is, the compliers perceived less susceptibility than the dropouts. The predictive ability of the health belief model was found to be very small. Thus, the authors concluded that the results of the study provided limited evidence for the usefulness of the health belief model in accounting for compliance behavior. Not surprisingly, there are few contemporary tests of the health belief model and

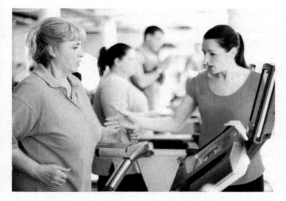

© Gilaxia/E+/Getty Images.

limited use of the model in physical activity interventions. Given the disease-based focus of the model, there has also been limited application of the model to understand sedentary behavior.

Protection Motivation Theory

Television advertisements often attempt to instill fear in observers in order to change their attitudes and behavior. For example, a dramatic car crash is followed by the observation that drinking and driving do not mix. But appeals based on fear do not consistently result in attitude and behavior changes. The protection motivation theory was originally developed to explain inconsistencies in research on fear appeals and attitude change (Rogers, 1983), but since this time, it has been used primarily as a model to explain health decision making and action. Protection motivation theory is concerned with the decision to protect oneself from harmful or stressful life events, although it can also be viewed as a theory of coping with such events. In the protection motivation theory, decisions to engage (or not engage) in health-related behaviors are thought to be influenced by two primary cognitive processes: (1) threat appraisal, which is an evaluation of the factors that influence the likelihood of engaging in an unhealthy behavior (e.g., smoking, sedentary lifestyle), and (2) coping appraisal, which is an evaluation of the factors that influence the likelihood of engaging in a recommended preventive response (e.g., physical activity). The most common index of protection motivation is a measure of intentions to perform the recommended preventive behavior, with behavior as the ultimate outcome. **Figure 15-2** provides an illustration of the constructs of protection motivation theory.

The **threat appraisal** component depends on (1) **perceived vulnerability**, which is a person's estimate of the degree of personal risk for

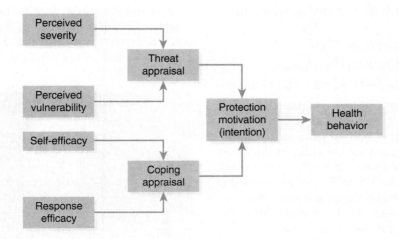

Figure 15-2 Protection Motivation Theory.

Data from Rogers, R. W. (1983). Cognitive and physiological processes in fear appeals and attitude change: A revised theory of protection motivation. In J. T. Cacioppo, & R. E. Petty (Eds.), *Social psychophysiology* (pp. 153–176). New York, NY: Guilford Press.

a specific health hazard if a current unhealthy behavior continues (e.g., risk for developing lung cancer if one continues smoking), and (2) perceived severity, which is a person's estimate of the threat of the disease (e.g., perceived severity of lung cancer). It is assumed that as perceptions of vulnerability and severity increase, the likelihood of engaging in the unhealthy behavior decreases.

Coping appraisal consists of (1) response efficacy, which is the person's expectancy that complying with recommendations will remove the threat (e.g., quitting smoking will reduce one's risk for lung cancer), and (2) self-efficacy, the person's belief in their ability to implement the recommended coping behavior or strategy (e.g., belief that one can quit smoking). As response efficacy and self-efficacy increase, so does the likelihood of engaging in the recommended preventive behavior.

Protection motivation theory assumes that the motivation to protect oneself from danger is a positive linear function of four cognitive beliefs. That is, when the individual perceives that (1) the threat is severe, (2) they are personally vulnerable to the threat, (3) the coping response is effective to avert the threat, and (4) they have the ability to perform the coping response, then motivation to implement the coping response is at its maximum. Thus, the emotional state of fear is thought to influence threat and change behavior indirectly through the appraisal of the severity.

Application of the Protection Motivation Theory to Physical Activity

Two meta-analytic reviews on protection motivation theory representing over 20 health issues, including exercise and physical activity, have found some support for the utility of the theory (Floyd, Prentice-Dunn, & Rogers, 2000; Milne, Sheeran, & Orbell, 2000). Specific reviews of protection motivation theory and physical activity (Plotnikoff & Trinh, 2010; Bui et al., 2013) also identified some support for the theory.

The meta-analysis carried out by Donna Floyd and her colleagues (2000) on 65 studies (with 29,650 participants) found that, in accordance with the theory, increases in threat severity, threat vulnerability, response efficacy, and self-efficacy facilitated adaptive intentions and behaviors. The magnitude of the effect sizes obtained was in the moderate range.

In the meta-analysis undertaken by Sarah Milne and her colleagues (2000), more stringent criteria for including studies were used. As a result, only 29 studies with approximately 7,700 participants were analyzed. Nonetheless, Milne et al. obtained results that were similar to those of Floyd et al. (2000) of effect sizes in the small to moderate range. Specifically, Milne et al. (2000) found that the threat and coping appraisal components of the protection motivation theory were useful in predicting ongoing behavior.

The reviews by Plotnikoff and Trinh (2010) and Bui and colleagues (2013) concluded relatively similar findings for protection motivation theory and physical activity as other health behaviors. Overall, the authors found little support for the threat component of the model but did find support for the coping constructs as predictors of both physical activity intention and behavior. For example, Plotnikoff and Higginbotham (1998) examined the relative contributions of the protection motivation theory to predict intentions to engage in both a low-fat diet and exercise for the prevention of further cardiovascular heart disease in 151 patients who had recently suffered a heart attack. The participants completed baseline measures of threat appraisal (i.e., vulnerability and susceptibility) during their hospital stay following a heart attack. Six months

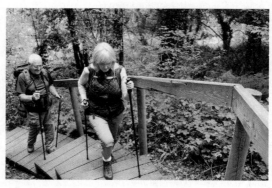

© Dean Mitchell/E+/Getty Images.

later, the participants completed measures of threat appraisal and coping appraisal (i.e., self-efficacy and response efficacy) via mail. It was found that self-efficacy was the strongest predictor of exercise and diet intentions and behaviors. The authors concluded that health education for this population should promote self-efficacy-enhancing activities for such behaviors.

Protection Motivation Theory and Physical Activity Intervention

The application of protection motivation theory to intervening upon actual physical activity behavior has had limited attention and mixed results (Bui et al., 2013). Typically, researchers use persuasive communications to manipulate the threat of a disease, and the subsequent effectiveness of physical activity can aid in coping. For example, Sandy Wurtele and James Maddux (1987) examined the relative effectiveness of threat (i.e., severity and vulnerability) and coping (i.e., self-efficacy and response efficacy) appraisals for increasing exercise behavior in 160 nonexercising undergraduate females. Nonexercisers were defined as engaging in fewer than two bouts of exercise per week. Each participant received a written persuasive message containing none, one, two, three, or four of the protection motivation theory components (see **Table 15-2** for examples of the persuasive messages). After reading the message, all participants completed a post-experiment questionnaire. Participants were then given a list of suggested means of achieving aerobic fitness. Two weeks later, the

Table 15-2 **Persuasive Messages Read by the Participants of Wurtele and Maddux's Experiment on Protective Motivation Theory**

Appraisal Construct	Message Focus	Example
Severity	The seriousness of remaining sedentary by describing the immediate and long-term effects of having a heart attack or stroke.	"Suddenly, the victim is overwhelmed with a crushing pain in the chest as if the ribs were being squeezed in a vise. . . . Nauseated, the victim vomits; pink foam comes out of the mouth. The face turns an ashen gray, sweat rolls down the face, and the victim, very weak, staggers to the floor."
Vulnerability	The susceptibility to developing heart disease and circulatory problems.	"Because you do not exercise regularly, your cardiovascular system has already begun deteriorating, which puts the health of your body in jeopardy."
Response efficacy	The importance and efficacy of exercising in preventing health problems by presenting evidence that the physiologic changes in the body resulting from a regular exercise program serve vital protection functions.	"Since exercise leads to higher levels of high-density lipoprotein, which in turn lowers the level of cholesterol, exercising thus prevents heart attacks."
Self-efficacy	Reasons why women would be able to begin and continue with a regular exercise program.	"We all have a built-in urge for physical activity, and this basic human physical need will serve as an energizer. . . . At your age, you now have the cognitive abilities to commit yourself to a long-term exercise program."

Data from Wurtele, S. K., & Maddux, J. E. (1987). Relative contributions of protection motivation theory components in predicting exercise intentions and behavior. *Health Psychology, 6,* 453–466.

participants reported on any changes in their exercise behavior since the initiation of the study.

It was found that perceptions of both vulnerability and self-efficacy enhanced exercise intentions and behaviors. Furthermore, intentions predicted changes in exercise behavior. It was also found that the participants adopted a "precaution strategy"; that is, they intended to adopt physical activity behavior even though they held weak beliefs about its effectiveness and were not convinced of their at-risk status.

This result was not replicated, however, by Milne and colleagues (2002). Their intervention using threat and coping messages in a persuasive communication among 248 undergraduates resulted in higher intentions to exercise but not actual exercise compared with a control group. Gaston and Harry Prapavessis (2009) also examined protection motivation threat and coping messaging among 208 pregnant women and found that intention and exercise 1 week later were significantly higher than the control group or a group that received nutritional information. The results suggest that protection motivation information was at least successful in producing very short-term changes in behavior. Still, this limited and mixed research on the usefulness of protection motivation theory suggests that very little is known about whether it has usefulness in the maintenance of physical activity.

Application of the Protection Motivation Theory to Sedentary Behavior

Like the health belief model, there have been limited applications of protection motivation theory to understand sedentary behavior. In one of the only applications, Wong and colleagues (2016) explored protection motivation theory to predict self-reported general sitting behavior or leisure-time sedentary behavior among a sample of 596 undergraduate students. Coping constructs, but not threat constructs, had small effects on intention to limit sedentary behavior (generally and leisure-specific). General sitting

behavior was not explained by the model, yet intention to limit leisure-time sitting had a small effect on leisure-time sedentary behavior. The study provided some tenability of protection motivation theory for explaining leisure-time sedentary behavior.

Limitations of the Health Belief Model and Protection Motivation Theory

An important construct in both the health belief model (Rosenstock, 1974) and protection motivation theory (Rogers, 1983) is perceived severity; that is, an individual's feelings about the seriousness of a health condition if it is contracted or not treated. However, researchers have been unable to consistently find that perceived severity is an important construct for motivation to engage in physical activity, and emerging evidence now suggest this extends to motivation to limit sedentary behavior. People may agree that being physically inactive can contribute to severe coronary problems, but there is a limited link between perceptions of the severity of the problem and the tendency to adopt a physically active lifestyle.

One of the problems that has plagued both the health belief model and protection motivation theory is the fundamental assumption that people engage in health behaviors such as regular physical activity for its protective health benefits. To be fair, it should be noted that the models were originally designed for risk-avoiding, not health-promoting, behaviors. A behavior such as physical activity has several other reasons for its performance beyond health, such as social aspects, physical appearance enhancement, and pure enjoyment (Symons Downs & Hausenblas, 2005). Indeed, the affective reasons for physical activity, such as enjoyment, have been shown to be a much larger and more reliable correlate of physical activity performance than health (Rhodes, Fiala, & Conner, 2009). The disease focus, rather than enjoyment focus, also explains why the models have not been readily applied to understand sedentary behavior. It is enjoyment for performing physical activity compared with outside interests that forms the basis for the theory that concludes this chapter.

Self-Determination Theory

Historically, motivational psychology has understood human motivation as a means to fulfilling a drive, based on an idea of deficits, or as a conditioning process by pairing a stimulus with an outcome (Freud, 1923; Hull, 1943). In the late 1950s, this understanding of drive-based theories began to shift, with a focus on an organismic approach, which assumes that human beings act on their internal and external environments to be effective and to satisfy a full range of their needs (Deci & Ryan, 1985; Heider, 1958). This approach deviates considerably in scope from the narrow, health-focused theories in the earlier part of this chapter, as the development to meet fundamental needs can be inclusive of many different factors.

The most commonly applied theory from this organismic perspective of growth and development in physical activity is *self-determination theory* (Deci & Ryan, 1985, 2000). Self-determination theory is composed of five mini-theories, including *causality orientations theory, goal contents theory, cognitive evaluation theory, basic psychological needs theory*, and *organismic integration theory* (Deci & Ryan, 2002; See also Rhodes et al., 2019 for an historical review of its role in physical activity). The two most commonly employed mini-theories that have been used to examine physical activity include basic psychological needs theory and organismic integration theory.

Self-determination theory (Deci & Ryan, 1985) has its origins in the search for understanding the relative influence of intrinsic interest and extrinsic rewards on human behavior. As a consequence, attention was directed toward understanding the function of rewards. A generalization that resulted from the earliest work was that extrinsic rewards can be perceived by a recipient in one of two ways. One way pertains to receiving information about competence. Thus, for example, a young child who receives a special treat for playing well in a competition likely would perceive that reward as an affirmation that they are competent. Another pertains to receiving information about control. If that same young child is given the special treat as an inducement to participate in the competition, that reward could be perceived to be a bribe to have them compete. Rewards that convey information to the individual that they are highly competent enhance intrinsic motivation. Conversely, however, rewards that convey information that the recipient is no longer fully in control of the reasons for behavior reduce intrinsic motivation.

Sources of Motivation

Early research emphasized the independence of intrinsic and extrinsic motivation; if one was present, it was assumed that the other could not be. However, when research showed that this approach did not adequately explain human behavior, Deci and Ryan (1985, 2000) developed organismic integration theory. In the micro-theory, extrinsic and intrinsic motivation are assumed to fall along a continuum (see **Figure 15-3**). At one end of the continuum is **amotivation**—the absence of motivation toward an activity.

In the middle of the continuum lies **extrinsic motivation**. According to self-determination theorists, extrinsic motivation is best viewed as multidimensional in nature. One dimension is called **external regulation**, the "purest" form of extrinsic motivation. The individual engages in a behavior solely to receive a reward or to avoid punishment. Consider the case of a person who

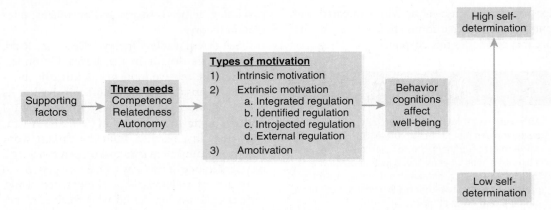

Figure 15-3 Self-Determination Theory.

Data from Deci, E. L., & Ryan, R. M. (1985). *Intrinsic motivation and self-determination in human behavior.* New York, NY: Plenum Press.

has been told by their physician that an immediate consequence of continued inactivity could be hospitalization. So, grudgingly, a program of physical activity is initiated. That person could be considered to be motivated through external regulation.

A dimension that is slightly further along the continuum is called **introjected regulation**. It represents the incomplete internalization of a regulation. Returning to our example, the individual might eventually progress to where they were no longer at high risk. However, if the physical activity program was maintained because of a sense of "should" or "must," the source of motivation would be introjected regulation. The distinction between external and introjected regulation lies in the fact that in the latter case, the individual has begun to internalize the motivation for the behavior.

A third extrinsic motivation dimension that is slightly further along the continuum is called **identified regulation**. Here, the individual freely chooses to carry out an activity that is not considered to be enjoyable per se, but which is thought to be important to achieve a personal goal. The individual internalizes the sentiment "I need to." Identified regulation would be illustrated by an individual who is regularly physically active, does not enjoy the activity in the least, but views it as essential for weight control.

The final extrinsic regulation construct is called **integrated regulation**. When identified regulations are well coordinated with other values, it is said to be integrated regulation, which can be a powerful form of regulation because it represents a choice to carry out the activity congruent with other behaviors and choices in one's life.

At another extreme on the continuum is **intrinsic motivation**, which is the motivation to do an activity for its own sake or the pleasure it provides. Vallerand and his colleagues (Vallerand, 1997; Vallerand, Deci, & Ryan, 1987; Vallerand et al., 1993) have proposed that intrinsic motivation is also multidimensional in nature. One form is reflected in intrinsic motivation toward knowledge—the pleasure of engaging in an activity to learn something new or about the activity. An individual who chooses to run a marathon to learn how their body will respond under that stress would be an example of this form of intrinsic motivation. A second type is intrinsic motivation toward accomplishment. The same would-be marathoner used in our earlier example might also want to have the satisfaction of completing such a long distance. Finally, the third type is reflected in intrinsic motivation toward stimulation. It represents motivation to experience the pleasant sensations derived from the activity itself. An individual

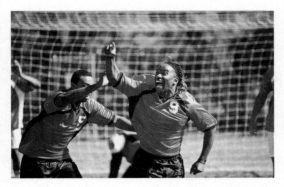

© SDI Productions/E+/Getty Images.

who is physically active because of the bodily sensations accompanying physical activity—sweating, elevated heart rate, muscles responding to the increased load—would be an example of intrinsic motivation toward stimulation.

The Antecedents of Intrinsic and Extrinsic Motivation

Figure 15-3 provides an overview of self-determination theory. According to Deci and Ryan (1985), the various motives that individuals have for an activity are driven by psychological needs that have as their basis a striving toward growth and the actualization of personal potential. This micro-theory is known as basic psychological needs theory (Deci & Ryan, 2000, 2002).

The need for autonomy refers to the desire to be self-initiating in the regulation of personal behavior. If a sense of autonomy is present, intrinsic motivation is facilitated. The need for competence reflects the fact that individuals want to interact effectively within their environment. As is the case with autonomy, if an activity provides the individual with a sense of competence, intrinsic motivation is facilitated. Thus, for example, if exercisers begin to attend a step class and discover that they are never able to coordinate their actions with the rest of their classmates, they are likely to seek out another form of physical activity. Finally, the need for relatedness reflects the fact that individuals want to feel connected to others. When relatedness is perceived

to be present, intrinsic motivation is facilitated. So, for example, if exercisers began to make friends with others in the step class, they would be more likely to continue to engage in the class in the future.

According to Deci and Ryan (1985), the various types of motivation are intimately related to perceptions of self-determination (refer back to Figure 15-3). When self-determination is absent, amotivation (i.e., an absence of motivation) exists. Also, when an activity is undertaken for extrinsic motives, minimal perceptions of self-determination are present. Finally, at the extreme end of the continuum, complete self-determination is associated with the various manifestations of intrinsic motivation.

CRITICAL THINKING ACTIVITY 15-3

The three needs outlined in self-determination theory are based on sound research and validation. Still, think about the behaviors you will perform this week, from watching TV to taking a nap. Are there other needs that these behaviors may meet? What other needs can you think of that might also drive behavior?

Research on Self-Determination Theory in Physical Activity Settings

Research using self-determination theory to understand sedentary behavior is scant at this point, but self-determination theory is now one of the most popular models applied to understand physical activity. Several reviews and meta-analyses on self-determination theory applied to the setting of physical activity have been published (e.g., Hagger & Chatzisarantis, 2007; Owen et al., 2014; Ryan, Williams, Patrick, & Deci, 2009; Teixeira, Carraça, Markland, Silva, & Ryan, 2012; Vasconcellos et al., 2020). Much of the earliest research into intrinsic and extrinsic motivation was observational and carried out in laboratory, school, and sport settings. However, researchers have begun to assess the applicability of the theory in physical activity and exercise settings.

In a seminal systematic review, Teixeira and colleagues (2012) analyzed 66 studies that have applied the model to understand physical activity. The findings showed clear support for more autonomous forms of motivation (intrinsic, integrated, identified) and a correlation with physical activity performance over more controlled forms of motivation (introjected, external). Interestingly, however, not all of the three psychological needs were associated with physical activity. Indeed, the need for relatedness was often null in its relationship with physical activity and need for autonomy was inconsistent. Only the need for competence has been a consistent correlate of physical activity (Teixeira et al., 2012).

Similar findings were reported in meta-analyses of self-determination theory applied amongst adolescents (Owen et al., 2014) and within the physical education context. For example, Vasconcellos and colleagues (2020) meta-analyzed data from 252 relevant studies using self-determination theory in physical education. In line with theory, autonomous motivation (an amalgam of intrinsic motivation, identified and integrated regulation) was positively correlated with various adaptive outcomes ($b = 0.32$) and negatively correlated with maladaptive outcomes ($b = -0.17$). Introjected regulation was correlated with maladaptive outcomes ($b = 0.41$) but not adaptive outcomes. External regulation was negatively associated with maladaptive outcomes ($b = -0.21$) but not associated with adaptive outcomes. Finally, amotivation showed a negative relationship with adaptive outcomes ($b = -0.16$), and a positive relationship with maladaptive outcomes ($b = 0.41$). Support of autonomy ($b = 0.19$) and competence ($b = 0.23$) are needed but not relatedness ($b = 0.08$); satisfactions were meaningfully associated with autonomous student motivation, and weak negative correlations were found between autonomy, competence, and relatedness and external regulation, which provides general support for the theory.

The measurement of self-determination theory constructs has generally been obtained through use of the Behavioral Regulation in Exercise Questionnaire (Markland & Tobin, 2004) or the exercise motivation scale. For example, Li (1999) used the exercise motivation scale to examine 371 male and female college students who varied in their frequency of exercise. Interestingly, Li found differences between males and females in underlying motivations for exercise. Females reported higher levels of intrinsic motivation and the self-determined forms of motivation illustrated in Figure 15-3. Frequent exercisers (i.e., individuals who were active two or more times per week) also showed higher levels of intrinsic motivation and self-determined forms of motivation than infrequent exercisers (i.e., individuals who were active either one or no times per week).

Li also tested self-determination theory to determine how perceptions of competence, autonomy, and relatedness about physical activity were related to the various forms of motivation illustrated in Figure 15-3. He found that consistent with what would be predicted from self-determination theory, perceptions of competence, autonomy, and relatedness were positively related to the three types of intrinsic motivation (i.e., to learn, to accomplish tasks, and to experience sensations) and negatively related to amotivation.

Similarly, Wilson and colleagues (Wilson, Rodgers, Blanchard, & Gessell, 2003) used the Behavioral Regulation in Exercise Questionnaire to assess 53 community-dwelling adults in Western Canada. The results suggested that identified and intrinsic regulation were large correlates of exercise behavior, while identified regulation

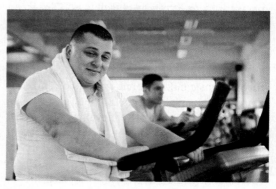

© hoozone/iStock/Thinkstock.

correlated with autonomy and competence and intrinsic regulation correlated with competence. The results lend some support to the importance of self-determined motivation and the potential impact of autonomy and competence.

Self-Determination Theory in Physical Activity Intervention

Like the popularity of research using self-determination theory to predict physical activity in different contexts, there are now several studies that have applied the theory to change physical activity through intervention. Evaluations of this research have been summarized in several recent reviews and meta-analyses (Gillison et al., 2019; Gourlan et al., 2016; Juwono & Szabo, 2020; Ntoumanis et al., 2021; Rhodes et al., 2021; Sheeran et al., 2020; Stewart and Sharma, 2020; Teixeira et al., 2012; Vasconcellos et al. 2020).

One of the largest and most sophisticated of these reviews was a meta-analysis undertaken by Sheeran and colleagues (2020). Their review identified 50 physical activity interventions that could be meta-analyzed to quantify their impact on physical activity changes and test whether changes in self-determination theory constructs (e.g., autonomous motivation, need for competence) accounted for these behavior changes. They found that self-determination theory interventions had a small, but meaningful effect on change in physical activity ($d = 0.25$). The authors also included an analysis of 10 studies that had been designed to change sedentary behavior through self-determination theory and these studies showed a comparable effect on lessening sedentary behavior ($d = 0.22$). Secondly, the authors found support for the premise that changes in autonomous motivation ($b = 0.04$) and competence ($b = 0.03$) from the intervention were linked to these changes in behavior but not controlled motivation (an amalgam of external and introjected regulation). Although these effects were very small, they are comparable to the intervention effectiveness of other popular theories in physical activity such as theory of planned

behavior (Chapter 14), social cognitive theory (Chapter 14), and the transtheoretical model of behavior change (Chapter 16) (Gourlan et al., 2016; Rhodes et al., 2021).

CRITICAL THINKING ACTIVITY 15-4

Self-determination theory intervenes on three needs (autonomy, competence, relatedness) in order to affect the quality of motivation toward a behavior. As these needs are met, the behavior is likely to become more self-determined. One challenge with this approach may be limits to the extent that a behavior can meet certain needs. For example, running may not meet the need for relatedness as well as team sports or going to the local pub. Think of your favorite leisure activities. Are there some that meet your three needs more than others? Do you think this would be likely to change with modifications to that behavior?

Summary

This chapter examined the health belief model, protection motivation theory, and self-determination theory and the research utilizing these models to explain and predict physical activity behavior. The components of the health belief model are perceived susceptibility, perceived seriousness or severity, perceived benefits of taking action, self-efficacy, perceived barriers to take action, and cues to action. In comparison, the premise for protection motivation theory is that decisions to engage in exercise are influenced by threat appraisals and coping appraisals. Despite limitations of both theories, they provide unique insights into physical activity behaviors, in particular perceived severity (i.e., an individual's feelings about the seriousness of a health condition if it is contracted or not treated). In short, the health belief model and protection motivation theory have provided a compass to guide research to explain physical activity.

Self-determination theory is based on the premise that activities are more likely to be selected and maintained if they satisfy three psychological needs: competence, self-determination, and relatedness. Behavior occurs as a result of extrinsic motivation (external regulation, introjected regulation, identified regulation, or integrated regulation) or intrinsic motivation. The various types of motivation are associated with perceptions of self-determination, and perceptions of self-determination are associated with satisfaction and behavior. Research has shown support for the theory as a means of understanding and intervening upon behavior in the context of exercise and physical activity.

Vignette: Bryan

I was sitting on my couch with a half-eaten ice cream cake and an overflowing ashtray on my coffee table when I got the call. My mother never contacted anyone after 10:00 p.m., so I assumed something was very wrong. She didn't even say hello when I answered. When I picked up, all I heard was, "Dad's in the emergency room. Again."

My father was a lifelong smoker, having begun around age 12. I picked up his bad habit during my first year of high school, during which time I'd also learned to mimic his pure aversion to all things physical. In his opinion, time spent playing sports was time wasted. (Better to rally your friends for a trip to the library or look for an after-school job than whittle away hours getting sweaty.)

To call dad a workaholic would have been an understatement. He got up early in the morning to drive from our suburban home to his city law office, often came home late (unless he booked a hotel for the night to be closer to work), and made it clear to me that if I didn't get into an Ivy League college he wouldn't pay for my education. (Thanks to the fortitude of my SAT scores and high school resume, I ended up making the mark. But I nearly had a nervous breakdown midway through freshman year due to all the pressure.)

In a typical day, dad would go through a pack and a half of menthols. Cheeseburgers, pizza, and steak topped his list of favorite meal choices. And, as I'd come to find out only after graduating from college, he frequently polished off a bottle of gin every week.

It wasn't surprising to anyone that he had his first heart attack at age 47. Because he only followed his cardiologist's orders to take up a thrice-weekly walking regimen for a month—and moderated his diet only by asking for an extra tomato with his usual burger orders—he was back in the hospital for a second heart attack about a year later. He got a stent put in during that visit and left the cardiac rehabilitation center with a new prescription for blood thinners atop an even stronger admonishment from his doctor to alter a lifestyle that was bound to keep his health mired in disaster.

Still, my dad didn't heed the doctors' advice. "They don't understand how I operate," he would say to mom and me, referring to his unstoppable work ethic—without which, he claimed, he'd never have founded his own successful law firm. Maybe he could see the link between his lack of adequate exercise and poor eating habits—not to mention the steady stream of alcohol and cigarettes into his bloodstream. But he didn't believe that starting a regular physical activity regimen or swapping French fries for salad would make a worthwhile impact on his well-being.

My grandfather—also a lawyer—led a lifestyle similar to my dad's. (Go figure that his behaviors got handed down one generation.) Grandpa suffered comparable medical issues but remained professionally successful well into his late 60s, when he finally succumbed to cardiac arrest. My father admired him more than anyone and endorsed the same attitude toward not making lifestyle changes that my grandfather did when he was ill: "I'd rather leave on a high note, without slacking," my father would often say, reiterating his belief that because exercise got in the way of work, it was a futile endeavor.

I had a feeling that the fourth time he landed in the ER—this time from complications due to the colon cancer he'd been diagnosed with shortly after his 58th birthday—it might be a red flag indicating his precipitous end. He was 63 at the time. On that fateful phone call mom told me the cancer had metastasized to his lungs. Though heartbroken, I wasn't surprised.

After a night of little to no sleep due to worrying, I arranged to meet my parents at the hospital the following morning. (This required me to call in sick to work, a decision I knew dad would decry.) On my way there in the car I could no longer avoid a horrifying reality. I was living an inactive lifestyle riddled with poor nutrition and tobacco. I wasn't as inflexible as my father in the belief that work should be the be all and end all of a man's existence, nor was I as much of a boozer as he was; however, in terms of lifestyle, we were strikingly similar. I was on track to end up cycling through hospital doors in about a decade, just like him. And at 32 years of age, if I didn't do anything to change my habits, I might already be halfway done with my life.

Dad finally succumbed to lung cancer before I turned 33. It was a devastating loss, but one neither my mother nor I could say we didn't expect. Up until his final days, he remained unaccepting—despite the morphine and other drugs he was on to numb his chronic pain and keep him alive—that the nurses wouldn't let him work from his hospital room.

I visited him each day in that hospital. And though it took a chunk out of my stamina at work, those months I spent with him toward the end of his life were the most meaningful time I think we ever had together. What's more, that was a period where I started walking each morning for 15 to 30 minutes, bought a couple of weights, and hired a personal trainer to show me some basic weight training exercises I could do in my own home after work.

Once I shed enough pounds to feel comfortable entering a gym without the stigma of being the largest one in there, I committed to spending at least 30 minutes on machines there every other day. I was bound and determined not to end up like my dad. Watching the decline of his health throughout my early adult life and seeing him die before he was even old enough to retire was more incentive than I could have ever asked for. (Not that it made pushing myself to be active after decades of laziness any easier. But I was convinced that I could actually take charge of my own health and thereby live longer, perhaps much longer, than dad.)

I've been exercising regularly for the past decade. (I'm turning 44 next month.) I can comfortably say it hasn't, as dad feared, negatively interfered with my work. I'm currently a partner at an impressive law firm. And, if anything, exercise has made me sharper, more energized, and less burnt out on the job.

I'd say smoking has been the hardest habit to give up. But I periodically attend a smoking-cessation support group and I've cut back to a few cigarettes a week. Of course, what helps keep me on track with my diet and fitness goals isn't just the knowledge that I might, in so doing, have a different life outcome from my dad. I can't deny that the influence of my wife—a part-time yoga teacher and special education instructor who I (can you believe it?) met at the gym!—has also been immensely helpful.

That we anticipate the arrival of our baby daughter in about 4 months is probably the most enormous motivator of all. I plan on being an available father for her. And that means doing whatever it takes for my health so as to be alive when she herself has children.

Key Terms

amotivation The absence of motivation toward a behavior.

coping appraisal An evaluation of the preventive response of a behavior.

cues to action Events and strategies that activate a readiness.

external regulation Engaging in a behavior to receive a reward or to avoid punishment.

extrinsic motivation Multidimensional concept whereby a person is motivated by external factors, such as rewards or punishments, to accomplish a particular task or engage in a certain behavior.

identified regulation Engaging in a behavior to achieve a personal goal.

integrated regulation Engaging in a behavior because it aligns with other behaviors and choices in one's life.

intrinsic motivation Engaging in a behavior for its own sake or the pleasure it provides.

introjected regulation Engaging in a behavior to relieve or prevent guilt.

perceived barriers A person's opinion of the physical and psychological costs of the advised action.

perceived benefits A person's opinion of the efficacy of the advised action to reduce risk or seriousness of impact.

perceived severity A person's opinion of the seriousness of a condition and its consequences.

perceived susceptibility/vulnerability A person's opinion of their chances of getting a particular disease.

self-efficacy Belief in one's capabilities to organize and execute the course of action required to produce a certain outcome.

threat appraisal An evaluation of the consequences of engaging in an unhealthy behavior (e.g., smoking, sedentary lifestyle).

Review Questions

1. According to the health belief model, what are the two main reasons one would engage in health behaviors?

2. People may perceive severe consequences from a health condition, consider they are susceptible, and see clear benefits to engaging in a health behavior, but not take action. According to the health belief model, what additional construct is needed to take action?

3. Protection motivation theory outlines two key appraisals needed to initiate health behavior intentions. What are these appraisals?

4. Self-determination theory suggests that a behavior is performed based on whether it satisfies three basic needs. What are these needs?

Applying the Concepts

1. What constructs of the health motivation model did Bryan's decision to change his diet and exercise behaviors illustrate?

2. How does the protection motivation theory help explain Bryan's motivational shift toward physical activity?

References

Aho, W. R. (1979). Smoking, dieting, and exercise: Age differences in attitudes and behavior to selected health belief model variables. *Rhode Island Medical Journal, 62*(3), 85–92.

Bandura, A. (1997). *Self-efficacy, the exercise of control.* New York, NY: Freeman.

Bandura, A. (2004). Health promotion by social cognitive means. *Health Education & Behavior, 31*(2), 143–164.

Becker, M. H., Kaback, M. M., Rosenstock, I. M., & Ruth, M. V. (1975). Some influences on public participation in a genetic screening program. *Journal of Community Health, 1*, 3–14.

Bui, L., Mullan, B., & McCaffery, K. (2013). Protection motivation theory and physical activity in the general population: A systematic literature review. *Psychology, Health & Medicine, 18*(5), 522–542.

Carico, R., Jr., Sheppard, J., & Thomas, C. B. (2021). Community pharmacists and communication in the time of COVID-19: Applying the health belief model. *Research in Social and Administrative Pharmacy, 17*(1), 1984–1987.

Chen, C-Y, Strecker Neufeld, P., Feely, C. A., & Sugg Skinner, C. (1998). Factors influencing compliance with home exercise programs among patients with upper-extremity impairment. *American Journal of Occupational Therapy, 153*(2), 171–180.

Cummings, K. M., Jette, A. M., Brock, B. M., & Haefner, D. P. (1979). Psychological determinants of immunization behavior in a swine influenza campaign. *Medical Care, 17*(6), 639–649.

Deci, E. L., & Ryan, R. M. (1985). *Intrinsic motivation and self-determination in human behavior.* New York, NY: Plenum Press.

Deci, E. L., & Ryan, R. M. (2000). The "what" and "why" of goal pursuits: Human needs and the self-determination of behavior. *Psychological Inquiry, 11*(4), 227–268.

Deci, E. L., & Ryan, R. M. (2002). *Handbook of self-determination research.* Rochester, NY: University of Rochester Press.

Floyd, D. L., Prentice-Dunn, S., & Rogers, R. W. (2000). A meta-analysis of research on protection motivation theory. *Journal of Applied Social Psychology, 30*(2), 407–429.

Fortier, M. S., Sweet, S. N., O'Sullivan, T. L., & Williams, G. C. (2007). A self-determination process model of physical activity adoption in the context of a randomized controlled trial. *Psychology of Sport and Exercise, 8*(5), 741–757.

Freud, S. (1923). *The Ego and the Id: Vol. XIX.*

Frewen, S., Schomer, H., & Dunne, T. (1994). Health belief model interpretation of compliance factors in a weight loss and cardiac rehabilitation programme. *South African Journal of Psychology, 24*(1), 39–43.

Gillison, F. B., Rouse, P., Standage, M., Sebire, S. J., & Ryan, R. M. (2019). A meta-analysis of techniques to promote motivation for health behaviour change from a self-determination theory perspective. *Health Psychology Review, 13*(1), 110–130.

Gourlan, M., Bernard, P., Bortolon, C., Romain, A. J., Lareyre, O., Carayol, M., Ninot, G., & Boiché, J. (2016). Efficacy of theory-based interventions to promote physical activity. A meta-analysis of randomised controlled trials. *Health Psychology Review, 10*(1), 50–66.

Haefner, D. P., & Kirscht, J. P. (1970). Motivational and behavioral effects of modifying health beliefs. *Public Health Reports, 85*(6), 478–484.

Hagger, M., & Chatzisarantis, N. L. (Eds.). (2007). *Intrinsic motivation and self-determination in exercise and sport.* Champaign, IL: Human Kinetics.

Harrison, J. A., Mullen, P. D., & Green, L. W. (1992). A meta-analysis of studies of the health belief model with adults. *Health Education Research, 7*(1), 107–116.

Hayslip, B., Jr., Weigand, D., Weinberg, R., Richardson, P., & Jackson, A. (1996). The development of new scales for assessing health belief model constructs in adulthood. *Journal of Aging and Physical Activity, 4*(4), 307–323.

Heider, F. (1958). *The psychology of interpersonal relations.* Wiley.

Hochbaum, G., Rosenstock, I., and Kegels, S. (1952). "Health Belief Model," United States Public Health Service, 1952.

Hull, C. L. (1943). *Principles of behavior: An introduction to behavior theory.* Appleton-Century.

Janz, N. K., & Becker, M. H. (1984). The health belief model: A decade later. *Health Education Quarterly, 11*(1), 1–47.

Juwono, I., & Szabo, A. (2020). The efficacy of self determination theory-based interventions in increasing students' physical activity: A systematic review. *Physical Activity Review, 8*(1), 74–86.

Kerlinger, F. N. (1973). *Foundations of behavioral research.* (2nd ed.). New York, NY: Holt, Rinehart & Winston.

Kirscht, J. P. (1974). The health belief model and illness behavior. *Health Education Monograph, 2*(4), 387–408.

Li, F. (1999). The Exercise Motivation Scale: Its multifaceted structure and construct validity. *Journal of Applied Sport Psychology, 11*(1), 97–115.

Markland, D., & Tobin, V. (2004). A modification to the Behavioural Regulation in Exercise Questionnaire to include an assessment of amotivation. *Journal of Sport and Exercise Psychology, 26*(2), 191–196.

Milne, S., Sheeran, P., & Orbell, S. (2000). Prediction and intervention in health-related behavior: A meta-analytic review of Protection Motivation Theory. *Journal of Applied Social Psychology, 30*(1), 106–143.

Ntoumanis, N., Ng, J. Y., Prestwich, A., Quested, E., Hancox, J. E., Thøgersen-Ntoumani, C., Deci, E. L., Ryan, R. M., Lonsdale, C., & Williams, G. C. (2021). A meta-analysis of self-determination theory-informed intervention studies in the health domain: Effects on motivation, health behavior, physical, and psychological health. *Health Psychology Review, 15*(2), 214–244.

O'Connell, J. K., Price, J. H., Roberts, S. M., Jurs, S. G., & McKinely, R. (1985). Utilizing the health belief model to predict dieting and exercising behavior of obese and nonobese adolescents. *Health Education Quarterly, 12*(4), 343–351.

Oldridge, N. B., & Streiner, D. L. (1990). The health belief model: Predicting compliance and dropout in cardiac rehabilitation. *Medicine & Science in Sports & Exercise, 22*(5), 678–683.

Owen, K. B., Smith, J., Lubans, D. R., Ng, J. Y., & Lonsdale, C. (2014). Self-determined motivation and physical activity in children and adolescents: A systematic review and meta-analysis. *Preventive Medicine, 67*, 270–279.

Plotnikoff, R. C., & Higginbotham, N. (1998). Protection motivation theory and the prediction of exercise and low-fat diet behaviors among Australian cardiac patients. *Psychology & Health, 13*(3), 411–429.

Plotnikoff, R. C., & Trinh, L. (2010). Protection motivation theory: Is this a worthwhile theory for physical activity promotion? *Exercise and Sport Sciences Reviews, 38*(2), 91–98.

Rhodes, R. E., Fiala, B., & Conner, M. (2009). Affective judgments and physical activity: A review and meta-analysis. *Annals of Behavioral Medicine, 38*(3), 180–204.

Rhodes, R. E., Boudreau, P., Weman Josefsson, K., & Ivarsson, A. (2021). Mediators of physical activity behavior change interventions among adults: A systematic review and meta-analysis. *Health Psychology Review, 15*(2), 272–286.

Rhodes, R. E., McEwan, D., & Rebar, A. (2019). Theories of physical activity behavior change: A history and synthesis of approaches. *Psychology of Sport & Exercise, 42*, 100–109.

Rogers, R. W. (1983). Cognitive and physiological processes in fear appeals and attitude change: A revised theory of protection motivation. In J. T. Cacioppo, & R. E. Petty (Eds.), *Social psychophysiology* (pp. 153–176). New York, NY: Guilford Press.

Rosenstock, I. M. (1974). Historical origins of the health belief model. *Health Education Monographs, 2*(4), 328–335.

Rosenstock, I. M. (1990). The health belief model: Explaining health behavior through expectancies. In K. Glanz, F. Lewis, & B. Rimer (Eds.), *Health behavior and health education* (pp. 39–62). San Francisco, CA: Jossey-Bass.

Rosenstock, I. M., Stretcher, V. J., & Becker, M. (1988). Social learning theory and the health belief model. *Health Education Quarterly, 15*(2), 175–183.

Ryan, R. M., Williams, G. C., Patrick, H., & Deci, E. L. (2009). Self-determination theory and physical activity: The dynamics of motivation in development and wellness. *Hellenic Journal of Psychology, 6,* 107–124.

Scarinci, I. C., Pandya, V. N., Kim, Y. I., Bae, S., Peral, S., Tipre, M., . . . & Baskin, M. L. (2021). Factors associated with perceived susceptibility to COVID-19 among urban and rural adults in Alabama. *Journal of Community Health, 46,* 1–10.

Sheeran, P., Wright, C. E., Avishai, A., Villegas, M. E., Lindemans, J. W., Klein, W. M., Rothman, A. J., Miles, E., & Ntoumanis, N. (2020). Self-determination theory interventions for health behavior change: Meta-analysis and meta-analytic structural equation modeling of randomized controlled trials. *Journal of Consulting and Clinical Psychology, 88*(8), 726–737.

Stewart, T., & Sharma, M. (2020). Physical activity among school-aged children and intervention programs using self-determination theory (SDT): A scoping review. *Journal of Health and Social Sciences, 5*(4), 457–470.

Symons Downs, D., & Hausenblas, H. A. (2005). Elicitation studies and the theory of planned behavior: A systematic review of exercise beliefs. *Psychology of Sport and Exercise, 6*(1), 1–31.

Teixeira, P. J., Carraça, E. V., Markland, D., Silva, M. N., & Ryan, R. M. (2012). Exercise, physical activity, and self-determination theory: A systematic review. *International Journal of Behavioral Nutrition and Physical Activity, 9*(78).

Tirrell, B. E., & Hart, L. K. (1980). The relationship of health beliefs and knowledge to exercise compliance in patients after coronary bypass. *Heart Lung, 9*(3), 487–493.

Vasconcellos, D., Parker, P. D., Hilland, T., Cinelli, R., Owen, K. B., Kapsal, N., Lee, J., Antczak, D., Ntoumanis, N., Ryan, R. M., & Lonsdale, C. (2020). Self-determination theory applied to physical education: A systematic review and meta-analysis. *Journal of Educational Psychology, 112*(7), 1444–1469.

Vallerand, R. J. (1997). Toward a hierarchical model of intrinsic and extrinsic motivation. In M. J. Zanna (Ed.), *Advances in experimental and social psychology* (pp. 271–360). New York, NY: Plenum.

Vallerand, R. J., Deci, E., & Ryan, R. (1987). Intrinsic motivation in sport. In K. B. Pandolf (Ed.), *Exercise and sport science reviews* (pp. 389–425). New York, NY: Macmillan.

Vallerand, R. J., Pelletier, L. G., Blais, M. R., Brière, N. M., Senécal, C. B., & Vallières, E. F. (1993). On the assessment of intrinsic, extrinsic, and amotivation in education: Evidence on the concurrent and construct validity of the Academic Motivation Scale. *Educational and Psychological Measurement, 53*(1), 159–172.

Venema, T. A., & Pfattheicher, S. (2021). Perceived susceptibility to COVID-19 infection and narcissistic traits. *Personality and Individual Differences, 175,* 110696.

Walrave, M., Waeterloos, C., & Ponnet, K. (2020). Adoption of a contact tracing app for containing COVID-19: A health belief model approach. *The Journal of Medical Internet Research Public Health and Surveillance, 6*(3), e20572.

Warburton, D. E., & Bredin, S. S. (2017). Health benefits of physical activity: A systematic review of current systematic reviews. *Current Opinion in Cardiology, 32*(5), 541–556.

Wilson, P. M., Rodgers, W. M., Blanchard, C. M., & Gessell, J. (2003). The relationships between psychological needs, self-determined motivation, exercise attitudes, and physical fitness. *Journal of Applied Social Psychology, 33*(11), 2373–2392.

Wong, T. S., Gaston, A., DeJesus, S., & Prapavessis, H. (2016). The utility of a protection motivation theory framework for understanding sedentary behavior. *Health Psychology and Behavioral Medicine, 4*(1), 29–48.

Wurtele, S. K., & Maddux, J. E. (1987). Relative contributions of protection motivation theory components in predicting exercise intentions and behavior. *Health Psychology, 6*(5), 453–466.

CHAPTER 16

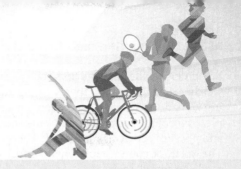

Stage-Based and Action Control Theories

LEARNING OBJECTIVES

After completing this chapter, you will be able to:

* Describe the constructs of the transtheoretical model.
* Discuss the physical activity research that has applied the transtheoretical model.
* Explain the intention-behavior gap in physical activity.
* Describe the structure and function of control theory, the health action process approach, and the multi-process action control framework.
* Discuss current research that has applied control theory, the health action process approach, and the multi-process action control framework to understand physical activity and sedentary behavior.

Introduction

For most people, changing unhealthy behaviors to healthy behaviors is often challenging. Change usually does not occur all at once; it may be a lengthy process. In this chapter, we overview models that emphasize a process of behavior change, whether this involves the process of forming and then translating an intention into behavior or progressing through several stages.

Transtheoretical Model of Behavior Change

The concept of stages—or a "one size does not fit all" philosophy (Marcus, King, Clark, Pinto, & Bock, 1996)—forms the basis for the transtheoretical model of behavior change (also sometimes referred to as the stages of change model) developed by Prochaska and his colleagues at the University of Rhode Island (Prochaska & DiClemente, 1982; Prochaska & Velicer, 1997). This model emerged from a comparative analysis of leading theories of psychotherapy and behavior change. In developing the model, the goal was to provide a systematic integration of a field that had fragmented into more than 300 theories of psychotherapy (Marcus et al., 1996). The transtheoretical model includes five constructs—stages of change, decisional balance, processes of change, self-efficacy, and temptation—that are considered important in understanding the process of volitional change. After its initial application with smoking cessation, the model was extended in an attempt to better understand a broad range of health behaviors such as nutrition, weight control, alcohol abuse, eating disorders, unplanned pregnancy protection, mammography screening, sun exposure, substance abuse, and physical activity (Prochaska & Velicer, 1997). The latter, of course, represents the focus on the model in this chapter.

Constructs of the Transtheoretical Model

Stages of Change

One of the major contributions of the transtheoretical model to the health field is the suggestion that behavior change unfolds slowly over time through a series of stages.

The **stages of change** construct has three aspects. First, stages fall somewhere between traits and states. Traits are stable and are not open to immediate change. States, in contrast, are readily changeable and typically lack stability. Thus, for example, an individual who is chronically anxious would be characterized as having high-trait anxiety. Conversely, an individual who has severe butterflies before a race would be known to possess high-state anxiety. Stages of change are trait-like in that they aren't quick to change and are driven by what's around us, but state-like in that it is theorized that people shift from one to another over time.

Second, stages are both stable and dynamic; that is, although stages may last for a considerable period, they are susceptible to change. Prochaska and DiClemente (1982, 1986) have hypothesized that as individuals change from an unhealthy to a healthy behavior they move through stages at varying rates and in a cyclical fashion, with periods of progression and relapse. For example, an inactive person may begin to think about the benefits (e.g., have more energy) and costs (e.g., time away from watching television) of physical activity. Then, a few months later, they may buy a pair of walking shoes. Six months later they may go walking three times a week. After a year of walking regularly, however, this individual may become overwhelmed with the stress of work and stop walking. The cessation of physical activity would represent a regression to an earlier stage. In short, individuals going through the process of behavioral change are thought to cycle (or progress and relapse) through a series of stages as they recognize the need to change, contemplate making a change, make the change, and, finally, sustain the new behavior. **Figure 16-1** provides a graphic illustration of the stages of change.

Third, people are hypothesized to pass through six stages in attempting any health behavior change: (1) precontemplation (not intending to make changes); (2) contemplation (intending to make changes within the foreseeable future, which is defined as the next 6 months); (3) preparation (intending to change in the immediate future, which is defined as within 1 month); (4) action (actively engaging in the new behavior); (5) maintenance (sustaining change over

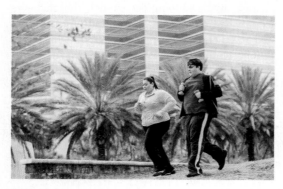
© kali9/E+/Getty Images.

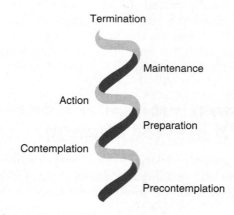
Figure 16-1 The Stages of Change.

Table 16-1 **Operational Definitions of the Stages of Exercise Change**

Stage	Operational Definition
Precontemplation	I do not intend to begin exercising in the next 6 months.
Contemplation	I intend to begin exercising in the next 6 months.
Preparation	I intend to begin exercising regularly in the next 30 days.
Action	I have been exercising, but for less than 6 months.
Maintenance	I have been exercising for more than 6 months.

Data from Reed, G. R., Velicer, W. F., Prochaska, J. O., Rossi, J. S., & Marcus, B. H. (1997). What makes a good staging algorithm: Examples from regular exercise. *American Journal of Health Promotion, 12*(1), 57–66.

time); and (6) termination (the probability of relapse is eliminated) (Reed, Velicer, Prochaska, Rossi, & Marcus, 1997). Operational definitions for the various stages are outlined in **Table 16-1**.

Precontemplation ("I won't" or "I can't")

People in the precontemplation stage are not considering change or do not want to change their behavior. The so-called "couch potato" is an example of someone who may fall into the precontemplation stage for shifting out of sedentary behavior. The hallmark of precontemplation is a lack of intention to take action, regardless of the reason or excuse (Reed et al., 1997). Insofar as adopting physical activity is concerned, an individual may be in precontemplation because they do not think it is valuable or think it is valuable but may be overwhelmed by barriers such as lack of time.

Interestingly, Reed (1999) reported the existence of two types of precontemplators. Precontemplation nonbelievers either do not believe in regular physical activity or do not see the value of engaging in it. Precontemplation believers do believe that physical activity is a worthwhile behavior; however, they cannot seem to start intending to participate in it. The precontemplation nonbelievers would conceivably need to become aware of and learn to appreciate the "pros," or benefits, of physical activity, such as improving mood states and energy levels.

By contrast, precontemplation believers need help overcoming the "cons," or costs, of exercising, such as taking time away from other activities (Reed, 1999).

Contemplation ("I might")

Individuals in the contemplation stage are thinking about changing their behavior sometime within the next 6 months. They see a need for change because they are aware of the costs and benefits of changing their behavior. For example, they may realize that physical activity reduces their risk of developing heart disease, or that too much sedentary behavior is contributing to depressive symptoms. However, they also acknowledge that there are many barriers to changing their lifestyle. Contemplators are conceived as being open to new information and interested in knowing more about the benefits of change. At this stage, however, people are not committed to the change; they are only contemplating or thinking about it. Therefore, they may become "chronic contemplators," never moving beyond the information-gathering phase (Prochaska & Velicer, 1997; Reed, 1999).

Preparation ("I will")

In the preparation stage, people are seriously considering to change their activity level in the near future, usually within the next month. The preparation stage has both a behavioral and an intentional component. For example, preparers may have bought a pair of running shoes, joined a running club, and even gone for a half hour walk once a week. Preparation is a relatively unstable stage because people in this stage are more likely than precontemplators or contemplators to progress over the next 6 months. Not surprisingly, this stage is the most controversial in terms of measurement because it can represent a hybrid of behavioral (e.g., some physical activity, but not regular activity) and/or intentional properties (e.g., intend to act within the month but not doing physical activity) (Reed et al., 1997).

Action ("I am")

Individuals who have recently changed their behavior (i.e., within the last 6 months) are considered to be in the action stage. To be classified within the action stage insofar as physical activity is concerned, the individual must meet the minimal physical activity recommendations developed by public health agencies (Ross et al., 2020; USDHHS, 2018). For example, in Canada and the United States, recommendations state that adults should accumulate 150 minutes or more of at least moderate-intensity (e.g., brisk walking) physical activity each week. Because the person in the action stage has only recently established the new activity pattern, attentiveness is necessary because relapse is probable (Reed, 1999).

Maintenance ("I have")

Once the individual has been regularly active for 6 consecutive months, they are deemed to have progressed into the maintenance stage. Although the new behavior has become better established, lapses in motivation or self-control could become a danger to relapse. It is at this time that a person works to reinforce the gains made through the various stages of change and strives to prevent lapses and relapses (Nigg et al., 2011; Reed, 1999).

Termination

Once a behavior has been maintained for more than 5 years, the individual is considered to have exited from the cycle of change, and a fear of relapse is eliminated. This stage is the ultimate goal for all people searching for a healthier lifestyle. Termination is the stage in which the person has no temptation to engage in the old behavior and shows 100% self-efficacy in all previously tempting situations.

CRITICAL THINKING ACTIVITY 16-1

The termination stage seems relevant for cessation behaviors where a person is trying to stop a behavior, such as smoking, but does it make sense for acquisition behaviors, where the goal is to keep on going? Can you ever really be "invulnerable" to missing physical activity?

Decisional Balance

Decision making was first conceptualized by Janis and Mann (1977) as a decisional "balance sheet" that assesses the importance that an individual places on the potential advantages, or pros, and disadvantages, or cons, of a behavior. According to the transtheoretical model, the balance between the pros and cons varies, depending on which stage of change the individual is in. When the cons of exercise (e.g., takes time away from other activities) are of greater importance than the pros of exercise (e.g., improves psychological well-being), motivation to change behavior (i.e., to move from being inactive to engaging in physical activity) is thought to be low. Thus, for example, in the precontemplation and contemplation stages, the cons are assumed to outweigh the pros. In the preparation stage, the pros and cons are believed to be relatively equal. Finally, in the action, maintenance, and termination stages, the pros are thought to outweigh the cons. DiClemente and his colleagues (1991) proposed that assessing the pros and cons is relevant for understanding and predicting transitions among the first three stages of change (i.e., precontemplation, contemplation, and preparation). During the action and maintenance stages, however, these **decisional balance** measures are thought to be much less important.

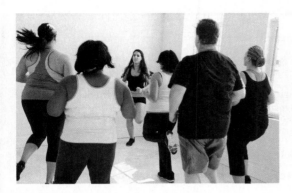

© Monkey Business Images/Shutterstock.

Processes of Change

According to the transtheoretical model, the 10 **processes of change** represent the behaviors, cognitions, and emotions that people engage in during the course of changing a behavior. These have been proposed to collapse into five experiential processes and five behavioral processes (Prochaska & Velicer, 1997). The experiential processes include: (1) consciousness raising (gathering information and determining the pros and cons of the positive behavior), (2) counterconditioning (substituting a positive behavior for a negative one), (3) dramatic relief (experiencing and expressing feelings about the consequences of the positive behavior), (4) environmental reevaluation (being a role model and considering how the negative behavior impacts significant

others), and (5) self-reevaluation (instilling the positive behaviors as an integral component of self-image). The behavioral processes include: (1) helping relationships (getting social support and using significant others to affect change), (2) reinforcement management (being rewarded by the self or others for engaging in the positive behavior), (3) social liberation (taking advantage of social situations that encourage the positive behavior), (4) stimulus control (using cues as a catalyst for the positive behavior), and (5) self-liberation (becoming committed to the positive behavior). It is postulated that the experiential processes are more important to the earlier three stages, whereas the later stages rely on the behavioral process of change to move to the next stage. **Table 16-2** outlines the various processes of change and provides a description for each. The processes of change provide information on how shifts in behavior occur.

CRITICAL THINKING ACTIVITY 16-2

The processes of change represent behavioral and mental strategies that people use to change their behavior. Think of some behaviors you have changed in the past. What strategies did you employ to make the change, if any? Do they resemble the processes of change outlined in the transtheoretical model, or were they different?

Table 16-2 The Processes of Change

Classic Term	Description
Consciousness raising	Gathering information about regular physical activity (learning the pros and cons of exercising)
Counterconditioning	Substituting sedentary behavior with activity
Dramatic relief	Experiencing and expressing feelings about the consequences of the positive behavior
Environmental reevaluation	Consideration and assessment of how inactivity affects friends, family, and citizens
Helping relationships	Getting support to implement your intention to exercise

(continues)

Table 16-2 **The Processes of Change**   (continued)

Classic Term	Description
Self-reevaluation	Appraising one's self-image as a healthy regular exerciser
Social liberation	Taking advantage of social policy, customs, and mores that enhance physical activity (e.g., New Year's resolutions)
Reinforcement management	Rewarding oneself or being rewarded by others for making changes
Stimulus control	Using cues to remember to engage in physical activity
Self-liberation	Committing oneself to becoming or remaining a regular exerciser

Data from Reed, G. R. (1999). Adherence to exercise and the transtheoretical model of behavior change. In S. Bull (Ed.), Adherence issues in sport and exercise (pp. 19–46). New York, NY: John Wiley & Sons.

Self-Efficacy

Self-efficacy is a judgment regarding one's ability to perform a behavior required to achieve a certain outcome. Not surprisingly, it is believed to be critical to behavior change (see also Chapter 14; Bandura, 1997). Self-efficacy is proposed to change with each stage, presumably increasing as the individual gains confidence (Prochaska & DiClemente, 1982). Conversely, self-efficacy may decrease if an individual falters and spirals back to an earlier stage.

Temptation

Temptation represents the intensity of the urges to engage in a specific behavior when in the midst of difficult situations (Grimley, Prochaska, Velicer, Blais, & DiClemente, 1994). Temptation and self-efficacy function inversely across the stages of change, with temptation proposed as a predictor of relapses and self-efficacy as a predictor of progression.

Advantages and Limitations of the Transtheoretical Model

Advantages

The advantages of the transtheoretical model to understanding physical activity behavior change have been detailed in various commentaries over the years (Armitage, 2009; Nigg et al., 2011; Reed, 1999; Romain et al., 2018). Nigg and colleagues (2011) have commented on the intuitive appeal of the model for allied health professions when understanding readiness for change, and this was also noted by Reed (1999) in earlier work. The staging construct provides for the opportunity to match interventions to the different needs of individuals. As a consequence, researchers and healthcare professionals are able to target specific interventions for the total population (i.e., those who have not yet made a behavior change and are at risk, as well as those who have changed but may be at risk of relapse).

For example, limited success has been observed for traditional interventions in terms of promoting the adoption and maintenance of a physically active lifestyle. According to the transtheoretical model, this lack of success may be attributed, in part, to the fact that an educational focus has been used rather than a behavioral and motivational focus. Many inactive individuals are not ready to adopt regular exercise because they are unmotivated. Thus, providing them with advice and a physical activity prescription is unlikely to lead to behavior change. Therefore, the traditional physical activity intervention may fail to recruit the vast majority of inactive individuals because they have no intention of becoming active. This reflects an incongruity between what is typically offered (action-oriented programs) and population motivational readiness to change (inactive and not intending to become active).

Armitage (2009) has also noted the innovation present in the processes of change constructs. Most models applied to understanding physical activity behavior use constructs that attempt to explain "why" people will perform the behavior. The transtheoretical model employs constructs that attempt to explain "why" people change or are resistant to change with constructs such as self-efficacy, decisional balance, and temptation, but it also includes constructs that attempt to understand "how" people change with the processes of change. These were relatively unique to the model at the time of its inception (Armitage, 2009).

Limitations

Despite some of the strengths of the model, the validity of the transtheoretical model has been a frequent source of debate for 20 years (Adams & White, 2003; Bandura, 1998; Brug et al., 2005; Weinstein, Rothman, & Sutton, 1998). Interested readers are encouraged to seek out these original papers, but the main points of critique are focused on whether a stage of change actually has validity and whether the constructs of the model represent a meaningful theoretical framework for behavior change in physical activity and sedentary behavior.

Most of the tests conducted with the stages of change model are descriptive, as opposed to explanatory, and involve cross-sectional designs (Nigg et al., 2011; Jiménez-Zazo et al., 2020). These descriptive designs have been successful at showing that constructs such as self-efficacy are significantly different across people who report they are at different stages of change. There is far less evidence to demonstrate that people actually go through these stages of change in longitudinal designs. It may be that these stages just describe the population more than they explain the change process. For example, Bandura (1998) stated that stages should reflect qualitative change and provide an invariant and nonreversible sequence. People's progression, however, through the stages of change of the transtheoretical model is reversible (i.e., people can relapse), and advancing from one stage to the next does not reflect a qualitative change (Weinstein, Rothman, & Sutton, 1998).

Another related critique of the model is from the sequential differences of the same constructs across the stages rather than different constructs showing importance at single stages but not others. For example, mean values for self-efficacy increase across the stages, but more compelling evidence would be where self-efficacy is only important for one stage transition. Finally, the stages of change construct has been criticized for the time frames attached to each stage (e.g., the action stage is the first 6 months). Certainly, some people could move from action to maintenance much faster than 6 months or move from contemplation to preparation to action in time frames different from that of the current staging (Rhodes & Sui, 2021). Nigg and colleagues (2011), recognizing the arbitrariness of the time frames, have called for the abandonment of them in favor of other criteria.

The stages of change construct has received the most criticism in the model, but the other constructs and their interrelationships have also received critique. Support for the relationship between the processes of change and decisional balance and the stages of change is equivocal. There is not a consistent pattern for how these constructs change across the stages and whether they have differential predictive utility (Spencer, Adams, Malone, Roy, & Yost, 2006; Romain et al., 2018). Finally, the integration of various theories (e.g., self-efficacy, decisional balance) to develop the transtheoretical model places these theories at odds with each other within the model. An understanding of the ordering for how these constructs interact is not defined, and too often, these constructs are treated as single (univariate) variables rather than as a complex (multivariate) theory.

CRITICAL THINKING ACTIVITY 16-3

The stages of change construct suggests a deliberative and ongoing progression to change behavior, with 6 months to contemplate, additional time to prepare, and then 6 months to move from action to maintenance. This raises the question about people who change cold turkey. The transtheoretical model does not explain this type of rapid change. Have you ever just changed a behavior very quickly?

Physical Activity Research Examining the Transtheoretical Model

Research that uses the transtheoretical model to understand sedentary behavior or sedentary-limiting behaviors (e.g., resisting screen time) is scant at this time (Han et al., 2015, 2017), but the model has considerable application in understanding physical activity. Over the last 3 decades, the model has been used to examine physical activity in cross-sectional studies, and to a lesser extent, in longitudinal and quasi-experimental intervention studies. The application of the transtheoretical model to physical activity was reviewed in the form of a meta-analysis several years ago (Marshall & Biddle, 2001), followed by systematic reviews (Hutchison, Breckon, & Johnston, 2009; Spencer et al., 2006) and a critical review with future research practices (Nigg et al., 2011). Two more recent reviews further summarize prior research evidence (Romaine et al, 2018; Pennington, 2021).

Observational Studies

Most of the existing research on the transtheoretical model has been conducted with cross-sectional or short longitudinal designs (Marshall & Biddle, 2001; Spencer et al., 2006). In general, these studies have shown that mean differences occur across stage membership for the constructs

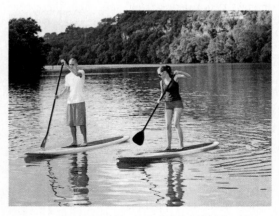

© Jodi Jacobson/E+/Getty Images.

of self-efficacy, decisional balance, and processes of change (Marshall & Biddle, 2001; Spencer et al., 2006). Probably, the most consistent construct to show differences by stages of change is self-efficacy. For example, Gorely and Godon (1995), in a study of Australian adults 50 to 65 years of age, found that self-efficacy to overcome barriers to exercise increased systematically from precontemplation to contemplation to preparation to action to maintenance.

Some research has demonstrated possible deviations of the transtheoretical model from smoking research compared with physical activity. For example, research on the termination stage for physical activity is limited and generally suggests that it may not be applicable to many people. Courneya and Bobick (2000) found no evidence for this stage. Cardinal (1999) also examined if a termination stage exists for physical activity, surveying 551 adults, and found that only 16.6% were classified within the termination stage.

Similar findings have been identified with the temptation construct. For example, Nigg and colleagues recently showed that the temptation construct was not predictive of stage of change after considering self-efficacy in the prediction equation (Nigg, McCurdy, et al., 2009). It may be that temptation is more relevant to smoking cessation.

Perhaps the biggest deviation from its relevancy for smoking compared with physical activity has been with the processes of change construct. Reviews and specific analyses show that the currently conceived processes of change do not work well with physical activity in their proposed structure (i.e., five behavioral and five experiential) or potentially, their content (Marshall & Biddle, 2001; Nigg, Norman, Rossi, & Benisovich, 1999; Nigg, Lippke, & Maddock, 2009; Rhodes, Berry, Naylor, & Wharf Higgins, 2004). This would make sense because different strategies for changing physical activity compared with smoking seem possible. Continued work on creating relevant constructs for the processes of change has been recommended (Nigg et al., 2011).

CRITICAL THINKING ACTIVITY 16-4

The transtheoretical model suggests that different people need different types of intervention, depending on their readiness for physical activity. This model suggests that these differences are based on decisional balance, self-efficacy, and the processes of change; however, there may be other aspects of an intervention: Consider culture, health status, age, gender, and physical activity background aspects. What might you change for people who differ on these variables? Would those changes be limited to just the constructs of the transtheoretical model?

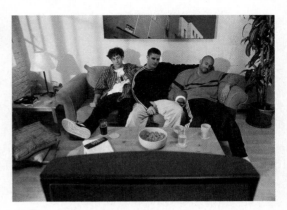

© Ryan McVay/Photodisc/Getty Images.

Intervention Research

Spencer and colleagues (2006) outlined 38 interventions from which to draw conclusions about the model, while Hutchinson and colleagues (2009) used 34 studies. Hutchinson and colleagues (2009) point out that many of the interventions have not focused on trying to change all of the constructs in the model, which could limit its ability to change physical activity. They note that all interventions have used the stages of change in intervention development, but more interventions have used the processes of change (71%) and pros/cons (63%) than self-efficacy (33%) in interventions. They further note that 86% of the interventions that used all of the transtheoretical model constructs in the intervention were successful at showing physical activity change, whereas only 71% of the studies that applied a few of the constructs were successful a point that has also been made more recently by Romaine and colleagues (2018).

The most compelling validation for the transtheoretical model comes from experimental tests to attempt to "match" or "mismatch" people on their interventions, corresponding to their stage of change. For example, people who are in the contemplation stage receive either an intervention package targeting the contemplation stage (match) or a package targeting the maintenance stage (mismatch), and the success of the intervention in moving people to preparation is then evaluated. To this end, Spencer and colleagues (2006) identified 15 studies in their systematic review that had examined this procedure. Nine of these studies showed some evidence for the superiority of the stage-matched intervention, indicating some support for the internal validity of the transtheoretical model. These effects were within the small effect size range, but they spanned all stages (Nigg et al., 2011). Thus, there is enough evidence to continue research on the stages of change construct, but more of these tests are recommended before any definitive conclusions can be drawn as to whether the stages of change construct is valid for understanding change of physical activity behavior.

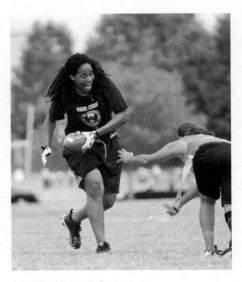

© Blulz60/iStock/Getty Images Plus/Getty Images.

Action Control Theories

The transtheoretical model highlights how people may progress through stages of behavior change. Many other models also highlight a potential progression sequence in behavioral performance. The most common of these types of models involves separating 1) the formation of an intention from 2) the translation of that intention into behavior, also known as **action control** (Kuhl, 1984). These models build from one of the central criticisms of social cognitive approaches (Chapter 14); specifically, there is often a modest association between intention and behavior, demonstrating a sizeable "intention-behavior gap" (Sheeran & Webb, 2016; Sniehotta, 2009). For example, experimental manipulations that increase physical activity intention ($d = 0.45$ or $r = 0.22$) result in much lower, and clinically less meaningful, increases in physical activity ($d = 0.15$ or $r = 0.075$) (Rhodes & Dickau, 2012). A meta-analysis of the dichotomization (e.g., those who intended to engage in regular physical activity but did not follow through, those who did not intend to engage in physical activity and subsequently followed through, etc.) of the intention and PA relationship around public health guidelines also showed that 48% of intenders failed to follow through with PA (see **Figure 16-2**. Rhodes & de Bruijn). Perhaps most important is the lowered practical value of theories that place intention as the proximal antecedent of health behavior. It is extremely common for inactive participants starting physical activity programs to already have high intentions at baseline, an implication of volunteering to change behavior in the first place (Rhodes & Rebar, 2017).

There are many different action control theories (Rhodes and Yao, 2015) and an even larger number of theories based on self-regulation of goals (Inzlicht, Werner, Briskin, & Roberts, 2021). Below, we briefly highlight three approaches that have received considerable research in physical activity.

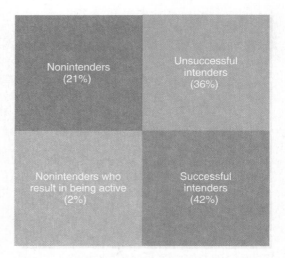

Figure 16-2 Relationship Between Intention and Physical Activity.

Data from Rhodes, R. E., & de Bruijn, G. J. (2013). How big is the physical activity intention-behaviour gap? A meta-analysis using the action control framework. *British Journal of Health Psychology, 18*(2), 296–309.

Control Theory

One of the most well-known general models of self-regulation is control theory (sometimes referred to as Cybernetic Control Theory) (Carver & Scheier, 1982, 1998). The model is based on a simple loop that contains four key constructs: (*a*) a goal (or intention); (*b*) input about the current state compared with that goal; (*c*) a monitoring system of discrepancies between the goal and the current state; and (*d*) a system that implements changes to reduce the discrepancy between current and desired state (see **Figure 16-3**). Control theory works as a continuous looping system where the current state is compared with the goal state by the monitoring system, and the process is repeated until the discrepancy between the goal state and the current state is reduced to the acceptable level (or the goal itself is changed).

For example, a person sets a goal to run twice a week (goal) and evaluates this goal every Sunday evening (input) using a journal of the week's activity (monitoring system). When there is a discrepancy (e.g., no running that week) that is detected between the goal and the evaluation,

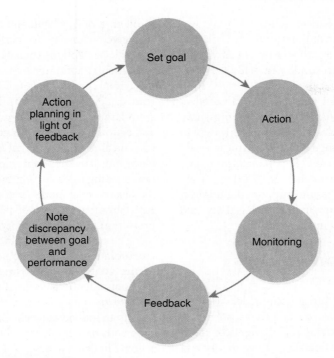

Figure 16-3 Control Theory Model.

Gould, N. J., Lorencatto, F., During, C., Rowley, M., Glidewell, L., Walwyn, R., & Francis, J. J. (2018). How do hospitals respond to feedback about blood transfusion practice? A multiple case study investigation. *PloS one, 13*(11), e0206676.

the person then responds to the discrepancy with a new behavioral course or a change in the goal until there is harmony within the feedback loop.

Control Theory, Physical Activity, and Sedentary Behavior

Specific, isolated tests of control theory are rare in physical activity and sedentary behavior research, yet the constructs are regularly imbedded in health behavior interventions as part of other theories and with various behavior change approaches. For example, the use of planning as the implementation system to modify intention is a core construct in the Health Action Process Approach highlighted later in this chapter.

The core construct of control theory is the presence of a self-monitoring system. While any monitoring system can, in concept, be applied to the context of physical activity (e.g., diaries,

calendars, notepads), the sophistication of physical activity trackers (e.g., Apple watch, Fitbit), allow for a more integrated and seamless application of control theory (see also Chapter 5). Evidence with physical activity trackers from randomized control trials generally support small gains in physical activity (Effect size $d = 0.27$) (Brickwood, Watson, O'Brien, & Williams, 2019). Similar findings for positive physical activity changes have been identified in reviews with trackers on mobile phones (Hosseinpour & Terlutter, 2019). However, there is also much broader evidence for the effectiveness of control theory on physical activity interventions beyond digital health applications. Evidence from a large meta-analysis of 122 diet and physical activity studies that have applied control theory has also shown similar results to wearable trackers (Michie, Abraham, Whittington, McAteer, & Gupta, 2009).

Of particular importance, self-monitoring was the construct of control theory, which explained the greatest amount of variance (in effectiveness), and interventions that combined self-monitoring with at least one other component derived from control theory, which proved the most effective in changing behavior. These findings have since been replicated with an updated review of physical activity change strategies (Knittle et al., 2018) and early research supports control theory in reducing sedentary behavior (Gardner et al., 2016). Overall, the results support the application of control theory in physical activity and potentially sedentary intervention.

Health Action Process Approach

The health action process approach (HAPA; Schwarzer, 2008) was developed as an action control theory to extend social cognitive models such as Bandura's social cognitive theory and theory of planned behavior (see Chapter 14). The framework includes two phases of behavior change that encompass preintentional constructs (known as the motivational phase), and postintentional constructs (known as the volitional phase) (see **Figure 16-4**). The motivational phase includes three constructs proposed to determine the formation of an intention. Specifically, outcome expectancies (beliefs that the behavior will result in a desired outcome), action self-efficacy (perceived capacity to perform the behavior), and risk perceptions (beliefs about susceptibility to particular conditions or associated with non-behavioral performance). For those who have read Chapters 14 and 15, these constructs will seem familiar. Specifically, outcome expectancies and action self-efficacy are nearly identical to the constructs residing in social cognitive theory; risk perception is a more specified outcome expectation residing in protection motivation theory and the health belief model, and intention is the construct from the theory of planned behavior and protection motivation theory.

The innovative contribution of HAPA is the incorporation of two components that operate in the volitional phase involved in the enactment of intentions: self-efficacy and planning. **Maintenance (or coping) self-efficacy** reflects an individual's beliefs in their capability to cope with barriers that might derail the intended action. Similarly, **recovery self-efficacy** reflects an individual's ability to overcome setbacks and recover from previously failed attempts to enact the behavior. Maintenance and recovery self-efficacy are proposed to directly affect behavior and result partly from action efficacy and the intention to act.

The HAPA also identifies two forms of planning relevant to intention enactment. **Action planning** assists individuals in identifying salient

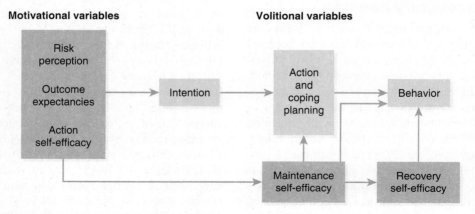

Figure 16-4 Health Action Process Approach.

Data from Schwarzer, R. (2008). Modeling health behavior change: How to predict and modify the adoption and maintenance of health behaviors. *Applied Psychology, 57*(1), 1–29.

cues that lead to action. These plans relate to the situation (when, where), the activity (what), and the sequence of actions (how) needed to perform the behavior. In exercise, for example, this may be the time (after work), place (at the recreation center), type of exercises (aerobic, strength, flexibility), and the steps (pack gym bag, secure transportation, arrange workout partner) that are required to perform the behavior. Action plans are also synonymous with a construct known as **implementation intentions** (Gollwitzer, 1999; Hagger & Luszczynska, 2014; Michie et al., 2013), although the theorizing for how they work to influence behavior differs (see box on Implementation Intentions).

The other type of planning in HAPA is known as coping planning. **Coping planning** entails the identification of barriers that might derail intended actions, and the generation of backup plans to manage or overcome them (Schwarzer, 2016). Action and coping planning are proposed to mediate the intention-behavior relationship in the HAPA. Specifically, it is proposed that individuals enact their intentions by making specific plans and managing contingencies that may derail actions.

Health Action Process Approach, Physical Activity, and Sedentary Behavior

The application of HAPA to physical activity has seen increasing research attention over the last decade, and two meta-analyses have summarized its effectiveness in observational research (Choi et al., 2018; Zhang et al., 2019). The most comprehensive review of HAPA and physical activity thus far was conducted by Zhang et al. (2019), who included 41 studies in their meta-analysis. Overall, the research team found that action self-efficacy ($\beta = 0.44$) and outcome expectancies ($\beta = 0.22$) had positive effects on physical activity intention. In turn, intention ($\beta = 0.18$), self-efficacy (maintenance and recovery self-efficacy were combined; $\beta = 0.16$) and coping planning ($\beta = 0.15$) had small effects on physical activity. Action planning ($\beta = 0.05$) did not have a sizeable effect on physical activity after controlling for these other variables. Taken together, there is some evidence that the volitional phase leads to understanding physical activity, particularly when coping planning and maintenance/recovery self-efficacy are considered.

Implementation Intentions

Implementation intentions are specific "if-then" action plans, whereby a link is forged between a cue and subsequent behavioral response (Gollwitzer & Brandstatter, 1997). Implementation intentions arose from the development of the model of action phases (Gollwitzer, 1990; Heckhausen & Gollwitzer, 1987) which, like HAPA, is also a two phase model with a motivational and a subsequent volitional phase. Implementation intentions are thought to be particularly suitable for behaviors where the motivation to enact the desired behavior is stable, but inaction may occur due to forgetting to recall the intention or failing to seize an appropriate moment to act (Gollwitzer & Sheeran, 2006). The theory behind implementation intentions suggests that the process of specifying cues to a behavioral response (e.g., if it is 3pm, I will exercise) helps build a link that is below conscious awareness and makes the appropriate behavioral response more accessible when the cue is presented (see also habits in Chapter 17). This distinction shows how it can vary from action planning because action planning can be both a conscious, deliberative process or an unconscious process (Hagger & Luszczynska, 2014).

Two meta-analyses (da Silva et al., 2018; Bélanger-Gravel et al., 2013) have shown that the effect of implementation intentions on physical activity is small ($d = 0.24$ to 0.25) but meaningful, and a recent review showed that having strong intention and self-efficacy already in place assists in maximizing the effectiveness of implementation intentions (Kompf, 2020). This supports the two-phase (motivational, volitional) approach taken in theories like HAPA. At present, the evidence is too limited to assess whether implementations affect reducing sedentary behavior, although the approach warrants exploration in future research (Gardner et al., 2016).

Experimental evidence for HAPA has also begun to accumulate in physical activity research, particularly when focused on action and coping planning. For example, Carraro and Gaudreau (2013) showed a small effect of action plans on changes in physical activity behavior compared with control groups among 19 eligible studies, suggesting the technique is effective in changing behavior above no intervention. Kwasnicka et al. (2013) conducted a systematic review of coping planning applied to five physical activity studies. The authors concluded that coping planning is an effective technique to increase health behaviors and is particularly effective in augmenting action planning. Carraro and Gaudreau's (2013) meta-analysis of coping planning in physical activity identified a small effect on behavior change when compared with no-treatment controls, and a medium-sized effect when coping planning was combined with action planning.

There has been less research applying HAPA to sedentary behavior compared with physical activity, yet current evidence has been mixed. In a sophisticated multi-group intervention of coping planning and action planning on sedentary behavior, Schroé et al. (2020) showed no effect of action planning and coping planning, alone or together, on reducing sedentary behavior. By contrast, Sui and Prapevessis (2018) examined a planning intervention to increase sedentary break times in 52 university students over 8 weeks. The researchers found a significant effect in break frequency favoring the HAPA intervention over the control group. A follow-up study using a similar HAPA intervention, this time with text messaging among university students, also yielded similar positive findings of reducing sedentary behavior (Dillon et al., 2021). Thus, more research on HAPA and its utility with reducing sedentary behavior is needed.

Multi-Process Action Control

The multi-process action control (M-PAC; Rhodes, 2017, 2021) framework was constructed as a meta-theory extension of the reasoned action approach and other similar social cognitive models (see Chapter 14) by including a focus on the translation of intentions into behavior and the subsequent sustainability of intention-behavior coupling (see **Figure 16-5**). Briefly, M-PAC suggests that sustained behavior change involves three developing processes that determine behavior through the repeated successful translation of intention into action. The formative level is called **reflective processes**, which represent the consciously deliberated and expected consequences of performing a behavior (Rhodes, 2017). The specific constructs include affective (expected pleasure) and instrumental (expected utility) attitudes, and perceived capability (ability to perform a behavior) and opportunity (social/environmental access to perform a behavior), which are nearly identical to the domain representation of the reasoned action approach's attitude and perceived behavioral control constructs (See Chapter 14). When reflective processes are positive and strong, the net result is a decision to perform physical activity (i.e., intend/do not intend) (Rhodes & Rebar, 2017).

In the M-PAC framework, however, reflective processes of perceived opportunity and affective attitude may also predict the translation of an intention into behavior, to the extent that they represent a proxy for the affective and logistical factors that challenge one's competing daily decisions. By contrast, instrumental attitude and perceived capability are not considered antecedents of the translation of an intention because they are expected to vary little from day to day and situation to situation (Rhodes, La, et al., 2021). Thus, a focus on strong affective experiences with the behavior and social and environmental opportunities to perform the behavior are needed to promote sustainability long after the initial decision to start.

Still, the translation of intention into behavior is primarily marked by the emergence of regulatory processes. **Regulatory processes** represent the behavioral, cognitive, and affective tactics that are used to translate a formulated intention into behavior. These can be prospective

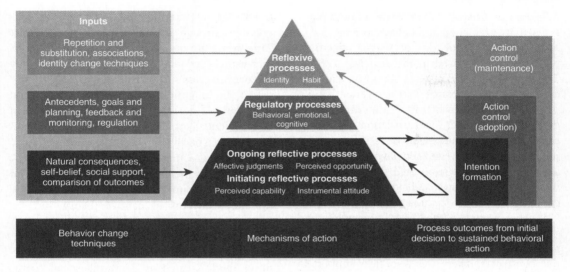

Figure 16-5 The Multi-Process Action Control Framework.

Rhodes, R. E. (2021). Multi-process action control in physical activity: A primer. *Frontiers in Psychology, 12,* 797484.

(e.g., planning, self-monitoring, restructuring the built and physical environment) or reactive (e.g., emotion regulation, attentional focus) in their implementation. Furthermore, engaging in regulatory processes may be a seamless consequence for some people when forming an intention (i.e., spontaneous behavioral regulation), or through the result of outside intervention. Thus, for those challenged by following through on an intention, interventions that focus on these types of regulatory processes are considered the first step in promotion.

Finally, continuance of a behavior is thought to rely upon reflexive processes. **Reflexive processes** represent impulsive constructs that influence action control most often through learned associations and are triggered through particular circumstances and stimuli (see Chapter 17). M-PAC highlights the development of two critical reflexive processes: habit (i.e., behavior performed from stimulus-response bonds) and identity (behavior performed to minimize the dissonance between self-categorization and behavior) as one begins to perform the behavior more regularly. Like regulatory processes, habit and identity are proposed to arise as a natural consequence of repeated successful

behavioral outcomes and can be intervened upon through specific external behavior change techniques (e.g., associations, repetition, identity formation strategies). Overall, the formation of habit and identity are proposed to engender sustained translation of intentions to behavior through greater enactment efficiency, in part by replacing the use of regulatory processes and lessening the cognitive demands of reflective processes (Rhodes & Sui, 2021).

M-PAC, Physical Activity, and Sedentary Behavior

M-PAC was specifically developed for regular physical activity, and thus tests of the approach with other behaviors, including sedentary behavior, have not seen much research attention. By contrast, there have been several narrative reviews of M-PAC when applied to physical activity (Rhodes & de Bruijn, 2013b; Rhodes & Yao, 2015; Rhodes et al., 2021). Because M-PAC is a high-level meta-construction of many other theories applied to physical activity, there are also general reviews that support the importance of reflective (see Chapter 14), regulatory (see HAPA and control theory earlier in this chapter), and reflexive (see Chapter 17) processes in both physical activity prediction and behavior change.

The multivariate tests of M-PAC constructs were recently reviewed in Rhodes et al. (2021). The authors reported on 29 studies that had used either a full M-PAC framework or a variant (>75% of the variables present). Eleven studies specifically tested the tenet that translation of physical activity intention into behavior is a function of reflective, regulatory, and reflexive processes and seven of these tests supported that assumption, while four tests showed reflexive and regulatory constructs as key determinants. The results provide some support of the M-PAC framework, and certainly support the additions of the regulatory and reflexive layers in the model over the reflective constructs. There was also clear support in the review that the affective property of an attitude was predictive of the follow-through of intention but the instrumental component was not. Experimental research using M-PAC to promote physical activity change has not seen as much research attention as observational research. Thus, the utility of intervening on all three layers/processes in the framework over one specific process cannot be appraised at present.

Summary

This chapter examined models that emphasize a process of behavior change, whether this involves the process of forming and then translating an intention into behavior or progressing through several stages. Over the last 2 decades, the transtheoretical model has been increasingly applied to examine physical activity behavior in cross-sectional studies and, to a lesser extent, in longitudinal and quasi-experimental intervention studies. One of the most well-known general models of self-regulation is control theory. While specific research on control theory with physical activity and sedentary behavior is scant, parts of the theory are often integrated in many different interventions. The results show that key concepts of control theory, such as self-monitoring, are reliably associated with behavior change. The health action process approach was developed to extend social cognitive models, such as Bandura's social cognitive theory and theory of planned behavior. Its constructs of action and coping planning have shown some evidence for mediation and moderating the relationship between intention and physical activity, and application of the model has promise for changing both physical activity and sedentary behavior. Multi-process action control is a theoretical framework that highlights reflective, regulatory, and reflexive processes that are proposed to influence the formation and enactment of intentions across initiation to maintenance. Observational research shows support for the framework and research testing its effectiveness in interventions for physical activity and sedentary behavior is ongoing.

Vignette: Gina

The way I saw it, the sole purpose of going to the gym or forcing yourself to run, walk, or bike outdoors was just to be skinny. Because I was never a fan of the outdoors and the idea that one could engage in sustained physical activity for pleasure struck me as absurd. And since I could always shimmy into a size 4 dress, I didn't see why I'd have to start an exercise program—especially since I'd made it to my 30s maintaining a healthy weight.

But then during an annual physical, my doctor discovered that I had high blood pressure, high blood sugar, and high cholesterol. I was floored. "Doesn't this only happen to people who are overweight?" I asked her. Apparently not.

During that visit—and after a fair bit of Googling "normal weight obesity"—I learned that even if a person (such as myself) has a normal BMI and thin frame, she could still be at risk for cardiovascular disease, hypertension, and metabolic syndrome. It comes down to how much body fat she has on her—not just her weight.

Apparently, my body fat levels were higher than I wanted to admit. And because a few of my maternal aunts and uncles suffered from heart disease, my doctor urged me to try walking or biking to and from work, possibly joining a gym, or investing in some kind of cardio trainer for my home.

My initial reaction was "yeah, right." I thought maybe I could cut back on the penne al forno and other cheesy pasta dishes that had been staples of my diet since my Italian grandmother taught me how to make them when I was a kid. But join a gym? I barely owned a functional pair of sneakers.

The doctor thought maybe yoga or a stationary bike would be better alternatives. I decided to give the former a shot but after three agonizing classes where I could barely hold a "downward-facing dog" for 15 seconds, I called it quits. Exercise simply wasn't for me.

But then the recession hit and I was laid off from my full-time high school teaching position. For many months, I was only able to secure part-time work, and I ended up facing long stretches of free time that I truly didn't know what on earth I'd do with.

A girlfriend of mine implored me to come take some dance class with her called Zumba that she'd grown increasingly obsessed with. I refused countless times until she promised to take me for gelato afterwards if I came with her on a Saturday. I acquiesced and ended up humiliating myself in a roomful of women far more adept at moving to a beat than I was.

When that same friend suggested we go for a hike the following week, my initial reaction was a resounding "no." But she offered to make it more about photography and brought along her fancy XLR digital camera. Because there was something artistic involved, I thought, fine.

I enjoyed the hike. Mostly because it was with my friend and there weren't any intimidating fitness instructors barking orders at us to keep moving. (Nor was there a gaggle of women far fitter than myself who might judge me for being out of sync with any music.)

Over the next few months, we'd regularly meet on weekend mornings to lightly trek the trails and state parks within a reasonable driving distance from our homes in Cincinnati. It got to the point where I even had to buy a new pair of sneakers in order to sustain the growing habit. And eventually, I was really coming to look forward to these hikes—sometimes even doing them on my own on days when I didn't have work or my friend wasn't available.

My doctor was pretty pleased with my progress as well. When I returned to her for my next annual physical, my cholesterol and blood sugar levels had come down a bit and my body fat percentage had gone down.

And then I was offered a full-time teaching job at a charter school in Indiana, requiring me to relocate away from my friend and away from our stomping grounds.

I took the job. I had to. I desperately needed the money, and the position was one I'd been hoping to land for months. I planned on staying active after I'd settled into my new (thankfully, larger) home, an apartment within walking distance of the new school. But once classes began and the stresses of adapting to a new environment piled up, my interest in finding a new hiking trail and recommitting to regular walks vastly diminished. By the end of my first year on the new job, I'd gone back to spending weekends cooking high-fat, high-carb recipes; avoiding physical activity; and feeling my body succumb to fatigue.

I've been working in Indiana for over a year now. And periodically, I get back in the habit of exercising. (Usually, during the summers, when I don't have to teach full time.) I have a gym membership to a fitness center, and every so often I'll go there to watch television while I cycle on a stationary bike or elliptical machine. But I'm sorry to say that it's harder to maintain my interest in fitness when I don't have a friend motivating me or an innate love of physical activity.

To help keep myself moving (not because I love to but because I feel like I should for my health—and my new doctor agrees), I did, however, take a measure that's proven to be quite effective. A few months ago, I adopted a rambunctious Boston terrier from my local humane society.

Having to take this adorable pup out in the morning, afternoon, and evening forces me to be on my feet. And as soon as he gets accustomed to his new abode, like I had to, I plan on taking him with me on some of the nearby hiking trails I've been researching. (I will, of course, be sending my former friend back in Ohio any and all pictures I end up snapping on the refurbished XLR she sent me for my birthday several weeks ago.)

Key Terms

action control The pursuit of translating an intention into behavior.

action planning Formulation of an articulated set of procedures to assist in behavioral action.

coping planning Formulation of plans to overcome important barriers when action initiation and/or maintenance is challenged.

decisional balance The importance that an individual places on the potential advantages, or *pros*, and disadvantages, or *cons*, of a behavior and the subsequent evaluation of these factors.

implementation intentions "If-then" action plans, whereby a link is forged between a cue and subsequent behavioral response.

maintenance self-efficacy An individual's beliefs in their capability to cope with barriers that might derail the intended action.

processes of change The behaviors, cognitions, and emotions that people engage in during the course of changing a behavior. In the transtheoretical model, these are proposed as five behavioral and five experiential processes.

recovery self-efficacy An individual's ability to overcome setbacks and recover from previously failed attempts to enact the behavior.

reflective processes Consciously deliberated and expected consequences of performing a behavior.

reflexive processes Influences on behavior that are triggered through particular circumstances and stimuli.

regulatory processes Behavioral, cognitive, and affective tactics that are employed to translate a formulated intention into behavior.

self-efficacy Belief in one's capabilities to organize and execute the course of action required to produce a certain outcome.

stages of change Six stages that people pass through in attempting any health behavior change, according to the transtheoretical model: precontemplation, contemplation, preparation, action, maintenance, and termination.

temptation The intensity of urges to engage in a specific behavior.

Review Questions

1. List and describe each of the six stages of change in the transtheoretical model.
2. Explain how self-efficacy, decisional balance, and the processes of change are expected to operate across the stages of change, according to Prochaska and DiClemente (1982).
3. Outline some of the potential advantages of the transtheoretical model.
4. Which construct in the transtheoretical model has the most validation? Which construct has received the most criticism?
5. How big is the physical activity intention gap? What proportion of people are typically unsuccessful intenders? What proportion are nonintenders?
6. What are the key constructs of control theory? How do they make a feedback loop?
7. How do action plans and implementation intentions work in translating intentions into behavior?
8. What are the three processes highlighted in multi-process action control? How do they relate to each other and what are example constructs found in each process?

Applying the Concepts

1. From her first visit to the doctor to her second, what stages of change did Gina progress through?

2. By the end of her story, had Gina arrived at the termination stage of the transtheoretical model? Why or why not?

References

Adams, J., & White, M. (2003). Are activity promotion interventions based on the transtheoretical model effective? A critical review. *British Journal of Sports Medicine, 37*(2), 106–114.

Armitage, C. J. (2009). Is there utility in the transtheoretical model? *British Journal of Health Psychology, 14*(2), 195–210.

Bandura, A. (1997). *Self-efficacy, the exercise of control.* New York, NY: Freeman.

Bandura, A. (1998). Health promotion from the perspective of social cognitive theory. *Psychology & Health, 13*(4), 623–649.

Bélanger-Gravel, A., Godin, G., & Amireault, S. (2013). A meta-analytic review of the effect of implementation intentions on physical activity. *Health Psychology Review, 7*(1), 23–54.

Brickwood, K. J., Watson, G., O'Brien, J., & Williams, A. D. (2019). Consumer-based wearable activity trackers increase physical activity participation: Systematic review and meta-analysis. *Journal of Medical Internet Research, 7*(4), e11819.

Brug, J., Conner, M., Harré, N., Kremers, S., McKellar, S., & Whitelaw, S. (2005). The transtheoretical model and stages of change: A critique. Observations by five commentators on the paper by Adams, J. and White, M. (2004) Why don't stage-based activity promotion interventions work? *Health Education Research, 20*(2), 244–258.

Cardinal, B. J. (1999). Extended stage model for physical activity behavior. *Journal of Human Movement Studies, 37*(1), 37–54.

Carraro, N., & Gaudreau, P. (2013). Spontaneous and experimentally induced action planning and coping planning for physical activity: A meta-analysis. *Psychology of Sport and Exercise, 14*(2), 228–248.

Carver, C. S., & Scheier, M. F. (1998). *On the Self-Regulation of Behavior.* New York: Cambridge University Press.

Carver, C. S., & Scheier, M. F. (1982). Control theory: A useful conceptual framework for personality–social, clinical, and health psychology. *Psychological Bulletin, 92*(1), 111–135.

Choi, Y., Yang, S. J., & Song, H. Y. (2018). Effects of the variables related to the health action process approach model on physical activity: A systematic literature review and meta-analysis. *Journal of the Community Academy of Community Health Nursing, 29,* 359–370.

Courneya, K. S., & Bobick, T. M. (2000). No evidence for a termination stage in exercise behavior change. *Avante, 6,* 75–85.

da Silva, M. A., São-João, T. M., Brizon, V. C., Franco, D. H., & Mialhe, F. L. (2018). Impact of implementation intentions on physical activity practice in adults: A systematic review and meta-analysis of randomized clinical trials. *PLoS One, 13,* e0206294.

Dillon, K., Rollo, S., & Prapavessis, H. (2021). A combined health action process approach and mHealth intervention to reduce sedentary behaviour in university students – a randomized controlled trial. *Psychology and Health.*

DiClemente, C. C., Prochaska, J. O., Fairhurst, S. K., Velicer, W. F., Velasquez, M. M., & Rossi, J. S. (1991). The process of smoking cessation: An analysis of precontemplation, contemplation, and preparation states of change. *Journal of Consulting and Clinical Psychology, 59*(2), 295–304.

Gardner, B., Smith, L., Lorencatto, F., Hamer, M., & Biddle, S. J. (2016). How to reduce sitting time? A review of behaviour change strategies used in sedentary behaviour reduction interventions among adults. *Health Psychology Review, 10*(1), 89–112.

Gollwitzer, P. M. (1990). Action phases and mind-sets. In E. T. Higgins & R. M. Sorrentino (Eds.), *Handbook of motivation and cognition: Foundations of social behavior* (Vol. 2, pp. 53–92). New York: Guilford Press.

Gollwitzer, P. M., & Brandstätter, V. (1997). Implementation intentions and effective goal pursuit. *Journal of Personality & Social Psychology, 73*(1), 186–199.

Gollwitzer, P. M. (1999). Implementation intentions: Strong effects of simple plans. *American Psychologist, 54*(7), 493–503.

Gollwitzer, P. M., & Sheeran, P. (2006). Implementation intentions and goal achievement: A meta-analysis of effects and processes. *Advances in Experimental Social Psychology, 38,* 69–119.

Gorely, T., & Gordon, S. (1995). An examination of the transtheoretical model and exercise behavior in older adults. *Journal of Sport & Exercise Psychology, 17*(3), 312–324.

Gould, N. J., Lorencatto, F., During, C., Rowley, M., Glidewell, L., Walwyn, R., & Francis, J. J. (2018). How do hospitals respond to feedback about blood transfusion practice? A multiple case study investigation. *PLoS one, 13*(11), e0206676.

Grimley, D., Prochaska, J. O., Velicer, W. F., Blais, W. F., & DiClemente, C. C. (1994). The transtheoretical model of change. In T. M. Brinthaupt, & R. P. Lipka (Eds.), *Changing the sell: Philosophies, techniques, and experiences* (pp. 201–227). Albany, NY: State University of New York.

Hagger, M. S., & Luszczynska, A. (2014). Implementation intention and action planning interventions in health contexts: State of the research and proposals for the way forward. *Applied Psychology: Health and Well-Being, 6*(1), 1–47.

Han, H., Gabriel, K. P., & Kohl, H. W. (2015). Evaluations of validity and reliability of a transtheoretical model for sedentary behavior among college students. *American Journal of Health Behavior, 39*(5), 601–609.

Han, H., Gabriel, K. P., & Kohl, H. W. (2017). Application of the transtheoretical model to sedentary behaviors and its association with physical activity status. *PLoS One, 12*(4), e0176330.

Heckhausen, H., & Gollwitzer, P. M. (1987). Thought contents and cognitive functioning in motivational and volitional states of mind. *Motivation and Emotion, 11*, 101–120.

Hosseinpour, M., & Terlutter, R. (2019). Your personal motivator is with you: A systematic review of mobile phone applications aiming at increasing physical activity. *Sports Medicine, 49*, 1425–1447.

Hutchison, A. J., Breckon, J. D., & Johnston, L. H. (2009). Physical activity behavior change interventions based on the transtheoretical model: A systematic review. *Health Education & Behavior, 36*(5), 829–845.

Inzlicht, M., Werner, K. M., Briskin, J. L., & Roberts, B. W. (2021). Integrating models of self-regulation. *Annual Review of Psychology, 72*, 319–345.

Janis, I. L., & Mann, L. (1977). *Decision-making: A psychological analysis of conflict, choice, and commitment.* New York, NY: Free Press.

Jiménez-Zazo, F., Romero-Blanco, C., Castro-Lemus, N., Dorado-Suárez, A., & Aznar, S. (2020). Transtheoretical model for physical activity in older adults: Systematic review. *International Journal of Environment Research and Public Health, 17*(24), 9262.

Knittle, K., Nurmi, J., Crutzen, R., Hankonen, N., Beattie, M., & Dombrowski, S. U. (2018). How can interventions increase motivation for physical activity? A systematic review and meta-analysis. *Health Psychology Review, 12*(3), 211–230.

Kompf, J. (2020). Implementation intentions for exercise and physical activity: Who do they work for? A systematic review. *Journal of Physical Activity and Health, 17*(3), 349–359.

Kuhl, J. (1984). Motivational aspects of achievement motivation and learned helplessness: Towards a comprehensive theory of action control. In B. A. Maher, & W. B. Maher (Eds.), *Progress in Experimental Personality Research* (Vol. 13, pp. 99–171). New York: Academic Press.

Kwasnicka, D., Presseau, J., White, M., & Sniehotta, F. F. (2013). Does planning how to cope with anticipated barriers facilitate health-related behaviour change? A systematic review. *Health Psychology Review, 7*(2), 129–145.

Marcus, B. H., King, T. K., Clark, M. M., Pinto, B. M., & Bock, B. C. (1996). Theories and techniques for promoting physical activity behaviours. *Sports Medicine, 22*, 321–331.

Marshall, S. J., & Biddle, S. J. (2001). The transtheoretical model of behavior change: A meta-analysis of applications to physical activity and exercise. *Annals of Behavioral Medicine, 23*, 229–246.

Michie, S., Abraham, C., Whittington, C., McAteer, J., & Gupta, S. (2009). Effective techniques in healthy eating and physical activity interventions: A meta-regression. *Health Psychology, 28*(6), 690–701.

Michie, S., Richardson, M., Johnston, M., Abraham, C., Francis, J., Hardeman, W., . . . Wood, C. E. (2013). The behavior change technique taxonomy (v1) of 93 hierarchically clustered techniques: Building an international consensus for the reporting of behavior change interventions. *Annals of Behavioral Medicine, 46*(1), 81–95.

Nigg, C. R., Geller, K. S., Motl, R. W., Horwath, C. C., Wertin, K. K., & Dishman, R. K. (2011). A research agenda to examine the efficacy and relevance of the transtheoretical model for physical activity behavior. *Psychology of Sport and Exercise, 12*(1), 7–12.

Nigg, C. R., Lippke, S., & Maddock, J. E. (2009). Factorial invariance of the theory of planned behavior applied to physical activity across gender, age, and ethnic groups. *Psychology of Sport and Exercise, 10*(2), 219–225.

Nigg, C. R., McCurdy, D. K., McGee, K. A., Motl, R. W., Paxton, R. J., Horwath, C. C., & Dishman, R. K. (2009). Relations among temptations, self-efficacy, and physical activity. *International Journal of Sport and Exercise Psychology, 7*(2), 230–243.

Nigg, C. R., Norman, G. J., Rossi, J. S., & Benisovich, S. V. (1999). Processes of exercise behavior change: Redeveloping the scale. *Annals of Behavioral Medicine, 21*(suppl), S79.

Pennington, C. G. (2021). Applying the transtheoretical model of behavioral change to establish physical activity habits. *Journal of Education and Recreation Patterns, 2*(1), 12–20.

Prochaska, J. O., & DiClemente, C. C. (1982). Transtheoretical therapy: Toward a more integrative model of change. *Psychotherapy: Theory, Research and Practice, 19*(3), 276–288.

Prochaska, J. O., & DiClemente, C. C. (1986). Toward a comprehensive model of change. In W. R. Miller, & N. Heather (Eds.), *Treating addictive behaviors: Processes of change* (pp. 3–27). New York, NY: Plenum.

Prochaska, J. O., & Velicer, W. F. (1997). The transtheoretical model of health behavior change. *American Journal of Health Promotion, 12*(1), 38–48.

Ross, R., Chaput, J., Giangregorio, L., Janssen, I., Saunders, T. J., Kho, M. E., . . . & Tremblay, M. S. (2020). Canadian 24-hour movement guidelines for adults aged 18–64 years and adults aged 65 years or older: An integration of physical activity, sedentary behaviour, and sleep. *Applied Physiology, Nutrition, and Metabolism, 45*(10, Suppl. 2), S57–S102.

Reed, G. R. (1999). Adherence to exercise and the transtheoretical model of behavior change. In S. Bull (Ed.), *Adherence issues in sport and exercise* (pp. 19–46). New York, NY: John Wiley & Sons.

Reed, G. R., Velicer, W. F., Prochaska, J. O., Rossi, J. S., & Marcus, B. H. (1997). What makes a good staging algorithm: Examples from regular exercise. *American Journal of Health Promotion, 12*(1), 57–66.

Rhodes, R. E., Berry, T., Naylor, P. J., & Wharf Higgins, S. J. (2004). Three-step validation of exercise processes of change in an adolescent sample. *Measurement in Physical Education and Exercise Science, 8*(1), 1–20.

Rhodes, R. E. (2017). The evolving understanding of physical activity behavior: A multi-process action control approach. In A. J. Elliot (Ed.), *Advances in Motivation Science* (Vol. 4, pp. 171–205). Cambridge, MA: Elsevier Academic Press.

Rhodes, R. E. (2021). Multi-process action control in physical activity: A primer. *Frontiers in Psychology, 12,* 797484.

Rhodes, R. E., & Dickau, L. (2012). Experimental evidence for the intention-behavior relationship in the physical activity domain: A meta-analysis. *Health Psychology, 31*(6), 724–727.

Rhodes, R. E., & de Bruijn, G-J. (2013). How big is the physical activity intention-behaviour gap? A meta-analysis using the action control framework. *British Journal of Health Psychology, 18*(2), 296–309.

Rhodes, R. E., & de Bruijn, G-J. (2013b). What predicts intention-behavior discordance? A review of the action control framework. *Exercise and Sports Sciences Reviews, 41*(4), 201–207.

Rhodes, R. E., & Rebar, A. (2017). Conceptualizing and defining the intention construct for future physical activity research. *Exercise and Sports Sciences Reviews, 45*(4), 209–216.

Rhodes, R. E., La, H., Quinlan, A., & Grant, S. (2021). Enacting physical activity intention: A multi-process action control approach. In C. Englert, & I. Taylor (Eds.), *Motivation and Self-regulation in Sport and Exercise* (pp. 8–20). New York: Taylor & Francis.

Rhodes, R. E., & Sui, W. (2021). Physical activity maintenance: A critical review and directions for future research. *Frontiers in Psychology, 12*(725671), 1–13.

Rhodes, R. E., & Yao, C. A. (2015). Models accounting for intention-behavior discordance in the physical activity domain: A user's guide, content overview, and review of current evidence. *International Journal of Behavioral Nutrition and Physical Activity, 12*(9), 1–15.

Romain, A. J., Caudroit, J., Hokayem, M., & Bernard, P. (2018). Is there something beyond stages of change in the transtheoretical model? The state of art for physical activity. *Canadian Journal of Behavioural Science, 50*(1), 42–53.

Schroé, H., Van Dyck, D., De Paepe, A., Poppe, L., Loh, W. W., Verloigne, M., Loeys, T., De Bourdeaudhuij, I., & Crombez, G. (2020). Which behaviour change techniques are effective to promote physical activity and reduce sedentary behaviour in adults: A factorial randomized trial of an e- and m-health intervention. *International Journal of Behavioural Nutrition and Physical Activity, 17*(127), 2–16.

Schwarzer, R. (2008). Modeling health behavior change: How to predict and modify the adoption and maintenance of health behaviors. *Applied Psychology, 57*(1), 1–29.

Schwarzer, R. (2016). Coping planning as an intervention component: A commentary. *Psychology & Health, 31*(7), 903–906.

Sheeran, P., & Webb, T. L. (2016). The intention-behavior gap. *Social & Personality Psychology Compass, 10*(9), 503–518.

Sniehotta, F. F. (2009). Towards a theory of intentional behaviour change: Plans, planning, and self-regulation. *British Journal of Health Psychology, 14*(2), 261–273.

Spencer, L., Adams, T. B., Malone, S., Roy, L., & Yost, E. (2006). Applying the transtheoretical model to exercise: A systematic and comprehensive review of the literature. *Health Promotion Practice, 7*(4), 428–443.

Sui, W., & Prapavessis, H. (2018). Standing Up for Student Health: An Application of the Health Action Process Approach for Reducing Student Sedentary Behavior—Randomised Control Pilot Trial. *Applied Psychology: Health and Well-Being, 10,* 87–107.

U.S. Department of Health and Human Services. (2018). *Physical Activity Guidelines for Americans* (2nd ed.). Washington, DC: US Department of Health and Human Services.

Weinstein, N. D., Rothman, A. J., & Sutton, S. R. (1998). Stage theories of health behavior: Conceptual and methodological issues. *Health Psychology, 17*(3), 290–299.

Zhang, C. Q., Zhang, R., Schwarzer, R., & Hagger, M. S. (2019). A meta-analysis of the Health Action Process Approach. *Health Psychology, 38*(7), 623–637.

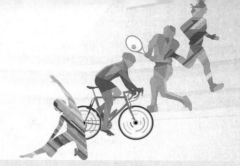

© Norbert/Shutterstock;
© sergeymansurov/Shutterstock.

CHAPTER 17

Dual Process Theories

LEARNING OBJECTIVES

After completing this chapter, you will be able to:

- Give three examples of how associative learning may impact your behavior.
- Understand the differences between habitual behavior and habit.
- Describe how automatic processes impact our behavior, even if it is outside of our awareness.
- Understand what effort minimization is and how it may influence people's motivation to engage in physical activity and sedentary behavior.

Introduction

Think about your day yesterday. How many different decisions did you make about the movement behaviors you were going to do? How many times did you decide to be sedentary or decide to be physically active? Think about it a different way now: How many times would you guess you changed from sitting or lying down to standing? Standing to moving? Moving to standing? Standing to sitting or lying down? We tend to transition among these movement behaviors a lot during the day but if you're like most people, these "decisions" to do movement or not don't feel like "decisions" because they just come naturally, by default. We automatically sit down to eat out of habit, or we automatically take the stairs instead of the elevator to get to the second floor of a building.

It turns out that a lot of the movement behavior we do on a daily basis is not the result of goals we have set or our beliefs about the values of physical activity or the health risks of sedentary behavior; rather, they are the result of more automatic influences on our behavior—our habits, automatic biases, and tendencies to approach or avoid movement behaviors. This chapter describes theories of physical activity and sedentary behavior that give voice to the idea that there are two types of influences on our behavior—the **controlled processes** that are the focus of the traditional theories of physical activity motivation, such as our goals, plans, and intentions, which are based on our values and expectations; and **automatic processes**, which are the more silent, spontaneous, unintentional influences on our behavior (See **Figure 17-1**; Evans, 2009; Evans & Frankish, 2009). Most of the chapters on motivation and theories discussed in Chapters 14–16 focus exclusively on controlled influences on behavior. In this chapter, we'll focus more on the other system—the automatic influences on behavior. There are many dual process models

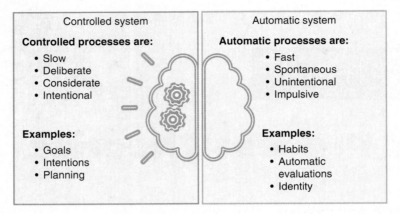

Figure 17-1 Controlled vs. Automatic Influences on Behavior.

and theories in psychology, and this chapter will focus only on some of the ways these approaches have been applied to understand physical activity and sedentary behavior. Generally, dual process theories tend to describe the automatic influences on our behavior as **automatic regulation**.

Automatic Regulation

Associative learning is a behavioral psychology tenet that learning occurs through the development and strengthening of mentally held links, or **automatic associations**, between cues and attributes such as "pleasant" or "unpleasant." For example, over time, people who were punished in sport by having to run may eventually learn to automatically associate cues related to running with the attribute of "unpleasant." Alternatively, people who have many pleasant experiences with running may associate cues

of running with the attribute of "pleasant." These automatic associations then influence our behavior through "automatic regulation"— the influences of automatic associations on our behavior (Bargh, 1994; Greenwald et al., 2002; Rebar, 2017).

Automatic regulation suggests that our understanding of the world around us is made up of a network of these automatic associations that have a range of influences on our behavior. The example of the association between "physical activity" and "pleasant" is an example of an **automatic evaluation**—a mentally held link between a cue and an attribute such as pleasant or unpleasant. The automatic process of habit is the influence of the automatic association between a cue and a behavioral response (e.g., the cue of "coming home from work" linked with the behavioral response of "sitting on the couch and watching *The Bachelor*"). **Automatic identity schemas** are links between a cue and our perception of ourselves or others. **Automatic pairings** are links between cues, such that the influence of automatic regulation may impact responses to related cues, such as different types of sedentary behavior. For example, if you have strong automatic identity schema as a gamer, and you automatically pair "gaming" with "scripting code," you may be more motivated to try your hand at programming (and spending more time being sedentary at a computer). Automatic

Table 17-1 **Types of Automatic Regulatory Processes and their Influences on Behavior and Decisions**

Construct	Automatic Association	Influence
Habit	Cue to behavior	Behavioral response to cue
Automatic evaluation	Cue to pleasant/unpleasant	Approach/avoid bias to cue
Automatic identity-schema	Cue to self/other	Approach/avoid bias to cue
Automatic pairing	Cue to cue	Shared response to both cues

Data from Rebar, A. L. (2017). Automatic regulation used in sport and exercise research. *Oxford Research Encyclopedia.* https://doi.org/10.1093/acrefore/9780190236557.013.231

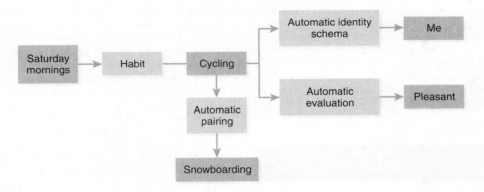

Figure 17-2 Hypothetical Network of Automatic Associations.

associations and their influences are described in **Table 17-1** and a depiction of a hypothetical network of automatic associations is shown in **Figure 17-2** (Rebar, 2017).

CRITICAL THINKING ACTIVITY 17-2

What do you think are some automatic associations that impact your life and how you behave? Do you think you automatically identify yourself as "physically active" or not? How might that automatic association come to be? How might you go about changing someone's automatic associations?

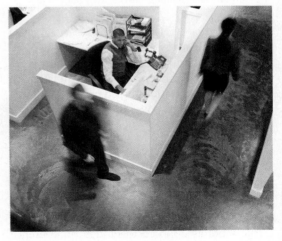

© XiXinXing/Shutterstock.

Implicit Association Tests

You might be thinking to yourself: If these automatic processes are unintentional and we may not be aware of them, how can they be accurately measured? You're not the only one grappling with this problem! For decades now, behavioral and psychological scientists have struggled with determining valid ways to assess automatic associations. One option is to use **implicit measures**. Rather than ask participants to self-report the automatic influences on their behavior, implicit measures score the strength of automatic associations indirectly. For example, for information on indirect assessments that do not require participants' subjective assessment, check out: https://implicit.harvard.edu/implicit/takeatest.html. This project allows you to take an assortment of implicit association tests, which arrive at a score of automatic evaluation strength based on your timing of responding to categorization tasks.

Implicit association tests require you to categorize a set of stimuli (usually words) into one of two categories (Greenwald et al., 1998). The categories each consist of a concept and an attribute such as "physical activity and good" or "sedentary behavior and bad." Then, halfway through the task, the concept-attribute pairings swap so that the categories are different: "physical activity and bad" or "sedentary behavior and good." The stimuli you categorize are a set of words representing the two concepts and the two attributes: physical activity (e.g., "run," "exercise"), sedentary behavior (e.g., "sitting," "watching TV"), good (e.g., "pleasant," "fun"), and bad (e.g., "unpleasant," "boring"). The concept behind implicit association tests is that you will be slower and less accurate when categorizing stimuli into categories of attributes that are different from your mentally held automatic associations compared with when you categorize stimuli into categories with attributes aligned with your own automatic associations (Greenwald et al., 1998). So, it would be harder for someone with favorable automatic associations of physical activity to do the task when categorizing into the options of "physical activity and bad" and "sedentary behavior and bad" compared with when categorizing into the options of "physical activity and good" and "sedentary behavior and bad."

CRITICAL THINKING ACTIVITY 17-3

Try out an implicit association test using the link provided and see what you think. Do you think the implicit association test is a good way to measure automatic associations? Why or why not?

There are many implicit measures used to assess automatic associations. Many of these types of measures make inferences about the strength of automatic associations based on people's accuracy and speed of response to the many trials of a task. There are advantages of these tasks, such as the low risk that they are influenced from social desirability and that people are less able to control the outcomes of these tasks compared with self-reported questionnaires (Gawronski, 2009). However, there are also limitations of these measures, including how much the scores represent a true score as opposed to random interference or measurement artifact. For example, Cope and colleagues (2018) revealed that people tended to more strongly associate images with exercise automatically if the images were of outdoor settings, presented as sport activities (as opposed to labor- or gym-based activity), and were of young adults. So, something as simple as using different images in an implicit measure may impact the outcome scores of these measures with added measurement error. There are many other important considerations needed when applying these types of measures such as intertrial reliability and scoring procedures (Rebar et al., 2015; Zenko & Ekkekakis, 2019). Although implicit measures are valuable for assessing the automatic processes that guide our behavior that are outside of our awareness, these types of measures can be burdensome for participants and are susceptible to different types of measurement artifact.

Habit

Anecdotally, we think of our behaviors as being habits, but in the context of the psychology of movement, we tend to define habit more as a precursor to behavior–something that influences our behavior rather than as a characteristic of the behavior itself. Instead of thinking about "having habits" think of it as doing something "out of habit." **Habit** is defined as the process by which a person's behavior is influenced from a prompt to act based on well-learned associations between cues and behaviors (Gardner, 2015; Wood & Neal, 2016). Presented differently, habit is the influence we experience as a result of the automatic associations between cues and behavioral responses (Rebar, 2017). Habit is experienced as an automatic "decision" to engage in the behavior without requiring much deliberation—you just do it. Although the way habit strength is being measured is expanding (Rebar et al., 2018), the most common assessment is through self-report of these felt symptoms of habit, including the Self-Report Habit Index that can be adapted to assess habits of different types of behavior (Verplanken & Orbell, 2003; see **Table 17-2**).

Because humans have a tendency for routine, we tend to do the same things at the same time of day, in the same place, with the same people (Epstein, 1979; Wood et al., 2002). Over time, as we repeat the behavioral response in the same context, our minds strengthen the association between the cue and behavior, and a habit develops (see **Figure 17-3**). Once established, the habit influences our behavior by triggering an urge to act in response to the cue. Because the urge to act is automatic and spontaneous, there is less need to deliberate about why and how to

Table 17-2 Self-Report Habit Index

"Behavior X is something . . .

Item	Question
1.	I do frequently.
2.	I do automatically.
3.	I do without having to consciously remember.
4.	That makes me feel weird if I do not do it.
5.	I do without thinking.
6.	That would require effort not to do.
7.	That belongs to my (daily, weekly, monthly) routine.
8.	I start doing before I realize I'm doing it.
9.	I would find hard not to do.
10.	I have no need to think about doing.
11.	That's typically "me."
12.	I have been doing for a long time.

Note. Response options: 1 (Strongly disagree) to 7 (Strongly agree); Habit strength is scored as calculated as mean to the 12 items.

Reproduced from Verplanken, B., & Orbell, S. (2003). Reflections on past behavior: A self-report index of habit strength. *Journal of Applied Social Psychology, 33*(6), 1313–1330. https://doi.org/10.1111/j.1559-1816.2003.tb01951.x

engage in habitual behaviors (Gardner & Rebar, 2019). Our habits become our defaults. So, there is benefit to your physical activity becoming

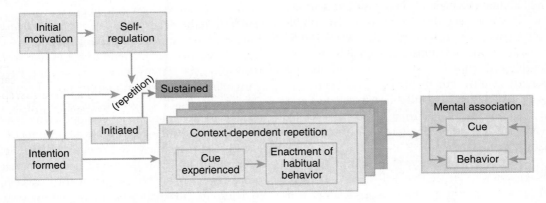

Figure 17-3 The Development of Habit.

habitual, in that it likely means you will be active long term and not give up as easily on physical activity, even when you're tired or not motivated.

Habit Influences on Physical Activity and Sedentary Behavior

For many people, physical activity or sedentary behavior can become habitual, occurring automatically in response to associated cues, rather than as the product of a thought-out decision based on values and expectancies (Rhodes & Rebar, 2018). Not surprisingly, the evidence supports that people with stronger physical activity habits tend to engage in more physical activity than people with weaker habits (Gardner et al., 2011; Rebar et al., 2016). For example, you may have the habit to drive your car to the university each time you have class, but someone else may have the habit to cycle to class. In these examples, the triggering "cues" is it being time for class and whether you drive or cycle is your behavioral response. If this is habitual for you, you won't think about what options you have to get to class and debate the pros and cons of each before making a decision; rather, you'll just do what comes naturally—you'll act out of habit. And most likely, a person with a habit for cycling will get more activity on the way to the University than someone with the habit for driving. If you have habits though, it doesn't mean you will always enact the habitual behaviors. When you have a strong motivation to act differently, you can inhibit or overrule your habit with self-control. Additionally, if your circumstances change or your routine is disrupted so that you don't come into contact with the cue that triggers the habit, you won't experience the influence from the habit at all. Your habit to drive to the University won't impact you on days you don't have class, for example.

There are now reviews of more than 30 studies providing evidence that self-reported strength of habit for physical activity is associated with how much physical activity you do ($r = 0.43$)

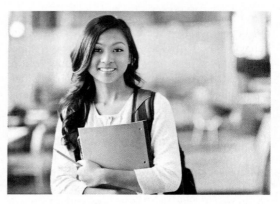

© Arekmalang/iStock/Getty Images Plus/Getty Images.

and that self-reported strength of habit for sedentary behavior is associated with time spent being sedentary ($r = 0.47$) (Gardner et al., 2011; Rebar et al., 2016). Supporting the idea that habit is an automatic influence on behavior is that most evidence shows that habit predicts physical activity, even after accounting for people's intentions to be physically active (Gardner et al., 2011; Rebar et al., 2016). Additionally, the evidence suggests that habit plays a role in determining whether or not people engage in the physical activity that they have intended to do (i.e., habit moderates the association between intention and behavior). Although the evidence has some mixed findings, in general, studies indicate that intentions are more strongly associated to behavior for people with weaker habits. Theoretically, this suggests that people with strong habits rely more on their automatic habitual responses to engage in physical activity and less on their controlled intentions. Evidence tracking intentions and behavior over repeated days shows that people tend to act in line with their physical activity habit unless they have particularly strong intentions to do otherwise (Rebar et al., 2014). Notably, however, there is some evidence that this moderation effect (and others as well) may be partially a byproduct of a statistical inaccuracy (Rebar et al., 2019). So, before we can say with confidence how these processes work together, more work is needed to determine how habit and intention interact to impact physical activity behavior.

Identity

Two very similar constructs have been circulating in distinct physical activity behavior research literatures for many years: *identity* (Stryker & Burke, 2000) and *schema* (Markus, 1977). **Identities** are considered components of a multi-dimensional self-concept, hierarchically organized by how one categorizes themselves in a given role (sometimes called role identity) (Burke, 2006) (see also Chapter 12). Each person has slightly different identities, based on past experiences, and we use our identities to serve as personal standards of behavior (Stryker & Burke, 2000). **Schema** is considered a heuristic cognitive generalization about the self, derived from past experiences and used to process self-related information (Markus, 1977). The schema concept is more heavily based on information processing efficiency, while identity is more focused on personal and social standards. However, the two concepts are extremely similar in description. The constructs are so similar that Markus and Wurf (1987) suggested that the schema and identity concepts are completely convergent. While there is limited research in sedentary behavior on identity and schema (e.g., Berry & Strachan, 2012), research in physical activity supports the notion

that these are basically the same construct (Berry, Strachan, & Verkooijen, 2013; Rhodes, Kaushal, & Quinlan, 2016). Based on this evidence, Rhodes and colleagues (2016) recommended that the two literatures (identity, schema) be merged under the identity label to unify the area of research.

Identity Influences on Physical Activity and Sedentary Behavior

Identities have been described as a dynamic, reflexive, self-regulating control system (Burke, 2006) (see also Control Theory in Chapter 16). As detailed in **Figure 17-4**, the identity standard acts as comparator to actual behavior and is activated automatically by relevant situational cues (e.g., social, environmental, performance) where the identity is either aligned or mismatched with one's behavior. Alignment experiences serve to

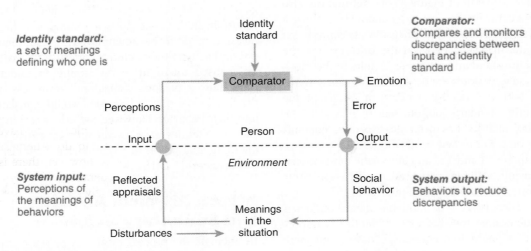

Figure 17-4 Identity Standard.

Data from from Burke, P. J., & Stets, J. E. (2009). Identity Theory. New York: Oxford University Press.

strengthen the identity while discrepancies challenge an identity. For example, if you hold the identity of an excellent basketball player, and you are performing well in a basketball game compared with the other players on the court, these cues serve to support this identity. By contrast, if you are with a group who are all performing better than you at basketball, your identity will be activated through the interpretation of these social, environmental, and behavioral performance cues as a challenge to that identity. This challenge creates negative affect and dissonance that serve to motivate identity-consistent behaviors (Burke & Stets, 2009). In the basketball example above, this will likely mean that you dig deeply and try harder in the game, giving your absolute best effort.

Over time, reflected appraisals between one's identity standard and identity incongruent experiences will change the identity, however, either by lessening its importance (i.e., the identity becomes less important compared with your other identities) or modifying the standard (i.e., you modify your identity to that congruent with your experiences) (Burke, 2006). In this way, identity has a complex relationship with behavior. Identity has an automatic component to its operation based on the cues that trigger its activation and the emotion the identity standard will evoke (top half of Figure 17-4). Yet identity also has a controlled aspect to its operation because a person will reflect on the negative affect produced by the mismatch between the behavior and the identity standard and either 1) initiate the motivation to perform the behavior to remain congruent with the identity standard or 2) change the identity standard (bottom half of Figure 17-4). Thus, identity has been described as containing both controlled motivational elements (See Chapters 14 and 15) and automatic motivational elements (Michie, van Stralen, & West, 2011; Rhodes, La, Quinlan, & Grant, 2021).

There is yet to be enough research conducted to determine to what extent identity is important for predicting sedentary behavior, but there is a much larger evidence base considering physical activity and identity. A review considered evidence from 62 studies and meta-analyzed data from 32 studies to determine that there is a medium-sized association between identity/schema and physical activity behavior ($r = 0.44$), such that people who strongly identified as being physically active engaged in more physical activity behavior than those who did not identify as strongly as being physically active. Interestingly, evidence from the review also suggests that the link between identity and physical activity behavior may partially be because people with strong physical activity identities tend to have more commitment, perceived ability, and motivation for physical activity and that people with physical activity identities tend to experience physical activity to be pleasant. It's amazing how much our expectations about how pleasant an activity will or will not be influences our behavior. The next section focuses more specifically on the role of pleasure in motivation for physical activity and sedentary behavior.

Affect and Hedonic Motivation

Psychology has long recognized that the way we feel influences our behavior. The scientific term for the idea that humans have a tendency to pursue pleasure and avoid displeasure is **psychological hedonism** (Cabanac, 1992; Johnston, 2003). The drive for humans to find pleasure tends to be downplayed in traditional physical activity motivation theories. In the past, we focused much more on aiming to understand how a person's values and awareness of the benefits of physical activity would translate into their behavior. However, the tide is turning, and our theories are now far more attentive to the influential power of psychological hedonism (Williams et al., 2018).

Affect, Physical Activity, and Sedentary Behavior

To untangle the process by which pleasure and behavior are linked, researchers have parsed **affect** (i.e., the way we feel) in many ways.

For example, there has been differentiation among **integral affect**—affect felt as a response to the behavioral task, **incidental affect**—affect felt beyond that of the response to the behavioral task, and **anticipated affective reactions**—the way we think it will feel to do something (Bodenhausen, 1993; Williams & Evans, 2014). It is theorized that these aspects of affect impact our future physical activity and sedentary behavior through both automatic and reflective motivation processes. For example, integral affect is thought to influence behavior through shaping our automatic evaluations and through changing how we expect future behavior to feel (e.g., Brand & Ekkekakis, 2018; Conroy & Berry, 2017). Anticipated affective reactions are theorized as influencing our behavior by impacting whether we intend to do a behavior or not and how strongly we are motivated to do the behavior (Richard et al., 1996; Williams & Evans, 2014). Generally, if we think something will feel pleasant, we strongly intend to do it; whereas if we think something will feel unpleasant, we either don't intend to do it or, if we do intend to do it, we may not have strong motivation underlying that intention.

Anticipated affective responses have been shown to partially determine whether people are motivated or not to engage in physical activity in the future. For example, Williams and colleagues (2012) found that how pleasant or unpleasant inactive adults felt during a treadmill walk predicted physical activity 6- and 12-months later, whereas how they felt after the treadmill walk did not predict their future behavior. Supporting this early evidence, a systematic review looked over studies testing relations between affective responses to physical activity and future physical activity behavior (Rhodes & Kates, 2015). They found 24 relevant studies and upon review determined, that a positive change in how people felt during moderate intensity physical activity was linked to future physical activity, but post-exercise affect was not associated with future behavior. Now, let's consider the automatic process by which affect is theorized to impact behavior.

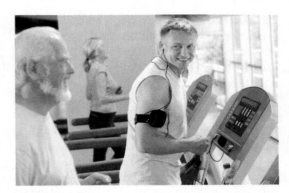

© bounce/Cultura/Getty Images.

Automatic Evaluations, Physical Activity, and Sedentary Behavior

Automatic evaluations are theorized to originate from both direct and observed experiences with that behavior to help us process and react to threats and rewards in our environment (Rudman et al., 2007). Conroy and Berry (2017) propose that automatic evaluations can influence physical activity behavior automatically through elicitation of approach or avoidance of behavioral impulses and by influencing anticipated affective reactions or affective attitudes about physical activity. That is, if people have favorable automatic evaluations toward physical activity, when opportunities arise, they may have automatic impulses to engage in physical activity as well as positive anticipations about what the physical activity will feel like.

Evidence shows support for the notion of Conroy and Berry that automatic evaluations are associated with physical activity behavior and controlled affective attitudes about physical activity. People vary in how favorable or unfavorable their automatic evaluations are for physical activity, and these differences tend to align with our behavior: people with more favorable automatic evaluations toward physical activity tend to be more physically active than those with less-favorable automatic evaluations toward physical activity (Chevance et al., 2019; Rebar et al., 2016; Schinkoeth & Antoniewicz, 2017). A 2019 meta-analysis reviewed 55 effects from

26 independent studies and found that there was a small, but statistically significant, association between automatic evaluations and physical activity (Chevance, Bernard, et al., 2019). This effect was found across a variety of study designs, automatic evaluation and physical activity behavior measurements, and in a range of populations of different ages and characteristics. Additionally, there is generally small-medium associations found between automatic evaluations and self-reported attitudes of other target behaviors and concepts (Hofmann et al., 2005), although notably, evidence of an association between automatic evaluations and self-reported attitudes toward physical activity remains elusive (Conroy & Berry, 2017). That automatic and controlled affective processes may not always align brings to light interesting considerations for what happens when our automatic evaluations oppose our controlled motivation for a behavior.

Self-Control Situations

When someone has favorable automatic evaluations toward physical activity and also values the health benefits of physical activity, it is likely they'll make the decision to regularly engage in physical activity without much use of self-control. However, sometimes, people's automatic evaluations may oppose their controlled motivation. For example, it may be that someone has automatic evaluations that are unfavorable toward physical activity, despite their values for physical activity, and therefore, they constantly face what the theory of hedonic motivation refers to as **self-control situations** (Williams et al., 2018). When hedonic motivation and controlled motivation are opposing, you will need to use self-control to act in line with controlled motivation and overcome the spontaneous influence of your automatic evaluations. By becoming aware of the potential that our automatic urges may be influencing our behavior in ways we don't want, we can use self-control when we want to engage in physical activity more often, although notably that solution usually does not work in the long term—think about how many

New Years' resolutions you've given up on over the years! Ideally, your controlled motivation and automatic motivation have the same direction of influence on your behavior so that they lead you in the same direction. Although the research is still quite fresh, there is some evidence that there are direct ways to change people's automatic evaluations toward physical activity or sedentary behavior.

CRITICAL THINKING ACTIVITY 17-5

Can you give an example of when a person's hedonic motivation opposes their controlled motivation? What about an example of when a person's hedonic motivation aligns with their controlled motivation?

Priming and Evaluative Conditioning

Priming is the nonconscious influence on responses to a cue as a result of recent experience with or exposure to the same cue. Priming can change the way we feel, think, or act in response to a cue, but the effects tend to last only a short time (Molden, 2014). **Evaluative conditioning** has been used in efforts to manipulate affective processes toward a target by repeatedly exposing a person to the target paired with pleasant or unpleasant stimuli (Hofmann et al., 2010). The underlying premise of evaluative conditioning is that through repeated exposures, people will learn to associate the target with pleasantness or unpleasantness, and the outcome will be shifts in their automatic evaluations toward the target. Unlike many of the approaches used to intervene with physical activity or sedentary behavior, these approaches directly target automatic processes and aim to do so without necessarily engaging reflective processing at all. Priming and evaluative conditioning may be used without even letting people know that an intervention is occurring.

There have been some efforts to utilize evaluative conditioning and priming to enhance

The Controversy of Priming Effects Research

In an early experiment of priming effects, Bargh and colleagues (1996) primed a group of people with stereotypes of "elderly" by having them complete a scrambled-sentence task containing words such as *Florida, old, lonely, grey*, and *knits*. They were told that the purpose of the study was to test language proficiency and were given language-related tasks to complete. Once the experiment was over, the speed by which participants walked down the hall to the elevator was monitored. Compared with the control group who were not primed, those primed with elderly stereotypes walked significantly slower. Primed participants took 8.28 seconds to get to the elevator, whereas control participants took 7.30 seconds. For several decades, this study was a key reference for evidence of the behavioral effects of priming.

In 2012, the study was replicated using the same methods but with a larger sample and automated tools for timing walking speed (Doyen et al., 2012). No significant priming effects were evident. Then, in a follow-up study, these researchers manipulated the beliefs of the experimenters. This study revealed that the priming effect was present but only when the experimenters believed that the effect would occur. This finding, as well as the revelation that a significant leader in research of priming, Diederik Stapel, had committed large-scale data fraud in some of his studies, raised a lot of skepticism about the strength of evidence of priming effects. There remain strong doubts about whether priming effects are robust and replicable (Molden, 2014; Sherman & Rivers, 2021). In large part, from the controversy of psychology research on priming, researchers have begun an initiative to evaluate the replicability of psychological science: https://osf.io/ezcuj/. So, while the verdict is still out as to whether priming has a reliable effect on behavior, there is no doubt that research on priming has made the field of psychology more robust.

automatic affective processes of physical activity vs. sedentary behavior. Conroy and Kim (2021) developed HeartPhone—an app for conditioning associations between physical activity and pleasure. It worked through regularly exposing users to pleasant images of physical activity as background images on their smartphone lock screen. Development studies revealed that through using lock screens led to about 2 min/day of exposure to the intervention and proof-of-concept support, and after 8 weeks of using the intervention app, 19 adults reported improved affective judgements and more physical activity than before the intervention. It may be that such interventions could use evaluative conditioning to enhance physical activity behavior with low burden; however, further research is needed with larger samples in randomized controlled trials to rule out alternative explanations for these findings.

Rasera and colleagues (2022) tested whether a gamified smartphone app that implemented features of priming and automatic evaluation strategies would enhance people's automatic evaluations to be more favorable toward physical activity compared with sedentary behavior (measured with an implicit association test). In the intervention condition, the app included games with physical activity-related avatars and words, whereas in the control condition, the app included avatars and words unrelated to physical activity. Unlike most physical activity interventions, participants were initially unaware that the intervention's aim was on physical activity. Although there were no immediate between-group differences found, a day after exposure to the app, there were significant differences in automatic evaluations found between the

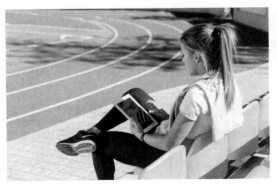

intervention and control groups. Unfortunately, this between-group difference was not from an enhancement of automatic evaluations of physical activity from the intervention. Rather, the effect was from a significant change in the control group's having more favorable automatic evaluations toward sedentary behavior (relative to physical activity)—and this effect was even stronger for people who used the app more. The app may have inadvertently enhanced automatic evaluations for sedentary behavior!

Other efforts have also been taken to enhance automatic evaluations of physical activity to no avail. Chevance and colleagues (2019) tested whether exposing pulmonary rehabilitation patients to posters of physical activity or sedentary behavior with pleasant stimuli would enhance automatic evaluations of physical activity vs. sedentary behavior and lead to more accelerometer-assessed physical activity. Participants were not informed of the aim of the intervention until after the study. Automatic evaluations of physical activity vs sedentary behavior were assessed pre- and post-intervention with an implicit association test. There were no significant effects of the interventions on automatic evaluations or behavior. Clearly, these initial studies do not provide much support for the effects of evaluative conditioning or priming to enhance people's physical activity behavior, but there are still very few studies out there with a range of limitations, so more is needed in this area before ruling out these approaches of behavior change.

Effort Minimization

There are evolutionary theories arguing that our ancestors would have benefited greatly from a tendency to avoid unnecessary physical exertion when food was more scarce and physical activity more essential for survival (Lee et al., 2016; Lieberman, 2015; Pontzer et al., 2016). Slowly, over generations, our bodies have changed to conserve energy, so that the same behaviors do not require as much energy as they used to for humans. Why would our minds be any different? The theory of effort minimization posits that people have an always-present impulse to avoid movement because it requires effort and comes at the cost of energy expenditure. The main tenet of the theory of effort minimization is that humans have an innate, automatic attraction to **physical effort minimization**—a tendency to avoid moving and using energy (Cheval & Boisgontier, 2021). The theorists of effort minimization suggest that cues of movement are constantly around us, as are our aversion to them—even breathing requires energy expenditure so our efforts to minimize energy expenditure are always "on" and impacting our behavior. So, unlike many other theories of physical activity motivation, this theory proposes that our decision to engage in movement behavior or not is largely dictated by how much effort we perceive the action to require. If something seems like a lot of effort, we are more likely to avoid it. And our perceptions of how much effort a behavior requires can vary, depending on how we're feeling and what's going on around us. Think about it—sometimes even getting up off the couch to get a snack can seem like an insurmountable effort.

Notably, the theory of effort minimization gives credence to the notion that there is a **feedback loop**—a system where the results of a process impacts the start of the next one. Within this theory, the feedback loop is that once we actually experience how much effort a movement behavior took, the actual experienced effort of the movement behavior is "categorized" and is used to inform the perceived effort in the next opportunity to engage in that movement behavior again. So, for example, if you decide to run up a hill during your jog around the neighborhood and realize halfway up that it was much more difficult than you thought it would be, you'll remember how much effort it actually required the next time you are faced with that hill on your next jog.

CRITICAL THINKING ACTIVITY 17-6

Do you think humans evolved to conserve energy? What might you use as evidence to support your argument?

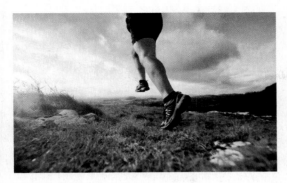

© BrianAJackson/iStock/Getty Images Plus/Getty Images.

To translate into the movement behavior, the theory of effort minimization that the controlled and automatic precursors encouraging movement must be strong enough in aggregate to overcome the inhibitory influence of effort minimization, which is magnified if it is perceived that the action requires much effort. Said plainly, the theory argues that if something seems like a lot of effort, we tend not to do it unless we are highly motivated. The relative impact of controlled precursors vs. automatic precursors on movement behavior is moderated by factors such as habit, fatigue, cognitive load, and pain experienced by the person at that particular moment in time. **Moderation** is when the impact of one factor on another depends on a third variable, the *moderator*. For example, whether your attitudes about dancing influence your decision to get out on the dance floor with your friends depends on how much your shoes are hurting your feet in that moment. If your feet hurt a lot, you probably won't go dance, regardless of how much you enjoy dancing, but if your feet feel fine, your decision to dance may be largely dependent on how much fun you think dancing is. The link between attitudes about dancing and the decision to dance or not is *moderated* by your foot pain levels (see Figure 17-2).

Summary

Dual process theories propose that there are two types of influence on our behavior—controlled processes that are deliberate, intentional, and require cognitive resources such as self-regulation; and automatic processes, which are more spontaneous, unintentional, and require motivation to inhibit. Dual process theories have in common that they propose that behavior is partially regulated by automatic associations—the behavioral psychology notion that we learn through making mental pairings between concepts and attributes. Most theories of motivation that you've read to this point focus on controlled processes, but there is burgeoning evidence that automatic processes such as habit and identity are also important for our movement behaviors.

Habit theory proposes that behavior can become habitual with regular repetition of a behavioral response to a cue, as we make "cue" to "behavior" automatic associations. Once a habit forms, the perception of the triggering cue elicits the automatic urge to engage in the habitual behavior, which will be enacted unless motivation or other factors inhibit the response. It may be that habits are the key to helping people maintain physical activity long term. Identity is also thought to impact behavior through automatic means. Whether someone pictures themselves as an active or sedentary person may have major consequences for how likely it is they will take up opportunities for physical activity.

The pleasure that influences our behavior may seem pretty obvious, but psychological hedonism has largely been underutilized as a means to understand or intervene with movement behavior. Evidence suggests that the way we expect physical activity or sedentary behavior to feel has importance for our decisions to engage in these behaviors or not in the future. Some theories such as the theory of effort minimization suggests that our behavior may also be impacted by the perceived effort of those activities, an influence largely driven by human's innate urge to avoid energy expenditure.

There remains a lot that is not understood about the automatic influences on our behavior. There is work to do to understand how best to measure and intervene with these processes. However, as a body of evidence, the general consensus is there are some motivational processes at play that impact behavior outside of the intentions and goals we make. The more we are aware of these and the potential impact they have on us, the better chance we have to ensure these influences work for us instead of against us.

Vignette: Quinlee

Journal Entry January 2: It's the start of a new year and I'm ready for a change. I know heart disease runs in my family and regular exercise is one of the best ways to reduce the chances that I'll end up sick like Mom. I just wish I didn't hate the gym so much. But I have to go, no more excuses. I'll set my alarm for 6:00 am every day and just get up and go.

Journal Entry January 10: Ok. Well, it's been a week and I've made it the gym 4 times! I'm not going to lie: it's pretty terrible. I'm so tired when I wake up and it's so cold. But I just think about my mom, and how I don't want to end up with heart disease and then I get out the door and go do my workout at the gym. I can do this!

Journal Entry January 25: I would love to keep going to the gym in the morning but things just keep coming up. It snowed last week and the roads were bad. And then I got this headache that I just couldn't kick. Then last week the exam was on and I really needed to study. It just wasn't a good month. February is my month though—I'm going to the gym every day!

Journal Entry February 14: I hate the gym. I hate getting up early and going. I don't like working out on the elliptical and it's just not for me. For Valentine's Day, I'm giving myself a gift though— I've decided that I can get exercise another way.

Jerry-Lyn has agreed to do yoga with me every day after our morning class. I love Jerry-Lyn and I think that will be really fun. And it will be a great way to relax too!

Journal Entry March 20: I'm loving yoga with Jerry-Lyn and I'm getting better at it too! It's so nice to have someone there with me and it's just part of our routine. I don't feel like it's a chore like I did with exercising at the gym in the mornings. I think this works better for me.

Journal Entry April 26: Yesterday, after class while Jerry-Lyn and I were getting ready for yoga, we realized that we don't even think about our goals about exercise anymore. I don't have to talk myself into going and I don't think about the fact that I started doing this because I wanted to avoid heart disease. We just do it. It feels so natural and just part of our routine. We learned in our exercise psychology class that habits are our mind's shortcuts to responding to cues. I think we did it! I think Jerry-Lyn and I have formed physical activity habits! Our "cue" is that we are done with our morning class, and our "behavioral response" is doing yoga. Having a habit doesn't make the yoga any easier—trust me! It's still really intense. But it's like the effort was taken out of the decision of whether or not to do the yoga. We just do it! ☺

Key Terms

affect Subjective feeling states at a global level.

anticipated affective reactions Expectations of how it will feel to experience something or do a behavior.

associative learning Behavioral psychology notions that learning occurs through developments and strengthening of mentally held automatic associations between stimuli and attributes.

automatic associations Mentally held associations between stimuli such as "physical activity" and attributes such as "pleasant" or "unpleasant."

automatic evaluation Mentally held link between a cue and attributes (pleasant vs. unpleasant) that manifest into behavioral impulses to approach or avoid the cue.

automatic identity schema Mentally held links between a cue and our perception of ourselves vs. others.

automatic pairings Mentally held links between cues, such that the influence of automatic regulation may impact responses to related cues.

automatic processes Influences on behavior that are spontaneous, unintentional, uncontrollable, and do not require high cognitive load.

automatic regulation The influence of automatic associations on behavior.

controlled processes Influences on behavior that are slow, deliberate, and intentional, and are cognitively demanding.

evaluative conditioning The manipulation of affective processes toward a target through repeated exposure to a target paired with pleasant or unpleasant stimuli.

feedback loop A system where the results of a process impacts the start of the next one.

habit The process by which a person's behavior is influenced from a prompt to act based on well-learned associations between cues and behaviors.

identities Components of a multi-dimensional self-concept, hierarchically organized by how one categorizes themselves in a given role.

implicit measures Indirect assessments that do not require participants' subjective assessment.

incidental affect Affect felt beyond that of a response to the behavior or event.

integral affect Affect felt as a response to the behavior or event.

moderation When the degree to which two variables are associated depends on a third variable, the moderator.

physical effort minimization The tendency to avoid moving and using energy.

priming The non-conscious influence on responses to a cue as a result of recent experience with or exposure to the same cue.

psychological hedonism The human tendency to pursue pleasure and avoid displeasure.

schema A heuristic cognitive generalization about the self, derived from past experiences and used to process self-related information.

self-control situation Occurs when hedonic motivation and controlled motivation conflict and self-control is needed to enact controlled motivation and inhibit the automatic influences of hedonic motivation.

Review Questions

1. Compare and contrast controlled vs. automatic processes and their influence on our behavior.
2. Give an example of how associative learning could impact physical activity behavior.
3. What is an implicit association test and what does it measure?
4. What is the difference between a habit and a habitual behavior?
5. Describe how habit may influence physical activity and sedentary behavior.
6. What is an identity and how does it influence our choices in day to day life?
7. What does the term hedonic motivation mean in the context of physical activity and sedentary behavior?
8. Describe three types of affect.
9. Give an example of a self-control situation.

Applying the Concepts

1. What automatic processes of physical activity motivation do you see at play in Quinlee's experiences?
2. On which days was Quinlee most likely to give up on physical activity? What type of intervention may have been useful then and why?

References

Bargh, J. A. (1994). The four horsemen of automaticity: Intention, awareness, efficiency, and control as separate issues. In R. S. Wyer, & T. K. Srull, *Handbook of social cognition* (pp. 1–40). Psychology Press.

Bargh, J. A., Chen, M., & Burrows, L. (1996). Automaticity of social behavior: Direct effects of trait construct and stereotype activation on action. *Journal of Personality and Social Psychology, 71*(2), 230–244. https://doi.org/10.1037/0022-3514.71.2.230

Berry, T. R., & Strachan, S. M. (2012). Implicit and explicit exercise and sedentary identity. *Research Quarterly for Exercise and Sport, 83*(3), 479–484. https://doi.org/10.1080/02701367.2012.10599883

Berry, T. R., Strachan, S. M., & Verkooijen, K. T. (2014). The relationship between exercise schema and identity. *International Journal of Sport and Exercise Psychology, 12*, 49–63.

Bodenhausen, G. V. (1993). Emotions, arousal, and stereotypic judgments: A heuristic model of affect and stereotyping. In D. M. Mackie, & D. L. Hamilton (Eds.), *Affect, cognition and stereotyping* (pp. 13–37). Academic Press. https://doi.org/10.1016/B978-0-08-088579-7.50006-5

Brand, R., & Ekkekakis, P. (2018). Affective–reflective theory of physical inactivity and exercise. *German Journal of Exercise and Sport Research, 48*(1), 48–58. https://doi.org/10.1007/s12662-017-0477-9

Burke, P. J. (2006). Identity change. *Social Psychology Quarterly, 69*(1), 81–96. https://doi.org/10.1177/019027250606900106

Burke, P. J., & Stets, J. E. (2009). *Identity theory*. Oxford University Press.

Cabanac, M. (1992). Pleasure: The common currency. *Journal of Theoretical Biology, 155*(2), 173–200. https://doi.org/10.1016/S0022-5193(05)80594-6

Cheval, B., & Boisgontier, M. P. (2021). The theory of effort minimization in physical activity. *Exercise and Sport Sciences Reviews, 49*(3), 168–178. https://doi.org/10.1249/JES.0000000000000252

Chevance, G., Bernard, P., Chamberland, P. E., & Rebar, A. (2019). The association between implicit attitudes toward physical activity and physical activity behaviour: A systematic review and correlational meta-analysis. *Health Psychology Review, 13*(3), 248–276. https://doi.org/10.1080/17437199.2019.1618726

Chevance, G., Berry, T., Boiché, J., & Heraud, N. (2019). Changing implicit attitudes for physical activity with associative learning. *German Journal of Exercise and Sport Research, 49*, 156–167. https://doi.org/10.1007/s12662-018-0559-3

Conroy, D. E., & Berry, T. R. (2017). Automatic affective evaluations of physical activity. *Exercise and Sport Sciences Reviews, 45*(4), 230–237. https://doi.org/10.1249/JES.0000000000000120

Conroy, D. E., & Kim, I. (2021). Heartphone: Mobile evaluative conditioning to enhance affective processes and promote physical activity. *Health Psychology, 40*(12), 988–997. https://doi.org/10.1037/hea0000886

Cope, K., Vandelanotte, C., Short, C. E., Conroy, D. E., Rhodes, R. E., Jackson, B., Dimmock, J. A., & Rebar, A. L. (2018). Reflective and non-conscious responses to exercise images. *Frontiers in Psychology, 8*, 2272. https://doi.org/10.3389/fpsyg.2017.02272

Doyen, S., Klein, O., Pichon, C-L., & Cleeremans, A. (2012). Behavioral priming: It's all in the mind, but whose mind? *PLOS ONE, 7*(1), e29081. https://doi.org/10.1371/journal.pone.0029081

Epstein, S. (1979). The stability of behavior: I. On predicting most of the people much of the time. *Journal of Personality and Social Psychology, 37*(7), 1097–1126. https://doi.org/10.1037/0022-3514.37.7.1097

Evans, J. S. B. T. (2009). How many dual-process theories do we need? One, two, or many? In J. S. Evans, & K. Frankish (Eds.), *In two minds: Dual processes and beyond* (pp. 33–54). Oxford University Press. https://doi.org/10.1093/acprof:oso/9780199230167.003.0002

Gardner, B. (2015). Defining and measuring the habit impulse: Response to commentaries. *Health Psychology Review, 9*(3), 318–322. https://doi.org/10.1080/17437199.2015.1009844

Gardner, B., de Bruijn, G-J., & Lally, P. (2011). A systematic review and meta-analysis of applications of the self-report habit index to nutrition and physical activity behaviours. *Annals of Behavioral Medicine, 42*(2), 174–187. https://doi.org/10.1007/s12160-011-9282-0

Gardner, B., & Rebar, A. L. (2019). Habit formation and behavior change. *Oxford Research Encyclopedia of Psychology.* https://oxfordre.com/psychology/view/10.1093/acrefore/9780190236557.001.0001/acrefore-9780190236557-e-129

Gawronski, B. (2009). Ten frequently asked questions about implicit measures and their frequently supposed, but not entirely correct answers. *Canadian Psychology/Psychologie Canadienne, 50*(3), 141–150. https://doi.org/10.1037/a0013848

Greenwald, A. G., Banaji, M. R., Rudman, L. A., Farnham, S. D., Nosek, B. A., & Mellott, D. S. (2002). A unified theory of implicit attitudes, stereotypes, self-esteem, and self-concept. *Psychological Review, 109*(1), 3–25. https://doi.org/10.1037/0033-295X.109.1.3

Greenwald, A. G., McGhee, D. E., & Schwartz, J. L. (1998). Measuring individual differences in implicit cognition: The implicit association test. *Journal of Personality and Social Psychology, 74*(6), 1464–1480.

Hofmann, W., De Houwer, J., Perugini, M., Baeyens, F., & Crombez, G. (2010). Evaluative conditioning in humans: A meta-analysis. *Psychological Bulletin, 136*(3), 390–421. https://doi.org/10.1037/a0018916

Hofmann, W., Gawronski, B., Gschwendner, T., Le, H., & Schmitt, M. (2005). A meta-analysis on the correlation between the Implicit Association Test and explicit self-report measures. *Personality and Social Psychology Bulletin, 31*(10), 1369–1385. https://doi.org/10.1177/0146167205275613

Johnston, V. (2003). The origin and function of pleasure. *Cognition and Emotion, 17*(2), 167–179. https://doi.org/10.1080/02699930302290

Lee, H. H., Emerson, J. A., & Williams, D. M. (2016). The exercise–affect–adherence pathway: An evolutionary perspective. *Frontiers in Psychology, 7*(1285), 1–11. https://doi.org/10.3389/fpsyg.2016.01285

Lieberman, D. E. (2015). Is exercise really medicine? An evolutionary perspective. *Current Sports Medicine Reports, 14*(4), 313–319. https://doi.org/10.1249/JSR.0000000000000168

Markus, H. (1977). Self-schemata and processing information about the self. *Journal of Personality and Social Psychology, 35*(2), 63–78. https://doi.org/10.1037/0022-3514.35.2.63

Markus, H., & Wurf, E. (1987). The dynamic self-concept: A social psychological perspective. *Annual Review of Psychology, 38*(1), 299–337.

Michie, S., van Stralen, M. M., & West, R. (2011). The behaviour change wheel: A new method for characterising and designing behaviour change interventions. *Implementation Science, 6*, 42.

Molden, D. C. (2014). Understanding priming effects in social psychology: An overview and integration. *Social Cognition, 32*(Suppl), 243–249. https://doi.org/10.1521/soco.2014.32.supp.243

Pontzer, H., Durazo-Arvizu, R., Dugas, L. R., Plange-Rhule, J., Bovet, P., Forrester, T. E., Lambert, E. V., Cooper, R. S., Schoeller, D. A., & Luke, A. (2016). Constrained total energy expenditure and metabolic adaptation to physical activity in adult humans. *Current Biology, 26*(3), 410–417. https://doi.org/10.1016/j.cub.2015.12.046

Rasera, M., Jayasinghe, H., Parker, F., Short, C. E., Conroy, D. E., Jackson, B., Dimmock, J. A., Rhodes, R. E., de Vries, H., Vandelanotte, C., & Rebar, A. L. (2022). An early phase trial testing the proof of concept for a gamified smartphone app in manipulating automatic evaluations of exercise. *Sport, Exercise, and Performance Psychology, 11*(1), 61–78. https://doi.org/10.1037/spy0000278

Rebar, A. L. (2017). Automatic regulation used in sport and exercise research. *Oxford Research Encyclopedias.* https://doi.org/10.1093/acrefore/9780190236557.013.231

Rebar, A. L., Dimmock, J. A., Jackson, B., Rhodes, R. E., Kates, A., Starling, J., & Vandelanotte, C. (2016). A systematic review of the effects of non-conscious regulatory processes in physical activity. *Health Psychology Review, 10*(4), 395–407. https://doi.org/10.1080/17437199.2016.1183505

Rebar, A. L., Elavsky, S., Maher, J. P., Doerksen, S. E., & Conroy, D. E. (2014). Habits predict physical activity on days when intentions are weak. *Journal of Sport & Exercise Psychology, 36*(2), 157–165.

Rebar, A. L., Gardner, B., Rhodes, R. E., & Verplanken, B. (2018). The measurement of habit. In *The psychology of habit* (pp. 31–49). Bath, UK: Springer.

Rebar, A. L., Ram, N., & Conroy, D. E. (2015). Using the EZ-diffusion model to score a single-category implicit association test of physical activity. *Psychology of Sport and Exercise, 16*(3), 96–105. https://doi.org/10.1016/j.psychsport.2014.09.008

Rebar, A. L., Rhodes, R. E., & Gardner, B. (2019). How we are misinterpreting physical activity intention – behavior relations and what to do about it. *International Journal of Behavioral Nutrition and Physical Activity, 16*(1), 71. https://doi.org/10.1186/s12966-019-0829-y

Rhodes, R. E., & Kates, A. (2015). Can the affective response to exercise predict future motives and physical activity behavior? A systematic review of published evidence. *Annals of Behavioral Medicine, 49*(5), 715–731. https://doi.org/10.1007/s12160-015-9704-5

Rhodes, R. E., Kaushal, N., & Quinlan, A. (2016). Is physical activity a part of who I am? A review and meta-analysis of identity, schema and physical activity *Health Psychology Review, 10*, 204–225.

Rhodes, R. E., La, H., Quinlan, A., & Grant, S. (2021). Enacting physical activity intention: A multi-process action control approach. In C. Englert & I. Taylor (Eds.), *Motivation and Self-regulation in Sport and Exercise* (pp. 8–20). New York: Taylor & Francis.

Rhodes, R. E., & Rebar, A. L. (2018). Physical activity habit: Complexities and controversies. In *The psychology of habit* (pp. 91–109). Bath, UK: Springer.

Richard, R., Van Der Pligt, J., & De Vries, N. (1996). Anticipated affect and behavioral choice. *Basic and Applied Social Psychology, 18*(2), 111–129. https://doi.org/10.1207/s15324834basp1802_1

Rudman, L. A., Phelan, J. E., & Heppen, J. B. (2007). Developmental sources of implicit attitudes. *Personality and Social Psychology Bulletin, 33*(12), 1700–1713. https://doi.org/10.1177/0146167207307487

Schinkoeth, M., & Antoniewicz, F. (2017). Automatic evaluations and exercising: Systematic review and implications for future research. *Frontiers in Psychology, 8*(2103). https://doi.org/10.3389/fpsyg.2017.02103

Sherman, J. W., & Rivers, A. M. (2021). There's nothing social about social priming: derailing the "train wreck". *Psychological Inquiry, 32*(1), 1–11. https://doi.org/10.1080/1047840X.2021.1889312

Stryker, S., & Burke, P. J. (2000). The past, present, and future of an identity theory. *Social Psychology Quarterly*, 284–297. https://doi.org/10.2307/2695840

Verplanken, B., & Orbell, S. (2003). Reflections on past behavior: A self-report index of habit strength. *Journal of Applied Social Psychology, 33*(6), 1313–1330. https://doi.org/10.1111/j.1559-1816.2003.tb01951.x

Williams, D. M., Dunsiger, S., Jennings, E. G., & Marcus, B. H. (2012). Does affective valence during and immediately following a 10-min walk predict concurrent and future physical activity? *Annals of Behavioral Medicine, 44*(1), 43–51. https://doi.org/10.1007/s12160-012-9362-9

Williams, D. M., & Evans, D. R. (2014). Current emotion research in health behavior science. *Emotion Review, 6*(3), 277–287. https://doi.org/10.1177/1754073914523052

Williams, D. M., Rhodes, R. E., & Conner, M. T. (2018). *Affective determinants of health behavior*. Oxford University Press.

Wood, W., & Neal, D. T. (2016). Healthy through habit: Interventions for initiating & maintaining health behavior change. *Behavioral Science & Policy, 2*(1), 71–83. https://doi.org/10.1353/bsp.2016.0008

Wood, W., Quinn, J. M., & Kashy, D. A. (2002). Habits in everyday life: Thought, emotion, and action. *Journal of Personality and Social Psychology, 83*(6), 1281–1297. https://doi.org/10.1037/0022-3514.83.6.1281

Zenko, Z., & Ekkekakis, P. (2019). Critical review of measurement practices in the study of automatic associations of sedentary behavior, physical activity, and exercise. *Journal of Sport and Exercise Psychology, 41*(5), 271–288. https://doi.org/10.1123/jsep.2017-0349

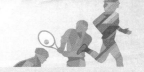

Glossary

accelerometer A device that detects and quantifies physical activity and movement via an electronic sensor. Records body acceleration minute to minute, providing detailed information about the frequency, duration, intensity, and pattern of movement. The data provided often are used to estimate energy expenditure.

action control The pursuit of translating an intention into behavior.

action planning Formulation of an articulated set of procedures to assist in behavioral action.

active control groups Study groups in which a comparable standard treatment is applied. Active control groups are usually used to test whether the intervention treatment is better than other forms of known effective treatments.

active travel An approach to travel that focuses on physical activities, such as walking and cycling, as opposed to car travel, to get to work, school, and other destinations.

activity trait A disposition toward a fast lifestyle. Individuals with this trait are high energy, fast talking, and tend to keep busy.

affect Subjective feeling states at a global level.

agreeableness Tendency to be kind, cooperative, altruistic, trustworthy, and generous.

Alzheimer's disease A neurodegenerative disease characterized by a progressive deterioration of higher cognitive functioning in the areas of memory, problem solving, and thinking.

amotivation The absence of motivation toward a behavior.

analytical psychology The psychoanalytic system of psychology developed and practiced by Carl Jung.

anorexia nervosa Eating disorder characterized by an intense and unrealistic fear of becoming fat and engaging in behaviors intended to produce distinct weight loss.

anticipated affective reactions Expectations of how it will feel to experience something or do a behavior.

anxiety A cognitive and emotional stress response that includes anticipation of a future threat.

anxiety disorders Diagnosable health conditions, distinct from feelings of anxiety or stress, characterized by a range of psychological and physiologic symptoms, including excessive rumination, worrying, uneasiness, and fear about future uncertainties.

apneas Pauses or reductions in breathing during sleep usually lasting between 20–40 seconds.

associative learning Behavioral psychology notions that learning occurs through developments and strengthening of mentally held automatic associations between stimuli and attributes.

attention deficit/hyperactivity disorder (ADHD) One of the most common childhood disorders and can continue through adolescence and into adulthood with symptoms including difficulty staying focused and paying attention, difficulty controlling behavior, and/or hyperactivity.

attitude An individual's positive or negative evaluation of performing a behavior.

automatic associations Mentally held associations between stimuli such as "physical activity" and attributes such as "pleasant" or "unpleasant."

automatic evaluation Mentally held link between a cue and attributes (pleasant vs. unpleasant) that manifest into behavioral impulses to approach or avoid the cue.

automatic identity schema Mentally held links between a cue and our perception of ourselves vs. others.

automatic pairings Mentally held links between cues, such that the influence of automatic regulation may impact responses to related cues.

automatic processes Influences on behavior that are spontaneous, unintentional, uncontrollable, and do not require high cognitive load.

automatic regulation The influence of automatic associations on behavior.

barrier efficacy An individual's beliefs about possessing the capability to overcome obstacles to physical activity.

basal sleep The amount of sleep we need on a regular basis for optimal performance.

behavioral activation A form of psychotherapy in which operant conditioning strategies are used through scheduling in order to encourage reconnection with environmental positive reinforcement.

behavioral beliefs Perceived consequences of carrying out a specific action and a person's evaluation of each of these consequences.

behavioral medicine An interdisciplinary field of medicine concerned with the development and integration of knowledge in the biological, behavioral, psychological, and social sciences relevant to health and illness.

benchmarking A way of interpreting effect sizes that does not rely on the arbitrariness of effect size descriptives.

binge eating Eating a large amount of food in a discrete period of time.

biomedical model of illness A model traditionally used to understand health and disease that excludes psychological and social factors and focuses only on biological risk factors.

bipolar disorder A psychological condition in which a person has periods of depression and periods of being extremely happy or being cross or irritable.

body image The self-perceptions and attitudes an individual holds with respect to their body and physical appearance.

brain hemispheres The two symmetrical halves of the brain.

brain-derived neurotrophic factor (BDNF) A protein found in the brain that is related to nerve survival and growth.

built environment The part of the physical environment that includes the human-made surroundings that provide the setting for human activity.

bulimia nervosa Eating disorder characterized by recurrent overeating and use of inappropriate measures to prevent weight gain afterward, such as purging, fasting, or exercising excessively.

cancer A broad group of diseases characterized by unregulated cell growth.

cancer survivor A person with cancer of any type who is still living.

cognition Mental processes that reflect a person's knowledge or awareness, including thinking, knowing, remembering, reasoning, decision making, learning, judging, and problem solving.

cognitive behavioral therapy A form of psychotherapy that helps people to identify and change inaccurate perceptions that may exacerbate symptoms.

cohesion a dynamic process that is reflected in the tendency for a group to stick together and remain united in pursuit of its instrumental objectives and/or for the satisfaction of member affective needs.

comorbid depression and anxiety The shared experience of a clinical anxiety disorder with major depressive disorder. It is more common to have comorbid depression and anxiety than either disorder in isolation.

conscientiousness Tendency to be ordered, dutiful, self-disciplined, and achievement oriented.

control beliefs Perceived presence or absence of required resources and opportunities, the anticipated obstacles or impediments to behavior, and the perceived power of a particular control factor to facilitate or inhibit performance of the behavior.

controlled processes Influences on behavior that are slow, deliberate, and intentional, and are cognitively demanding.

coping appraisal An evaluation of the preventive response of a behavior.

coping planning Formulation of plans to overcome important barriers when action initiation and/or maintenance is challenged.

corpus callosum The connective flat neural fibers that relay information between the brain's hemispheres.

correlate A variable that is associated with either an increase or decrease of another variable, such as physical activity.

cues to action Events and strategies that activate a readiness.

daylight saving time Adjustment of the time to achieve longer evening daylight, especially in summer, by setting the clocks an hour ahead of the standard time.

decisional balance The importance that an individual places on the potential advantages, or *pros*, and disadvantages, or *cons*, of a behavior and the subsequent evaluation of these factors.

delayed gratification The ability to reject immediately available smaller rewards in favor of later larger rewards.

delayed sleep phase syndrome A disorder of sleep timing where people tend to fall asleep at very late times and have difficulty waking up in time for daily living activities.

dementia A non-specific illness syndrome characterized by a serious loss of global cognitive ability in a previously unimpaired person, beyond what might be expected from normal aging.

depressed mood A transient mental state characterized by feeling unhappy, sad, miserable, down in the dumps, or blue.

determinant A variable that has a causal association with an outcome, such as physical activity.

diabetes A group of diseases that affect how the body uses blood glucose.

digital age Refers to an economy based on the digitization of information and widespread use of computers. Also known as the computer age or information age.

digital health the general use of information and communication technologies for health.

digital native A person who was born during or after the general introduction of digital technologies and is therefore familiar with computers and the internet from an early age.

disability-adjusted life years (DALYs) The combination of years of life lost to premature death and years of life lost to time lived in poor health or in disability.

drive for muscularity Individual's perception that they are not muscular enough and that bulk should be added to their body frame in the form of muscle mass (irrespective of a person's percentage of actual muscle mass or body fat).

dynamic A characteristic of a variable that describes change over time.

dysthymia A depressed mood that occurs for most of the day, for more days than not, for at least 2 years (at least one year for children and adolescents).

early onset dementia Dementia that occurs before the age of 65 years.

ecological model The integration of ideas from several theories, including interrelations between individuals and their social and physical environments.

ecological momentary assessment (EMA) A study design in which the target variables are assessed as they occur (in real time) and assessments are dependent upon a strategic timing schedule, intensively repeated over many observations, and made in the environment they occur in. It is also known as experience sampling methodology.

eHealth literacy The users' competence needed to engage with digital health services; digital health literacy.

enacted support The support given by the provider of a social exchange.

evaluative conditioning The manipulation of affective processes toward a target through repeated exposure to a target paired with pleasant or unpleasant stimuli.

event-contingent A type of ecological momentary assessment study in which participants respond to assessments when a specific event occurs.

executive functioning The cognitive process that regulates the ability to organize thoughts and activities, prioritize tasks, manage time efficiently, and make decisions.

exercise addiction Craving for leisure-time physical activity that results in uncontrollably excessive exercise behavior that manifests itself in physiological (e.g., tolerance) and/or psychological (e.g., withdrawal) symptoms.

exercise identity The extent that exercise is descriptive of one's self-concept.

exergames Video games in which gameplay requires the player to move in order to interact with the avatar on screen.

exergaming Technology-driven physical activity.

external regulation Engaging in a behavior to receive a reward or to avoid punishment.

extraversion Tendency to be sociable, assertive, energetic, seek excitement, and experience positive affect.

extrinsic motivation Multidimensional concept whereby a person is motivated by external factors, such as rewards or punishments, to accomplish a particular task or engage in a certain behavior.

feedback loop A system where the results of a process impacts the start of the next one.

fight-or-flight response The response of the sympathetic nervous system to a stressful event, preparing the body to fight or flee, and associated with the release of stress hormones.

first trimester Begins on the first day of a woman's last period and lasts until the end of week 12.

fitspiration A message, usually in the form of an image with a quote included, designed to inspire people to attain a fitness goal.

genesis The progression of the onset and development of symptoms throughout a disorder.

green space An area of grass, trees, or other vegetation set apart for recreational or aesthetic purposes in an otherwise urban environment.

grit The tendency to persevere and be passionate about long-term goals.

group dynamics The nature of groups, individual relationships within groups, and the group members' interactions with each other.

habit The process by which a person's behavior is influenced from a prompt to act based on well-learned associations between cues and behaviors.

happiness A state of mind or a feeling characterized by contentment, love, satisfaction, pleasure, or joy.

health A state of complete physical, mental, and social wellbeing.

health psychology The study of the psychological and behavioral processes in health, illness, and health care.

health-related quality of life (HRQoL) An assessment of how an individual's quality of life affects their physical, mental, and social health.

heritability The proportion of disorder risk attributable to genetics.

heritable Something that tends to run in families, shared through common genes.

homeostasis The natural state of our body and mind, characterized by calmness and balance that is disrupted by stress responses.

identified regulation Engaging in a behavior to achieve a personal goal.

identities Components of a multi-dimensional self-concept, hierarchically organized by how one categorizes themselves in a given role.

implementation intentions "If-then" action plans, whereby a link is forged between a cue and subsequent behavioral response.

implicit measures Indirect assessments that do not require participants' subjective assessment.

inactive behavior Performing insufficient amounts of moderate and/or vigorous physical activity (i.e., not meeting specified physical activity guidelines).

incidence The proportion of the population who have experienced their first episode of a condition at a particular time.

incidental affect Affect felt beyond that of a response to the behavior or event.

income inequality An unequal distribution of resources based on income.

industriousness-ambition Tendency toward achievement-striving and self-discipline.

insomnia Sleeplessness; a clinical sleep disorder characterized by long-term difficulties with initiating or maintaining sleep.

integral affect Affect felt as a response to the behavior or event.

integrated regulation Engaging in a behavior because it aligns with other behaviors and choices in one's life.

intention Person's willingness and how much effort they are planning to exert to perform a behavior.

intrinsic motivation Engaging in a behavior for its own sake or the pleasure it provides.

introjected regulation Engaging in a behavior to relieve or prevent guilt.

isotemporal substitution modelling A way of statistically testing how outcomes are impacted by substitution of one type of behavior for another.

jet lag Excessive sleepiness and a lack of daytime alertness in people who travel across time zones.

just-in-time adaptive interventions Intervention programs aiming to provide the right type and amount of support at the time when the support is most needed.

land use mix The diversity or variety of land uses, such as residential, commercial, industrial, and agricultural.

maintenance self-efficacy An individual's beliefs in their capability to cope with barriers that might derail the intended action.

major depressive disorder A psychological disorder characterized by persistent feelings of sadness and/or loss of interest that can interfere with your daily functioning.

mastery experiences Personal experiences with carrying out a task successfully; thought to be the most important cause of self-efficacy beliefs.

memory consolidation A process in which recently encoded memory representations are reactivated and transformed into long-term memory.

meta-analysis A statistical method of reviewing a body of research evidence that is both systematic and quantitative.

meta-synthesis Meta-analytic approach to synthesizing results of meta-analyses using quantitative methods.

metabolic equivalent (MET) A physiological measure used to express the energy cost of physical activities. It is the ratio of metabolic rate (i.e., the rate of energy consumption) during a specific physical activity to a reference metabolic rate.

mHealth Health promotion using mobile phones as the primary mechanism.

mild cognitive impairment An intermediate stage between the expected cognitive decline of normal aging and the more pronounced decline of dementia that involves problems with memory, language, thinking, and judgment that are greater than typical age-related changes.

moderation When the degree to which two variables are associated depends on a third variable, the moderator.

modernization The transformation of a society from rural and agrarian to an urban and industrial one.

mood disorders Psychiatric disorders characterized by a distorted mood that is inconsistent with your circumstances and interferes with daily functioning.

mood states A source of self-efficacy beliefs whereby previous successes and failures are stored in memory (and recalled) with associated feelings.

muscle dysmorphia Psychological disorder characterized by the preoccupation with the idea that one's body is not lean and muscular.

neurogenesis New nerve cell generation.

neuroticism Tendency to be emotionally unstable, anxious, self-conscious, and vulnerable.

neurotransmitters Chemical substances that transmit nerve impulses across a synapse, the tiny communication gap between the neurons in the brain.

non-active control groups Study groups in which the participants receive no comparison treatment during the study. These are usually used to test whether the intervention treatment is effective at all.

nonclinical populations Consisting of people who have not been diagnosed with a clinical disorder.

normative beliefs Perceived expectations of important significant others or groups and the individual's motivation to comply with the expectations of these important significant others.

Old Order Amish Religious community that emphasizes humility, nonviolence, and traditional values rather than advancement and technology.

openness to experience/intellect Tendency to be perceptive, creative, and reflective, and to appreciate fantasy and aesthetics.

outcome expectations Expectations an individual has about the outcomes of a particular behavior.

perceived barriers A person's opinion of the physical and psychological costs of the advised action.

perceived behavioral control Perceived ease or difficulty of performing a behavior.

perceived benefits A person's opinion of the efficacy of the advised action to reduce risk or seriousness of impact.

perceived severity A person's opinion of the seriousness of a condition and its consequences.

perceived support An individual's cognitive appraisal of support.

perceived susceptibility/vulnerability A person's opinion of their chances of getting a particular disease.

perfectionism Striving for flawlessness and perfection and accompanied by critical self-evaluations.

peripheral A device that is connected to a host architecture but is not an integral part.

personality traits Enduring and consistent individual-level differences in tendencies to show consistent patterns of thoughts, feelings, and actions.

physical activity An umbrella term for any body movement produced by skeletal muscles that requires energy expenditure.

physical activity psychology The study of psychological issues and theories related to physical activity.

physical effort minimization The tendency to avoid moving and using energy.

physical environment The part of the environment that includes all of a person's indoor and outdoor surroundings, both those that have been designed (e.g., neighborhoods and parks) and those that occur naturally (e.g., oceans and mountains).

physical inactivity The absence of physical activity, usually reflected as the proportion of time not engaged in physical activity of a predetermined intensity.

Physical Self-Perception Profile An assessment tool based on a hierarchical, multidimensional theoretical model of self-esteem in which self-perceptions can be categorized as superordinate, domain, subdomain, facet, subfacet, and state.

physiological state Bodily sensations, such as increased heart rate, increased sweating, and increased respiratory rate.

point-of-choice prompt Informational or motivational signs near where alternative behavioral options are available and where decisions to act are likely.

polar climate Climate characterized by a lack of warm summers. Every month a polar climate has an average temperature of less than 10°C (50°F).

polysomnography Comprehensive recording of biophysiological changes that occur during sleep.

positive psychology The study of happiness and how people can become happier and more fulfilled.

postpartum depression Moderate to severe depression in a woman after she has given birth.

prevalence The proportion of the population who have experienced their first episode of the condition at a particular time.

primary exercise addiction Meeting the criteria for exercise addiction and exercising solely for the psychological gratification resulting from the exercise behavior itself.

priming The non-conscious influence on responses to a cue as a result of recent experience with or exposure to the same cue.

processes of change The behaviors, cognitions, and emotions that people engage in during the course of changing a behavior. In the transtheoretical model, these are proposed as five behavioral and five experiential processes.

processing speed The speed at which the brain processes information. Faster processing speed means more efficient thinking and learning.

productivity loss Loss of revenue as a result of unavailability of employees.

psychological hedonism The human tendency to pursue pleasure and avoid displeasure.

psychoticism Tendency toward risk taking, impulsiveness, irresponsibility, manipulativeness, sensation-seeking, tough-mindedness, and nonpragmatism.

quality of life A broad, multidimensional term that encompasses a person's perceived quality of his or her daily life.

quantitative research The systematic empirical investigation of a phenomenon via statistical, mathematical, or numerical data or computational techniques.

racial discrimination Different treatment from people or organizations/systems between people of different races or ethnicities.

received support The support received from the recipient of a social exchange.

reciprocal determinism The interdependency and codetermination of behavior, internal personal factors, and external environmental factors.

recovery self-efficacy An individual's ability to overcome setbacks and recover from previously failed attempts to enact the behavior.

recreational screen time Activities such as watching television, playing video games, using the computer, or using other screens during discretionary time (i.e., nonschool or work-based use) that are practiced while sedentary.

reflective processes Consciously deliberated and expected consequences of performing a behavior.

reflexive processes Influences on behavior that are triggered through particular circumstances and stimuli.

regulatory processes Behavioral, cognitive, and affective tactics that are employed to translate a formulated intention into behavior.

restless leg syndrome A neurological disorder characterized by an irresistible urge to move one's body to stop uncomfortable or odd sensations.

restoration Sleep that allows the body and mind to repair itself and regulate cellular functioning that can deteriorate through waking periods.

scheduling efficacy An individual's beliefs about possessing the capability to schedule physical activity into a daily or weekly routine.

schema A heuristic cognitive generalization about the self, derived from past experiences and used to process self-related information.

screen time The amount of time people spend in sedentary behaviors such as playing video games, using the computer, watching television, or using mobile devices.

season A division of the year marked by changes in weather, ecology, and hours of daylight.

secondary exercise addiction Meeting the criteria for exercise addiction, but using excessive exercise to accomplish some other end (e.g., weight loss or body composition changes) that is related to an eating disorder.

sedentarism Engagement in sedentary behaviors characterized by minimal movement, low energy expenditure, and rest.

sedentary behavior Any waking activity characterized by an energy expenditure of less than or equal to 1.5 metabolic equivalents (METs) in a sitting or reclining posture.

self-concept The multitude of attributes and roles through which a person evaluates themselves to establish self-esteem judgments.

self-control situation Occurs when hedonic motivation and controlled motivation conflict and self-control is needed to enact controlled motivation and inhibit the automatic influences of hedonic motivation.

self-efficacy Belief in one's capabilities to organize and execute the course of action required to produce a certain outcome.

self-esteem A stable global positive or negative evaluative of one's own worth.

self-presentation The process by which people attempt to control and monitor how they are perceived and evaluated by others.

shift work A work roster that involves recurring periods in which different groups of workers do the same job at different times, including overnight.

sleep A naturally recurring state of rest for the mind and body, in which the eyes usually close and consciousness is either completely or partially lost.

sleep debt The accumulated sleep that is lost each night.

sleep disorder Medical conditions that prevent you from sleeping well on a regular basis.

sleep hygiene A set of behavioral and environmental recommendations intended to promote healthy sleep.

sleep latency Amount of time spent asleep.

sleep spindles Bursts of electricity in the brain characteristic of the second stage of sleep, which play a pivotal role in information processing and memory storage.

sleepwalking disorder Repeated episodes of sleepwalking that results in distress or problems with daily functioning.

social environment The physical surroundings, social relationships, and cultural milieu within which people function and interact.

social identity The degree to which a person identifies with a social group.

social inequality An unequal distribution of resources based on social status.

social integration The degree to which the individual participates and is involved in family life, the social life of the community and has access to resources and support services.

social networks A person's connectedness to other people.

social physique anxiety Anxiety related to the public presentation of one's image.

social support The perception and actuality that one is cared for by others, has assistance available from other people, and that one is part of a supportive social network.

spatial-visual processes How we sense the interrelations of things in space around us, including navigating where we are going, and representing a concept through drawing.

sport psychology The study of the how psychological factors affect athletes' performance and well-being.

stages of change Six stages that people pass through in attempting any health behavior change, according to the transtheoretical model: precontemplation, contemplation, preparation, action, maintenance, and termination.

standard of living Refers to the level of wealth, comfort, material goods, and necessities available to a certain socioeconomic class in a certain geographic area.

state anxiety Temporary state of high anxiety.

stigma When people have negative views of a person as a result of associations between characteristics of that person and negative attributes.

street connectivity How often streets or roadways intersect.

stress The process by which we perceive and respond to events, called stressors, that we appraise as threatening or challenging.

stress hormones Hormones such as cortisol and epinephrine released by the body in situations that are interpreted as being potentially dangerous.

stressor Any event or situation that triggers coping adjustments.

subjective norm Perceived social pressure that individuals feel to perform or not perform a particular behavior.

support network An individual's social network from a functional perspective. Also known as network resources.

supportive climate The quality of social relationships and systems.

systematic review A review of scientific literature focused on a particular research question to identify, appraise, select, and synthesize all high-quality research evidence relevant to that question.

tailored interventions Intervention programs that include features and content made specifically to be relevant to the people who will be using it.

task efficacy An individual's beliefs about possessing the capability to perform a behavioral act.

temptation The intensity of urges to engage in a specific behavior.

theory of planned behavior A theory about the link between beliefs and behavior.

theory of reasoned action A theory about the link between volitional behavior and intention.

threat appraisal An evaluation of the consequences of engaging in an unhealthy behavior (e.g., smoking, sedentary lifestyle).

trait anxiety Individual differences in tendencies to experience frequent high levels of state anxiety.

type A personality Personality type characterized by a blend of competitiveness and hostility with agitated behavior and continual movement patterns.

type D personality Personality type that experiences distress in the form of higher levels of negative affect and social inhibition.

umbrella review A systematic review summarizing evidence from other reviews (review of reviews).

urban sprawl The expansion of auto-oriented, low-density development outside of city centers. Also known as suburban sprawl.

verbal persuasion A source of self-efficacy beliefs whereby positive verbal statements ("you can do it") increase self-efficacy. Greatest impact on self-efficacy is found in those individuals who have some reason to believe that they could be successful with a task if they persist.

vicarious experiences Observational learning from the successful or unsuccessful behavior of others used as a comparative standard; thought to be a powerful cause of self-efficacy beliefs.

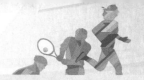

Index

Note: Page numbers followed by *f* or *t* indicate materials in figures or tables, respectively.